YOUR B

This invaluable volun al
direction of distingu ov,
M.D., M.S., F.A.A.P., and ac-
tical wisdom of more than 100 pediatric subspecialists and an editorial review board. Written in a warm, accessible style and richly illustrated with helpful drawings and diagrams, this book gives you the information you need to safeguard your child's most precious asset: his or her health.

In *Your Baby's First Year* you'll find:

- A month-by-month guide to your baby's first year that lets you know what to expect in terms of growth, behavior, and development
- "Health Watch" features that alert you to potential medical problems at each stage
- "Safety Check" reminders for home, outdoors, and car travel
- A discussion of family issues—from grandparents to single parenting and stepfamilies

Plus reliable information on:

- Nutrition, with advice on breastfeeding and bottle-feeding, and when to introduce solid foods
- All common infectious diseases, from chickenpox and measles to flu and ear infections
- Developmental disabilities, such as congenital abnormalities, cerebral palsy, hearing loss, and autism
- Emergencies, including bites, poisoning, choking, and CPR
- Car safety seats
- Child care programs
- Sleep habits and challenges

Additional Parenting Books from the American Academy of Pediatrics

Heading Home with Your Newborn: From Birth to Reality

Mommy Calls: Dr. Tanya Answers Parents' Top 101 Questions About Babies and Toddlers

The Wonder Years: Helping Your Baby and Young Child Negotiate the Major Developmental Milestones

Raising Twins: From Pregnancy to Preschool

Your Baby's First Year (*English and Spanish*)

New Mother's Guide to Breastfeeding (*English and Spanish*)

Food Fights: Winning the Nutritional Challenges of Parenthood Armed with Insight, Humor, and a Bottle of Ketchup

A Parent's Guide to Childhood Obesity: A Road Map to Health

Guide to Your Child's Nutrition

ADHD: A Complete and Authoritative Guide

Waking Up Dry: A Guide to Help Children Overcome Bedwetting

A Parent's Guide to Building Resilience in Children and Teens: Giving Your Child Roots and Wings

Sports Success Rx!—Your Child's Prescription for the Best Experience

Less Stress, More Success: A New Approach to Guiding Your Teen Through College Admissions and Beyond

Mental Health, Naturally: The Family Guide to Holistic Care for a Healthy Mind and Body

Caring for Your School-Age Child: Ages 5 to 12

Caring for Your Teenager

Guide to Your Child's Allergies and Asthma

Guide to Toilet Training (*English and Spanish*)

YOUR BABY'S FIRST YEAR

Steven P. Shelov, M.D., M.S., F.A.A.P.
Editor-in-Chief
Associate Chief of Staff
Schneider Children's Hospital
North Shore Long Island
Jewish Health System
Professor of Pediatrics, SUNY-Downstate
School of Medicine

BANTAM BOOKS
NEW YORK

A note about revisions: Every effort is made to keep *Your Baby's First Year* consistent with the most recent advice and information available from the American Academy of Pediatrics. In addition to major revisions identified as "Revised Editions," the text has been updated as necessary for each additional reprinting listed below.

2010 Bantam Books Mass Market Edition

Published in the United States by Bantam Books, an imprint of The Random House Publishing Group, a division of Random House, Inc., New York.

BANTAM BOOKS and the rooster colophon are registered trademarks of Random House, Inc.

Your Baby's First Year is abridged from the American Academy of Pediatrics' *Caring for Your Baby and Young Child: Birth to Age Five* (5th Edition) and published by arrangement with the American Academy of Pediatrics.

ISBN 978-0-553-59300-6

Cover design: Beverly Leung
Cover photographs: © Barbara Peacock (top), © FPG International Corp. (center), © The Image Bank/Elyse Lewin (bottom)

Printed in the United States of America

www.bantamdell.com

2 4 6 8 9 7 5 3 1

REVIEWERS AND CONTRIBUTORS

Editor-in-Chief
Steven P. Shelov, M.D., M.S., F.A.A.P.

Associate Medical Editor
Tanya Remer Altmann, M.D., F.A.A.P.

Associate Editor Emeritus
Robert E. Hannemann, M.D., F.A.A.P.

Editorial Board
Phyllis F. Agran, M.D., M.P.H., F.A.A.P.
Paul H. Dworkin, M.D., F.A.A.P.
Andrew Garner, M.D., F.A.A.P.
Frank Greer, M.D., F.A.A.P.
Laura Jana, M.D., F.A.A.P.
H. Cody Meissner, M.D., F.A.A.P.
Regina Milteer, M.D., F.A.A.P.

AAP Board of Directors Reviewer
Myles B. Abbott, M.D., F.A.A.P.

American Academy of Pediatrics
Executive Director: Errol R. Alden, M.D., F.A.A.P.
Associate Executive Director: Roger F. Suchyta, M.D., F.A.A.P.
Director, Department of Marketing and Publications: Maureen DeRosa, M.P.A.

Director, Division of Product Development: Mark T. Grimes
Manager, Consumer Publishing, Division of Product Development: Carolyn Kolbaba

Project Coordinator, Division of Product Development: Holly L. Kaminski

Contributors
Henry Adams, M.D., F.A.A.P.
Lisa Albers, M.D., F.A.A.P.
Susan Aronson, M.D., F.A.A.P.
Diane L. Atkins, M.D., F.A.A.P.
Richard G. Azizkhan, M.D., F.A.A.P.
Susan S. Baker, M.D., Ph.D., F.A.A.P.
Miriam Bar-On, M.D., F.A.A.P.
Robert Beekman III, M.D., F.A.A.P.
Roger L. Berkow, M.D., F.A.A.P.
Dana Best, M.D., M.P.H., F.A.A.P.
Jatinder J. S. Bhatia, M.D., F.A.A.P.
Carol Jean Blaisdell, M.D., F.A.A.P.
David A. Bloom, M.D., F.A.A.P.
Thomas Bojko, M.D., M.S., F.A.A.P.
Suzanne C. Boulter, M.D., F.A.A.P.
Lawrence W. Brown, M.D., F.A.A.P.
Marilyn Bull, M.D., F.A.A.P.
Susan Buttross, M.D., F.A.A.P.
Anthony J. Casale, M.D., F.A.A.P.
William J. Cochran, M.D., M.P.H., F.A.A.P.
George J. Cohen, M.D., F.A.A.P.
William L. Coleman, M.D., F.A.A.P.
Donald E. Cook, M.D., F.A.A.P.
James J. Corrigan, M.D., F.A.A.P.
David Howard Darrow, M.D., D.D.S., F.A.A.P.
Catherine DeAngelis, M.D., F.A.A.P.
Ellen Sue Deutsch, M.D., F.A.A.P.
William H. Dietz, M.D., Ph.D., F.A.A.P.
Elaine Donoghue, M.D., F.A.A.P.
Joanna Douglass, B.D.S., D.D.S.
John C. Duby, M.D., F.A.A.P.
Roselyn Epps, M.D., F.A.A.P.
Maria Escolar, M.D., F.A.A.P.

Stephen A. Feig, M.D., F.A.A.P.
Margaret Fisher, M.D., F.A.A.P.
Paul Graham Fisher, M.D., F.A.A.P.
Laura Sue Fitzmaurice, M.D., F.A.A.P.
John William Foreman, M.D., F.A.A.P.
Lawrence W. Gartner, M.D., F.A.A.P.
Robert Gatehouse, D.D.S.
James Gern, M.D., F.A.A.P.
Peter A. Gorski, M.D., M.P.A., F.A.A.P.
David Albert Gremse, M.D., F.A.A.P
Ann P. Guilot, M.D., F.A.A.P.
Joseph Hagan, M.D., F.A.A.P.
Robert J. Haggerty, M.D., F.A.A.P.
Kevin Hale, D.D.S.
Christopher Endom Harris, M.D., F.A.A.P.
Peter Lucas Havens, M.D., F.A.A.P.
Melvin Bernard Heyman, M.D., F.A.A.P.
Pamela C. High, M.D., M.S., F.A.A.P.
Marjorie Joan Hogan, M.D., F.A.A.P.
Douglas N. Homnick, M.D., M.P.H., F.A.A.P.
Paul Stephen Horowitz, M.D., F.A.A.P.
James Nelson Jarvis, M.D., F.A.A.P.
Chet D. Johnson, M.D., F.A.A.P.
Christine L. Johnson, M.D., F.A.A.P.
Steven W. Kairys, M.D., F.A.A.P.
Ronald J. Kallen, M.D., F.A.A.P.
Julie Pamela Katkin, M.D., F.A.A.P.
John Kattwinkel, M.D., F.A.A.P.
Celia I. Kaye, M.D., Ph.D., F.A.A.P.
Jonathan D. Klein, M.D., M.P.H., F.A.A.P.
Ronald Ellis Kleinman, M.D., F.A.A.P.
Mark W. Kline, M.D., F.A.A.P.
David M. Krol, M.D., M.P.H., F.A.A.P.
Marian E. Kummer, M.D., F.A.A.P.
Shantanu Lal, D.D.S.
Kevin Patrick Lally, M.D., F.A.A.P.
Ruth A. Lawrence, M.D., F.A.A.P.
Jessica Y. Lee, D.D.S., M.P.H., Ph.D.
Steven J. Lichtenstein, M.D., F.A.A.P.
Michael J. Light, M.D., F.A.A.P.
Gregory Stephen Liptak, M.D., F.A.A.P.
M. Jeffrey Maisels, M.D., F.A.A.P.
Teri Metcalf McCambridge, M.D., F.A.A.P.
Joan Younger Meek, M.D., M.S., R.D., I.B.C.L.C., F.A.A.P.
Andrew P. Mezey, M.D., F.A.A.P.
Peter M. Miller, M.D., F.A.A.P.
Howard Mofenson, M.D., F.A.A.C.T., F.A.A.P.
Rachel Y. Moon, M.D., F.A.A.P.
John W. Moore, M.D., M.P.H., F.A.A.P.
Brigitta Ursula Mueller, M.D., F.A.A.P.
Suhas M. Nafday, M.D., M.R.C.P. (Ire), D.C.H., F.A.A.P.
Scott Needle, M.D., F.A.A.P.
Steven Neish, M.D., F.A.A.P.
Ian Michael Paul, M.D., F.A.A.P.
Jerome A. Paulson, M.D., F.A.A.P.
James Perrin, M.D., F.A.A.P.
Nancy Powers, M.D., F.A.A.P.
Ellen Marie Raney, M.D., F.A.A.P.
Michael Ian Reiff, M.D., F.A.A.P.
Leonard Rome, M.D., F.A.A.P.
Paul James Sagerman, M.D., F.A.A.P.
Scott R. Schoem, M.D., F.A.A.P.
Richard Schwartz, M.D., F.A.A.P.
Richard Michael Schwend, M.D., F.A.A.P.
Gwendolyn Scott, M.D., F.A.A.P.
Robert C. Shamberger, M.D., F.A.A.P.
Henry L. Shapiro, M.D., F.A.A.P.
William Thomas Shearer, M.D., F.A.A.P.
Donald L. Shifrin, M.D., F.A.A.P.
Scott Howard Sicherer, M.D., F.A.A.P.
Benjamin S. Siegel, M.D., F.A.A.P.
Irene N. Sills, M.D., F.A.A.P.
Janet Silverstein, M.D., F.A.A.P.
Deborah Mulligan Smith, M.D., F.A.A.P.
Gary Smith, M.D., F.A.A.P.
Michael Smith, M.D., F.A.A.P.
Martin Stein, M.D., F.A.A.P.
John Stirling, Jr., M.D., F.A.A.P.
Janice E. Sullivan, M.D., F.A.A.P.
Jack T. Swanson, M.D., F.A.A.P.
David E. Tunkel, M.D., F.A.A.P.
Dennis L. Vickers, M.D., F.A.A.P.
Sunita Vohra, M.D., F.A.A.P.
Robert Gerard Voigt, M.D., F.A.A.P.
Robert Walker, M.D., F.A.A.P.
Richard Walls, M.D., Ph.D., F.A.A.P.
Jeffrey C. Weiss, M.D., F.A.A.P.
Mark Widome, M.D., F.A.A.P.
Catherine Wilfert, M.D., F.A.A.P.
Modena Hoover Wilson, M.D., M.P.H., F.A.A.P.

This book is dedicated to
all the people who recognize that children
are our greatest inspiration in the present
and our greatest hope for the future.

We also appreciate the contributions of the late
Leonard P. Rome, M.D., F.A.A.P.,
to the original publication of this book.

Acknowledgments

Writer:
Richard Trubo

Writer, first edition:
Aimee Liu

Illustrators:
Wendy Wray/Morgan Gaynin, Inc.
Alex Grey

Administrative Support:
Marilyn Rosenfeld
Joan Ruddy
Carrie Peters

Additional Assistance:
Jeanne M. Anderson
Martha Cook, M.S.
Eileen Glasstetter, M.S.
Jeanne Christensen Lindros
Becky Levin-Goodman, M.P.H.
Tammy Piazza Hurley
Bonnie Kozial
Elizabeth Sobczyk, M.S.W., M.P.H.
Gina Ley Steiner

Designer:
Richard Oriolo

Special thanks to Marc Weissbluth, M.D., F.A.A.P., for his review and consultation on the "Sleep" chapter.

PLEASE NOTE

The information contained in this book is intended to complement, not substitute for, the advice of your child's pediatrician. Before starting any medical treatment or medical program, you should consult with your child's pediatrician, who can discuss your child's individual needs and counsel you about symptoms and treatment. If you have questions regarding how the information in this book applies to your child, speak to your child's pediatrician.

Products mentioned in this book are for informational purposes only. Inclusion in this publication does not constitute or imply a guarantee or an endorsement by the American Academy of Pediatrics.

The information and advice in this book apply equally to children of both sexes (except where noted). To indicate this, we have chosen to alternate between masculine and feminine pronouns throughout the book.

The American Academy of Pediatrics constantly monitors new scientific evidence and makes appropriate adjustments in its recommendations. For example, future research and the development of new childhood vaccines may alter the regimen for the administration of existing vaccines. Therefore, the schedule for immunizations outlined in this book is subject to change. These and other potential situations serve to emphasize the importance of always checking with your child's pediatrician for the latest information concerning the health of your child.

CONTENTS

Foreword

This fifth edition of *Your Baby's First Year* is the first in a three-volume series of child care books developed by the American Academy of Pediatrics (AAP). The other books in this series include *Caring for Your School-Age Child: Ages 5 to 12* and *Caring for Your Teenager.* The Academy also has published books for parents on topics ranging from breastfeeding, nutrition, and toilet training to sleep, allergies and asthma, and attention-deficit/hyperactivity disorder.

The AAP is an organization of 60,000 primary-care pediatricians, pediatric medical subspecialists, and pediatric surgical specialists dedicated to the health, safety, and well-being of all infants, children, adolescents, and young adults. This book is part of the ongoing educational efforts of the Academy to provide parents and caregivers with high-quality information on a broad spectrum of children's health issues.

What distinguishes this book from the many others in bookstores and on library shelves is that it has been developed and extensively reviewed by physician members of the American Academy of Pediatrics. A six-member editorial board developed the initial material with the assistance of more than one hundred contributors and reviewers. Because medical information is constantly changing, every effort has been made to ensure that this book contains the most up-to-date findings. Readers can visit the AAP website at www.aap.org to keep current on the latest information.

It is the Academy's hope that this book will become an invaluable resource and reference guide for parents and caregivers. We believe it is the best comprehensive source of information on matters of children's health and well-being.

We are confident that parents and caregivers will find the book extremely valuable. We encourage its use along with the advice and counsel of our readers' own pediatricians, who will provide individual guidance and assistance related to the health of children.

Errol R. Alden, M.D., F.A.A.P.
Executive Director
American Academy of Pediatrics

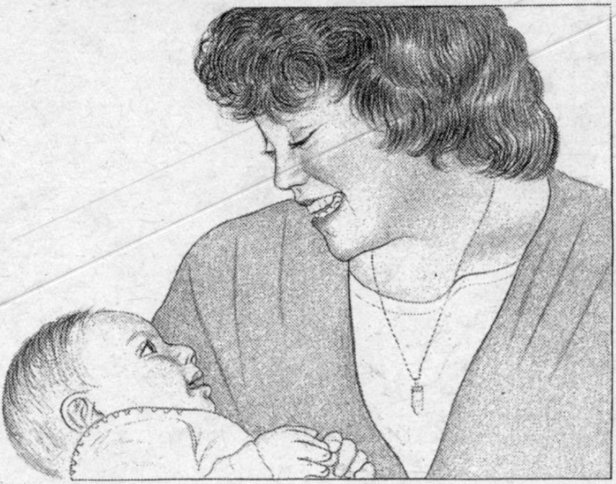

INTRODUCTION: THE GIFTS OF PARENTHOOD

Your baby is the greatest gift you will ever receive. From the moment you first hold this miracle of life in your arms, your world will be broader and richer. You will experience a flood of feelings, some of wonder and joy and others of confusion and of being overwhelmed and wondering whether you can ever measure up to the needs of your new baby. These are feelings you could barely imagine before—feelings that no one can truly experience without having a child.

Even describing them can be difficult because the bond between parent and baby is so intensely personal. Why do tears come to your eyes the first time your baby smiles or reaches for you? Why are you so

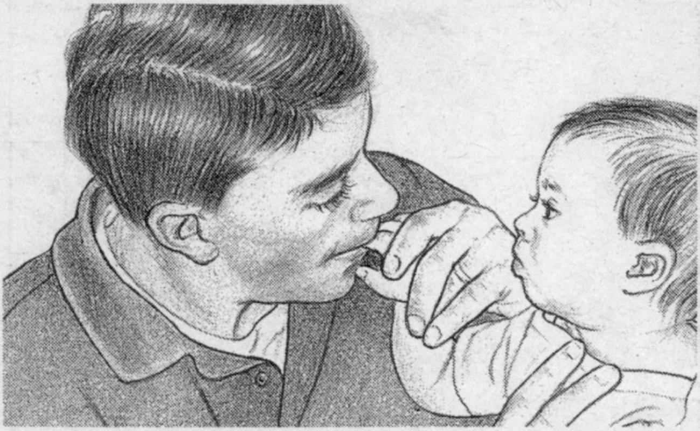

proud of her first words? Why does your heart suddenly start to pound the first time you watch her stumble and fall? The answer lies in the unique two-way giving relationship between you and your baby.

Your Baby's Gifts to You

Although simple, your baby's gifts to you are powerful enough to change your life positively.

Unqualified Love. From birth, you are the center of your infant's universe. He gives you his love without question and without demand. As he gets older, he will show this love in countless ways, from showering you with his first smiles to

Your Baby's Gifts to You

- Unqualified love
- Absolute trust
- The thrill of discovery
- The heights of emotion

giving you his handmade Valentines. His love is filled with admiration, affection, loyalty, and an intense desire to please you.

Absolute Trust. Your child believes in you. In her eyes, you are strong, capable, powerful, and wise. Over time, she will demonstrate this trust by relaxing when you are near, coming to you with problems, and proudly pointing you out to others. Sometimes she also will lean on you for protection from things that frighten her, including her own sensitivities. For example, in your presence she may try out new skills that she would never dare to try alone or with a stranger. She trusts you to keep her safe.

The Thrill of Discovery. Having a baby gives you a unique chance to rediscover the pleasure and excitement of childhood. Although you cannot relive your life through your child, you can share in his delight as he explores the world. In the process, you probably will discover abilities and talents you never dreamed you possessed. Feelings of empathy mixed with growing self-awareness will help shape your ability to play and interact with your growing child. Discovering things together, whether they are new skills or words or ways to overcome obstacles, will add to your experience and confidence as a parent and will better prepare you for new challenges that you never even envisioned.

The Heights of Emotion. Through your baby, you will experience new heights of joy, love, pride, and excitement. You probably also will experience anxiety, anger, and frustration. For all those delicious moments when you hold your baby close and feel her loving arms around your neck, there are bound to be times when you feel you cannot communicate. The extremes sometimes become sharper as your baby gets older and seeks to establish her independence. The same child who at three dances across the room with you may at four have a rebellious and active period that surprises you. The extremes are not contradictions, but simply a reality of growing up. For you as a parent, the challenge is to accept and appreciate all the feelings with which your baby expresses himself and arouses in you, and to use them in giving him steady guidance.

The Gifts You Give Your Baby

- Unconditional love
- Self-esteem
- Values and traditions
- Joy in life
- Good health
- Secure surroundings
- Skills and abilities

The Gifts You Give Your Baby

As his parent, you have many vital gifts to offer your baby in return. Some are subtle, but all are very powerful. Giving them will make you a good parent. Receiving them will help your baby become a healthy, happy, capable individual.

Unconditional Love. Love lies at the core of your relationship with your child. It needs to flow freely in both directions. Just as she loves you without question, you must give her your love and acceptance absolutely. Your love shouldn't depend on the way she looks or behaves. It shouldn't be used as a reward or withheld as a threat. Your love for your baby is constant and indisputable, and it's up to you to convey that, especially when she misbehaves and needs to have limits set or behavior corrected. Love must be held separate and above any fleeting feelings of anger or frustration over her conduct. Never confuse the actions with the child. The more secure she feels in your love, the more self-assurance she will have as she grows up.

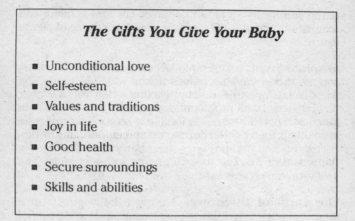

Self-Esteem. One of your most important gifts as a parent is to help your child develop self-esteem. It's not an easy or quick process. Self-respect, confidence, and belief in oneself, which are the building blocks of self-esteem, take years to become firmly established. Beginning in infancy your child needs your steady support and encouragement to discover his strengths. He needs you to believe in him as he learns to believe in himself. Loving him, spending time with him, listening to him, and praising his accomplishments are all part of this process. On other occasions, helping him modify his troubling behaviors in ways that aren't punitive or hurtful, but constructive, is just as important to building a firm self-esteem. If he is confident of your love, admiration, and respect, it will be easier for him to develop the solid self-esteem he needs to grow up happy and emotionally healthy.

Values and Traditions. Regardless of whether you actively try to pass on your values and beliefs to your baby, she is bound to absorb some of them just by living with you. She'll notice how disciplined you are in your work, how deeply you hold your beliefs, and whether you practice what you preach. She'll participate in family rituals and traditions and think about their significance. You can't expect or demand that your child subscribe to all your opinions, but you can present your beliefs honestly, clearly, and thoughtfully, in keeping with the child's age and maturity level. Give her guidance and encouragement, not only commands. Encourage questions and discussions, when age and language permit, instead of trying to force your values on your child. If your beliefs are well reasoned and if you are true to them, she probably will adopt many of them. If there are inconsistencies in your actions—something we all live with—often your child will make that clear to you, either subtly by his behavior or, when he is older, more directly by disagreeing with you. The road to developing values is not straight and unerring. It demands flexibility built on firm foundations. Self-awareness, a willingness to listen to your child and change when appropriate, and, above all, a demonstration of your commitment to traditions will best serve your relationship with your child. While the choice of values and principles ultimately will be hers to make, she depends on you to give her the foundation through your thoughts, shared ideas, and, most of all, your actions and deeds.

Joy in Life. Your baby doesn't need to be taught to be joyful, but he does need your encouragement and support to let his natural enthusiasm fly free. The more joyful you are, particularly when you are with him, the more delightful life will seem to him and the more eagerly he will embrace it. When he hears music, he'll dance. When the sun shines, he'll turn his face skyward. When he feels happy, he'll laugh. This exuberance often is expressed through his being attentive and curious, willing to explore new places and things, and eager to take in the world around him and incorporate the new images, objects, and people into his own growing experience. Remember, different babies have different temperaments—some are more apparently exuberant than others, some are more noisily rambunctious, some are more playful, some are more reserved and quiet. Still others are more even-keeled, mixtures of the two extremes. But all babies demonstrate their joy in life in their own ways, and you as the parent will discover what those ways are and will nurture your child's joy.

Good Health. Your child's health depends significantly on the care and guidance you offer her during these early years. You begin during pregnancy by taking good care of yourself and by arranging for obstetric and pediatric care. By taking your baby to the doctor regularly for checkups and consultations, keeping her safe from injuries, providing a nutritious diet, and encouraging exercise throughout childhood, you help protect and strengthen her body. You'll also need to maintain good health habits yourself, while avoiding unhealthy ones, such as smoking, excessive drinking, drug use, and lack of adequate physical activity. In this way, you'll give your child a healthy example to follow as she grows up.

Secure Surroundings. You naturally want to give your baby a safe, comfortable home. This means more than a warm place to sleep and a collection of toys. As important as it is to provide shelter that is physically safe and secure, it is even more important to create a home that is emotionally secure with a minimum of stress and a maximum of consistency and love. Your child can sense problems between other family members and may be very troubled by them, so it's important that all family problems, even minor conflicts, be dealt with directly and resolved as quickly as possible through cooperation. This may entail seeking advice, but remember, your family's well-being helps maintain an environment that promotes your baby's development and will allow him to achieve his potential. The family's dealing effectively with conflicts or differences ultimately will help him feel secure in his ability to manage conflicts and disagreements and will provide him with a positive example for resolving his own challenges.

Skills and Abilities. As your child grows up, she'll spend most of her time developing and polishing a variety of skills and abilities in all areas of her life. You should help her as much as possible by encouraging her and providing the equipment and instruction she needs. Books, magazines, play groups, and preschool will quickly take on a central role as your toddler becomes a preschooler. But it's important not to forget some of the most important learning tools: Your child will learn best when she feels secure, confident, and loved; she will learn best when information is presented in a way that she will respond to positively. Some information is best presented through play—the language of children. Young children learn a tremendous amount through play, especially when with parents or playmates. Other information is best learned or incorporated through actual experience. This may mean learning through exposure to diverse places, people, activities, and experiences. Other things are learned through stories, picture books, magazines, and activity books. Still other things are learned by watching—sometimes just watching you, sometimes watching other children or adults. Preschool experiences also promote socialization.

If you enjoy learning and making discovery fun for your baby, she soon will recognize that achievement can be a source of personal satisfaction as well as a way to please you. The secret is to give her the opportunities and let her learn as best fits her style and at her own rate.

How to Make Giving a Part of Your Daily Family Life

The back-and-forth sharing of these gifts between you and your child will foster your relationship and nurture your child's development. Much like learning a new dance, working out the actual steps in giving is not always going to be easy. But it will happen with time and patience, and with your own commitment to strengthen the parent-child relationship.

Giving your baby the guidance and support that he needs to grow up healthy involves all the skills of parenthood: nurturing, guiding, protecting, sharing, and serving as an example or model. Like other skills, these must be learned and perfected through practice. Some will be easier for you than others. Some will seem easier on certain days than on others. These variations are a normal part of raising a child, but they do make the job challenging. The following suggestions will help you make the most of your natural parenting skills so you can give your child the best possible start.

Enjoy Your Baby as an Individual. Recognize that your baby is unique—different from everyone else—and appreciate her special qualities. Discover her special needs and strengths, her moods and vulnerabilities, and especially her sense of humor, which starts to show itself early in infancy. Let her show you the joy of play. The more you enjoy your baby and appreciate her individuality, the more successful you'll be in helping her develop a sense of trust, security, and self-esteem. You'll also have a lot more fun being a parent!

Educate Yourself. You probably know much more than you think you do about being a parent. You spent years observing your own parents and other families. Perhaps you've cared for other children. And you have many instinctive responses that will help make you a giving parent. In other times, this probably would have been all the preparation you needed to raise a baby. However, our society is extremely complex and is constantly changing. In order to guide their children in this new world, parents often benefit from some extra education. Talk to your pediatrician and other parents, and ask questions. Get to know other families with children the same age, and watch how these parents raise their children (for example, when are they protective and when do they let go, and how much responsibility do they expect of their children at various ages?). Also, read about issues and problems that affect your family. Contact your local religious organizations, school systems and PTAs, child care programs, parent education classes, and other groups that specialize in child-related concerns. Often these groups serve as networks for concerned and interested parents. These networks will help you feel more comfortable and secure when issues seem puzzling or frustrating.

As you gather advice, sift through it for information that is right for you and your baby. Much of what you receive will be very valuable, but not all of it. Because child rearing is such a personal process, there is bound to be disagreement. You are not obligated to believe everything you hear or read. In fact, one of the purposes of educating yourself is to protect your baby from advice that does not fit your family. The more you know, the better equipped you'll be to decide what works best for your family.

Be a Good Example. One of the ways your infant shows her love for you is by imitating you. This is also one of the ways she learns how to behave, develop new skills, and take care of herself. From her earliest moments, she watches you closely and patterns her own behavior and beliefs after yours. Your examples become permanent images, which will shape her attitudes and actions for the rest of her life. Setting a good example for your child means being responsible, loving, and consistent not only with her but with all members of the family. Show your affection and nurture your relationships. If your child sees her parents communicating openly, cooperating, and sharing household responsibilities, she'll bring these skills to her own future relationships.

Setting good examples also means taking care of yourself. As an eager, well-meaning parent, it's easy to concentrate so hard on your family that you lose sight of your own needs. That's a big mistake. Your baby depends on you to be physically and emotionally healthy, and she looks to you to show her how to keep herself healthy. By taking care of yourself, you demonstrate your self-esteem, which is important for both you and your baby. Getting a sitter and resting when you're overtired or ill teaches your child that you respect yourself and your needs. Setting aside time and energy for your own work or hobbies teaches your child that you value certain skills and interests and are willing to pursue them. By giving yourself some personal time (at least once a week), the easier it will be for you and your child to develop your own identities. That needs to occur as she grows older. She also will benefit from getting to know other trusted grown-ups by having them babysit, and at times involving your entire family in group activities with other families. Ultimately she will pattern some of her own habits after yours, so the healthier and happier you keep yourself, the better it will be for both of you.

You can set an example in still another important area, too, and that's in demonstrating tolerance and acceptance in an increasingly multicultural society. As the United States has become a melting pot of nationalities and cultures, it is more important than ever to teach tolerance to your child when relating to people of other racial, ethnic, and religious groups and alternate lifestyles. Make an effort to help your child understand and even celebrate diversity. No boy or girl is born prejudiced, but it can be learned at a very young age. The way you relate to people in your life will provide a foundation for how your child will treat her peers and others throughout her childhood and adulthood. As your child grows, let her know that there are many similarities among people and make an effort to dispel stereotypes that she is exposed to, replacing them with the belief that all people deserve to be respected and valued.

Show Your Love. Giving love means more than just saying "I love you." Your child can't understand what the words mean unless you also treat him with love. Be spontaneous, relaxed, and affectionate with him. Give him plenty of physical contact through hugging, kissing, rocking, and playing. Take the time to talk, sing, and read with him every day. Listen and watch as he responds to you. By paying attention and freely showing your affection, you make him feel special and secure and lay a firm foundation for his self-esteem.

Communicate Honestly and Openly. One of the most important skills you teach your child is communication. The lessons begin when she is a tiny baby gazing into your eyes and listening to your soothing voice. They continue as she watches and listens to you talking with other members of the family and, later, as you help her sort out her concerns, problems, and confusions. She needs you to be understanding, patient, honest, and clear with her. Good communication within a family is not always easy. It can be especially difficult when both parents are working, overextended, or under a great deal of stress, or when one person is depressed, ill, or angry. Preventing a communications breakdown requires commitment, cooperation among family members, and a willingness to recognize problems as they arise. Express your own feelings, and as your child grows, encourage her to be equally open with you. Look for changes in her behavior—such as frequent or constant crying, irritability, sleep problems, or appetite loss—that may signal sadness, fear, frustration, or worry, and show her that you're aware of and understand these emotions. Ask questions, listen to the responses, and offer constructive suggestions.

Listen to yourself, as well, and consider what you say to your child before the words leave your mouth. It's sometimes easy to make harsh, even cruel, statements in anger or frustration that you don't really mean but that your child (depending on her age) may never forget. Thoughtless comments or jokes that seem incidental to you may be hurtful to your child. Phrases like "That's a dumb question" or "Don't bother me" make your child feel worthless and unwanted and may seriously damage her self-esteem. If you constantly criticize or put her off, she also may back away from you. Instead of looking to you for guidance, she may hesitate to ask questions and may mistrust your advice. Like everyone else, children need encouragement to ask questions and speak their minds. The more sensitive, attentive, and honest you are, the more comfortable she'll feel being honest with you.

Spend Time Together. You cannot give your child all that he needs if you only spend a few minutes a day with him. In order to know you and feel confident of your love, he has to spend a great deal of time with you, both physically and emotionally. Spending this time together is possible even if you have outside commitments. You can work full-time and still spend some intimate time with your baby every day. The important thing is that it be time devoted just to him, meeting his needs and your needs together. Is there any fixed amount? No one can really say. One hour of quality time is worth more than a day of being in the same house but in different rooms. You can be at home full-time and never give him the undivided attention he requires. It's up to you to shape your schedule and direct your attention so that you meet his needs.

It may help to set aside a specific block of time for your child each day and devote it to activities he enjoys. Also make an effort to include him in all family activities—meal preparation, mealtimes, and so forth. Use these times to talk about each other's problems (do be attentive, however, to overburdening your child with adult problems; kids don't need to shoulder your anxieties), personal concerns, and the day's events.

If you're a working parent, your attentiveness to your child when you're together will help ensure that he is well adjusted and well loved. If your child is well taken care of when you're at work, he will thrive regardless of your hours spent away on the job.

Nurture Growth and Change. When your child is a newborn, it may be difficult for you to imagine her ever growing up, and yet your main purpose as a parent is to encourage, guide, and support her growth. She depends on you to provide the food, protection, and healthcare her body needs to grow properly, as well as the guidance her mind and spirit need to make her a healthy, mature individual. Instead of resisting change in your baby, your job is to welcome and nurture it.

Guiding your child's growth involves a significant amount of discipline, both for you and for your child. As she becomes increasingly independent, she needs rules and guidelines to help her find what she can do and grow from there. You need to provide this framework for her, establishing rules that are appropriate for each stage of development and adjusting them as your child changes so they encourage growth instead of stifling it.

Confusion and conflict do not help your child to mature. Consistency does. Make sure that everyone who cares for her understands and agrees on the way she is being raised and the rules she's expected to follow. Establish policies for all her care providers to observe when she misbehaves, and adjust these policies along with the rules as she becomes more responsible.

You also should create an environment that encourages the healthy brain development of your baby. Her world—including where she lives and plays and whom she interacts with—will affect how her brain grows. Your baby's environment and experiences need to be nurtured constantly, with warm and loving care providers who give her the freedom to explore and learn safely. (Throughout this book, you'll find guidelines on ensuring the optimal development of your child's brain.)

Minimize Frustrations and Maximize Success. One of the ways your child develops self-esteem is by succeeding. The process starts in the crib with his very first attempts to communicate and use his body. If he achieves his goals and receives approval, he soon begins to feel good about himself and eager to take on greater challenges. If, instead, he's prevented from succeeding and his efforts are ignored, eventually he may become so discouraged that he quits trying and either withdraws or becomes angry and even more frustrated.

As a parent, you must try to expose your child to challenges that will help him discover his abilities and achieve successes while simultaneously preventing him from encountering obstacles or tasks likely to lead to too great a series of frustrations and defeats. This does not mean doing his work for him or keeping him from tasks you know will challenge him. Success is meaningless unless it involves a certain amount of struggle. However, too much frustration in the face of challenges that really are beyond your child's current abilities can be self-defeating and perpetuate a negative self-image. The key is to moderate the challenges so they're within your child's reach while asking him to stretch a bit. For example, try to have toys that are appropriate for his age level, neither too basic for him nor too difficult for him to handle. See if you can find a variety of playmates, some older and some younger. Invite your child to help you around the house and have him do chores as he gets older, but don't expect more of him than he realistically can manage.

As you raise your baby, it's easy to get carried away by your hopes and dreams for him. You naturally want him to have the best education, all possible opportunities, and eventually a successful career and lifestyle. But be careful not to confuse your own wishes with his choices. In our highly competitive society, a great deal of pressure is placed on children to perform. Some preschools have entrance requirements. In some professions and sports, children are considered out of the running if they haven't begun training by age ten. In this atmosphere, the popularity of programs that promise to turn "ordinary babies" into "super babies" is understandable. Many well-meaning parents want desperately to give their children a head start on lifetime success. Unfortunately, this is rarely in the children's best interests. In fact, there is a lack of evidence that these rigorous, early-training programs can actually produce "super babies." Achieving a balanced, moderate approach is the key to meeting expectations and avoiding frustration and disappointment for both you and your child.

Children who are pressured to perform early in life do not learn better or achieve higher skills over the long run than do other children. On the contrary, the effects of psychological and emotional pressures may be so negative that the child develops learning or behavioral problems. If a child is truly gifted, he might be able to handle the early-learning barrage and develop normally, but most gifted children require less pressure, not more. If their parents push them, they may feel overloaded and become anxious. If they don't live up to their parents' expectations, they may feel like failures and worry that they'll lose their parents' love. This kind of chronic stress and so-called "adverse childhood experiences" can even have a negative impact on brain development and keep children from reaching their own innate potential.

Your child needs understanding, security, and opportunity geared to his own special gifts, needs, and developmental timetable. These things cannot be packaged in a program and they don't guarantee the future, but they will make him a success on his own terms.

Offer Coping Strategies. Some disappointment and failure are inevitable, so your child needs to learn constructive ways to handle anger, conflict, and frustration. Much of what she sees in movies and on television teaches her that violence is the way to solve disputes. Her personal inclination may be either to erupt or to withdraw when she's upset. She may not be able to distinguish the important issues from the insignificant ones. She needs your help to sort out these confusing messages and find healthy, constructive ways to express her negative feelings.

Building Resilience

As a parent, one of your greatest challenges is to protect your child from danger and discomfort throughout her younger years and beyond. But no matter how skilled and conscientious you are, you can't shield your child from all of the misfortunes she'll encounter during childhood. Eventually, as she goes out into the world—spending time in preschool and in the homes of playmates and care providers—she'll encounter stresses and setbacks that are simply part of life. She may also experience a divorce, a serious family illness, or a death, any of which can have a profound effect on her.

So how should you react? Can you insulate your child from every misfortune, from being teased or bullied to being excluded from a group activity? And even if you could protect her, should you always do so?

Most pediatricians agree that it may not be a good idea to protect her from every negative experience that the world puts in her path. So, as she grows and within the safe and supportive environment of your family, you need to nurture in her the resilience that can help her bounce back from the upsets and disappointments that are part of life.

By definition, resilience is the capacity to rebound from setbacks. It is the opposite of vulnerability, or the risk of being temporarily or permanently scarred by those same setbacks. Researchers have focused considerable attention on the home environment and the powerful impact it can have on how children develop emotionally. Studies have shown that by two to three years old, a child's early life experiences are already shaping her level of resilience or vulnerability to adverse life events.

To help strengthen your child's resilience, she needs your nurturing beginning at birth and continuing throughout childhood. She needs to know that there are parents and other adults in her life who believe in her and love her unconditionally. Provide her with a secure environment at home. Even when an uncontrollable event like a major family illness takes place, try keeping your child's life as predictable as you can, and make her feel secure and protected.

The American Academy of Pediatrics is strongly committed to having children grow up with caring adults and in safe places. But if you're feeling overloaded with the stresses in your own life—from work-related anxieties to financial or marital concerns—it can rub off on your child. So don't hesitate to ask your doctor for a referral to a therapist for yourself. Family stresses and changes can influence your child's psychological well-being, and major problems such as domestic violence or parental depression need prompt attention for your child's resilience to thrive during difficult times.

Begin by handling your own anger and unhappiness in a mature fashion so that she learns from your example. Encourage her to come to you with problems she can't solve herself, and help her work through them and understand them. Set clear limits for her so that she understands that violence is not permissible, but at the same time let her know it's normal and okay to feel sad, angry, hurt, or frustrated.

Recognize Problems and Get Help When Necessary. Although it is an enormous challenge, parenthood can be more rewarding and enjoyable than any other part of your life. Sometimes, though, problems are bound to arise, and occasionally you may not be able to handle them alone. There is no reason to feel guilty or embarrassed about this. Healthy families accept the fact and confront difficulties directly. They also respect the danger signals and get help promptly when it's needed.

Sometimes all you need is a friend. If you're fortunate enough to have parents and relatives living nearby, your family may provide a source of support. If not, you could feel isolated unless you create your own network of neighbors, friends, and other parents. One way to build such a network is by joining organized parent-child groups at your local YM/YWCA, religious center, or community center. The other parents in these groups can be a valuable source of advice and support. Allow yourself to use this support when you need it.

Occasionally you may need expert help in dealing with a specific crisis or ongoing problem. Your personal physician and pediatrician are sources of support and referral to other health professionals, including family and marriage counselors. Don't hesitate to discuss family problems with your pediatrician. If not resolved, eventually many of these problems can adversely affect your family's health. Your pediatrician should know about them and be interested in helping you resolve them.

If your baby has special needs, you and your family may face particularly difficult challenges. Families whose children have chronic illnesses or disabilities often deal with and conquer everyday obstacles in order to ensure that their children have access to optimal care to support their well-being and proper development. In such situations, one of your immediate goals is to find a pediatrician who is accessible and knowledgeable, can coordinate your infant's treatment with other healthcare providers, and can help you navigate the conflicting advice that you may encounter. The term "medical home" often is used to describe care that is accessible, family-centered, continuous, comprehensive, coordinated, compassionate, and culturally effective. This is the optimal system of medical care for all children, particularly those with special healthcare needs. Creating a medical home is a partnership between pediatric healthcare professionals, parents, and child care providers, and is a goal you should strive for in helping your child lead a fulfilling life that is as normal and healthy as possible.

Your journey with your child is about to begin. It will be a wondrous time filled with many ups and downs, times of unbridled joy and times of sadness or frustration. The chapters that follow provide a measure of knowledge intended to make fulfilling the responsibilities of parenthood a little easier and, it is hoped, a lot more fun.

PART I

1

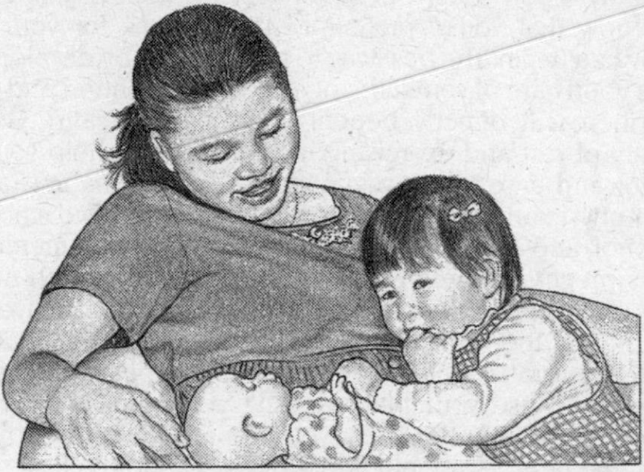

Preparing for a New Baby

Pregnancy is a time of anticipation, excitement, preparation, and, for many new parents, uncertainty. You dream of a baby who will be strong, healthy, and bright—and you make plans to provide her with everything she needs to grow and thrive. You probably also have fears and questions, especially if this is your first child, or if there have been problems with this or a previous pregnancy. What if something goes wrong during the course of your pregnancy, or what if labor and delivery are difficult? What if being a parent isn't everything you've always dreamed it would be? These are perfectly normal feelings and fears to have. Fortunately, most of these worries are needless. The nine months of pregnancy will give you time to have your questions answered, calm your fears, and prepare yourself for the realities of parenthood.

Some of your initial concerns may have been raised

and addressed if you had difficulty becoming pregnant, particularly if you sought treatment for an infertility problem. But now that you're pregnant, preparations for your new baby can begin. The best way to help your baby develop is to take good care of yourself, since medical attention and good nutrition will directly benefit your baby's health. Getting plenty of rest and exercising moderately will help you feel better and ease the physical stresses of pregnancy. Talk to your physician about prenatal vitamins, and avoid smoking, alcohol, and eating fish containing high levels of mercury.

As pregnancy progresses, you're confronted with a long list of related decisions, from planning for the delivery to decorating the nursery. You probably have made many of these decisions already. Perhaps you've postponed some others because your baby doesn't yet seem "real" to you. However, the more actively you prepare for your baby's arrival, the more real that child will seem, and the faster your pregnancy will appear to pass.

Eventually it may seem as if your entire life revolves around this baby-to-be. This increasing preoccupation is perfectly normal and healthy and actually may help prepare you emotionally for the challenge of parenthood. After all, you'll be making decisions about your child for the next two decades—at least! Now is a perfect time to start.

Here are some guidelines to help you with the most important of these preparations.

Giving Your Baby a Healthy Start

Virtually everything you consume or inhale while pregnant will be passed through to the fetus. This process begins as soon as you conceive. In fact, the embryo is most vulnerable during the first two months, when the major body parts (arms, legs, hands, feet, liver, heart, genitalia, eyes, and brain) are just starting to form. Chemical substances such as those in cigarettes, alcohol, illegal drugs, and certain medications can interfere with the developmental process and with later development, and some can even cause congenital abnormalities.

Take smoking, for instance. If you smoke cigarettes during pregnancy, your baby's birth weight may be significantly decreased. Even inhaling smoke from the cigarettes of

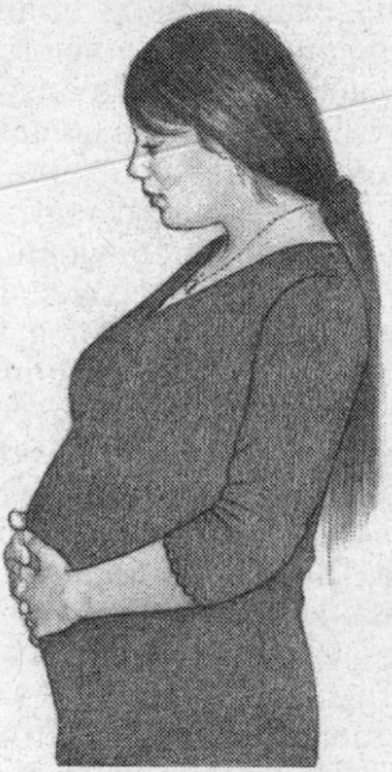

others (passive smoking) can affect your baby. Stay away from smoking areas and ask smokers not to light up around you. If you smoked before you got pregnant and still do, this is the time to stop—not just until you give birth, but forever. Children who grow up in a home where a parent smokes have more ear infections and more respiratory problems during infancy and early childhood. They also have been shown to be more likely to smoke when they grow up.

There's just as much concern about alcohol consumption. Alcohol intake during pregnancy increases the risk for a condition called fetal alcohol syndrome (FAS), which is responsible for birth defects and below-average intelligence. A baby with fetal alcohol syndrome may have heart defects, malformed limbs (e.g., club foot), a curved spine, a small head, abnormal facial characteristics, small body size, and low birth weight. Fetal alcohol syndrome is also the leading cause of mental retardation in newborns. Alcohol consumption during pregnancy increases the likelihood of a miscarriage or preterm delivery, as well.

There is evidence that the more alcohol you drink during pregnancy, the greater the risk to the fetus. It is safest not to drink *any* alcoholic beverages during pregnancy.

You also should avoid all medications and supplements except those your physician has specifically recommended for use during pregnancy. This includes not only prescription drugs that you may have already been taking, but also nonprescription or over-the-counter products such as aspirin, cold medications, and antihistamines. Even vitamins can be dangerous if taken in high doses. (For example, excessive amounts of vitamin A have been known to cause congenital [existing from birth] abnormalities.) Consult with your physician before taking drugs or supplements of any kind during pregnancy, even those labeled "natural."

Fish and shellfish contain high-quality protein and other essential nutrients, are low in saturated fat, and contain fatty acids called omega-3's. They can be an essential part of a balanced diet for pregnant women.

At the same time, you should be aware of the possible health risks from eating fish while you're pregnant. You should avoid raw fish during pregnancy because it may contain parasites such as flukes or worms. Cooking and freezing are the most effective ways to kill the parasite larvae found in fish. For safety reasons, the U.S. Food and Drug Administration (FDA) recommends cooking fish at 140 degrees Fahrenheit. The fish should appear opaque and flaky when done. Certain types of cooked sushi such as eel and California rolls are safe to eat when pregnant.

The most worrisome contaminant in both freshwater and ocean fish is mercury (or more specifically, a form of mercury called methyl mercury). Mercury in a pregnant woman's diet has been shown to be damaging to the development of the brain and nervous system of the fetus. The FDA advises pregnant women, women who may become pregnant, nursing mothers, and young children to avoid eating shark, swordfish, king mackerel, and tilefish due to high levels of mercury in these fish. According to the FDA, pregnant women can safely eat an average of 12 ounces (two average meals) of other types of *cooked* fish each week. Five of the most commonly eaten fish that are low in mercury are shrimp, canned light tuna, salmon, pollock, and catfish: Albacore tuna tends to be high in mercury, so canned chunk light tuna is a better choice. If local health agencies have not issued any advisories about the safety of fish caught in your area, you can eat up to 6 ounces (one average meal) per week of fish you catch from local waters, but don't consume any other fish during that week.

While no adverse effects from minimal caffeine intake (one cup of caffeinated coffee per day) have yet been proven, you may want to limit or avoid caffeine when you are pregnant. Remember, caffeine is also found in many soft drinks and foods such as chocolate.

Another cause of congenital abnormalities is illness during

pregnancy. You should take precautions against these dangerous diseases:

German measles (*rubella*) can cause mental retardation, heart abnormalities, cataracts, and deafness. Fortunately, this illness now can be prevented by immunization, although *you must not get immunized against rubella during pregnancy.* If you're not sure whether you're immune, ask your obstetrician to order a blood test for you. In the unlikely event that the test shows you're not immune, you must do your best to avoid sick children, especially during the first three months of your pregnancy. It is then recommended that you receive this immunization after giving birth to prevent this same concern in the future.

Chickenpox is particularly dangerous if contracted shortly before delivery. If you have not already had chickenpox, avoid anyone with the disease or anyone recently exposed to the disease. You also should receive the preventive vaccine when you are not pregnant.

Herpes is an infection that newborns can get at the time of birth. Most often, it occurs as the infant moves through the birth canal of a mother infected with genital herpes. Babies who get a herpes viral infection may develop fluid-filled blisters on the skin that can break and then crust over. A more serious form of the disease can progress into a severe and potentially fatal inflammation of the brain called encephalitis. When a herpes infection occurs, it is often treated with an antiviral medication called acyclovir. Women may reduce their risk of contracting the herpes virus by following safer sexual practices.

Toxoplasmosis is primarily a danger for cat owners. This illness is caused by a parasitic infection common in cats, but it also is found in uncooked meat and fish. The infected animal excretes a form of the parasite in its stools, and people who come in contact with infected stools could become infected themselves. To guard against this disease, see the box *Protecting Against Toxoplasmosis* on page 9.

Getting the Best Prenatal Care

Throughout your pregnancy, you should work closely with your obstetrician to make sure that you stay as healthy as possible. Regular doctor's visits up until the birth of your

Tdap Vaccine: Protection for You and Baby

In their first 4 to 6 months, babies are more prone to infections because their immune systems are not fully developed. That is why it is important that moms are protected against many things, including tetanus, diphtheria, and pertussis. The vaccine for these three serious diseases is known as Tdap and it stands for:

- **T**etanus—also called lockjaw, a painful tightening of the muscles, including the jaw, which gets "locked" shut making it impossible to open the mouth or swallow and can lead to death.
- **D**iphtheria—a severe throat infection caused by a germ that makes it difficult to breathe and can affect the heart and nervous system and can lead to death.
- **P**ertussis—also called whooping cough, which causes severe coughing, vomiting, and trouble sleeping for months in adults. In infants this infection can cause sleep problems, severe cough, and pneumonia that last for months and can even lead to brain damage or death.

Bacteria cause all these diseases. Diphtheria and pertussis are spread from person to person. Tetanus enters the body through cuts, scratches, or wounds.

Since newborns haven't gotten their first few doses of the vaccine that protects them from these diseases, moms who were never immunized or moms who may have lost their immunity from earlier immunizations could pick up these diseases and pass them on to their babies.

Before Tdap is recommended, your doctor will review your immunization history and decide if and when you should get the vaccine. It is also recommended that anyone who will be in close contact with your baby should be vaccinated as well. This includes dads, grandparents, other relatives, and child-care providers younger than sixty-four years of age. They should ask their doctor if Tdap vaccine is needed. Other children in the family should be sure their tetanus, diphtheria, and pertussis immunizations are up to date also.

Protecting Against Toxoplasmosis

According to the Centers for Disease Control and Prevention (CDC), the best way to protect your unborn child is by protecting yourself against toxoplasmosis.

- Have someone who is healthy and not pregnant change your cat's litter box daily. If this is not possible, wear gloves and clean the litter box every day. Wash your hands well with soap and water afterward.
- Also, wash your hands with soap and water after *any* exposure to soil, sand, raw meat, or unwashed vegetables. Wear gloves when gardening or handling sand from a sandbox.
- Cook all meat thoroughly. Do not taste meat before it is fully cooked.
- Freeze meat for several days before cooking to greatly reduce the chance of infection.
- Wash all cutting boards and knives thoroughly with hot, soapy water after each use.
- Wash and/or peel all fruits and vegetables before eating them.
- Avoid drinking untreated water, particularly when traveling in less developed countries.

Where We Stand

Drinking alcohol during pregnancy is one of the leading preventable causes of birth defects, mental retardation, and other developmental disorders in newborns. There is no known safe amount of alcohol consumption during pregnancy. For that reason, the American Academy of Pediatrics recommends that women who are pregnant, or who are planning to become pregnant, abstain from drinking alcoholic beverages of any kind.

Where We Stand

The American Academy of Pediatrics's message is clear—don't smoke when pregnant, and protect yourself and your children from secondhand tobacco smoke. Many studies have shown that if a woman smokes or is exposed to secondhand smoke during pregnancy, her child may be born too early (prematurely) or be smaller than normal. Other effects caused by smoking during pregnancy may include sudden infant death syndrome (SIDS), depressed breathing movements while in the uterus, learning problems, respiratory disorders, and heart disease as an adult.

After birth, children exposed to secondhand tobacco smoke have more respiratory infections, bronchitis, pneumonia, poor lung function, and asthma than children who aren't exposed. Smoke exposure is most dangerous for younger children because they spend more time in close proximity to parents or other smokers, and they have immature lungs.

If you smoke, quit. Ask your child's pediatrician or your primary care doctor for free help, or call 1-800-QUIT-NOW. If you can't quit, don't expose your child to smoke—make your home and car completely

> smoke-free. The Academy supports legislation that would prohibit smoking in public places, including outdoor public places that children frequent. The Academy also supports banning tobacco advertising, harsher warning labels on cigarette packages, attaching an "R" rating to movies depicting tobacco use, FDA regulation of nicotine, insurance coverage for smoking-cessation counseling, and increases in cigarette excise taxes. For more information, visit www.aap.org/ richmondcenter.

baby can significantly improve your likelihood of having a healthy newborn. During each doctor's visit, you will be weighed, your blood pressure will be checked, and the size of your uterus will be estimated to evaluate the size of your growing fetus.

Here are some areas that deserve attention during your pregnancy.

Nutrition

Follow your obstetrician's advice regarding your use of prenatal vitamins. As mentioned, you should take vitamins only in the doses recommended by your doctor. Perhaps more than any other single vitamin, make sure you have an adequate intake (generally, 400 micrograms a day) of folic acid, a B vitamin that can reduce the risk of certain birth defects, such as spina bifida. Your obstetrician may recommend a daily prenatal vitamin pill, which includes not only folic acid and other vitamins, but also iron, calcium, and other minerals, and the fatty acids docosahexaenoic acid (DHA) and arachidonic acid (ARA). Fatty acids are "good" fats, and DHA in particular accumulates in the brain and eyes of the fetus, especially during the last trimester of pregnancy. These fatty acids are also found in the fat of human breast milk. Make sure your doctor knows about any other supplements you may be taking, including herbal remedies.

Eating for Two

When it comes to your diet, do some planning to ensure that you're consuming balanced meals. Make sure that they contain protein, carbohydrates, fats, vitamins, and minerals. This is no time for fad or low-calorie dieting. In fact, as a general rule, you need to consume about 300 more calories per day than you did before you became pregnant. You need these extra calories and nutrients so your baby can grow normally.

Exercise

Physical activity is just as important when you're pregnant as at any other time of life. Discuss a fitness program with your doctor, including fitness DVDs or videotapes that you've found of interest. Particularly if you haven't been exercising regularly, your doctor may suggest a moderate walking or swimming regimen, or perhaps prenatal yoga or Pilates classes. Don't overdo it. Take it particularly slowly during the first few workouts—even just five to ten minutes a day is beneficial and a good place to start. Drink plenty of water while working out, and avoid activity with jumping or jarring movements.

Tests During Pregnancy

Whether your pregnancy is progressing normally or if concerns are present, your obstetrician may recommend some of the following tests.

- An *ultrasound* exam is a safe procedure and one of the most common tests given to pregnant women. It monitors your fetus's growth and the well-being of his internal organs by taking sonograms (images made from sound waves) of him. It can ensure that your baby is developing normally and will help determine any problems or fetal abnormality. It also can be used if your doctor suspects that your baby is in the breech position. Although most babies are in a head-down position in the uterus at the time of delivery, breech babies are positioned so that their buttocks or feet will move first through the birth canal, before the baby's head. Although some breech babies can safely be delivered vaginally, the risk of complications may be higher in many breech deliveries, and thus your doctor may recommend delivery by Cesarean section. (For further discussion of breech babies and Cesarean births, see *Delivery by Cesarean Section* in Chapter 2, pages 51–54.)

- A *nonstress test* electronically monitors the fetus's heart rate and movements. In this test, a belt is positioned around your abdomen. It is called a "nonstress" test because medications are not used to stimulate movement in your unborn baby or trigger contractions of the uterus.
- A *contraction stress test* is another means of checking the fetus's heart rate, but this time it is measured and recorded in response to mild contractions of the uterus that are induced during the test. For example, an infusion of the hormone oxytocin may be used to cause these contractions. By monitoring your baby's heart rate during the contractions, your doctor may be able to determine how your baby will react to contractions during the actual delivery; if your baby is not responding favorably during these contractions, the delivery of your baby (perhaps by Cesarean section) might be scheduled prior to your due date.
- A *biophysical profile* uses both a nonstress test plus an ultrasound. It evaluates the movement and breathing of the unborn baby, as well as the volume of amniotic fluid. Scores are given for each component of the profile, and the collective score will help determine whether there is a need for an early delivery.

Other tests may be recommended, depending on your own physical health and personal and family history. For example, particularly for women with a family history of genetic problems or for those who are age thirty-five or older, your obstetrician may advise tests that can detect genetic disorders. The most common genetic tests are *amniocentesis* and *chorionic villus sampling,* which are described in the box *Detecting Genetic Abnormalities* on pages 14–15.

Your doctor may recommend other screening tests. For example:

Detecting Genetic Abnormalities

Some tests can detect genetic abnormalities before birth. By learning about these problems before birth, you can help plan your child's healthcare in advance, and in some cases even treat the disorder while the baby is still in the womb.

- With *amniocentesis,* the doctor inserts a thin needle through the pregnant woman's abdominal wall and into the uterus, where a small sample of amniotic fluid is withdrawn from the sac surrounding the fetus. When the fluid is analyzed in the laboratory, it can indicate (or rule out) serious genetic and chromosomal disorders, including Down syndrome and spina bifida. Amniocentesis is usually performed during the second trimester (between the fifteenth and twentieth weeks of pregnancy), although it may be done later (typically after the thirty-sixth week) to test whether the baby's lungs are developed enough for birth. Results of most amniocentesis tests are available within about two weeks.

- With *chorionic villus sampling* (*CVS*), a long, slender needle is inserted through the abdomen to remove a small sample of cells (called chorionic villi) from the placenta. Or a catheter (a thin plastic tube) is placed into the vagina and then inserted through the cervix to withdraw cells from the placenta. This sample is then analyzed in the laboratory. CVS is usually performed earlier during the pregnancy than amniocentesis, most often between the tenth and twelfth week of pregnancy, and the test results are available within one to two weeks. It can be used to detect various genetic and chromosomal conditions, including Down syndrome, Tay-Sachs disease, and (especially in African American families) so-called "hemoglobinopathies" such as sickle cell disease and thalassemia (see page 542).

> Both amniocentesis and CVS are considered accurate and safe procedures for prenatal diagnosis, although they pose a small risk of miscarriage and other complications. You should discuss both the benefits and the risks with your doctor and, in some cases, with a genetic counselor.

- *Glucose screening* can check for high blood sugar levels, which could be an indication of gestational diabetes, a form of diabetes that can develop during pregnancy. To conduct the test, which is usually performed between the twenty-fourth and twenty-eighth week of pregnancy, you'll be asked to drink a sugar solution and then a sample of your blood will be collected. If a high level of glucose (a type of sugar used for energy) is in the blood, then additional testing should be done. This will determine if you do have gestational diabetes, which is associated with an increased likelihood of pregnancy complications.
- *Group B streptococcus (GBS) screening,* which will determine whether a type of bacteria is present that can cause a serious infection (such as meningitis or a blood infection) in your baby. While GBS bacteria are common and may be found in the mother's vagina or rectum—and are harmless in healthy adults—they can cause illness if they're passed to a newborn during childbirth. If GBS is detected in a pregnant woman, the doctor will prescribe antibiotics to be given through a vein (intravenously) during the birthing process; once the baby is born, she may be observed for a longer time in the hospital nursery. The GBS screening test is usually given between the thirty-fifth and thirty-seventh week of pregnancy.
- *HIV (or human immunodeficiency virus) testing* is now commonly done in pregnant women, preferably early in their pregnancy. HIV is the virus that causes AIDS, and when a pregnant woman is infected with the virus, it can be passed to her baby during pregnancy, delivery of her baby, or during breastfeeding.

Preparing for Delivery

As the weeks and months pass leading up to your delivery date, you're probably eagerly planning for the new addition to your family, and adjusting to what is going on in your own body. During the third trimester, you'll notice many changes that may affect how you feel:

- You'll gain weight, typically at a rate averaging about one pound a week during the last trimester.
- As your baby grows in size and places pressure on nearby organs, you may experience episodes of shortness of breath and back pain.
- You may urinate more frequently as pressure is placed on your bladder, and you might have episodes of incontinence.
- You may find it harder to get comfortable, and sleep may become more difficult. You may prefer to sleep on your side.
- You could experience more fatigue than usual.
- You may have heartburn, swelling in your feet and ankles, back pain, and hemorrhoids.
- You may have "false labor" contractions known as Braxton-Hicks contractions. These Braxton-Hicks contractions begin to soften and thin the cervix, preparing it for the delivery of the baby. But unlike true labor contractions, they are irregular, do not occur more often as time passes, and do not become stronger or more intense.

While you're pregnant, you and your spouse/partner may be participating in childbirth education classes, which will give you information about labor and birth, provide the chance to meet other parents-to-be, and help you prepare for the birth. Several types of classes are available in many communities. The Lamaze method, for example, uses approaches such as focused breathing, massage, and labor support that can be used during the actual childbirth process. The Bradley method emphasizes natural childbirth, and relies heavily on deep-breathing techniques. Many childbirth education classes discuss a combination of these as well as other methods to teach expectant parents about the birth process and ways to make the delivery successful, comfortable, and enjoyable.

Whatever class you're considering, ask in advance about the topics and methods of childbirth that will be emphasized, and whether the classes are primarily lectures or also involve your active participation. What is the instructor's philosophy about pregnancy and birth? Is he or she certified? Will you learn proper methods for breathing and relaxation? What will the classes cost? Is there a limit on class size?

At the same time, consider signing up for other classes that can help prepare you for the parenting challenges ahead. Ask your doctor for referrals to breastfeeding classes, infant care programs, or instructional courses on cardiopulmonary resuscitation (CPR).

Some education classes encourage their participants to develop a "birth plan," and may provide guidance in helping you do so. The birth plan is usually a written document for both you and your doctor in which you'll record your own preferences for labor and delivery. For example:

- Where will you be delivering your baby?
- Based on your doctor's instructions, do you plan to go directly to the hospital when labor begins, or will you call the office first? What arrangements have you made for transportation to the hospital or birthing center? Do you have a doula or want to participate in a doula program? (A doula provides various forms of nonmedical support in the childbirth process.)
- Who would you like to deliver your baby (an obstetrician or a nurse midwife)?
- Who do you want to be present to support you during the childbirth experience?
- What position would you prefer to be in during delivery?
- What are your preferences for pain medication (if any is going to be used)?

Last-Minute Activities

If you do have the time, consider these activities before delivery. For example:

- Make a list of people who will receive birth announcements. If you're ordering print announcements, select the announcement style, and address the envelopes in advance. Likewise, gather e-mail addresses or phone numbers for announcing your baby's arrival.
- Cook a number of meals and freeze them.
- Look for child care and/or housekeeping help if you can afford it, and interview candidates in advance. (See *Finding Help at Home,* page 209.) You can also take advantage of friends and family members who are available to help. Even if you don't think you'll need extra help, you should have a list of names to call in case the situation changes.

Before your ninth month, make last-minute preparations for delivery. Your checklist should include the following:

- Name, address, and phone number of the hospital.
- Name, address, and phone number of the doctor or nurse-midwife who will deliver your baby and of the person who covers the practice when your doctor is not available.
- The quickest and easiest route to the hospital or birthing center.
- The location of the hospital entrance you should use when labor begins.
- The phone number of an ambulance service, in case you need such assistance in an emergency.

- The phone number of the person who will take you to the hospital (if that individual does not live with you).
- A bag packed with essentials for labor and for the rest of your hospital stay, including toiletries, clothing, addresses and phone numbers of friends and relatives, reading material, and a receiving blanket and suit of clothes for the baby to wear home.
- A car safety seat for the vehicle so you can take your baby home safely. Make sure the seat meets all federal safety standards. (It should state this on the label.) Read and follow the manufacturer's instructions carefully. Install it in the backseat, facing the rear. (*Never* place a rear-facing car safety seat in front of an air bag.) It should stay in this position at least until your baby reaches one year of age *and* weighs at least 20 pounds (9 kg). According to safety experts, keeping her **facing the rear until she reaches the highest weight or height allowed by the car seat manufacturer is the safest way for her to ride.** Don't forget to have your car seat checked by a trained professional. Proper use and installation is key to protecting your little one during a crash. (See *Car Safety Seats,* page 406, for complete details.)
- If you have other children, arrange for their care during the time you will be at the hospital.

- What options would you consider if unexpected circumstances develop (e.g., the need for an episiotomy or a Cesarean section)?
- If you deliver prematurely, does the facility have adequate resources to take care of your prematurely born infant?

Not only should you talk about and share this document with your doctor, but also let your family members and friends know of your decisions. (Also see the *Last-Minute*

Activities checklist on page 18 for other ideas of what to include in your "birth plan.")

Choosing a Pediatrician

Sometime in the last trimester of pregnancy, you will choose a care provider for your baby. It is important to know that infants and young children have many more visits to the doctor's office than most adults.

The person you choose to be your child's healthcare provider may be a pediatrician, family physician, or a nurse practitioner. This is a personal decision for families, and you should consider what factors are most important to your family before choosing your baby's doctor.

- **Pediatricians** focus their care on infants, children, and teenagers. Children have different healthcare needs from adults—both medical and emotional. Pediatricians are specially trained to prevent and manage these health concerns. Older patients trust their pediatrician because they have known one another for many years. (For more information, see *A Pediatrician's Training,* below.) Family physicians have broad experience in caring for patients of all ages, and they are able to treat the entire family.
- **A nurse practitioner** is a nurse with advanced training that allows her/him to provide healthcare services similar to a doctor. Nurse practitioners focus on wellness, disease prevention, health education, and counseling.

In selecting a doctor, here are some specific considerations to help you make your choice.

A Pediatrician's Training

Pediatricians graduate from medical school and then take special courses solely in pediatrics for three or more years. This is called residency. Under supervised conditions, the pediatrician-in-training acquires the knowledge and skills necessary to treat a broad range of conditions, from the mildest childhood illnesses to the most serious diseases.

After completing residency training, the pediatrician is eligible to take a written exam given by the American Board of Pediatrics. Once she passes this exam, a certificate is issued, which you probably will see hanging on the pediatrician's office wall. If you see the initials "F.A.A.P." after a pediatrician's name, it means she has passed her board exam and is now a full Fellow of the American Academy of Pediatrics. Only board-certified pediatricians can add the designation "F.A.A.P." after their names, which means they have reached the highest status of membership in this professional organization.

Following their residency, some pediatricians elect an additional one to three years of training in a subspecialty, such as neonatology (the care of sick and premature newborns) or pediatric cardiology (the diagnosis and treatment of heart problems in children). These pediatric subspecialists generally are called on to consult with general pediatricians when a patient develops uncommon or special problems. If a subspecialist is ever needed to treat your child, your regular pediatrician will help you find the right one for your child's problem.

Finding a Pediatrician

The best way to start looking for a pediatrician is by asking other parents you know and trust. They are likely to know you, your style, and your needs. You also should consider asking your obstetrician for advice. She will know local pediatricians who are competent and respected within the medical community. If you're new to the community, you may decide to contact a nearby hospital, medical school, or county medical society for a list of local pediatricians. If you are a member of a managed care plan, you probably will be required to choose a pediatrician from among their approved network of doctors. (For more information about managed care, see *Managed Care Plans: Getting Good Care for Your Child* on pages 25–27).

Once you have the names of several pediatricians you wish to consider, start by contacting and arranging a personal interview with each of them during the final months of your pregnancy. Many pediatricians are happy to fit such preliminary interviews into their busy schedules. Before meeting with the pediatrician, the office staff should be able to answer some of your more basic questions:

- Is the pediatrician accepting new patients with my insurance or managed care plan?
- What are the office hours?
- What is the best time to call with routine questions?
- How does the office handle billing and insurance claims? Is payment due at the time of the visit?

Both parents should attend the interviews with pediatricians, if possible, to be sure you both agree with the pediatrician's policies and philosophy about child rearing. Don't be afraid or embarrassed to ask any questions. Here are a few suggestions to get you started.

- *How soon after birth will the pediatrician see your baby?*

  Most hospitals ask for the name of your pediatrician when you're admitted to deliver your baby. The delivery nurse will then phone that pediatrician or her associate on call as soon as your baby is born. If you had any complications during either your pregnancy or the delivery, your baby should be examined at birth, although this exam may be conducted by a staff pediatrician or neonatologist at the hospital if your pediatrician is not there at the time of delivery. Otherwise, the routine newborn examination can take place anytime during the first twenty-four hours of life. Ask the pediatrician if you can be present during that initial examination. This will give you an opportunity to learn more about your baby and get answers to any questions you may have. Your baby will undergo routine newborn tests that will screen for hearing and jaundice levels as well as thyroid and other metabolic disorders.

  Other tests may need to be done if your baby develops any problems after birth or to follow up on any unusual findings on your prenatal sonograms.

- *When will your baby's next exams take place?*

Pediatricians routinely examine newborns and talk with parents before the babies are discharged from the hospital. Many pediatricians will check the baby every day that the newborn is in the hospital, and then will conduct a thorough exam on the day of discharge. During these exams, the doctor can identify any problems that may have come up, while also giving parents a chance to ask questions that occurred to them during the hospital stay. Your pediatrician also will let you know when to schedule the first office visit for your baby and how to reach her if a medical problem develops before then.

All babies also should begin their immunizations before leaving the hospital. The first and most important "immunization" is starting to breastfeed your baby as soon as possible after the baby is born. This provides some early disease protection for your baby. The second recommended immunization is the first dose of the hepatitis B vaccine, which is given as a shot in the baby's thigh. Your baby will receive the next series of vaccinations when he is six to eight weeks old. (The American Academy of Pediatrics's immunization schedule appears in the Appendix on page 734.)

- *When is the doctor available by phone? E-mail?*

Some pediatricians have a specific call-in period each day when you can phone with questions, while others will return calls as they come in throughout the day. If members of the office staff routinely answer these calls, consider asking what their training is. Also ask your pediatrician for guidelines to help you determine which questions can be resolved with a phone call and which require an office visit. Some pediatricians prefer using e-mail to communicate. While you may have some concerns about discussing issues in this way, overall it can help foster your relationship with the doctor.

- *What hospital does the doctor prefer to use?*

Ask the pediatrician where to go if your child becomes seriously ill or is injured. If the hospital is a teaching hospital with interns and residents, find out who would actually care for your child if he were admitted.

- *What happens if there is an after-hours (nighttime or weekend) concern or emergency?*

  Find out if the pediatrician takes her own emergency calls at night. If not, how are such calls handled? Also, ask if the pediatrician sees patients in the office after regular hours, or if you must take your child to an emergency department or urgent care center. When possible, it's easier and more efficient to see the doctor in her office, because hospitals often require lengthy paperwork and extended waits before your child receives attention. However, serious medical problems usually are better handled at the hospital, where staff and medical equipment are always available.

- *Who "covers" the practice when your pediatrician is unavailable?*

  If your physician is in a group practice, it's wise to meet the other doctors, since they may treat your child in your pediatrician's absence. If your pediatrician practices alone, she probably will have an arrangement for coverage with other doctors in the community. Usually your pediatrician's answering service will refer you to the doctor on call automatically, but it's still a good idea to ask for the names and phone numbers of all the doctors who take these calls—just in case you have trouble getting through to your own physician.

  If your child is seen by another doctor at night or on the weekend, you should check in by phone with your own pediatrician the next morning (or first thing Monday, after the weekend). Your doctor probably will already know what has taken place, but this phone call will give you a chance to bring her up to date and reassure you that everything is being handled as she would recommend.

- *How often will the pediatrician see your baby for checkups and immunizations?*

  The American Academy of Pediatrics recommends a checkup within forty-eight to seventy-two hours after your newborn is discharged from the hospital. This is especially important in breastfed babies to evaluate feeding, weight gain, and any yellow discoloration of skin (jaundice). Your pediatrician may adjust this feeding schedule, particularly in the first weeks of life, depending on how your newborn is doing.

During your baby's first year of life, additional visits to your doctor's office should take place at about two to four weeks of age, and then at two, four, six, nine, and twelve months of age as well. During your baby's second year of life, she should be seen by your pediatrician at ages fifteen, eighteen, and twenty-four months, followed by annual visits from two to five years of age. If the doctor routinely schedules examinations more or less frequently than the Academy's guidelines, discuss the differences with her. Additional appointments can be scheduled any time that you have a concern or if your child is ill.

- *What are the costs of care?*

Your pediatrician should have a standard fee structure for hospital and office visits as well as after-hours visits and home visits (if she makes them). Find out if the charges for routine visits include immunizations. Be sure to familiarize yourself with the scope of your insurance coverage before you actually need services.

Managed Care Plans: Getting Good Care for Your Child

Many Americans receive their healthcare in managed care plans. These plans, typically offered by employers and state Medicaid programs, provide services through health maintenance organizations (HMOs) or preferred provider organizations (PPOs). The plans have their own networks of pediatricians and other physicians, and if you or your employer change from one managed care plan to another, you may find that the pediatrician you've been using and whom you like is not part of the new network. Once you have a pediatrician whom you like, ask what plans she is in, and see if you can join one of them if there's a need to switch from one HMO or PPO to another.

Managed care plans attempt to reduce their costs by having doctors control patient access to certain healthcare services. Your pediatrician may act as a "gatekeeper," needing to give approval before your child can be seen by a pediatric medical subspecialist or surgical specialist. Without this approval, you'll have to pay for part or all of these services out of pocket.

To help you maneuver effectively through your managed care plan, here are some points to keep in mind:

- To determine what care is provided in your managed care plan, carefully read the materials provided by the plan (often called a certificate of coverage). If you have questions, talk to a plan representative or your employer's benefits manager. All plans limit some services (e.g., mental healthcare, home healthcare), so find out what's covered and what's not.
- When you're part of a managed care plan, primary and preventive care visits usually will be covered, including well-child checkups, treatment for illnesses or injuries, and immunizations. In many plans, you'll have to pay a portion of the primary care services that your family receives, called a co-payment, for each doctor's visit.
- Once you've chosen a pediatrician, it's best to stay with her. But if you feel the need to switch, all plans allow you to select another doctor from among those who are part of their network. The plan administrator can give you information on how to make this change; some plans allow you to switch only during certain time periods called "open enrollment."
- If you feel that your child needs to see a pediatric subspecialist, work with your pediatrician to find one who is part of your plan, and obtain approval

to schedule an appointment with her. Check your plan contract for details about whether your insurer will pay at least a portion of these costs. Also, if hospital care is needed, use your pediatrician's guidance in selecting a hospital in your plan that specializes in the care of children. (Most hospital procedures and surgeries require prior approval.)

- Know in advance what emergency services are covered since you won't always have time to contact your pediatrician. Most managed care plans will pay for emergency room care in a true emergency, so in a life-threatening situation, go immediately to the nearest hospital. In general, follow-up care (e.g., removing stitches) should be done in your pediatrician's office.
- To file a complaint—for example, if coverage of certain procedures is denied—start by expressing your concern to your pediatrician. If she is unable to resolve the problem, contact your plan's member service representative or employee benefits manager about filing a complaint. If a claim has been denied, you typically have fifteen to thirty days to file an appeal, and you should receive a decision about the appeal within thirty to ninety days of the request. If you still are dissatisfied, you may decide to seek help from the office of your state insurance commissioner, or you can take legal action.

After these interviews, ask yourself if you are comfortable with the pediatrician's philosophy, policies, and practice. You must feel that you can trust her and that your questions will be answered and your concerns handled compassionately. You also should feel comfortable with the staff and the general atmosphere of the office.

Once your baby arrives, the most important test of the pediatrician you have selected is how she cares for your child and responds to your concerns. If you are unhappy with any aspect of the treatment you and your child are receiving, you should talk to the pediatrician directly about the problem. If the response does not address your concerns, or if the problem simply cannot be resolved, seek out another physician.

Issues to Discuss with Your Pediatrician

Once you have found a pediatrician with whom you feel comfortable, let her help you plan for your child's basic care and feeding. Certain decisions and preparations should be made before the baby arrives. Your pediatrician can advise you on such issues as the following.

When Should the Baby Leave the Hospital?

Each mother and baby should be evaluated individually to determine the best time of discharge. The timing of the discharge should be the decision of you and the physician caring for the infant, not the insurance company.

Should the Baby Be Circumcised?

If you have a boy, you'll need to decide whether to have him circumcised. Unless you are sure you're having a girl, it's a good idea to make a decision about circumcision ahead of time, so you don't have to struggle with it amid the fatigue and excitement following delivery.

Circumcision has been practiced as a religious rite for thousands of years. In the United States, most boys are circumcised for religious or social reasons. At present, there is controversy over whether circumcision is advisable from a medical standpoint. There are potential medical benefits to circumcision. Studies have concluded that circumcised infants have a slightly lower risk of urinary tract infections, although these are not common in boys and occur less often in circumcised boys mostly in the first year of life. Neonatal circumcision also provides some protection from penile cancer, a very rare condition. (See also *Circumcision*, page 29.)

Some research also suggests a reduced likelihood of developing sexually transmitted diseases and HIV infections in

Circumcision

At birth, most boys have skin that completely covers, or almost covers, the end of the penis. Circumcision removes some of this foreskin so that the tip of the penis (glans) and the opening of the urethra, through which the baby urinates, are exposed to air. Routine circumcisions are performed in the hospital within a few days of birth. When done by an experienced physician, circumcision takes only a few minutes and is rarely complicated. After consultation with you, your doctor will provide local anesthesia to reduce the pain the baby experiences during the procedure; the doctor should inform you in advance about the type of anesthesia she recommends.

circumcised men, and possibly a reduced risk for cervical cancer in female partners of circumcised men. However, while there are potential medical benefits, these data are not sufficient to recommend routine neonatal circumcision. (See *Where We Stand* box, page 30).

Circumcision does, however, pose certain risks, such as infection and bleeding. Although the evidence also is clear that infants experience pain, there are several safe and effective ways to reduce the pain. If the baby is born prematurely, has an illness at birth, or has congenital abnormalities or blood problems, he should not be circumcised immediately. For example, if a condition called *hypospadias* (see page 653) is present, in which the infant's urinary opening has not formed normally, your doctor will probably recommend that your baby boy *not* be circumcised at birth. In fact, circumcision should be performed only on stable, healthy infants.

Should I Breastfeed or Bottle-Feed?

Before your baby arrives, you'll want to consider whether you're going to breastfeed or use formula. The American Academy of Pediatrics advocates breastfeeding as the optimal form of infant feeding. Even though formula feeding is

Where We Stand

The American Academy of Pediatrics believes that circumcision has potential medical benefits and advantages, as well as risks. The existing scientific evidence is not sufficient to recommend routine circumcision. Therefore, because the procedure is not essential to a child's current well-being, we recommend that the decision to circumcise is one best made by parents in consultation with their pediatrician, taking into account what is in the best interests of the child, including medical, religious, cultural, and ethnic traditions. Your pediatrician (or your obstetrician if he or she would be performing the circumcision) should discuss the benefits and risks of circumcision with you and the forms of analgesia that are available.

not identical to breastfeeding, formulas do provide appropriate nutrition. Both approaches are safe and healthy for your baby, and each has its advantages.

The most practical benefits of breastfeeding are convenience and cost, but there are some real medical benefits, too. Breastmilk provides your baby with natural antibodies that help her resist some types of infections (including ear, respiratory, and intestinal infections). Breastfed babies also are less likely to suffer from allergies that occasionally occur in babies fed cow's milk formulas. Breastfed infants also may be

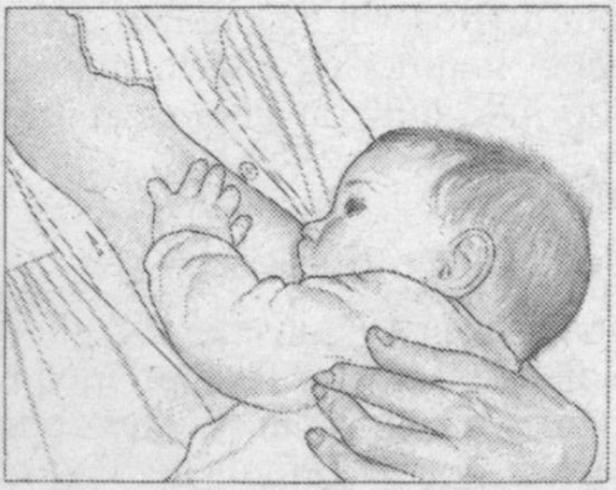

The American Academy of Pediatrics advocates breastfeeding as the optimal form of infant feeding.

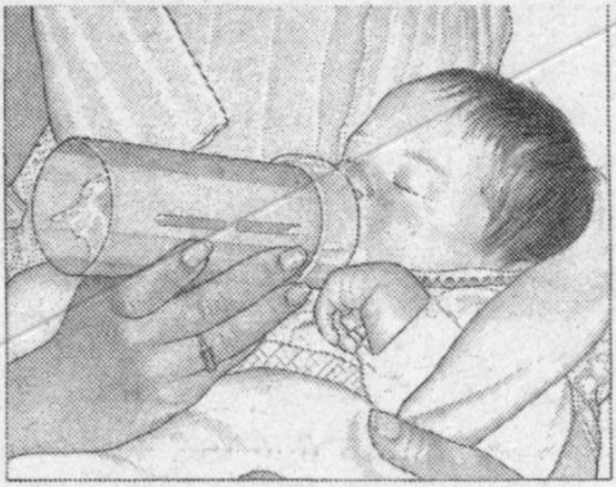

If you cannot breastfeed or you choose not to do so, you still can achieve similar feelings of closeness during bottle-feedings.

less likely to develop asthma and diabetes, or become overweight, than those who are bottle-fed (see also Chapter 4).

Mothers who nurse their babies feel there are many emotional rewards. Once the milk supply is established and the baby is nursing well, both mother and child experience a tremendous sense of closeness and comfort, a bond that continues throughout infancy. The first week or two can be challenging for some, but most pediatricians can offer guidance or refer you to a certified lactation consultant for assistance if needed.

If there is a medical reason you cannot breastfeed or you choose not to do so, you still can achieve similar feelings of closeness during bottle-feedings. Rocking, cuddling, stroking, and gazing into your baby's eyes will enhance the experience for both of you, regardless of the milk source.

Before making your decision on this issue, read Chapter 4, so that you thoroughly understand the advantages and disadvantages of breastfeeding and bottle-feeding, and you are aware of all the options available to you. If you decide upon breastfeeding, there are classes available in many communities to help you plan for breastfeeding and get your questions about it answered. Ask your doctor for a referral.

Should I Store My Newborn's Cord Blood?

Umbilical cord blood has been used successfully to treat a number of genetic, blood, and cancer conditions in children such as leukemia and immune disorders. Some parents are choosing to store their baby's cord blood for possible future use. However, there are no accurate statistics on the likelihood of children someday needing their own stored cells. In response, the American Academy of Pediatrics discourages storing cord blood at private banks for later personal or family use as a general "insurance policy." Rather, they encourage families to donate their newborn's cord blood, which is normally discarded at birth, to cord blood banks (if accessible in their area) for other individuals in need. (You should be aware, though, that your baby's cord blood would not be available as a stem cell source if your child developed leukemia later in life.)

Storing your child's cord blood is certainly an issue that you should discuss with your obstetrician and/or pediatrician *before* your baby is born, not during the emotionally stressful time of delivery. She may refer you to cord blood banks in your community. You will need to register ahead of time so that the appropriate collection kit can be sent to you or your obstetrician to be used at your delivery.

Preparing Your Home and Family for the Baby's Arrival

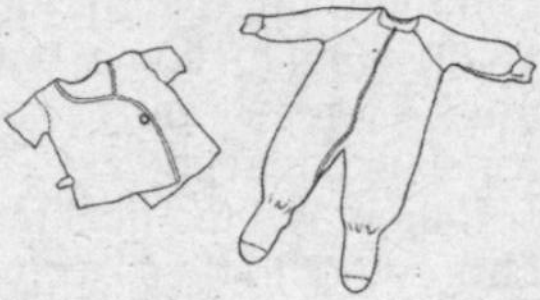

Choosing a Layette

As your due date nears, you'll need a layette, the basic collection of baby clothes and accessories that will get your newborn through his first few weeks. A suggested starting list includes:

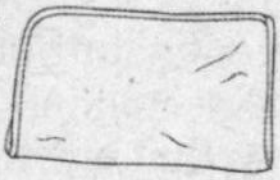

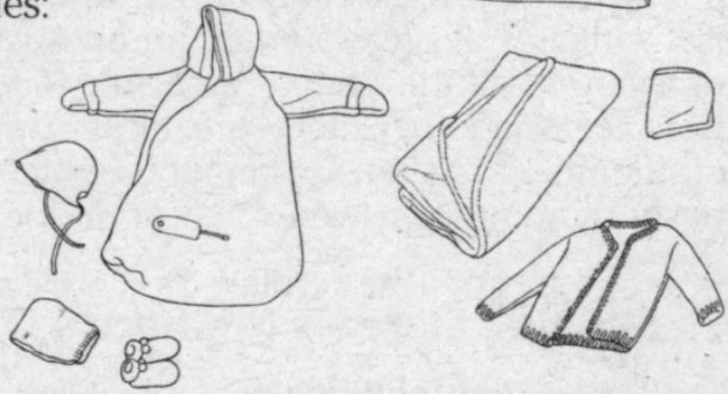

3 or 4 pajama sets (with feet)
6 to 8 T-shirts
3 newborn sleep sacks
2 sweaters
2 bonnets/hats
4 pairs of socks or booties
4 to 6 receiving/swaddle blankets
1 set of baby washcloths and towels (look for towels with hoods)

3 to 4 dozen newborn-size diapers
3 to 4 onesies/T-shirts with snaps between legs

For more information to help you make your selections for the rest of the items you need, see *Guidelines on Making Layette Choices* below.

Guidelines on Making Layette Choices

Here are some suggestions to keep in mind when selecting clothing for your newborn:

- Buy big. Unless your baby is born prematurely or is very small, she probably will outgrow "newborn" sizes in a matter of days—if she ever fits into them at all! Even three-month sizes may be outgrown within the first month. You'll want a couple of garments that your child can wear in the very beginning, but concentrate on larger sizes for the rest of the wardrobe. Your baby won't mind if her clothes are slightly large for a while, or if she wears the same outfit every day.
- To avoid injury from a garment that catches fire, all children should wear flame-retardant sleepwear and clothing. Make sure the label indicates this. These garments should be washed in laundry detergents, not soap, because soap will wash out the flame retardant. Check garment labels and product information to determine which detergents to use.
- Make sure the crotch opens easily for diaper changes.
- Avoid any clothing that pulls tightly around the neck, arms, or legs or has ties or cords. These clothes are not only safety hazards, but are also uncomfortable.

- Check washing instructions. Clothing for children of all ages should be washable and require little or no ironing.
- Do *not* put shoes on a newborn's feet. Shoes are not necessary until after she starts to walk. Worn earlier, they can interfere with the growth of her feet. The same is true of socks and footed pajamas if they're too small and worn for a prolonged period of time.

Buying Furniture and Baby Equipment

Walk into any baby store and you probably will be overwhelmed by the selection of equipment available. A few items are essential, but most things, while enticing, are not necessary. In fact, some are not even useful. To help you sort through the options, here is a list of the basic necessities you should have on hand when your baby arrives.

- **A crib** that meets all safety specifications (see *Safety Alert: Cribs,* below). New cribs sold today must meet these standards, but if you're looking at used cribs, check them carefully to make sure they meet the same standards and have not been recalled. Unless you have money to spare, don't bother with a bassinet. Your baby will outgrow it in just a few weeks.

Safety Alert: Cribs

Your baby usually will be unattended when in her crib, so this should be a totally safe environment. Falls are the most common injury associated with cribs, even though they are the easiest to prevent. Children are most likely to fall out of the crib when the mattress is raised too high for their height or when the side rail is left down.

If you use a new crib or one manufactured since 1985, it should meet current safety standards. Look for one with Juvenile Product Manufacturers Association (JPMA) certification. If you plan to use an older crib, inspect it carefully for the following features:

- Slats should be no more than 2⅜ inches (6 cm) apart so a child's head cannot become trapped between them.
- There should be no cutouts in the headboard or footboard, as your child's head could become trapped in them.
- If the crib has corner posts (sometimes called finials), unscrew them or cut them off. Loose clothing can become snagged on these and choke your baby.

You can prevent other crib hazards by observing the following guidelines:

1. If you purchase a new mattress, remove and destroy all plastic wrapping material that comes with it, because it can suffocate a child. If you cover the mattress with heavy plastic, be sure the cover fits tightly; zippered covers are best. The mattress should be firm, not soft.

2. As soon as your baby can sit, lower the crib mattress to the level where she cannot fall out either by leaning against the side or by pulling herself over it. Set the mattress at its lowest position before your child learns to stand (typically between ages six and nine months). The most common falls occur when a baby tries to climb out, so move your child to another bed when she is 35 inches (88.9 cm) tall, or the height of the side rail is at or below her nipple line while standing.

3. When fully lowered, the top of the crib's side rail should be at least 4 inches (10.16 cm) above the mattress, even when the mattress is set at its highest position. Be sure the locking latch that holds the side up is sturdy and can't be released by your child. Always leave the side up when your child is in the crib.

4. The mattress should fit snugly so your child cannot slip into the crack between it and the crib side. If you can insert two fingers between the mattress and the sides or ends of the crib, replace the mattress with one that fits snugly.

5. Periodically check the crib to be sure there are no rough edges or sharp points on the metal parts and no splinters or cracks in the wood.

6. If you use a crib bumper when your child is an infant, be sure it goes all the way around the crib and is secured with at least six straps or ties, to keep the bumper from falling away from the sides. To prevent strangulation, the ties should be no more than 6 inches (15.24 cm) long. Do not use pillowlike bumper pads or any other soft bedding.

7. As soon as your child can pull to a standing position, remove the crib bumpers, which could be used as a step for climbing out.

8. If you hang a mobile over your child's crib, be sure it is securely attached to the side rails. Hang it high enough so your baby cannot reach it to pull it down, and remove it when he starts to push up on his hands and knees or when he reaches five months, whichever comes first. Even before pushing up, some infants roll on their side and reach up to grab the mobile and pull it down.

9. Remove crib gyms (objects like bright balls affixed to the crib rail) as soon as your child can get up on all fours. Even though these gyms are designed to withstand a child's grabbing and tugging, she could fall forward onto the gym and become entangled.

10. To prevent the most serious falls, don't place a crib—or any other child's bed—beside a window. Do not hang pictures or shelves above the child's bed; they can pose hazards in the event of an earthquake.

- **Bedding for the crib,** including a flannel-backed, waterproof mattress cover (which is cooler and more comfortable for your baby than plain plastic or rubber covers), and tight fitted sheets. Never use infant cushions that have soft fabric coverings and are loosely filled with plastic foam beads or pellets. Remove all pillows, quilts, comforters, sheepskins, and other pillowlike soft products. Remember that the safest position for a baby to sleep in is on her back (see *Positioning for Sleep,* page 71).
- **A changing table** that meets all safety specifications (see *Changing Tables,* page 391). It should be placed on a carpet or padded mat and against a wall, not a window, so there is no danger of your child falling out the window. Put shelves or tables to hold diapers, wipes, and other changing equipment within immediate reach (but away from the baby's reach), so you will not have to step away from the table—even for a second—to get anything.
- **A diaper pail.** Keep the pail securely closed. If you are going to wash your own diapers, you'll need a second pail so you can separate wet diapers from "soiled" ones.
- **A large plastic washtub** for bathing the baby. As an alternative to the washtub, you can use the kitchen sink to bathe your newborn, provided the faucet swings out of the way and the dishwasher is off. (The water from the dishwasher could dump into the sink, resulting in scalding.) After the first month, it's safer to switch to a separate tub, because the baby will be able to reach and turn on

Safety Alert: Bassinets and Cradles

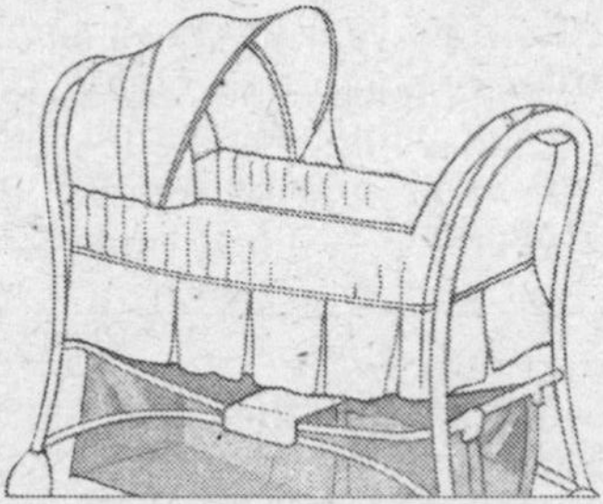

Many parents prefer to use a bassinet or cradle for the first few weeks, because it's portable and allows the newborn to sleep in the parents' room. But remember that infants grow very fast, so a cradle that is sturdy enough one month may be outgrown the next. To get the longest and safest possible use from your baby's first bed, check the following before buying:

1. The bottom of the cradle or bassinet should be well supported so it cannot possibly collapse.

2. The bassinet or cradle should have a wide base so it cannot tip over even if someone bumps against it. If the bassinet or cradle has folding legs, they should be locked straight whenever the bed is in use. Your baby should graduate to a crib around the end of the first month or by the time she weighs 10 pounds (4.5 kg).

Co-sleepers are infant beds or bassinets that can be attached to the parents' bed, and many mothers and fathers find them convenient to have their baby close by for nighttime feedings. However, the Consumer Product Safety Commission has not established safety standards for these products.

the faucet from the sink. Always make sure the bathing area is very clean before bathing your baby. Also, be sure the hottest temperature at the faucet is no more than 120 degrees Fahrenheit (48.9 degrees Celsius) to avoid burns. In most cases, you can adjust your water heater.

Everything in the nursery should be kept clean and dust-free. (See Chapter 11 for safety specifications.) All surfaces, including window and floor coverings, should be washable. So should all toys that are left out. Although stuffed animals look cute around newborns (they seem to be a favorite shower gift), they tend to collect dust and may contribute to stuffy noses. Since your baby won't actively play with them for many months, you might consider storing them until she's ready for them.

If the air in the nursery is extremely dry, your pediatrician may recommend using a cool mist humidifier. This also may help clear your child's stuffy nose when she has a cold. If you do use a humidifier, clean it frequently as directed in the package instructions and empty it when not in use. Otherwise, bacteria and molds may grow in the still water. Steam vaporizers are not recommended because of the danger of scalding.

One object that your baby is sure to enjoy is a mobile. Look for one with bright colors (the first color she'll see is red) and varied shapes. Some also play music. When shopping for a mobile, look at it from below so that you'll know how it appears from your baby's point of view. Avoid the models that look good only from the side or above—they were designed more for your enjoyment than for the infant's. Make sure you remove the mobile at five months of age or as soon as your baby can sit up, because that's when she'll be able to pull it down and risk injury.

Other useful additions to the nursery may include a rocking chair or glider, a music box or musical toy and a tape, CD, or MP3 player. The rocking motion of the chair will increase the soothing effect your baby feels when you hold her. Playing soft music for your baby will comfort her when you're not nearby and will help her fall asleep.

You will want to keep the lights in the nursery soft once your newborn has arrived and leave a night-light on after dark. The night-light will allow you to check on the baby more easily, and as she gets older, it will reassure her when she awakens at night. Make sure all lights and cords are kept safely out of the baby's reach.

Preparing Your Other Children for the Baby's Arrival

If you have other children, you'll need to plan carefully how and when to tell them about the new baby. A child who is four or older should be told as soon as you start telling friends and relatives. She should have a basic sense of how she is related to her new brother or sister. Fables about storks and such may seem cute, but they won't help your youngster understand and accept the situation. Using one of the picture books published on the subject may help you to explain "where babies come from." Too much detail can be scary for her. It's usually enough to say: "Like you, this baby was made from a little bit of Mommy and a little bit of Daddy."

If your child is younger than four when you become pregnant, you can wait awhile before telling her. When she's this young, she's still very self-centered and may have difficulty understanding an abstract concept like an unborn baby. But once you start furnishing the nursery, bringing her crib back into the house, and making or buying baby clothes, she should be told what's going on. Also take advantage of any questions she may ask about Mom's growing "stomach" to explain what's happening. Picture books about babies or about becoming a big sister or brother can be useful with very young children, too. Sharing ultrasound pictures with

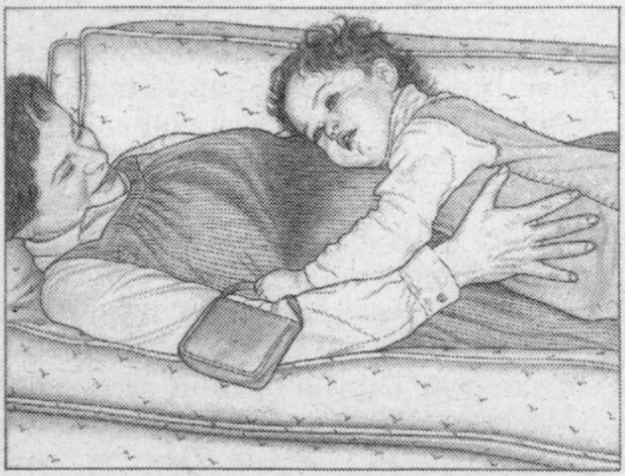

Take advantage of any questions your child may ask about Mom's growing "stomach" to explain what's happening.

her can be helpful, as well. Even if she doesn't ask any questions, start talking to your older child about the baby by the last few months of pregnancy. If your hospital offers a sibling preparation class, take her so that she can see where the baby will be born and where she can visit you. Point out other newborns and their older siblings, and tell her how she's going to be a big sister soon.

Don't promise that things will be the same after the baby comes, because they won't be, no matter how hard you try. But reassure your child that you will love her just as much, and help her understand the positive side of having a baby sibling.

Breaking the news is most difficult if your child is between two and three. At this age, she's still extremely attached to you and doesn't yet understand the concept of sharing time, possessions, or your affection with anyone else. She's also very sensitive to changes going on around her and may feel threatened by the idea of a new family member. The best way to minimize her jealousy is to include her as much as possible in the preparations for the new baby. Let her shop with you for the layette and the nursery equipment. Show her pictures of herself as a newborn, and if you're recycling some of her old baby equipment, let her play with it a bit before you get it in order for the newcomer.

Any major changes in your preschooler's routine, such as toilet training, switching from a crib to a bed, changing bedrooms, or starting preschool should be completed before the baby arrives. If that's not possible, put them off until after the baby is settled in at home. Otherwise, your child may feel overwhelmed when the upheaval caused by the baby's arrival is added to the stress of her own adjustments.

Don't be alarmed if news that a baby is coming—or, later, the baby's arrival—prompts your older child's behavior to regress a little. She may demand a bottle, ask to wear diapers again, cry for no apparent reason, or refuse to leave your side. This is her way of demanding your love and attention and reassuring herself that she still has it. Instead of protesting or telling her to act her age, simply grant her requests, and don't get upset about it. A three-year-old toilet-trained child who demands a diaper for a few days, or the five-year-old who wants her outgrown (you thought long-forgotten) security blanket for a week, will soon return to her normal routine when she realizes that she now has just as important a place in the family as her new sibling. Similarly, an older sibling who wants to try nursing again will quickly lose interest.

However busy or preoccupied you may be with your new arrival, make sure you reserve some special time each day just for you and your older child. Read, play games, listen to music, or simply talk together. Show her that you're interested in what she's doing, thinking, and feeling—not only in relation to the baby, but about everything else in her life. It

Preparing Dad for Delivery

If you're the father-to-be, remember that having a baby is a family event. You can help with the tasks and preparations for the baby's arrival described above. At the same time, you'll be making your own adjustments, which are challenging, too. Of course, your role during the nine-month pregnancy has been quite different, but you still have had adjustments to make. At times you've felt excited and elated; other times, fearful, exhausted, and perhaps just tired of waiting for the baby to arrive. There probably have been times when you've been an emotional anchor for your wife or partner during some of the more difficult moments of pregnancy, from periods of extreme fatigue to morning sickness.

When you attend prenatal visits to the obstetrician, discuss what role you'll play in the delivery room. Be sure to get all your questions answered about what will take place and how you can be most supportive. If you can do any advance planning in order to take off a few days or weeks from work once the baby arrives, make those arrangements now. And, of course, be ready to play a very active role in your child's life, not only in the first few days after her birth, but for the rest of your lives together. (For a further discussion about the unique role of fathers—and grandparents—in the birth of their baby, see Chapter 6, pages 215–220.)

takes only five or ten minutes a day of protected time—time when the baby is asleep or being cared for by another adult—to make your older child feel special.

For both parents, once your baby finally arrives, all the waiting and discomforts of pregnancy will seem like minor inconveniences. Suddenly you'll get to meet this new person who's been so close and yet so mysterious all these months. The rest of this book is about the child she will become and the job that awaits you as a parent.

There's only so much preparation you can do before you start any journey. We have discussed a lot of the supplies you will need as well as many of the dos and don'ts. Ultimately, the way you assume your role as a parent will be determined more by the way you prepare yourself spiritually and emotionally than by what color you choose for the nursery wallpaper or the style of crib you buy. Only you know how you respond to stress and change. Try to prepare yourself for parenthood in a way that feels most comfortable to you. Some parents find support groups helpful; others prefer to meditate, sketch, or write.

Preparing yourself might be more difficult for some soon-to-be parents than others, especially if you are the kind of person who likes spontaneity more than figuring everything out in advance, but preparation is important, since it gives rise to greater confidence. It takes a stunning amount of confidence for a child to begin to walk. Similarly, you will need that type of confidence to take your own first steps into parenting.

Finally—Delivery Day!

The duration of most pregnancies is between thirty-seven and forty-two weeks. Labor contractions are the clearest indication that your body is getting ready to deliver your baby. When labor starts, your cervix (the lower end of the uterus) will open, and the uterus will begin contracting or squeezing. The cervix must be effaced (or thinned out) in order for the baby's head to move into the birth canal. Each time a contraction occurs, your uterus and abdomen will become tighter and firmer. Between contractions, the uterus will soften, and you can relax for a short time while awaiting the next contraction.

Although most women know when they are nearing labor

or when labor has started, it isn't always easy to tell for sure when this process has begun. That's because "false labor" can occur, in which contractions are sporadic and relatively weak. Even so, don't be embarrassed to call your doctor or go to the hospital if you're uncertain whether this is the real thing!

With actual labor, you will experience:

- Repeated contractions, cramps, and increases in pain levels corresponding to the opening up (dilating) of your cervix and the baby's descent through the birth canal.
- A slightly bloody, pink, or clear vaginal discharge that is the mucus plug at the cervix.
- A breaking of your water, which is really a rupture in the amniotic sac that contains watery fluid that surrounds and protects your baby.

As labor progresses, the contractions will become stronger, they'll occur more often, and they'll continue for about thirty to seventy seconds each. The pain of the contractions will tend to start in your back, and then move forward to the lower abdomen.

When should you call your doctor or go to the hospital? Hopefully, you've already discussed this with your doctor. In general, you should head for the hospital or phone your doctor if your water breaks (even if you aren't having contractions yet), you're experiencing vaginal bleeding, or the pain is severe and persistent even between contractions.

The doctor may induce labor before you go into labor on your own. This induction may be chosen if your doctor determines that your health or the health of your baby is being threatened. Perhaps you have a chronic disease such as diabetes or high blood pressure that may pose risks to you or your child. Or your doctor may recommend inducing labor if tests indicate that your baby's growth is unusual. With certain medications (such as oxytocin or prostaglandin drugs that may be given intravenously in the hospital), the mother will have contractions and her cervix will start to open and efface. The doctor can also intentionally rupture the membranes that surround the fetus or use other means to get labor started.

What About the Pain?

Pain levels during delivery vary from one woman to another. For some, the process can be very painful, but women can often turn to relaxation and breathing techniques (taught in their childbirth classes) to help them deal with the discomfort. Massage on the lower back by a spouse or other labor coach often eases discomfort as well, as does taking a bath or shower (if allowed) or applying ice packs to the back.

If an episiotomy (surgical incision in vaginal area) is needed to ease the baby's head through the birth canal, a local anesthetic is injected ahead of time to make the area numb. Local anesthetics given in this manner almost never have any negative effects upon the baby.

As labor progresses, many women decide to have medication to ease the pain of the contractions. These include:

1. *Narcotic (opioid) medications given as a shot or through an intravenous catheter.* These medications make the labor pains more tolerable but can slow the baby's breathing if given very close to delivery.

2. *Numbing medicines given in the spinal region to reduce the intensity of the contractions.* This is generally referred to as epidural analgesia or an epidural block. A small tube called a catheter is placed into the epidural space, an area just outside of the spinal cord region. Medicines are then given through this catheter to decrease the feeling in your abdomen and make the contractions less painful. Pain relief generally begins within ten to twenty minutes. Most of the time these medications are given in small enough doses so that you are still alert, aware of the contractions (though they are not as painful), and still have enough strength to push the baby down the birth canal. Side effects or

complications are rare, but may include headaches or a drop in your blood pressure.

If your doctor decides that a Cesarean section is necessary, there are three options for pain relief/anesthesia:

1. *Additional numbing medicine can be given through an epidural catheter to make your entire lower body numb (from below your rib cage to your toes).* If you already had an epidural catheter placed to ease the labor pain, then extra medicine can be given through this catheter to make you numb enough for surgery. The advantage of this type of anesthesia is that the baby will not be as sleepy and you can be awake when the baby is born.

2. *If you are having a scheduled Cesarean section, your doctor may recommend a spinal block.* This is a single injection into the fluid surrounding the spinal cord. Spinal blocks are very quick and easy to perform and generally make you even more numb than an epidural block. Pain relief begins immediately. One difference between a spinal and an epidural block is that a spinal is a one-time shot of pain medication that wears off on its own in several hours, instead of being administered continuously through a catheter. Side effects or complications are rare, but are similar to an epidural.

3. *If the surgery needs to be performed as an emergency or you have a medical issue that would make an epidural or spinal block dangerous for you, medicines can be given that will make you lose consciousness or "go to sleep" (general anesthesia).* This can make the baby very sleepy when he/she is born and affect the baby's breathing. When general anesthesia is given, the baby must be delivered very quickly in order to decrease these effects, so epidural or spinal blocks are preferred when possible.

For more detailed information about routine vaginal deliveries and Cesarean sections, including procedures in hospital delivery rooms upon the birth of your baby, see Chapter 2, *Birth and the First Moments After,* pages 48–65.)

2

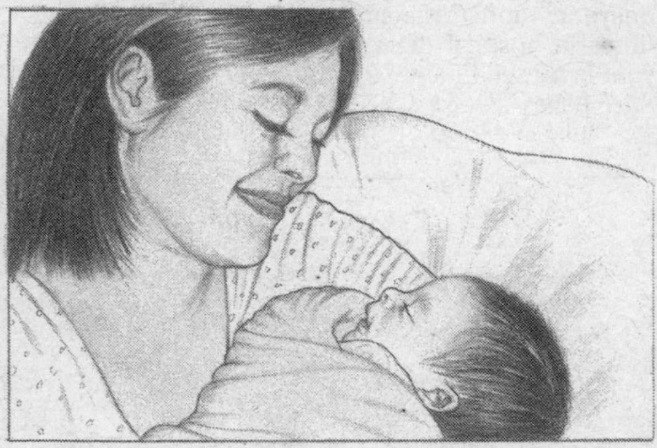

Birth and the First Moments After

Giving birth is one of the most extraordinary experiences of a woman's life. Yet after all the months of careful preparation and anticipation, the moment of birth is almost never what you had expected. Labor may be easier or more physically demanding than you had imagined. You may end up in a delivery room instead of the birthing room you'd wanted, or you could have a Cesarean section instead of a vaginal delivery. Your health, the condition of the fetus, and the policies of the hospital will all help determine what actually happens. But fortunately, despite what you may have thought when you were pregnant, these are not the issues that will make your child's birth a "success." What counts is the baby, here at last and healthy.

ROUTINE VAGINAL DELIVERY

In the days and weeks leading up to the birth of your baby, you'll probably feel a bit of apprehension along with your excitement, wondering when this much-anticipated event finally will happen. Then, usually between the thirty-seventh and forty-second week of your pregnancy, you'll go into labor. Although no one knows for certain what triggers this process, shifts in hormone levels appear to play a role. Your amniotic sac may seem to begin the process by rupturing, commonly referred to as "breaking your water." As you proceed through labor, your uterus will contract rhythmically, or squeeze, which will move your baby down the birth canal. At the same time, these contractions will fully open, or dilate, your cervix to an opening of about 10 centimeters (4 in.) so the baby can make his appearance through the vagina.

In a routine vaginal delivery, your first view of your child may be the top, or crown, of his head, seen with the help of a mirror. After the head is delivered, the obstetrician will suction the nose and mouth and your baby will take her first breath. She doesn't need to be slapped or spanked to begin breathing, nor will she necessarily cry; many newborns take their first breath quietly.

With the most difficult part of the birth now over, there is usually one last pause before the push that sends the rest of your child's body, which is smaller than his head, gliding smoothly into the doctor's or nurse midwife's waiting arms. After another, more thorough suctioning of his nose and mouth, your child may be handed to you to hold—and behold.

Even if you've seen pictures of newborns, you're bound to be amazed by the first sight of your own infant. When she opens her eyes, they will meet yours with curiosity. All the activity of birth may make her very alert and responsive to your touch, voice, and warmth. Take advantage of this attentiveness, which may last for the first few hours. Stroke her, talk to her, and look closely at this child you've created. The obstetrician or nurse midwife may place the baby on your abdomen or lower chest in those first few moments. Watch how the baby moves up toward your breast, seeking that first feeding. Those moments are magical for you and the baby. Those moments should not be hindered; they should be allowed to happen. The natural wonder of your baby looking at you, looking at your breasts and wriggling upward, will make you realize just how exciting those important first few minutes are. Attendants should not wash you, nor should they wash the baby or interfere. The smell and feel of the moment will guide the baby to her first feeding. As with many moms, you may find that putting your baby to your breast creates an intense emotional bond between you and your newborn.

Nursing After Delivery

We recommend that you plan to breastfeed your baby. If this is the decision you've made, ask ahead of time about the hospital's policies on nursing in the delivery area. Today, most hospitals encourage immediate breastfeeding following routine delivery unless the baby's scores on the Apgar test are low or she's breathing very rapidly, in which case nursing may need to be delayed temporarily. (See page 55 for detailed information on these tests.)

Breastfeeding right away benefits the mother by causing the uterus to contract, thus reducing the amount of uterine bleeding. (The same hormone that stimulates the milk ejection reflex, or letdown response, triggers the uterine contractions.)

The first hour or so after birth is a good time to begin breastfeeding, because your baby is very alert and eager. When put to the breast she may first lick it. Then, with a little help, she'll grasp and latch on to the areola, not the nipple, and suck vigorously for several minutes. If you wait until later, she may be sleepier and have more difficulty holding the nipple effectively.

For the first two to five days after delivery, your body produces colostrum, a thin, yellowish fluid that contains protein and antibodies to protect him from infection. Colostrum provides all the nutrients and fluids your baby needs in the first few days of life. (For a complete discussion of breastfeeding, see Chapter 4.)

Fresh from birth, your child may be covered with a white cheesy substance called vernix. This protective coating is produced toward the end of pregnancy by the sebaceous (oil-producing) glands in her skin. She'll also be wet with amniotic fluid. If there was an episiotomy (surgical cutting) or tearing of tissue in the vaginal area, she may have some of your own blood on her. Her skin, especially on the face, may be quite wrinkled from the wetness and pressure of birth.

Your baby's shape and size also may surprise you, especially if this is your first child. On one hand, it's hard to believe that a human being can be so tiny; on the other, it's incredible that this "enormous" creature could possibly have fit inside your body. The size and shape of her head in particular may alarm you. How could the head possibly have made it through the birth canal? The answer lies in its slightly elongated shape. The head was able to adapt to the contours of the passageway as it was pushed through, squeezing to fit. Now free, it may take up to several days to revert to its normal oval shape. Your baby's skin color may be a little blue at first, but gradually will turn pinker as her breathing becomes regular. Her hands and feet may be slightly blue and feel cool, and may remain so, on and off, for several weeks until her body is better able to adjust to the temperature around her.

You also may notice that your newborn's breathing is irregular and very rapid. While you normally take twelve to fourteen breaths per minute, your newborn may take as many as forty to sixty breaths per minute. An occasional deep breath may alternate with bursts of short, shallow breaths followed by pauses. Don't let this make you anxious. It's normal for the initial days after birth.

Delivery by Cesarean Section

More than one mother in three gives birth by Cesarean section in the United States (it is also called C-section or, simply, section). In a C-section, surgery is performed, with an incision made in the mother's abdomen and uterus, so the baby can be taken directly from the uterus instead of traveling through the birth canal.

Cesarean sections are done most often when:

- The mother has had a previous baby by Cesarean delivery
- The obstetrician feels that the baby's health might suffer if born vaginally
- The fetus's heartbeat slows abnormally or becomes irregular (in which case the obstetrician will perform an emergency C-section instead of taking the chance of allowing labor to progress)

While most babies are in a head-down position in the mother's uterus, about three in one hundred newborns have their buttocks, feet, or both positioned to come out first during birth (a breech presentation). If your baby has assumed a breech position, your obstetrician will recommend a Cesarean section as the best means of delivery. The reason is because breech babies are more difficult to deliver vaginally, and complications are more likely to occur with a vaginally delivered breech baby. A doctor can determine the baby's position by feeling the mother's lower abdomen at particular points; the physician may decide to confirm the breech position by ordering an ultrasound or other tests.

The birth experience with a C-section is very different from that of a vaginal delivery. For one thing, the whole operation ordinarily takes no more than an hour, and—depending on the circumstances—you may not experience any labor at all. Another important difference is the need to use medication that affects the mother and may affect the baby. If given a choice of anesthetic, most women prefer to have a regional anesthesia—an injection in the back that blocks pain by numbing the spinal nerves—such as an epidural or a spinal. Administration of a regional anesthesia numbs the body from the waist down, has relatively few side effects, and allows you to witness the delivery. But sometimes, especially for an emergency C-section, a general anesthetic must be used, in which case you are not conscious at all. Your obstetrician and the anesthesiologist in attendance will advise you which approach they think is best, based on the medical circumstances at the time.

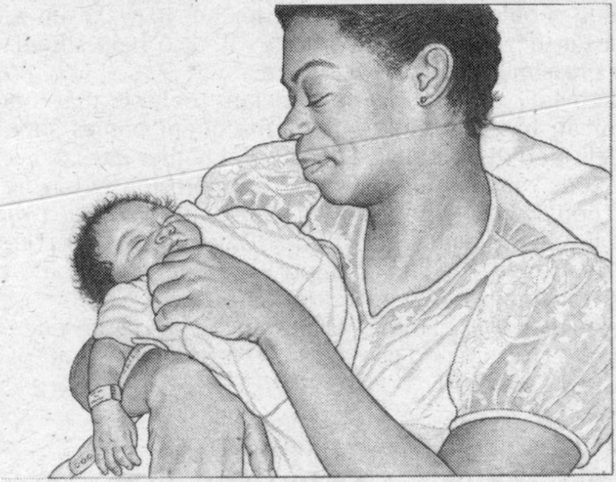

Because of the effects of the anesthesia and the way the baby is delivered, babies born by C-section sometimes have difficulty breathing in the beginning and need extra help. A pediatrician or other person skilled in newborn problems usually is present during a Cesarean section to examine and assist the baby's breathing, if necessary, immediately after birth.

If you were awake during the operation, you may be able to see your baby as soon as she's been examined and proclaimed healthy. She may then be taken to the nursery to spend several hours in a temperature-controlled crib or isolette. This allows the hospital staff to observe her while the anesthesia wears off and she adjusts to her new surroundings.

If general anesthesia was used during the delivery, you may not wake up for a few hours. When you do, you may feel groggy and confused. You'll probably also experience some pain where the incision was made. But you'll soon be able to hold your baby, and you'll quickly make up for lost time.

Don't be surprised if your baby is still affected by the anesthesia for six to twelve hours after delivery and appears a little sleepy. If you're going to breastfeed, try to nurse her as soon as you feel well enough. Even if she's drowsy, her first feeding should provide a reason for her to wake up and meet her new world—and you. It will also help stimulate your breastmilk production.

As mentioned, many obstetricians believe that once a woman has a C-section, her subsequent babies should be delivered the same way because of higher rates of complications with vaginal deliveries after previously having a C-section. However, many women are candidates for a vaginal birth after Cesarean section (VBAC). But a decision to do this will depend on a number of factors and should be made together with your doctor.

If you're the father-to-be, discuss your role and presence in the delivery room and ways you can best support your partner during the birth.

Delivery Room Procedures Following a Normal Vaginal Birth

As your baby lies with you following a routine delivery, her umbilical cord still will be attached to the placenta. The cord may continue to pulsate for several minutes, supplying the baby with oxygen while she establishes her own breathing. Once the pulsing stops, the cord will be clamped and cut. (Because there are no nerves in the cord, the baby feels no pain during this procedure.) The clamp will remain in place for twenty-four to forty-eight hours, or until the cord is dry and no longer bleeds. The stump that remains after the clamp is removed will fall off sometime between one and three weeks after birth.

Once you've had a few moments to get acquainted with your baby, she will be dried to keep her from getting too cold, and a doctor or nurse will examine her briefly to make sure there are no obvious problems or abnormalities. She will be given Apgar scores (see pages 55–56), which measure her overall responsiveness. Then she will be wrapped in a blanket and given back to you.

Depending on the hospital's routine, your baby also may be weighed and measured, and receive medication before leaving the delivery room. She will receive a dose of vitamin K as well, since all newborns have slightly low levels of this vitamin (which is needed for normal blood clotting). You should feel comfortable to suggest that all of these steps

Apgar Scores

As soon as your baby is born, a delivery nurse will set one timer for one minute and another for five minutes. When each of these time periods is up, a nurse or physician will give your baby her first "tests," called Apgars.

This scoring system (named after its creator, Virginia Apgar) helps the physician estimate your baby's general condition at birth. The test measures your baby's heart rate, breathing, muscle tone, reflex response, and color. It cannot predict how healthy she will be as she grows up or how she will develop; nor does it indicate how bright she is or what her personality is like. But it does alert the hospital staff if she is sleepier or slower to respond than normal and may need assistance as she adapts to her new world outside the womb.

Each characteristic is given an individual score; two points for each of the five categories if all is completely well; then all scores are totaled. For example, let's say your baby has a heart rate of more than 100, cries lustily, moves actively, grimaces and coughs in response to the syringe, but is blue; her one-minute Apgar score would be 8—two points off because she is blue and not pink. Most newborn infants have Apgar scores greater than 7. Because their hands and feet remain blue until they are quite warm, few score a perfect 10.

If your baby's Apgar scores are between 5 and 7 at one minute, she may have experienced some problems during birth that lowered the oxygen in her blood. In this case, the hospital nursing staff probably will dry her vigorously with a towel while oxygen is held under her nose. This should start her breathing deeply and improve her oxygen supply so that her five-minute Apgar scores total between 8 and 10.

A small percentage of newborns have Apgar scores of less than 5. For example, babies born prematurely or delivered by emergency C-section are more likely to have low scores than infants with normal births. These scores may reflect difficulties the baby experienced during labor or problems with her heart or respiratory system.

If your baby's Apgar scores are very low, a mask may be placed over her face to pump oxygen directly into her lungs. If she's not breathing on her own within a few minutes, a tube can be placed into her windpipe, and fluids and medications may be administered through one of the blood vessels in her umbilical cord to strengthen her heartbeat. If her Apgar scores are still low after these treatments, she will be taken to the special-care nursery for more intensive medical attention.

Apgar Scoring System

Score	**0**	**1**	**2**
Heart Rate	Absent	Less than 100 beats per minute	More than 100 beats per minute
Respiration	Absent	Slow, irregular; weak cry	Good; strong cry
Muscle Tone	Limp	Some flexing of arms and legs	Active motion
Reflex*	Absent	Grimace	Grimace and cough or sneeze
Color	Blue or pale	Body pink; hands and feet blue	Completely pink

*Reflex judged by placing a catheter or bulb syringe in the infant's nose and watching her response.

wait thirty minutes to an hour while you hold your new baby and allow her to move successfully to your breast for her first feeding. Once successful, and once your baby appears to be resting on your skin, then those other steps, including the vitamin K injection, can be performed. The

Bonding

If you have a delivery without complications, you'll be able to spend the first hour or so after birth holding, stroking, and looking at your baby. Because babies are usually alert and very responsive during this time, researchers have labeled this the sensitive period.

The first exchanges of eye contact, sounds, and touches between the two of you are all part of a process called bonding, which helps lay the foundation for your relationship as parent and child. Although it will take months to learn your child's basic temperament and personality, many of the core emotions you feel for her may begin to develop during this brief period immediately after birth. As you gaze at her and she looks back, following your movements and perhaps even mirroring some of your expressions, you may feel a surge of protectiveness, awe, and love. This is part of the attachment process.

It's also quite normal if you do *not* immediately have tremendously warm feelings for your baby. Labor is a demanding experience, and your first reaction to the birth may well be a sense of relief that at last it's over. If you're exhausted and emotionally drained, you may simply want to rest. That's perfectly normal. Give yourself until the strain of labor fades and then request your baby. Bonding has no time limit.

Also, if your baby must be taken to the nursery right away for medical attention, or if you are sedated during the delivery, don't despair. You needn't worry that your relationship will be harmed because you didn't "bond" during this first hour. You can and will love your baby just as much, even if you weren't able to watch her birth or hold her immediately afterward. Your baby also will be fine, just as loving of you and connected to you.

most important thing is to maximize the skin-to-skin contact between you and your baby as much as possible in those first minutes.

Because bacteria in the birth canal can infect a baby's eyes, your baby will be given antibiotic or antiseptic eye drops or ointment (erythromycin ointment is commonly used), either immediately after delivery or later in the nursery, to prevent an eye infection.

At least one other important procedure must be done before either you or your newborn leave the delivery room: Both of you (and the baby's father) will receive matching labels bearing your name and other identifying details. After you verify the accuracy of these labels, each will be attached to your wrist and to the father's, while the other will be placed on your baby's wrist (and often to her ankle as well). Each time the child is taken from or returned to you while in the hospital, the nurse will check these bracelets to make sure they match. Many hospitals also footprint newborns as an added precaution and attach a small security device to the baby's ankle.

Leaving the Delivery Area

If you've given birth in a birthing room or alternative birth center, you probably won't be moved right away. But if you've delivered in a conventional delivery room, you'll be taken to a recovery area where you can be watched for problems such as excessive bleeding. Once again, insist that this separation from your baby wait until the baby has been with you for a while, at least an hour. Your baby may then be taken to the nursery at that time, or she may receive her first physical examination by your side.

This exam will measure her vital signs: temperature, respiration, and pulse rate. The pediatrician or nurse will check your baby from head to toe, paying specific attention to her color, activity level, and breathing pattern. If she didn't receive her vitamin K and eye drops earlier, they will be administered now. And once she's warm, she'll be given her first bath, and the stump of her cord may be painted with a blue antibacterial dye or other medication to prevent infection. Then she'll be wrapped in a blanket and, if you wish, returned to you.

If Your Baby Is Premature

Premature birth occurs in about 11 to 13 percent of pregnancies in the U.S. Almost 60 percent of twins, triplets, and other multiple deliveries result in preterm births. A birth is considered "preterm" when a child is born before 37 weeks of pregnancy have been completed. Other categories of preterm birth include late preterm (34–36 weeks), moderately preterm (32–36 weeks), and very preterm (less than 32 weeks).

It is important to recognize that preterm deliveries, even if late preterm, should never be done for the convenience of the mother or obstetrician. Research has shown that late preterm babies have significantly greater risk for negative outcomes, and all efforts should be made to have babies reach full term.

If your baby is born prematurely, she may neither look nor behave like a full-term infant. While the average full-term baby weighs about 7 pounds (3.17 kg) at birth, a premature newborn might weigh 5 pounds (2.26 kg) or even considerably less. But thanks to medical advances, children born after twenty-eight weeks of pregnancy, and weighing more than 2 pounds 3 ounces (1 kg), have almost a full chance of survival; eight out of ten of those born after the thirtieth week have minimal long-term health or developmental problems, while those preterm babies born before twenty-eight weeks have more complications, and require intensive treatment and support in a neonatal intensive care unit.

The earlier your baby arrives, the smaller she will be, the larger her head will seem in relation to the rest of her body, and the less fat she will have. With so little fat, her skin will seem thinner and more transparent, allowing you actually to see the blood vessels beneath it. She also may have fine hair, called lanugo, on her back and shoulders. Her features will appear sharper and less rounded than they would at term, and she probably won't have any of the white, cheesy vernix protecting her at birth, because it isn't produced until late in pregnancy. Don't worry, however; in time she'll begin to look like a typical newborn.

Because she has no protective fat, your premature baby will get cold in normal room temperatures. For that reason, she'll be placed immediately after birth in an incubator (often called an isolette) or under a special heating device called a radiant warmer. Here the temperature can be adjusted to keep her warm. After a quick examination in the delivery room, she'll probably be moved to a special-care nursery (often called a neonatal intensive care unit [NICU]).

You also may notice that your premature baby will cry only softly, if at all, and may have trouble breathing. This is because her respiratory system is still immature. If she's more than two months early, her breathing difficulties can cause serious health problems, because the other immature organs in her body may not get enough oxygen. To make sure this doesn't happen, doctors will keep her under close

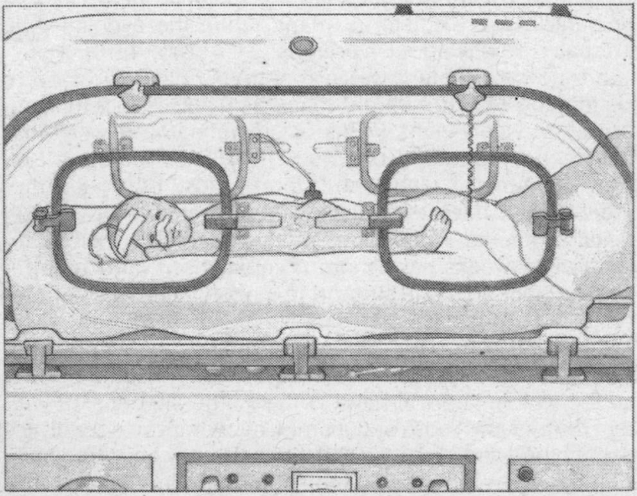

Your premature baby will be placed immediately after birth in an enclosed bed to keep her warm.

observation, watching her breathing and heart rate with equipment called a cardio-respiratory monitor. If she needs help breathing, she may be given extra oxygen, or special equipment such as a ventilator; or another breathing assistance technique called CPAP (continued positive airway pressure) may be used temporarily to support her breathing. As important as this care is for your baby's survival, her move to the special-care nursery may be wrenching for you. On top of all the worry about her health, you may miss the experience of holding, breastfeeding, and bonding with her right after delivery. You won't be able to hold or touch her whenever you want, and you can't have her with you in your room.

To deal with the stress of this experience, ask to see your baby as soon as possible after delivery, and become as active as you can in caring for her. Spend as much time with her in the special-care nursery as your condition—and hers—permit. Even if you can't hold her yet (until she's stable), touch her often. Many intensive care units allow parents to do "kangaroo care"—or skin-to-skin care—for their babies once the infants don't require major support to their organ systems.

You can also feed her as soon as your doctor says it's OK. The nurses will instruct you on either breast- or bottle-feeding techniques, whichever is appropriate for the baby's needs and your desires. Some premature babies may initially require fluids given intravenously or through a feeding tube that passes through the mouth or nose into the stomach. But your breastmilk is the best possible nutrition, and provides antibodies and other substances that enhance her immune response and help her resist infection. In some cases, if it's too difficult for your premature baby to nurse at the breast, you can pump breastmilk for feeding through a tube or bottle. Once you are able to start breastfeeding directly, your baby should nurse frequently to increase your milk supply. Even so, mothers of premature babies sometimes find it necessary to continue using a breast pump in addition to feeding frequently to maintain a good milk supply.

You may be ready to return home before your newborn is, which can be very difficult, but remember that your baby is in good hands, and you can visit her as often as you'd like.

You can use your time away from the hospital to get some needed rest and prepare your home and family for your baby's homecoming, and read a book or two for parents on caring for preterm babies. Even after you've returned home, if you participate in your infant's recovery and have plenty of contact with her during this time, the better you'll feel about the situation and the easier it will be for you to care for her when she leaves the special-care nursery. As soon as your doctor says it's OK, gently touch, hold, and cradle your newborn.

Health Issues of Premature Babies

Because premature babies are born before they are physically ready to leave the womb, they often have health problems. These newborns have higher rates of disabilities (such as cerebral palsy) and even death. African Americans and Native Americans have the highest neonatal death rate associated with prematurity.

Because of these health concerns, premature babies are given extra medical attention and assistance immediately after delivery. Depending on how early the baby has arrived, your pediatrician or obstetrician may call in a neonatologist (a pediatrician who specializes in the care of premature or very ill babies) to help determine what, if any, special treatment the infant needs. Here are some of the most common conditions that occur in premature infants:

- *Respiratory distress syndrome* is a breathing disorder related to the baby's immature lungs. It occurs because the lungs of preterm babies often lack surfactant, a liquid substance that allows the lungs to remain expanded. Artificial surfactants can be used to treat these babies, along with a ventilator to help them breathe better and maintain adequate oxygen levels in their blood. Sometimes, extremely preterm babies may need long-term oxygen treatment and occasionally may go home on supportive oxygen therapy.

- *Bronchopulmonary dysplasia*, or chronic lung disease, is a term used to describe babies who require oxygen for several weeks or months. They tend to outgrow this uncommon condition, which varies in severity, as their lungs grow and mature.
- *Apnea* is a temporary pause (more than fifteen seconds) in breathing that is common in preterm infants. It often is associated with a decline in the heart rate, called bradycardia. A drop in oxygen saturation as measured by a procedure called *pulse oximetry* is called desaturation. Most infants outgrow the condition by the time they leave the hospital for home.
- *Retinopathy of prematurity* (*ROP*) is an eye disease in which the retina is not fully developed. Most cases resolve without treatment, although serious cases may need treatment, including laser surgery in the most severe instances. Your infant may be examined by a pediatric ophthalmologist or retina specialist to diagnose and, if needed, recommend treatment for this condition.
- *Jaundice* happens when a chemical called bilirubin builds up in the baby's blood. As a result, the skin may develop a yellowish color. Jaundice can occur in babies of any race or color. Treating it involves placing the undressed baby under special lights (while her eyes are covered to protect them). For additional information about jaundice, see pages 173–175.
- Other conditions sometimes seen in preterm babies include *anemia of prematurity* (a low red blood cell count) and *heart murmurs*. For additional information on heart murmurs, see pages 674–676.

Newborn Screening Tests

Shortly after birth, and before you and your baby are discharged from the hospital to return home, she'll be given a number of screening tests to detect a variety of congenital conditions. These tests are designed to detect problems early in order to treat them promptly, prevent disabilities, and save lives. However, while laws mandate some tests, the tests required in one state are often different from those required in another (and they change periodically). Before your baby is born, talk to your pediatrician about which screening tests your baby will undergo, including their benefits and any risks, and ask if it is necessary for you to consent to this testing. Ask when you can find out the test results, and what they mean if your newborn is found to be out of the normal range (this may not necessarily mean that your baby actually has a congenital or genetic condition, so inquire about whether and when retesting would be done). Also, double-check to make certain the tests are actually performed before your baby leaves the hospital.

Your own pediatrician may participate in, or at least will be informed about, your infant's immediate care. Because of this, he will be able to answer most of your questions. Your baby will be ready to come home once she's breathing on her own, able to maintain her body temperature, able to be fed by breast or bottle, and gaining weight steadily.

For more resources and information on premature birth, contact the March of Dimes (www.marchofdimes.org; 1-914-997-4488) or the American College of Obstetricians and Gynecologists (www.acog.org; 1-202-638-5577).

Reflecting on Your Baby's Arrival

After all this activity during her first few hours of life, your baby probably will fall into a deep sleep, giving you time to rest and think back over the exciting things that have happened since labor began. If you have your baby with you, you may stare at her in wonder that you could possibly have produced such a miracle. Such emotions may wipe away your physical exhaustion temporarily, but don't fool yourself. You need to relax, sleep, and gather your strength. You have a very big job ahead of you—you're a parent now!

3

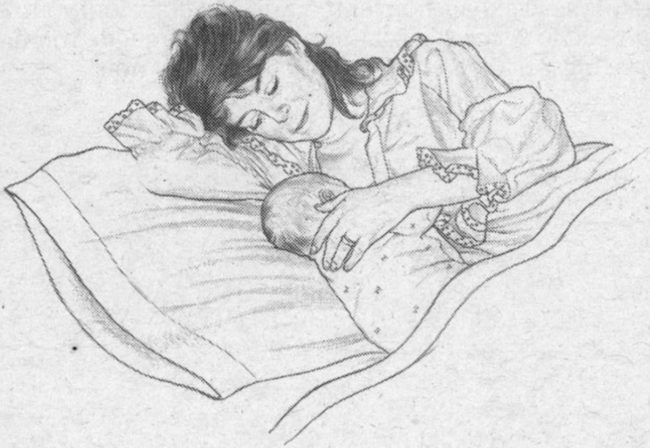

Basic Infant Care

When your baby first arrives, you may feel a bit overwhelmed by the job of caring for her. Even such routine tasks as diapering and dressing her can fill you with anxiety—especially if you've never spent much time around babies before. But it doesn't take long to develop the confidence and calm of an experienced parent, and you'll have help. While you are in the hospital, the nursery staff and your pediatrician will give you instructions and support your needs. Later, family and friends can be helpful; don't be bashful about asking for their assistance. But your baby will give you the most important information—how she likes to be treated, talked to, held, and comforted. She'll bring out parental instincts that will guide you automatically to many of the right responses, almost as soon as she's born.

The following sections address the most common questions and concerns that arise during the first months of life.

Day to Day

Responding to Your Baby's Cries

Crying serves several useful purposes for your baby. It gives her a way to call for help when she's hungry or uncomfortable. It helps her shut out sights, sounds, and other sensations that are too intense to suit her. And it helps her release tension.

You may notice that your baby has fussy periods throughout the day, even though she's not hungry, uncomfortable, or tired. Nothing you do at these times will console her, but right after these spells, she may seem more alert than before, and shortly thereafter she may sleep more deeply than usual. This kind of fussy crying seems to help babies get rid of excess energy so they can return to a more contented state.

Pay close attention to your baby's different cries. You'll soon be able to tell when she needs to be picked up, consoled, or tended to, and when she is better off left alone. You may even be able to identify her specific needs by the way she cries. For instance, a hungry cry is usually short and low-pitched, and it rises and falls. An angry cry tends to be more turbulent. A cry of pain or distress generally comes on suddenly and loudly with a long, high-pitched shriek followed by a long pause and then a flat wail. The "leave-me-alone" cry is usually similar to a hunger cry. It won't take long before you have a pretty good idea of what your baby's cries are trying to tell you.

Sometimes different types of cries overlap. For example, newborns generally wake up hungry and crying for food.

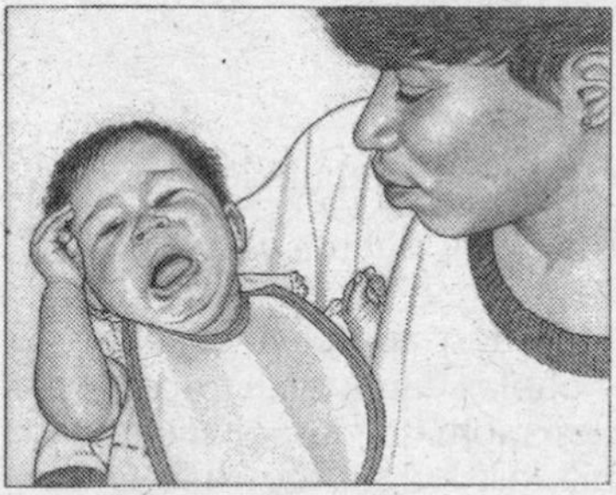

Respond promptly to your infant whenever he cries during his first few months. You cannot spoil a young baby by giving him attention.

If you're not quick to respond, your baby's hunger cry may give way to a wail of rage. You'll hear the difference. As your baby matures, her cries will become stronger, louder, and more insistent. They'll also begin to vary more, as if to convey different needs and desires.

The best way to handle crying is to respond promptly to your infant whenever she cries during her first few months. You cannot spoil a young baby by giving her attention, and if you answer her calls for help, she'll cry less overall.

When responding to your child's cries, try to meet her most pressing need first. If she's cold and hungry and her diaper is wet, warm her up, change her diaper, and then feed her. If there's a shrieking or panicked quality to the cry, consider the possibility that a piece of clothing or something else is making her uncomfortable. Perhaps a strand of hair is caught around a finger or toe. If she's warm, dry, and well fed but nothing is working to stop the crying, try the following consoling techniques to find the ones that work best for your baby:

- Rocking, either in a rocking chair or in your arms as you sway from side to side
- Gently stroking her head or patting her back or chest
- Swaddling (wrapping her snugly in a receiving blanket)
- Singing or talking
- Playing soft music
- Walking her in your arms, a stroller, or a carriage
- Riding in the car (Be sure to properly secure her in her car safety seat.)
- Rhythmic noise and vibration
- Burping her to relieve any trapped gas bubbles
- Warm baths (*Most* babies like this, but not all.)

Sometimes, if all else fails, the best approach is simply to leave the baby alone. Many babies cannot fall asleep without crying, and will go to sleep more quickly if left to cry for a while. The crying shouldn't last long if the child is truly

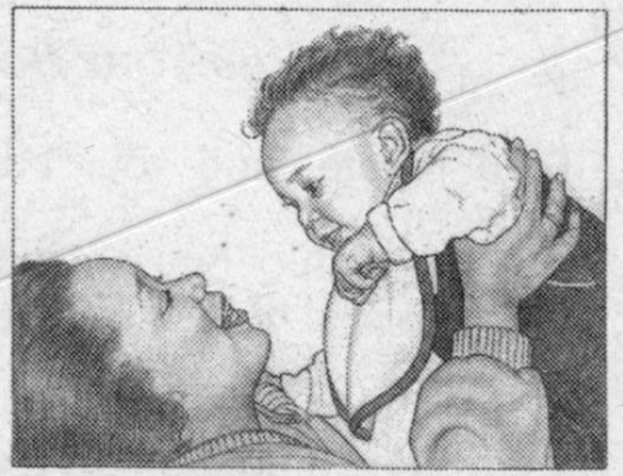

Enjoy all those wondrous moments with your child.

tired. If your baby is inconsolable no matter what you do, she may be sick. Check her temperature (see *Taking a Rectal Temperature,* page 87). If you take it rectally and it is over 100.4 degrees Fahrenheit (38 degrees Celsius), she could have an infection. Contact your pediatrician.

The more relaxed you remain, the easier it will be to console your child. Even very young babies are sensitive to tension around them and react to it by crying. Listening to a wailing newborn can be agonizing, but letting your frustration turn to anger or panic will only intensify your infant's screams. If you start to feel that you can't handle the situation, get help from another family member or a friend. Not only will this give you needed relief, but a new face sometimes can calm your baby when all your own tricks are spent. No matter how impatient or angry you feel, *do not* shake the baby. Shaking an infant hard can cause blindness, brain damage, or even death. Also, make sure to share this information on crying with other caretakers of your baby, including your spouse or partner.

Above all, don't take your newborn's crying personally. She's not crying because you're a bad parent or because she doesn't like you. All babies cry, often without any apparent cause. Newborns routinely cry a total of one to four hours a day. It's part of adjusting to this strange new life outside the womb.

No mother can console her child *every* time she cries, so don't expect to be a miracle worker with your baby. Instead, take a realistic approach to the situation, line up some help, get plenty of rest, and enjoy all those wondrous moments with your child.

How Your Baby Sleeps

Even before birth your baby's days were divided between periods of sleep and wakefulness. By the eighth month of pregnancy or earlier, her sleep periods consisted of the same two distinct phases that we all experience:

1. **Rapid eye movement (or REM) sleep,** the times during which she does her active dreaming. During these periods, her eyes will move beneath her closed lids, almost as if she were watching a dream take place. She also may seem to startle, twitch her face, and make jerking motions with her hands and feet. All are normal signs of REM sleep.
2. **Non-REM sleep,** which consists of four phases: drowsiness, light sleep, deep sleep, and very deep sleep. During the progression from drowsiness to deepest sleep, your baby becomes less and less active, and her breathing slows and becomes very quiet, so that in deepest sleep she is virtually motionless. Very little, if any, dreaming occurs during non-REM sleep.

At first your newborn probably will sleep about sixteen hours a day, divided into three- or four-hour naps evenly spaced between feedings.

Each of these sleep periods will include relatively equal amounts of REM and non-REM sleep, organized in this order: drowsiness, REM sleep, light sleep, deep sleep, and very deep sleep.

After about two to three months the order will change, so that as she grows older, she will cycle through all the non-REM phases before entering REM sleep. This pattern will last into and through adulthood. As she grows older, the amount of REM sleep decreases, and her sleep generally will become calmer. By the age of three, children spend one-third or less of total sleep time in REM sleep.

Helping Your Baby Sleep

Initially your infant doesn't know the difference between day and night. Her stomach holds only enough to satisfy her for three or four hours, regardless of the time, so there's no escaping round-the-clock waking and feeding for the first few weeks. But even at this age, you can begin to teach her that nighttime is for sleeping and daytime is for play. Do this by keeping nighttime feedings as subdued as possible. Don't turn up the lights or prolong late-night diaper changes. Instead of playing, put her right back down after feeding and changing her. If she's napping longer than three or four hours, particularly in the late afternoon, wake her up and play with her. This will train her to save her extra sleeping for nighttime. Also begin to develop a routine before bedtime. Repeatedly experiencing a strong sensation (like a sponge bath), followed by soothing time (like applying a bit of moisturizing lotion and reading or singing) and then a final feeding in the evening followed by a short bedtime story, can help signal to your baby that the "longer nap" is coming.

Positioning for Sleep

The American Academy of Pediatrics recommends that healthy infants be placed on their backs for sleep, as this is the safest position for an infant to sleep. Putting your baby to sleep on his back decreases his chance of *sudden infant death syndrome (SIDS), which is responsible for more infant deaths in the United States than any other cause during the first year of life (beyond the newborn period)*. The exact reason for this finding is not certain, but it may be related to findings that suggest that an infant who sleeps on her stomach gets less oxygen or gets rid of carbon dioxide less because she is "rebreathing" the air from a small pocket of bedding pulled up around the nose.

In addition, recent findings suggest that certain regions of the brain may be underdeveloped in babies who die from SIDS. When these sleeping babies encounter a situation challenging to their well-being, they may fail to wake up to remove themselves from danger. Since it is impossible to identify which babies may not arouse normally, and because the relationship between SIDS and sleep position is so strong, the Academy recommends that all infants be placed to sleep on their backs. Some doctors once thought that sleeping on the side might be a reasonable alternative to back positioning, but recent evidence has shown that side sleeping also should be avoided for safety reasons. (Please note that there are a few exceptions to this recommendation, including babies with certain medical conditions, which your pediatrician can discuss with you.)

This recommendation of putting the baby down on her back applies to infants throughout the first year of life. However, it is particularly important during the first six months, when the incidence of SIDS is the highest.

Even when you are sure your baby is lying on her back when going to sleep, it is also important to avoid placing her on soft, porous surfaces such as pillows, quilts, comforters, sheepskins, or bean bags—even soft materials used for stuffed toys—which may block her airway if she burrows her face in them. Also avoid having her sleep on waterbeds, sofas, or soft mattresses. A firm crib mattress covered by a sheet is the safest bedding. Keep all soft toys and stuffed animals out of your child's crib throughout infancy. Keep the temperature in your baby's room comfortable and do not place her near air-conditioning or heating vents, open windows, or other sources of drafts. Use sleep clothing (such as a one-piece sleeper) with no other covering, as an alternative to blankets. For an extra layer, a wearable blanket sleeper or sleepsack is a safe alternative.

Pacifiers also may help reduce the risk of SIDS. However, if your baby doesn't want the pacifier or if it falls out of her mouth, don't force it. If you are breastfeeding, wait until breastfeeding is well established, usually around three or four weeks of age, before using a pacifier.

While sleeping on the back is important, your baby also should spend some time on her stomach *when she is awake and being observed.* This will help to develop her shoulder muscles and her head control, and avoid the development of flat spots on the back of her head.

As she gets older and her stomach grows, your baby will be able to go longer between feedings. In fact, you'll be encouraged to know that more than 90 percent of babies sleep through the night (six to eight hours without waking) by three months. Most infants are able to last this long between feedings when they reach 12 or 13 pounds (5.44–5.89 kg), so if yours is a very large baby, she may begin sleeping through the night even earlier than three months. As encouraging as this sounds, don't expect the sleep struggle to end all at once. Most children swing back and forth, sleeping beautifully for a few weeks, or even months, then returning abruptly to a late-night wake-up schedule. This may have to do with growth spurts increasing the need for food, or, later, it may be related to teething or developmental changes.

From time to time, you will need to help your baby fall asleep or go back to sleep. Especially as a newborn, she probably will doze off most easily if given gentle continuous stimulation. Some infants are helped by rocking, walking, patting on the back, or by a pacifier in the mouth. For others, music from a radio or a CD player can be very soothing if played at moderate volume. Certain stimulation, however, is irritating to any baby—for example, ringing telephones, barking dogs, and roaring vacuum cleaners.

There is no reason to restrict your baby's sleeping to her crib. If, for any reason, you want her closer to you while she sleeps, use her bassinet as a temporary crib and move it

Where We Stand

Based on an evaluation of current sudden infant death syndrome (SIDS) data, the American Academy of Pediatrics recommends that healthy infants, when being put down to sleep, be placed on their backs. Despite common beliefs, there is no evidence that choking is more frequent among infants lying on their backs (the supine position) when compared to other positions, nor is there evidence that sleeping on the back is harmful to healthy babies. In some circumstances, there are still good reasons for placing certain infants on their stomachs for sleep. Discuss your individual circumstances with your pediatrician.

Since 1992, when the American Academy of Pediatrics began recommending this sleep position, the annual SIDS rate has declined more than 50 percent.

around the house with you. (She'll be perfectly happy in a padded basket if you don't have an "official" bassinet.)

Diapers

Since disposable diapers were introduced about forty years ago, these modern diapers are meeting the needs and expectations of most parents; however, diaper choice is a decision that every new parent faces. Ideally, you should make the choice between cloth and disposable diapers before the baby arrives, so you can stock up or make delivery arrangements ahead of time. In order to plan ahead, you should know that most newborns go through about ten diapers a day.

Disposable Diapers. Most disposable diapers today consist of an inner liner next to the baby to help keep wetness away from the skin, an absorbent core made of purified wood pulp and superabsorbent polymers, and an outer waterproof covering. Over the years, disposable diapers have become thinner and lighter, while continuing to meet the needs for containment, comfort, ease of use, and skin care. When changing a soiled diaper, dump loose stool into a toilet. Do not flush the diaper, because it can block your plumbing. Wrap the diaper in its outer cover, and discard in a waste receptacle.

Cloth Diapers. Like disposable diapers, reusable cloth diapers have improved in recent years, and are available in a variety of absorbencies and textures. If you want to use a diaper service, shop around; ideally, a diaper service should pick up dirty diapers and drop off clean ones twice a week. If you choose to wash diapers yourself, keep them separate from other clothes. After you dump stool into the toilet, rinse the diapers in cold water, then soak them in a mild detergent solution with bleach. Wring them out, then wash in hot water with a mild detergent.

Diaper Choice. Diaper choice has been complicated in recent years by the debate on the environmental effects of diapers, mostly centered on the effects of disposable diapers on landfill space. Actually, a number of scientific

How to Diaper Your Baby

Before you start to change your baby, make sure you have all the necessary supplies within arm's reach. Never leave your baby alone on the changing table—not even for a second. Babies wiggle and squirm and can easily fall off a changing table. In addition, it won't be long before she will be able to turn over, and if she does it when your attention is diverted, a serious injury could result.

When changing a newborn, you will need:

- a clean diaper (plus fasteners if a cloth diaper is used)
- a small basin (or a mug or bowl) with lukewarm water and a washcloth, soft paper towels or cotton balls (commercial diaper wipes also can be used, although some babies are sensitive to them; if any irritation occurs, discontinue use)
- diaper ointment or petroleum jelly

This is how you proceed:

1. Remove the dirty diaper and use the lukewarm water and cotton ball or soft paper towel to gently wipe your baby clean. (Remember to wipe front to back on female infants.)
2. Use the damp washcloth to wipe the diaper area.
3. Use the diaper rash preparation recommended by your pediatrician if needed.

studies have found that both cloth and disposable diapers have environmental effects, including raw material and energy usage, air and water pollution, and waste disposal. Disposable diapers add 1 to 2 percent to municipal solid waste, while cloth diapers use more energy and water in laundering and contribute to air and water pollution. In

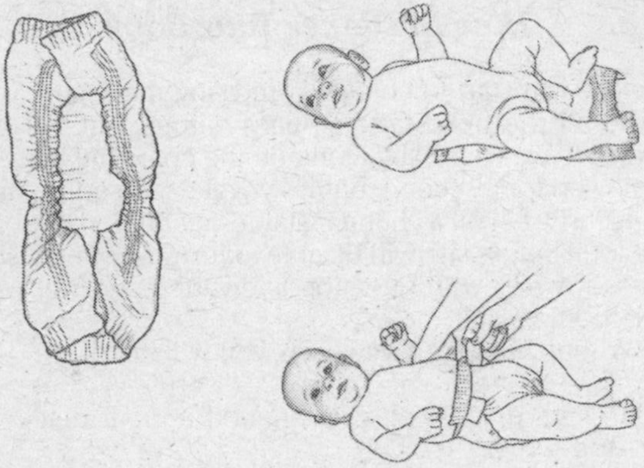

the end, it is up to individuals to make their own decisions about diaper type based on their own concerns and needs.

There are some health aspects to consider as well. Excessively wet skin and contact with urine and stool can cause diaper rash. Because cloth diapers can't keep wetness away from your baby's skin as effectively as disposables, it's especially important to change cloth diapers quickly after they become wet or soiled.

Urination

Your baby may urinate as often as every one to three hours or as infrequently as four to six times a day. If she's ill or feverish, or when the weather is extremely hot, her usual output of urine may drop by half and still be normal. Urination should never be painful. If you notice any signs of distress while your infant is urinating, notify your pediatrician, as this could be a sign of infection or some other problem in the urinary tract.

In a healthy child, urine is light to dark yellow in color. (The darker the color, the more concentrated the urine; the urine will be more concentrated when your child is not drinking a lot of liquid.) Sometimes you'll see a pink stain

Diaper Rash

Diaper rash is the term used to describe a rash or irritation in the area covered by the diaper. The first sign of diaper rash is usually redness or small bumps on the lower abdomen, buttocks, genitals, and thigh folds—surfaces that have been in direct contact with the wet or soiled diaper. This type of diaper rash is rarely serious and usually clears in three or four days with appropriate care. The most common causes of diaper rash include:

1. Leaving a wet diaper on too long. The moisture makes the skin more susceptible to chafing. Over time, the urine in the diaper decomposes, forming chemicals that can further irritate the skin.
2. Leaving a stool-soiled diaper on too long. Digestive agents in the stool then attack the skin, making it more susceptible to a rash.

Regardless of how the rash begins, once the surface of the skin is damaged, it becomes even more vulnerable to further irritation by contact with urine and stool and to subsequent infection with bacteria or yeast. Yeast infections are common in this area and often appear as a rash on the thighs, genitals, and lower abdomen, but they almost never appear on the buttocks.

Although most babies develop diaper rash at some point during infancy, it happens less often in babies who are breastfed (for reasons we still do not know). Diaper rash occurs more often at particular ages and under certain conditions:

- Among babies eight to ten months old
- If babies are not kept clean and dry
- When babies have diarrhea

- When a baby starts to eat solid food (probably due to changes in the digestive process caused by the new variety of foods)
- When a baby is taking antibiotics (because these drugs encourage the growth of yeast organisms that can infect the skin)

To reduce your baby's risk of diaper rash, make these steps part of your diapering routine:

1. Change the diaper as soon as possible after a bowel movement. Cleanse the diaper area with a soft cloth and water after each bowel movement. Avoid using diaper wipes, which may irritate the skin further.
2. Change wet diapers frequently to reduce skin exposure to moisture.
3. Expose the baby's bottom to air whenever feasible. When using plastic pants or disposable diapers with tight gathers around the abdomen and legs, make sure air can circulate inside the diaper.

If a diaper rash develops in spite of your efforts, begin using an oil-based barrier (ointment) to prevent further irritation from the urine or stool. The rash should improve noticeably within forty-eight to seventy-two hours. If it doesn't, consult your pediatrician.

on the diaper that you may mistake for blood. In fact, this stain is usually a sign of highly concentrated urine, which has a pinkish color. As long as the baby is wetting at least four diapers a day, there probably is no cause for concern, but if the pinkish staining persists, consult your pediatrician.

The presence of actual blood in the urine or a bloody spot on the diaper is never normal, and your pediatrician should be notified. It may be due to nothing more serious than a small sore caused by diaper rash, but it also could be a sign of a more serious problem. If this bleeding is accompanied by other symptoms, such as abdominal pain or bleeding in other areas, seek medical attention for your baby immediately.

Bowel Movements

Beginning with the first day of life and lasting for a few days, your baby will have her first bowel movements, which are often referred to as meconium. This thick black or dark-green substance filled her intestines before birth, and once the meconium is passed, the stools will turn yellow-green.

If your baby is breastfed, her stools soon should resemble light mustard with seedlike particles. Until she starts to eat solid foods, the consistency of the stools may range from very soft to loose and runny. If she's formula-fed, her stools usually will be tan or yellow in color. They will be firmer than in a baby who is breastfed, but no firmer than peanut butter.

Whether your baby is breastfed or bottle-fed, hard or very dry stools may be a sign that she is not getting enough fluid or that she is losing too much fluid due to illness, fever, or heat. Once she has started solids, hard stools might indicate that she's eating too many constipating foods, such as cereal or cow's milk, before her system can handle them. (Whole cow's milk is not recommended for babies under twelve months.)

Here are some other important points to keep in mind about bowel movements:

- **Occasional variations in** color and consistency of the stools are normal. For example, if the digestive process slows down because the baby has had a particularly large amount of cereal that day or foods requiring more effort to digest, the stools may become green; or if the baby is given supplemental iron, the stools may turn dark brown. If there is a minor irritation of the anus, streaks of blood may appear on the outside of the stools. However, if there are large amounts of blood, mucus, or water in the stool, call your pediatrician immediately. These symptoms may indicate an intestinal condition that warrants attention from your doctor.

- **Because an infant's** stools are normally soft and a little runny, it's not always easy to tell when a young baby has mild diarrhea. The telltale signs are a sudden increase in frequency (to more than one bowel movement per feeding) and unusually high liquid content in the stool. Diarrhea may be a sign of intestinal infection, or it may be caused by a change in the baby's diet. If the baby is breastfeeding, she can even develop diarrhea because of a change in the mother's diet.
- **The main concern** with diarrhea is the possibility that dehydration can develop. If fever is also present and your infant is less than two months old, call your pediatrician. If your baby is over two months and the fever lasts more than a day, check her urine output and rectal temperature; then report your findings to your doctor so he can determine what needs to be done. Make sure your baby continues to feed frequently. As much as anything else, if she simply looks sick, let your doctor know.

The frequency of bowel movements varies widely from one baby to another. Many pass a stool soon after each feeding. This is a result of the gastrocolic reflex, which causes the digestive system to become active whenever the stomach is filled with food.

By three to six weeks of age, some breastfed babies have only one bowel movement a week and still are normal. This happens because breastmilk leaves very little solid waste to be eliminated from the child's digestive system. Thus, infrequent stools are not a sign of constipation and should not be considered a problem as long as the stools are soft (no firmer than peanut butter), and your infant is otherwise normal, gaining weight steadily, and nursing regularly.

If your baby is formula-fed, she should have at least one bowel movement a day. If she has fewer than this and appears to be straining because of hard stools, she may be constipated. Check with your pediatrician for advice on how to handle this problem. (See *Constipation,* page 439.)

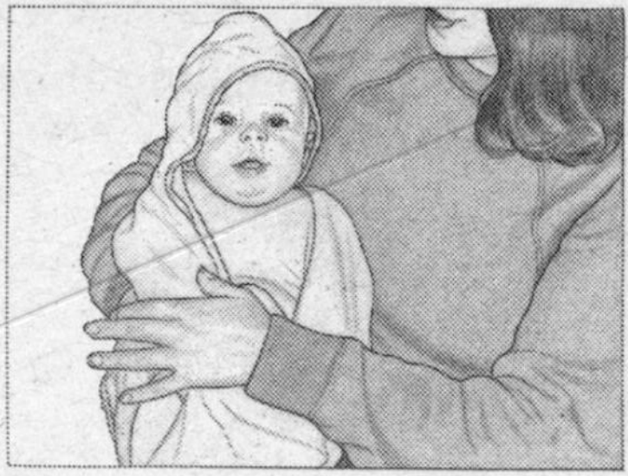

Baby towels with built-in hoods are a very effective way to keep your baby's head warm when she's wet.

Bathing

Your infant doesn't need much bathing if you wash the diaper area thoroughly during diaper changes. Three times a week during her first year may be enough. Bathing her more frequently may dry out her skin, particularly if soaps are used or moisture is allowed to evaporate from the skin. Patting her dry and applying a fragrance-free, hypoallergenic moisturizing lotion immediately after bathing can help prevent dry skin or worsening the skin condition called eczema (see page 470).

During her first week or two, until the stump of the umbilical cord falls off, your newborn should have only sponge baths. In a warm room, lay the baby anywhere that's flat and comfortable for both of you—a changing table, bed, floor, or counter next to the sink will do. Pad hard surfaces with a blanket or fluffy towel. If the baby is on a surface above the floor, use a safety strap or keep one hand on her *at all times* to make sure she doesn't fall.

Have a basin of water, a damp, double-rinsed washcloth (so there is no soap residue in it), and a supply of mild baby soap within reach before you begin. Keep your baby wrapped in a towel, and expose only the parts of her body you are actively washing. Use the dampened cloth first without soap to wash her face, so you don't get soap into her eyes or mouth. Then dip it in the basin of soapy water before washing the remainder of her body and, finally, the diaper area. Pay special attention to creases under the arms, behind the ears, around the neck, and, especially with a girl, in the genital area.

Bathing Your Baby

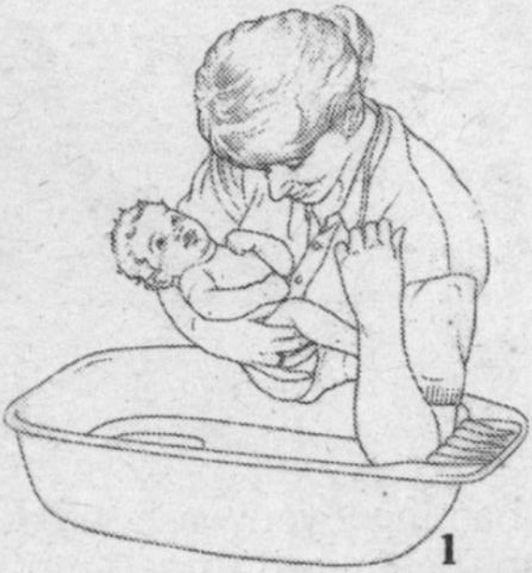
1

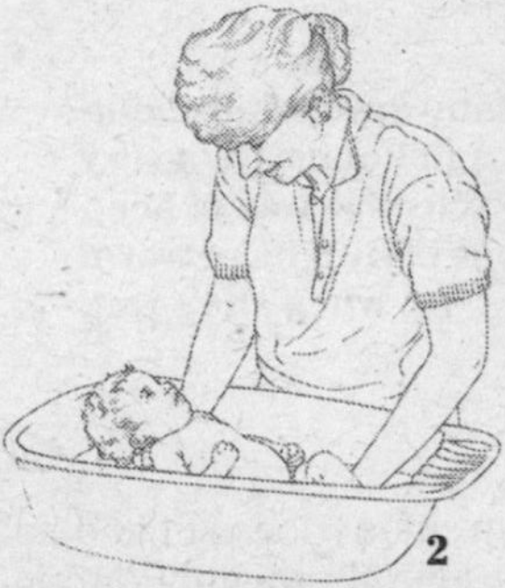
2

Once you've undressed your baby, place her in the water immediately so she doesn't get chilled. Use one of your hands to support her head and the other to guide her in, feet first. Speak to her encouragingly, and gently lower the rest of her body until she's in the tub. Most of her body and face should be well above the water level for safety, so you'll need to pour warm water over her body frequently to keep her warm.

Use a soft cloth to wash her face and hair, shampooing once or twice a week. Massage her entire scalp gently, including the area over her fontanelles (soft spots). When you rinse the soap or shampoo from her

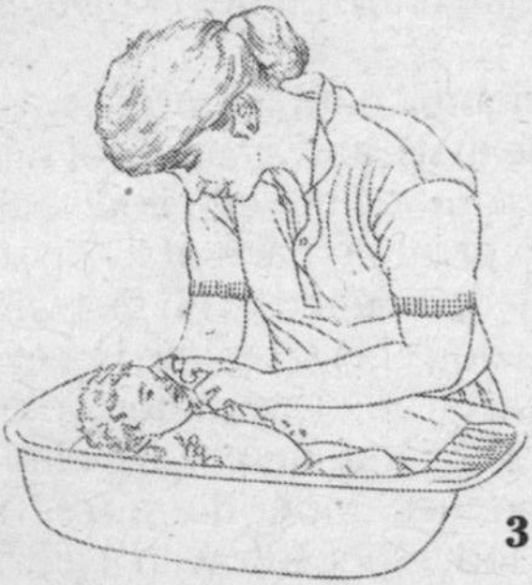
3

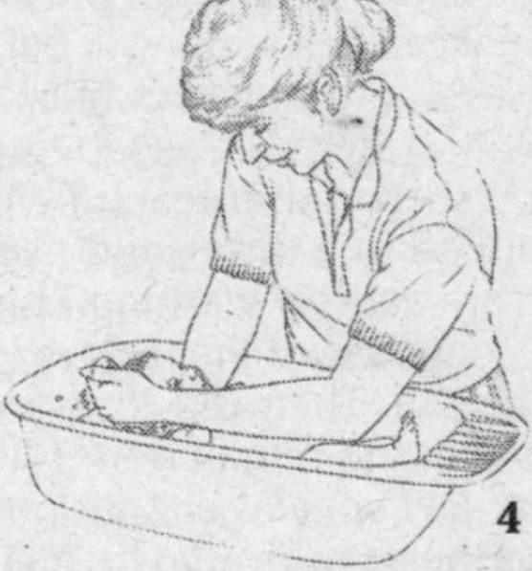
4

head, cup your hand across her forehead so the suds run toward the sides, not into her eyes. Should you get some soap in her eyes, and she cries out in protest, simply take the wet washcloth and liberally wipe her eyes with plain, lukewarm water until any remains of the soap are gone, and she will open her eyes again. Wash the rest of her body from the top down.

Once the umbilical area is healed, you can try placing your baby directly in the water. Her first baths should be as gentle and brief as possible. She probably will protest a little; if she seems miserable, go back to sponge baths for a week or two, then try the bath again. She will make it clear when she's ready.

Most parents find it easiest to bathe a newborn in a bathinette, sink, or plastic tub lined with a clean towel. Fill the basin with 2 inches (5.08 cm) of water that feels warm—not hot—to the inside of your wrist or elbow. If you're filling the basin from the tap, turn the cold water on first (and off last) to avoid scalding yourself or your child. The hottest temperature at the faucet should be no more than 120 degrees Fahrenheit to avoid burns. In many cases you can adjust your water heater.

Make sure that supplies are at hand and the room is warm before undressing the baby. You'll need the same supplies that you used for sponge bathing, but also a cup for rinsing with clear water. When your child has hair, you'll need baby shampoo, too.

If you've forgotten something or need to answer the phone or door during the bath, *you must take the baby with you,* so keep a dry towel within reach. *Never leave a baby alone in the bath, even for an instant.*

If your baby enjoys her bath, give her some extra time to splash and explore the water. The more fun your child has in the bath, the less she'll be afraid of the water. As she gets older, the length of the bath will extend until most of it is taken up with play. Bathing should be a very relaxing and soothing experience, so don't rush unless she's unhappy.

Bath toys are not really needed for very young babies, as

the stimulation of the water and washing is exciting enough. Once a baby is old enough for the bathtub, however, toys become invaluable. Containers, floating toys, even waterproof books make wonderful distractions as you cleanse your baby.

When your infant comes out of the bath, baby towels with built-in hoods are the most effective way to keep her head warm when she's wet. Bathing a baby of any age is wet work, so you may want to wear a terry-cloth apron or hang a towel over your shoulder to keep you dry.

The bath is a relaxing way to prepare her for sleep and should be given at a time that's convenient for you.

Skin and Nail Care

Your newborn's skin may be susceptible to irritation from chemicals in new clothing and from soap or detergent residue on clothes that have been washed. To avoid problems, double-rinse all baby clothes, bedding, blankets, and other washable items before exposing the child to them. (Wash her new layette, too, before she uses it.) For the first few months, do your infant's wash separately from the rest of the family's.

Contrary to what you may read in ads for baby products, your infant does not ordinarily need any lotions, oils, or powders. If her skin is very dry, you can apply a small amount of nonperfumed baby lotion or cream sparingly to the dry areas; the massage involved in applying the lotion will make your baby feel good. Never use any skin-care products that are not specifically made for babies, because they

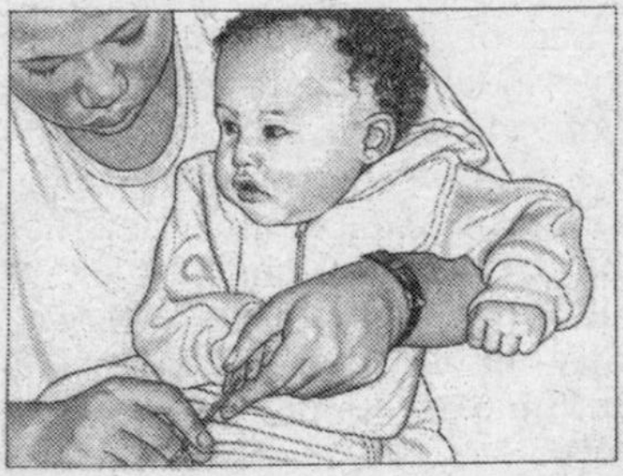

In the early weeks, your baby's fingers are so small and his nails grow so quickly you may have to trim them twice a week.

generally contain perfumes and other chemicals that can irritate an infant's skin. Also avoid baby oil, which does not penetrate or lubricate as well as baby lotion or cream. If the dryness persists, you may be bathing your child too often. Give her a bath just once a week for a while and see if the dryness stops. If not, consult your pediatrician.

The only care your child's nails require is trimming. You can use a soft emery board, baby nail clippers, or blunt-nosed toenail scissors, but be very careful when using clippers or scissors because accidentally cutting the tip of your baby's finger will cause pain and bleeding. A good time to trim nails is after a bath if your baby will lie quietly, but you may find it easiest to do when she's asleep. Keep her fingernails as short and smoothly trimmed as possible so she can't scratch herself (or you). In the early weeks, her fingers are so small and her nails grow so quickly you may have to trim them twice a week. Also, as odd as it may sound, some parents bite their child's nails as a way of trimming them, which they should avoid doing to prevent the risk of a condition called herpetic whitlow (a finger or thumb infection caused by the herpes simplex virus).

By contrast, your baby's toenails grow much more slowly and are usually very soft and pliable. They needn't be kept as short as the fingernails, so you may have to trim them only once or twice a month. Because they are so soft, they sometimes look as if they're ingrown, but there's no cause for concern unless the skin alongside the nail gets red, inflamed, or hard. As your baby gets older, his toenails will become harder and better defined.

Clothing

Unless the temperature is hot (over 75 degrees Fahrenheit [23.88 degrees Celsius]), your newborn will need several layers of clothing to keep her warm. It's generally best to dress her in an undershirt and diapers, covered by pajamas or a dressing gown, and then wrap her in a receiving blanket. If your baby is premature, she may need still another layer of clothing until her weight reaches that of a full-term baby and her body is better able to adjust to changes in temperature. In hot weather you can reduce her clothing to a single layer. A good rule of thumb is to dress the baby in one more

Dressing and Undressing Your Baby

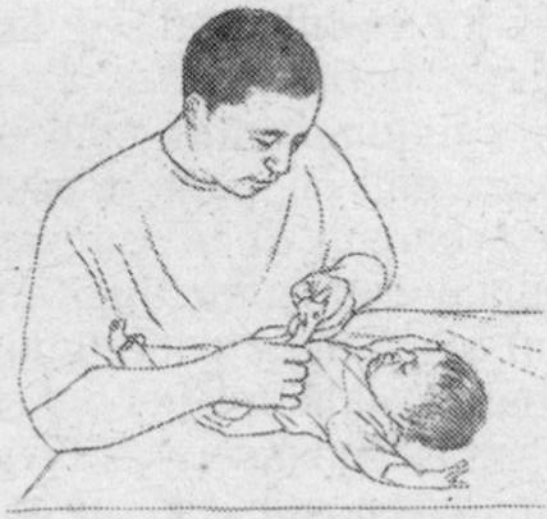

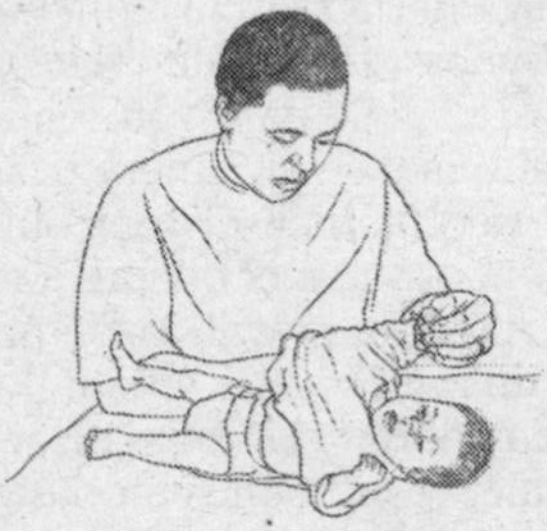

When dressing your baby, supporting her on your lap, stretch the garment neckline and pull it over your baby's head. Use your fingers to keep it from catching on her face or ears.

Don't try to push your baby's arm through the sleeve. Instead, put your hand into the sleeve from the outside, grasp your baby's hand, and pull it through.

When undressing, take off the sleeves one at a time while you support your baby's back and head.

Then stretch the neckline, lifting it free of your baby's chin and face as you gently slip it off.

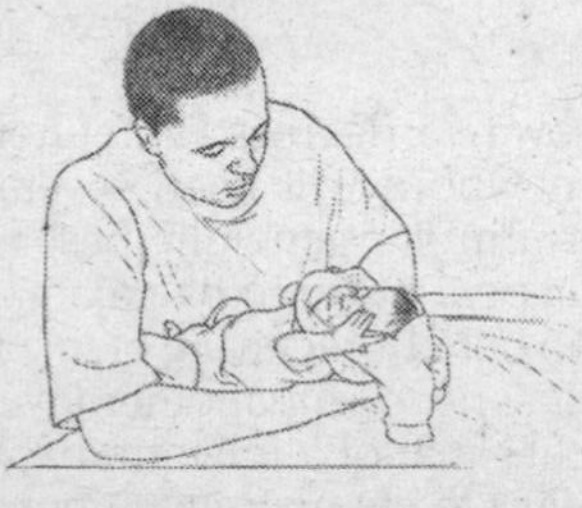

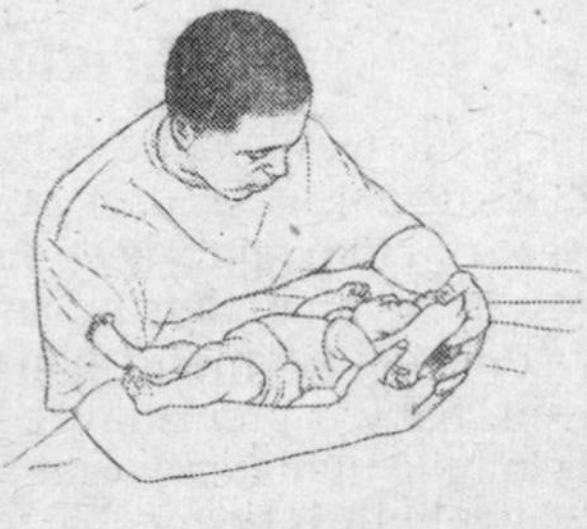

layer of clothing than you are wearing to be comfortable in the same environment.

If you've never taken care of a newborn baby before, the first few times you change her clothes can be quite frustrating. Not only is it a struggle to get that tiny little arm through the sleeve, but your infant may shriek in protest through the whole process. She doesn't like the rush of air against her skin, nor does she enjoy being pushed and pulled through garments. It may make things easier for both of you if you hold her on your lap while changing the upper half of her body, then lay her on a bed or changing table while doing the lower half. When you're dressing her in one-piece pajamas, pull them over her legs before putting on the sleeves. Pull T-shirts over her head first, then put one arm at a time through the sleeves. Use this opportunity to ask "Where's the baby's hand?" As she gets older this will turn into a game, with her pushing her arm through just to hear you say, "*There's* the baby's hand!"

Certain clothing features can make dressing much easier. Look for garments that

- Snap or zip all the way down the front, instead of the back
- Snap or zip down both legs to make diaper changes easier
- Have loose-fitting sleeves so your hand fits underneath to push the baby's arm through
- Have no ribbons or strings to knot up, unravel, or wrap around the neck (which could cause choking)
- Are made of stretchy fabric (avoid tight bindings around arms, legs, or neck)

Your Baby's Basic Healthcare

Taking a Rectal Temperature

Very few babies get through infancy without having a fever, which can be a sign of infection somewhere in the body. A fever often indicates that the immune system is actively fighting viruses or bacteria, so—in this respect—it is a positive

Swaddling

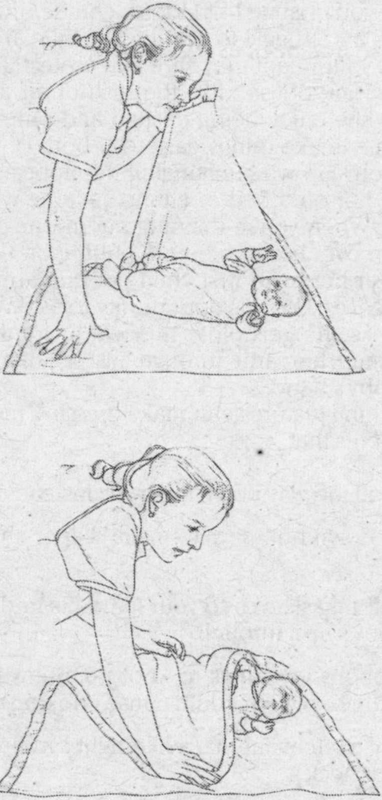

During the first few weeks, your baby will spend most of her time wrapped in a receiving blanket. Not only does this keep her warm, but the slight pressure around the body seems to give most newborns a sense of security. To swaddle, spread the blanket out flat, with one corner folded over. Lay the baby face-up on the blanket, with her head at the folded corner.

Wrap the left corner over her body and tuck it beneath her. Bring the bottom corner up over her feet, and then wrap the right corner around her, leaving only her head and neck exposed.

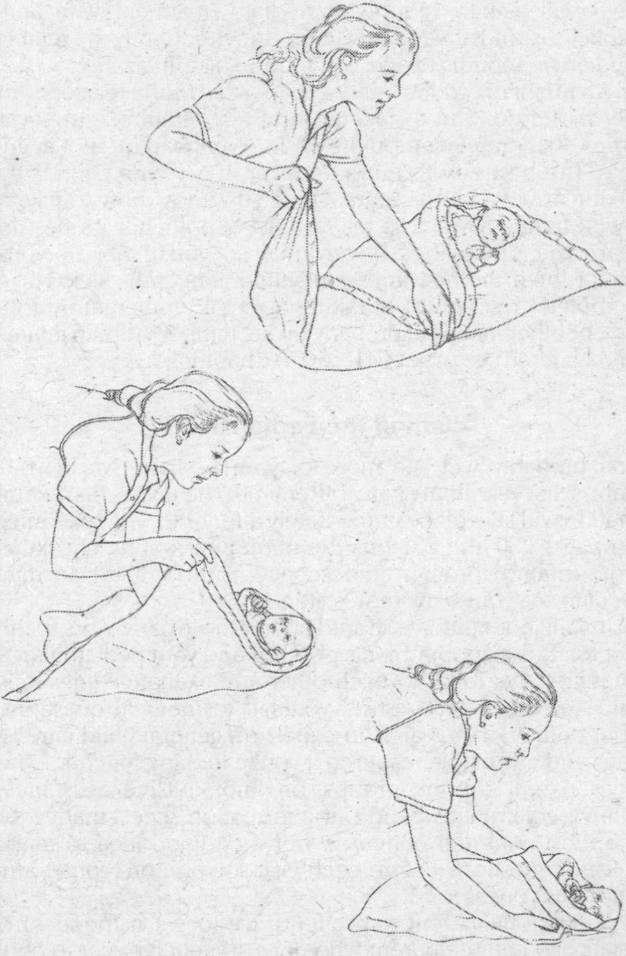

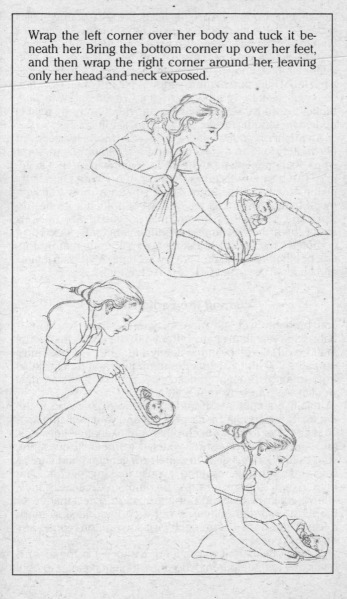

sign that the body is protecting itself. Because young babies have very few signs that they are ill, any child two months or younger with a fever needs an urgent evaluation by a physician to determine the cause of the fever; if it is due to a minor viral infection, it will usually resolve on its own, while a bacterial infection or more serious viral infection (e.g., herpes) will usually require immediate treatment with antibiotics or antiviral medications and frequently, in infants under two months of age, will require hospitalization.

An infant or toddler cannot hold a thermometer steady in her mouth for you to take an oral temperature, and "fever strips" that are placed on the child's forehead are not accurate. The best way to measure fever in a young child is by taking a rectal temperature. Once you know how to take a rectal temperature, it is really quite simple; but it's best to learn the procedures in advance so you're not nervous about them the first time your child is actually sick. For a complete description of taking a rectal temperature properly, or other means of properly taking temperatures in infants and children see pages 641–650 in Chapter 23, *Fever.*

Visiting the Pediatrician

You probably will see more of your pediatrician in your baby's first year than at any other time. The baby's first examination will take place immediately after birth. The schedules on pages 730 and 731 lists the minimum routine checkups from infancy through adolescence. Your pediatrician may want to see your baby more often.

Ideally, both parents should attend these early visits to the doctor. These appointments give you and your pediatrician a chance to get to know each other and exchange questions and answers. Don't restrict yourself to medical questions; your pediatrician is also an expert on general child care issues and a valuable resource if you're looking for child care help, parent support groups, or other outside assistance. Many pediatricians hand out information sheets that cover the most common concerns, but it's a good idea to make a list of questions before each visit so you don't forget any important ones.

If only one parent can attend, try to get a friend or a relative to join the parent who does. It's much easier to concentrate on your discussions with the doctor if you have a little help dressing and undressing the baby and gathering all of her things. While you're getting used to outings with your newborn, an extra adult also can help carry the diaper bag and hold doors. Grandparents can fulfill this role quite well if they live nearby. (For additional information about the role of grandparents in your baby's life, see pages 217, 345, and 429 in Chapters 6, 9, and 11.)

The purpose of these early checkups is to make sure your child is growing and developing properly and has no serious abnormalities. Specifically, the doctor will check the following areas.

Growth. You will be asked to undress your baby, and then she'll be weighed on an infant scale. Her length may be measured lying on a flat table with her legs stretched straight. A special tape is used to measure the size of her head. All of these measurements should be plotted on a graph in order to determine her growth curve from one visit to the next. (You can plot your baby's growth curve in the same way using the charts on pages 736–739.) This is the most reliable way to judge whether she's growing normally, and will show you her position on the growth curve in relation to other children her age.

Head. The soft spots (fontanelles) should be open (normal skin-covered openings in the skull) and flat for the first few months. By two to three months of age, the spot at the back should be closed. The front soft spot should close before your child's second birthday (around eighteen months of age).

Ears. The doctor will look inside both ears with an otoscope, an instrument that provides a view of the ear canal and eardrum. This tells him whether there is any evidence of fluid or infection in the ear. You'll also be asked if the child responds normally to sounds. Formal hearing tests are done in the newborn nursery and later if there is suspicion that a problem exists.

Eyes. The doctor will use a bright object or flashlight to catch your baby's attention and track her eye movements.

He also may look inside the baby's eyes with a lighted instrument called an ophthalmoscope—repeating the internal eye examination that was first done in the hospital nursery. This is particularly helpful in detecting cataracts (clouding of the lens of the eye). (See *Cataracts,* page 615.)

Mouth. The mouth is checked for signs of infection and, later, for teething progress.

Heart and Lungs. The pediatrician will use a stethoscope on the front and back of the chest to listen to your child's heart and lungs. This examination determines whether there are any abnormal heart rhythms, sounds, or breathing difficulties.

Abdomen. By placing his hand on the child's abdomen and gently pressing, the doctor makes sure that none of the organs are enlarged and there are no unusual masses or tenderness.

Genitalia. The genitalia are examined at each visit for any unusual lumps, tenderness, or signs of infection. In the first exam or two, the doctor pays special attention to a circumcised boy's penis to make sure it's healing properly. Pediatricians also check all baby boys to make certain both testes are down in the scrotum.

Hips and Legs. The pediatrician will move your baby's legs to check for problems with the hip joints. The movements your pediatrician will perform with your baby's legs are designed to detect dislocation or dysplasia of the hip joint. It is important to look for this early in life as early detection can lead to proper referral and correction. Later, after the baby starts to walk, the doctor will watch her take a few steps to make sure the legs and feet are properly aligned and move normally.

Developmental Milestones. The pediatrician also will ask about the baby's general development. Among other things, he'll observe and discuss when the baby starts to smile, roll over, sit up, and walk, and how she uses her hands and arms. During the exam, the pediatrician will test reflexes and general muscle tone. (See Appendix and Chapters 5 through 9 for details of normal development.)

Immunizations

Your child should receive most of his childhood immunizations before his second birthday. These will protect him against fourteen major diseases: hepatitis B, diphtheria, tetanus, pertussis (whooping cough), polio, *Haemophilus* (Hib) infections, pneumococcal infections, rotavirus, influenza, measles, mumps, rubella, chickenpox, and hepatitis A. (See Chapter 27, *Immunizations,* for more information on each of these diseases as well as the Appendix for the immunization schedule recommended by the American Academy of Pediatrics.)

This chapter has dealt in a general way with the topic of infant care. Your baby is a unique individual, however, so you will have some questions specific to her and her alone. These are best answered by your own pediatrician.

4

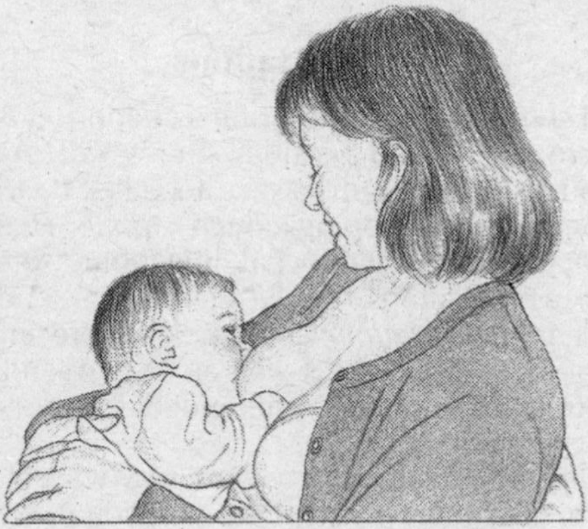

FEEDING YOUR BABY: BREAST AND BOTTLE

Your baby's nutritional needs during the rapid-growth period of infancy are greater than at any other time in his life. He will approximately triple his birth weight during his first year.

Feeding your infant provides more than just good nutrition. It also gives you a chance to hold your newborn close, cuddle him, and make eye contact. These are relaxing and enjoyable moments for you both, and they bring you closer together emotionally.

Before your baby arrives, you should consider how you are going to feed him. All major medical groups worldwide agree that breastfeeding is best for mother and baby. This chapter will provide the basic information you need to learn more about infant feeding and to feel comfortable with your feeding decision.

Because of its nutritional composition, human milk is the ideal food for human infants. Babies who are breastfed are at reduced risk of acquiring ear infections and severe diarrhea and of developing allergic reactions. Formula-fed babies are slightly more likely to need hospitalization for one of these problems. Recent information indicates that breastfeeding plays a significant role in the prevention of overweight and diabetes, both in childhood and in later years. In addition, there is some evidence that for mothers, breastfeeding helps to return to pre-pregnancy weight and reduces the incidence of certain types of cancers later in life. As a result, most pediatricians urge expectant and new mothers to breastfeed.

Many women are uncertain about breastfeeding for various reasons. Try to get more information from your prenatal care provider. Be sure someone knowledgeable discusses your specific concerns, doubts, or fears with you. If for some reason you decide not to breastfeed, infant formula is an acceptable and nutritious alternative to human milk. But you should thoughtfully weigh the many benefits of breastfeeding for yourself and your baby before making the

Where We Stand

The American Academy of Pediatrics believes that breastfeeding is the optimal source of nutrition through the first year of life. We recommend exclusively breastfeeding for a minimum of four months but preferably for six months, and then gradually adding solid foods while continuing breastfeeding until at least the baby's first birthday. Thereafter, breastfeeding can be continued for as long as both mother and baby desire it.

Breastfeeding should begin as soon as possible after birth, usually within the first hour. Newborns should be nursed whenever they show signs of hunger—approximately eight to twelve times every twenty-four hours. The amount of time for each feeding varies widely for each mother-baby pair: It may be anywhere from ten to forty-five minutes in the first few weeks.

choice to formula feed. It's important that you give it serious consideration before your baby arrives, because starting with formula and then switching to breastmilk can be difficult or even impossible if you wait too long. The production of milk by the breast (the process is called lactation) is most successful if breastfeeding begins immediately after delivery. If you begin breastfeeding and then, for any reason, decide that it's not right for you, you can always switch to formula.

The American Academy of Pediatrics, the World Health Organization (WHO), and many other experts encourage women to breastfeed as long as possible, one year or even longer, with a preference of up to six months of exclusive breastfeeding (see *Where We Stand* on page 95). That's because breastmilk provides optimal nutrition and protection against infections. Approximately 7 out of 10 newborns in the United States are breastfed at birth. By six months, only about 3 out of 10 are being breastfed. We know that the longer your baby is breastfed, the greater the benefits.

BREASTFEEDING

As we've already mentioned, human milk is the best possible food for any infant. Its major ingredients are sugar (lactose), easily digestible protein (whey and casein), and fat (digestible fatty acids)—all properly balanced to suit your baby and protect against such conditions as ear infections (otitis media), allergies, vomiting, diarrhea, pneumonia, wheezing, bronchiolitis, and meningitis. In addition, breastmilk contains numerous minerals and vitamins, as well as enzymes that aid the digestive and absorptive process. Formulas only approximate this combination of nutrients and don't provide the enzymes, antibodies, growth-promoting factors, and many other valuable ingredients of breastmilk.

There are many practical reasons to breastfeed, or nurse, your baby. Human milk is relatively low in cost. While maintaining a balanced diet yourself, you should increase slightly your own caloric intake, but that costs only a small percentage of what you would spend for formula. Also, human milk needs no preparation and is instantly available at any time, wherever you may be. As an added advantage to the nursing mother, breastfeeding may make it easier for some women to get back into shape physically after giving birth, by using about 500 calories a day to produce the milk. Breastfeeding also helps the uterus tighten up and return more quickly to its normal size.

The psychological and emotional advantages of breastfeeding are just as compelling, for both mother and child, as the physical benefits. Nursing provides direct skin-to-skin contact, which is soothing for your baby and pleasant for you. The same hormones that stimulate milk production and milk release also may promote feelings that enhance mothering. Almost all nursing mothers find that the experience of breastfeeding makes them feel more attached and protective toward their babies and more confident about their own abilities to nurture and care for their children. When breastfeeding is going well, it has no known disadvantages for the baby. The breastfeeding mother may feel that there is some increased demand on her time. Actually, studies show that breastfeeding and formula feeding take about the same total amount of time, but in breastfeeding all the time is spent with the baby. In bottle-feeding, more time is spent shopping, preparing formula, and cleaning feeding utensils. Time spent with the baby is an important component of infant nurturing and development and is pleasurable to mothers. Other family members can assist by assuming the responsibility for household tasks, especially during the first few weeks after delivery when the mother needs extra rest and the baby needs frequent feeding.

Keep in mind that other family members can actively share in all aspects of caring for the baby even though they do not directly feed milk to her. Remain sensitive to the needs of fathers and siblings. In fact, other members of the family can hold the baby during burping or change the diaper before or after feeding, for example. For the father of the breastfed infant, nonnutritive cuddling plays an important role. A father is invaluable when comforting is necessary for baby and mother. He can hold, diaper, bathe, and walk with the baby. As the baby gets older, and breastfeeding is well established (about three to six weeks of age), the father may feed a bottle of expressed milk or formula.

The best protection against miscommunication about matters surrounding feeding is for parents to discuss these issues openly and make sure both mother and father understand and support the choice before the baby arrives. Many parents and care providers want their children to receive the best possible nutrition from the start, and without question, that is mother's milk. Once breastfeeding is well established (usually between three to six weeks of age), if mothers are away from the baby for a period of time (to return to work, for example, or to go out with family or friends), they can continue to provide their milk to the baby by pumping and collecting breastmilk for feeding from a bottle by the father, other family members, or child care providers.

In rare medical circumstances, breastfeeding may not be recommended. A mother who is extremely ill may not have the energy or stamina to breastfeed without interfering with her own recovery. She also may be taking certain medications that would pass into her milk and be dangerous to her infant, although many medications are safe for breastfeeding.

If you are taking medications for any reason (prescription drugs or over-the-counter medications), let your pediatrician know before you start breastfeeding. She can advise you whether any of these drugs can pass through breastmilk and cause problems for your baby. Sometimes medicines can be switched to safer ones for your baby while you are nursing.

Some mothers may experience mild discomfort in the early days of breastfeeding. But significant discomfort is *not* normal. If you are experiencing pain, having difficulty getting the baby to latch on and feed well, or would like further support with nursing, seek help early in the first week from an experienced health professional (pediatrician, nurse, or lactation specialist).

Occasionally some mothers have breastfeeding problems that lead to untimely weaning from the breast (before the mother had intended). Most women feel disappointed and sad when breastfeeding does not work out as they had planned. Still, you should not feel that you have failed. Sometimes, despite the best attempts and with all available support, it just doesn't work. Fortunately, in those occasional times, infant formula is an acceptable source of nutrition. Providing this type of nutrition is safe, satisfying, and rewarding as well.

Getting Started: Preparing for Lactation

Your body starts preparing to breastfeed as soon as you become pregnant. The area surrounding the nipples—the areola—becomes darker. The breasts themselves enlarge as the cells that will manufacture the milk multiply, and the ducts that will carry the milk to the nipple develop. This increase in breast size is normal and is a sign that your breasts are preparing to produce milk for your baby. Meanwhile, your body starts storing excess fat in other areas to provide the extra energy needed for pregnancy and lactation.

As early as the sixteenth week of pregnancy, the breasts are ready to produce milk as soon as the infant is born. Early milk, called colostrum, is a rich, somewhat thick-appearing, orange-yellow substance that is produced for several days after delivery. Colostrum contains more protein, salt, antibodies, and other protective properties than later breastmilk, but less fat and calories. Your body will produce colostrum for several days after delivery, as it gradually changes into mature milk. Colostrum is a form of milk, even though people commonly say that the "milk comes in" two to five days after delivery. At this time, colostrum increases rapidly in volume, becomes milklike in color and thinner in consistency, and continues to adjust to the baby's needs

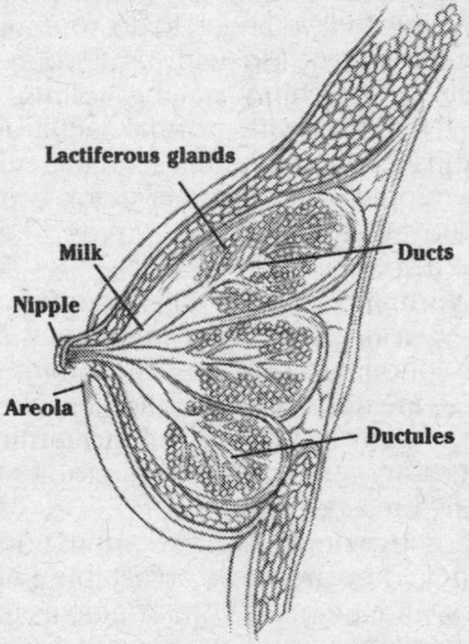

Milk is produced by the lactiferous glands. The milk then passes through the ductules into the ducts and out the nipple.

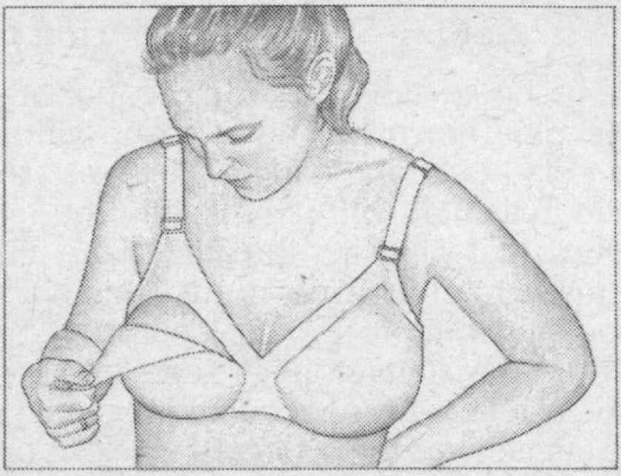

Nursing bras have flaps that allow easy access to the breast. If you wear a nursing bra, make sure it fits properly and is not constricting.

for the rest of the time that you breastfeed. The nutritional qualities of breastmilk change to match the changing needs of your growing infant. This is a characteristic that infant formula cannot duplicate.

As your body naturally prepares for breastfeeding, there is very little that you need to do. Your nipples do not need to be "toughened up" to withstand your baby's sucking. Tactics such as stretching, pulling, rolling, or buffing the nipples may interfere with normal lactation by harming the tiny glands in the areola that secrete a milky fluid that lubricates the nipples in preparation for breastfeeding. In short, it could make your nipples more likely to develop soreness and irritation.

Normal bathing and gentle drying is the best way to care for your breasts during pregnancy. Although many women rub lotions and ointments on their breasts to soften them, these are not necessary and may clog the skin pores. Salves, particularly those containing vitamins or hormones, are unnecessary and could cause problems for your baby if used while breastfeeding.

Some women start wearing nursing bras during pregnancy. They are more adjustable and roomier than normal bras, and are more comfortable as the breast size increases. Nursing bras also have flaps that can be opened for breastfeeding or expressing milk.

Preparing Inverted Nipples for Breastfeeding

Normally, when you press the areola (the darkened area around your nipple) between two fingers, the nipple should protrude and become erect. If the nipple seems to pull inward and disappear instead, it is said to be "inverted" or "tied." Inverted nipples are a normal variation. They may begin to move out more as the pregnancy progresses. If you have questions about your nipples, discuss the issue with your prenatal professional or with a lactation specialist.

At times, inverted nipples may be noticed only at the time of delivery. In this case, the postpartum staff will assist you with early feedings.

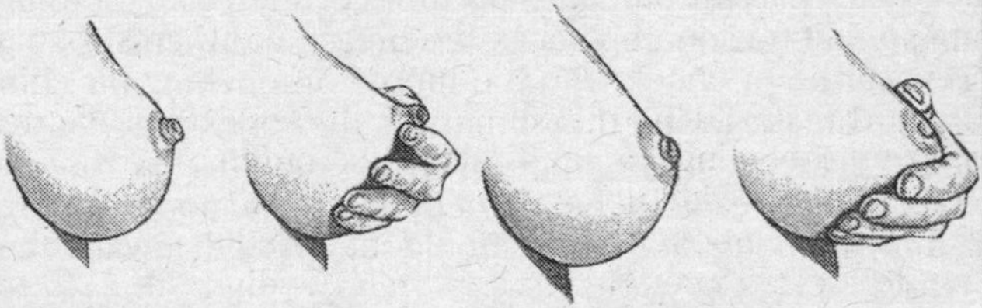

Normal nipple **Inverted nipple**

Letting Down and Latching On

By the time your baby is born, your breasts are already producing colostrum. As he nurses, your infant's actions will let your body know when to start and stop the flow of milk. The process of the baby going to the breast begins in those first moments after birth in the delivery room. This placement of the baby on your upper abdomen in the first moments after birth will allow your new baby to move up your chest and latch on during the first thirty minutes after birth. The process begins with the baby getting a good grip on the areola, not just on the nipple, and starting to suck. He will do this "latching on" instinctively as soon as he feels the breast against his mouth.

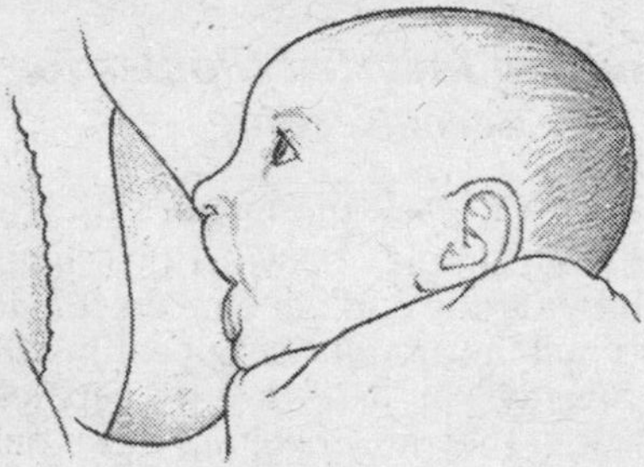

The baby has latched onto the breast correctly. The nose, lips, and chin are all close to the breast allowing for effective breastfeeding.

Once out of the delivery room, and the first real breast feed takes place, you can help him get started by holding him so that he squarely faces the breast and then stroking his lower lip or cheek with the nipple or touching his chin to your breast. Doing this stimulates the reflex that causes him to search for the nipple with his mouth (the rooting reflex). It will result in the infant opening the mouth widely; at that moment, the baby should be moved toward the breast.

As your baby takes the breast into his mouth, his jaws should close around the areola, *not* the nipple. His lips will separate and the gums will encircle the areola. His tongue will form a trough around the nipple and, in a wavelike motion, compress the milk reservoirs and empty the milk ducts. Putting your baby to the breast in the first hour after delivery will establish good breastfeeding patterns at a time when infants are usually alert and vigorous. Later in the first day he may get sleepy, but if he began nursing in the first hour, he is more likely to be a successful breastfeeder.

In some cases an infant will have trouble latching on. This occurs most often in newborns who have been given bottles or pacifiers. Suckling from the breast is different from sucking the nipple on a bottle or pacifier, and some infants are very sensitive to the difference. These babies may simply lick, nibble, or chew with their jaws instead of using the tongue. Others may show frustration by pulling away or cry-

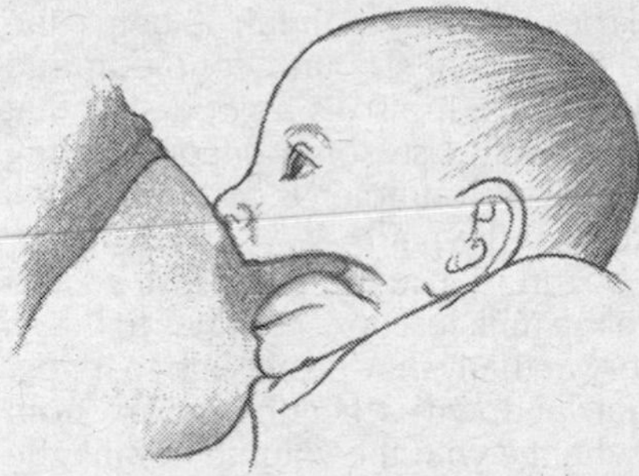

Most of the areola and nipple are in his mouth.

ing. This sensitivity has been called nipple confusion or nipple preference. Although nipple confusion has been considered controversial, there is now good evidence to show that starting artificial nipples early on is associated with decreased exclusive breastfeeding and decreased duration of breastfeeding. Researchers are still uncertain if the artificial nipples are the cause of breastfeeding problems or are just a response to a breastfeeding problem that already existed. *Experts generally recommend that you avoid bottles and pacifiers for the first several weeks until you feel that breastfeeding is going well.* During that time, if the baby seems to need more sucking, offer the breast again, or help him to find his own hand or fingers to soothe himself.

When your baby suckles effectively at the breast, his movements will stimulate the nerve fibers in the nipple. Breast stimulation also starts milk flowing through the milk ducts in what is known as the let-down reflex, which is associated with the release of another pituitary hormone, oxytocin. In turn, the release of the hormone prolactin from the pituitary gland (see box on page 104) and the removal of milk from the breast cause the breasts to make more milk.

Oxytocin causes many wonderful things to happen for you. It gives a feeling of euphoria and diminishes the sense of pain immediately after the birth. Some also say it enhances the feeling of love between you and your baby. It also causes the muscles of the uterus to contract. So, in the first days or weeks after delivery, you may feel "after pains," or cramping of the uterus, each time you nurse. Although this may be annoying and occasionally painful, it helps the uterus return quickly to its normal size and condition and reduces postpartum blood loss. It also is a good sign that your baby is feeding effectively. Use some deep-breathing techniques or pain medication (ibuprofen is commonly prescribed after delivery) to ease the pain.

Once lactation has begun, it usually takes just a brief period of sucking before the milk lets down (begins to flow). Just hearing your baby cry actually may be enough to trigger milk flow. The signs that let-down is occurring vary from woman to woman and change with the volume of milk the baby demands. Some women feel a subtle tingling sensation, while others experience a buildup of pressure that feels as if their breasts are swelling and overfull—sensations that are quickly relieved as the milk starts to flow. Some women

The Let-Down Process

As your baby sucks, several different hormones work together to produce milk and release it for feeding. From the moment she starts to nurse, here is what happens within your body:

1. Her sucking movements stimulate nerve fibers in the nipple.
2. These nerve fibers send a message to your brain to provide milk for your baby.
3. The pituitary gland, sometimes called the "master gland," in your brain responds to this message by releasing the hormones prolactin and oxytocin.
4. Prolactin stimulates the breasts to produce more milk.
5. Oxytocin stimulates contractions of the tiny muscles surrounding the ducts in the breasts. These contractions squeeze the ducts and eject the milk to make it readily available for your baby while nursing.

never feel these sensations, even though they are nursing successfully and the infant is getting plenty of milk. The way the milk flows also varies widely. It may spray, gush, trickle, or flow. Some women have leakage of milk with let-down or between feedings and others don't; either case can be normal. Flow or leakage also may be quite different in each breast—perhaps gushing on one side and trickling on the other. This is due to slight differences in the ducts on either side and is no cause for concern, as long as the baby is getting adequate milk and growing well.

The First Feeding

If you had a normal delivery, and you and your baby are alert and awake, he can be placed on your abdomen or chest to allow him access to the breast, so you can nurse him right away. If there were complications with the delivery, or if your newborn needs immediate medical attention, you may have to wait a few hours. If the first feeding takes place within the first day or two, you should have no physical difficulty nursing. If nursing must be delayed beyond the first few hours of life, the nursing staff will assist you with pumping or hand expression.

If you do nurse immediately after delivery, you might find it most comfortable to lie on your side, with the baby lying

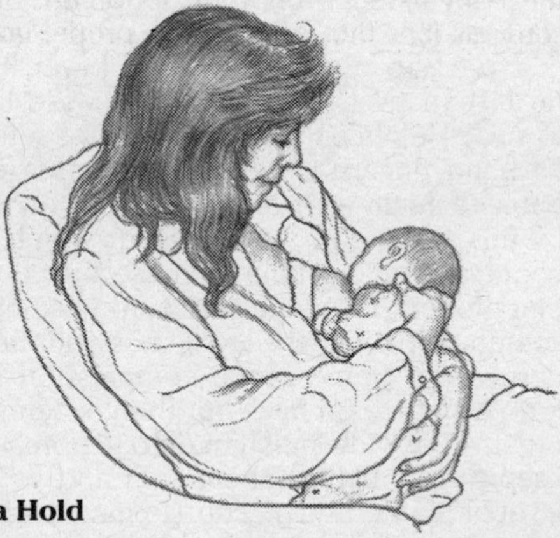

Cradle or Madonna Hold

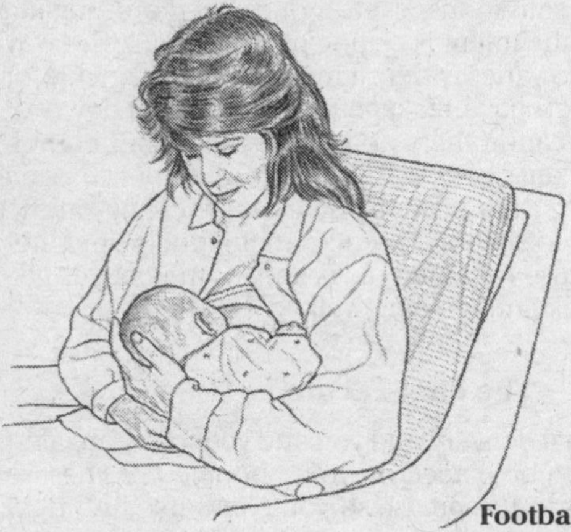

Football or Clutch Hold

facing you, opposite the breast. If you'd rather sit up, use pillows to help support your arms and cradle the baby slightly below breast level, making sure his entire body, not just his head, is facing your body. Following a Cesarean delivery, the most comfortable position may be a side hold, or what's also called a football hold, in which you sit up and the baby lies at your side facing you. Curl your arm underneath him and support and hold his head at your breast. This position keeps the baby's weight off your abdomen, but the infant must squarely face the breast for the proper grasp.

If you stroke your newborn's lower lip with the nipple, he'll instinctively open his mouth wide, latch on, and begin to suck. He's been practicing this for some time by sucking his hand, fingers, and possibly even his feet in utero. (Some babies actually are born with blisters on their fingers caused by this sucking in the uterus, or womb.) It takes little encouragement to get him to nurse, but you may need to help him properly grasp the areola. You can hold the breast with your thumb above the areola and your fingers and palm underneath it. Some gentle compression may be helpful to form a surface for latch-on. Then, when the baby opens his mouth very wide, pull him onto the breast. It is important to keep fingers behind the areola and be sure the nipple is level or pointed slightly up. No matter which technique you

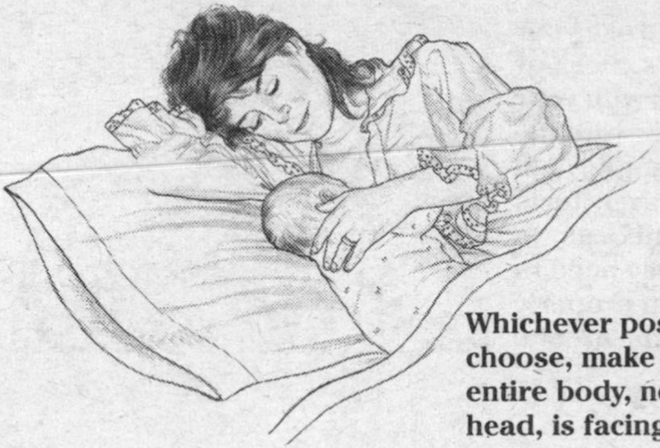

Whichever position you choose, make sure his entire body, not just his head, is facing your body.

try, you need to keep your fingers clear of the areola so the baby can grasp it. Be sure your fingers are no closer than two inches from the base of the nipple. Let your baby nurse at the first side as long as he wishes, then put him on the other side if he is still interested in feeding. It is more important to complete a feeding on one breast than to have brief feedings from both breasts. The longer your baby feeds, the more fat and calories he will consume. Let-down, uterine cramping, swallowing sounds, and return to sound sleep by the baby are all signs of successful breastfeeding. In the beginning, it may take one to two minutes for let-down to occur. Within a week or so, let-down will take place much more rapidly and your milk supply will increase dramatically.

If you are not sure you are experiencing a let-down sensation, just watch your baby. Following a let-down, he should be swallowing after every few sucks at the start of the feeding. After five or ten minutes, he may switch to what's called nonnutritive sucking—a more relaxed sucking that provides emotional comfort along with small amounts of creamier, fat-rich *hindmilk.* Other signs of let-down vary from woman to woman and already have been discussed: uterine cramps the first few days after delivery; sensations of let-down; leakage of milk from the opposite breast during breastfeeding; the breast feeling full before and soft after feeding; or the appearance of milk in or around the baby's mouth after feeding. The more relaxed and confident you feel, the quicker your milk will let down.

If you stroke your newborn's cheek or lower lip with your finger or with the nipple, he'll instinctively turn, latch on, and begin to suck. You may need to help him properly grasp the areola.

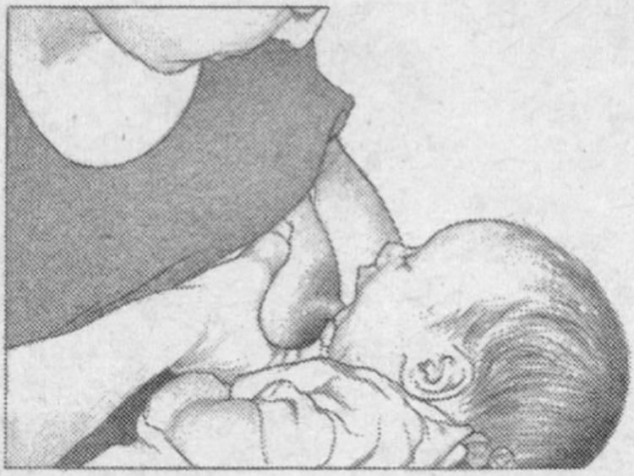

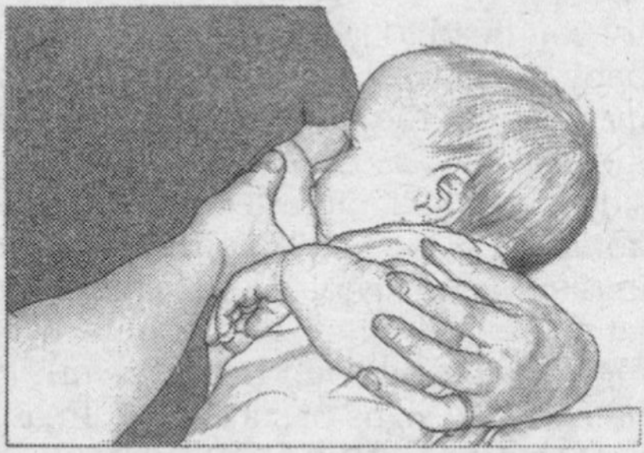

You may continue to provide some breast support while the baby is feeding, especially if the breasts are large.

You can slide your finger into the corner of your baby's mouth if you need to interrupt the feeding before the baby is finished.

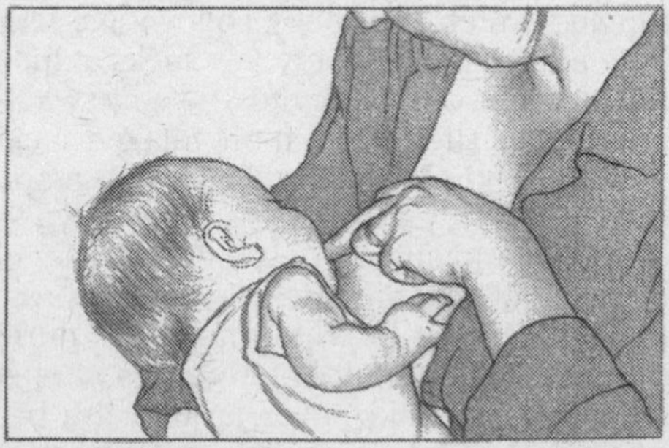

The first feedings in the hospital may be difficult because of excitement or, perhaps, your uncertainty about what to do. Breastfeeding should not cause sustained pain in the nipple, areola, or breast. If there is pain for more than a few moments at the beginning, ask the doctor, nurse, or lactation specialist to evaluate the breastfeeding and suggest changes. Ask the hospital staff for help; they are usually very experienced at assisting nursing mothers and babies.

Once you are back home, try the following suggestions to help the let-down reflex.

- Apply moist heat (i.e., warm, wet washcloths) to the breast several minutes before starting the feeding.
- Sit in a comfortable chair, with good support for your back and arms. (Many nursing mothers recommend rocking chairs.)
- Make sure the baby is positioned so he squarely faces the breast and is well latched on, as described earlier.
- Use some relaxation techniques, such as deep breathing or visual imagery.
- Listen to soothing music and sip a nutritious drink during feedings.
- If your household is very busy, find a quiet corner or room where you won't be disturbed during feedings.
- Do not smoke, and avoid secondhand smoke. Do not consume alcohol, or use illegal drugs (i.e., marijuana, cocaine, heroin, ecstasy, etc.), as all contain substances that can interfere with let-down, affect the content of breastmilk, and be harmful to the baby. Check with your obstetrician or pediatrician about any prescription or nonprescription drugs you may be taking.

If you still are not letting down after trying these suggestions, contact your pediatrician for additional help. If you continue to have difficulties, ask to be referred to a lactation expert.

When Your Milk Supply Increases

For the first few days after delivery, your breasts will be soft to the touch; but as the blood supply increases and milk-producing cells start to function more efficiently, the breasts will become firmer. By the second to fifth day following delivery, your breasts should be producing transitional milk (the milk that follows colostrum) and may feel very full. At the end of the baby's first week, you will see creamy white breastmilk; after ten to fourteen days, your milk may initially look like skimmed milk, but as the feeding continues, the amount of fat in the milk will increase and the milk will look creamier. This is normal and does not mean there is anything wrong with your milk. Nursing your baby frequently and massaging your breasts prior to and during feeding may help minimize the fullness.

Engorgement occurs when the breasts become overfilled with milk and excess body fluids. This can be very uncomfortable and at times painful. The best solution to this problem is to nurse your baby whenever she is hungry, feeding at both breasts about every two hours. Sometimes the breasts are so engorged that the baby has trouble latching on. If that happens, you can apply moist heat to soften the breasts, and if necessary, manually express some milk or use a mechanical breast pump before you start to nurse. Doing this may help the baby get a better grasp and nurse more efficiently. (See page 119 regarding milk expression.) You also can try several techniques to ease the pain of engorgement, such as the following.

- Soak a cloth in warm water and put it on your breasts. Or take a warm shower. These techniques, when used just before breastfeeding or expressing milk, will encourage milk flow.
- Warmth may not help cases of severe engorgement. In this case, you may want to use cool compresses in between or just after feeding.
- Express milk or pump just enough milk for comfort's sake.
- Try feeding your baby in more than one position. Begin by sitting up, then lying down. This changes the segments

of the breast that are drained most optimally at each feeding.

- Gently massage your breasts from under the arm and down the nipple. This will help reduce soreness and ease milk flow.
- The use of ibuprofen has been shown to be safe and effective for the treatment of engorgement. Take the dosage recommended by your doctor. Do not take any other medications without your doctor's approval.

Fortunately, engorgement lasts only a few days while lactation is getting established. However, it can occur anytime when feedings are skipped and the breasts are not emptied frequently.

Breastfeeding Twins

Twins present a unique challenge to the nursing mother. At first it may be easier to feed them one at a time, but after lactation is established, often it's more convenient to feed them simultaneously in order to save time. Feeding them together can also help to increase your milk supply. You can do this using the "football hold" to position one at each side, or cradle them both in front of you with their bodies crossing each other. Books and support groups for parents of twins can provide further information.

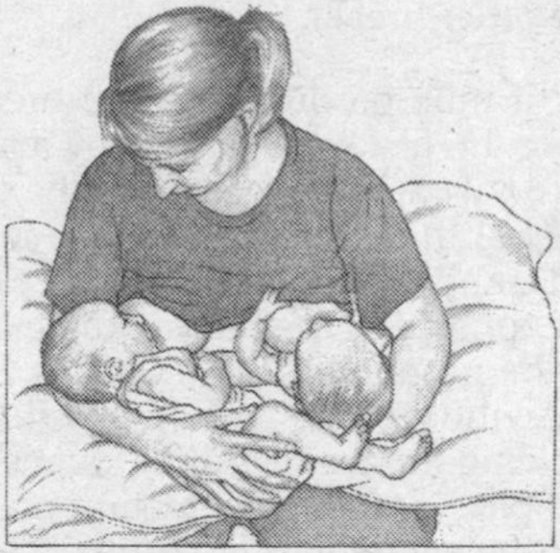

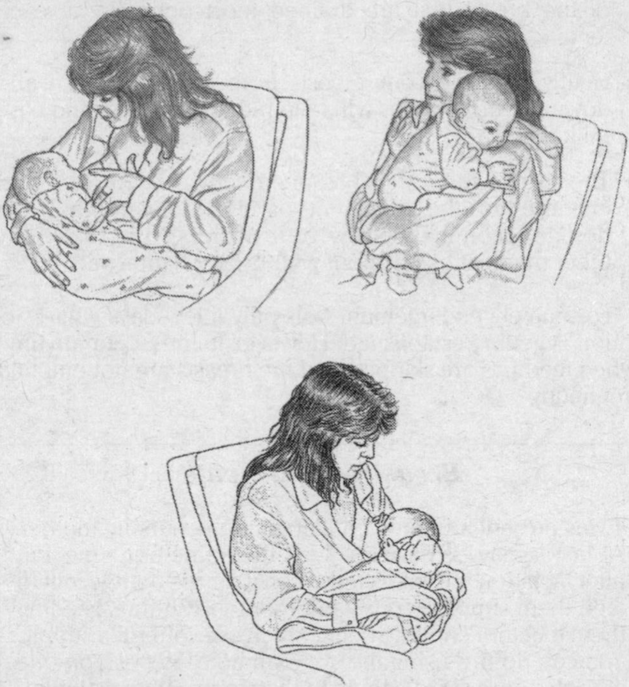

The baby will generally feed for about ten to fifteen minutes on the first breast. Then the baby can be burped and offered the other breast.

The volume of milk produced by the breasts increases dramatically over the first week. Your baby may take as little as 1 teaspoon (5 ml) at each feeding in the first couple of days. But by the fourth or fifth day, the volume may be up to 1 ounce (30 ml), and by the end of the week—depending on the size and appetite of the baby and the length of feedings—you may be producing 2 to 6 ounces (60–180 ml) at each feeding. At the end of your baby's first month, she should be receiving an average of 24 ounces (720 ml) of milk a day. See page 116 for information on how to tell if your baby is getting enough.

How Often and How Long?

Breastfed babies vary greatly in their feeding behaviors. They generally eat more frequently than formula-fed infants. Breastfed newborns typically feed eight to twelve or more times per twenty-four hours. As they get older, some may be able to go longer between feedings, because their stomach capacity enlarges and their mothers' milk production increases. Others continue to prefer frequent, smaller feeds.

What's the best feeding schedule for a breastfed baby? It's the one she designs herself. Your baby lets you know when she's hungry by waking and looking alert, putting hands toward her mouth, making sucking motions, whimpering and flexing arms and hands, moving fists to her mouth, becoming more active, and nuzzling against your breast. (She can smell its location even through your clothing.) It is best to start nursing the baby before crying starts. Crying is a late sign of hunger. Whenever possible, use these signals rather than the clock to decide when to nurse her. This way, you'll ensure that she's hungry when she eats. In the process, she'll stimulate the breast more efficiently to produce milk.

As stated earlier, breastfeeding for the healthy mother and infant is generally most successful when you start nursing immediately after delivery (in the first hour). Keep the baby with you as much as possible (rooming in with her in the hospital), and respond promptly to cues of hunger (a practice called demand feeding). Sleepy babies should be awakened to feed after every three to four hours during the first few weeks of life (or until they have regained their birth weight and your pediatrician says it's OK to let her sleep at night), so that they have a minimum of eight feedings in twenty-four hours.

Allow your baby to continue nursing on the first breast as long as desired. When she spontaneously stops for a prolonged period or withdraws from the breast, burp her. If your baby seems sleepy after the first breast, you may want to wake her up a bit by changing her diaper or playing with her a little before switching her to the second side. Since your infant sucks more efficiently on the first breast she uses, you should alternate from feeding to feeding the one she uses first. You might consider placing a safety pin or an extra nursing pad on the side where the baby last nursed as a

Getting to Know Your Baby's Feeding Patterns

Each baby has a particular style of eating. Years ago researchers at Yale University playfully attached names to five common eating patterns. See if you recognize your baby's dining behavior among them:

Barracudas get right down to business. As soon as they're put to the breast, they grasp the areola and suck energetically for ten to twenty minutes. They usually become less eager as time goes on.

Excited Ineffectives become frantic at the sight of the breast. In a frenzied cycle they grasp it, lose it, and start screaming in frustration. They must be calmed down several times during each feeding. The key to nourishing this type of baby is to feed him as soon as he wakes up, before he gets desperately hungry. Also, if the milk tends to spray from the breast as the baby struggles, it may help to manually express a few drops first to slow the stream.

Procrastinators can't be bothered with nursing until the milk supply increases, commonly referred to as "coming in." These babies shouldn't be given bottles of water or formula. Feeding them bottles may make it more difficult to get them to nurse at the breast. You should continue to put them to the breast regularly, whenever they appear alert or make mouthing movements. Reluctant nursers sometimes benefit from being placed naked on the reclining mother's bare abdomen and chest for a period of time. They may spontaneously move toward the breast, or they can be placed on the breast after a time. You may find advice on improved positioning and attachment from a lactation specialist helpful. For a baby who resists nursing for the first few days, you can use an electric pump between feedings to stimulate milk production. (See pages 119–122.) Just don't give up! Contact your pediatrician's office for assistance or referral to a lactation specialist.

Gourmets or *Mouthers* insist on playing with the nipple, tasting the milk first and smacking their lips before digging in. If hurried or prodded, they become furious and scream in protest. The best solution is tolerance. After a few minutes of playing, they do settle down and nurse well. Just be sure the lips and gums are on the areola and not on the nipple.

Resters prefer to nurse for a few minutes, rest a few minutes, and resume nursing. Some fall asleep on the breast, nap for half an hour or so, and then awaken ready for dessert. This pattern can be confusing, but these babies cannot be hurried. The solution? It's best just to schedule extra time for feedings and remain as flexible as possible.

Learning your own baby's eating patterns is one of your biggest challenges in the first few weeks after delivery. Once you understand his patterns, you'll find it much easier to determine when he's hungry, when he's had enough, how often he needs to eat, and how much time is required for feedings. It is generally best to initiate a feeding at the earliest signs of hunger and before the baby cries. Babies also have unique positions that they prefer and will even show preference for one breast over the other.

reminder to start first on the other side at the next feeding. Or you can start on the breast that feels the fullest.

Initially your newborn probably will nurse every couple of hours, regardless of whether it's day or night. By six to eight weeks of age, many newborns have one sleep period of four to five hours. Establish nighttime sleep patterns by keeping the room dark, warm, and quiet. Don't turn on a bright light for the nighttime feeding. If soiled or wet, change her diaper quickly and without fanfare before this feeding and put her right back to sleep afterward. By four months, many—but not all—babies are sleeping six hours or more at a stretch without awakening during the night. However, some breastfed babies may continue to awaken more frequently for feedings at night. (See *Helping Your Baby Sleep*, page 71.)

You'll also find that your infant may require long feedings at certain times of the day and be satisfied quickly at others. She'll let you know when she's finished by letting go or drifting off to sleep between spurts of nonnutritive sucking. A few babies want to nurse around the clock. If your baby falls into this category, check with your pediatrician's office. You may be referred to a lactation specialist. There are several reasons why infants behave this way, and the sooner the sit-

Is Your Baby Eating Enough?

Your baby's diapers will provide clues about whether he is getting enough to eat. During the first month, after your milk supply increases and if his diet is adequate, he should wet six or more times a day and generally have three to four or more bowel movements daily (often one little one after each feeding). Later he may have less frequent bowel movements, and there may even be a day or more between them. If the bowel movements are soft, and your baby is otherwise thriving, this is quite normal. Another clue about intake is whether you can hear your baby swallow, usually after several sucks in a row. Appearing satisfied for a couple of hours right after a feeding is also a sign that he is getting enough. On the other hand, a baby who is not getting enough to eat over several days may become very sleepy and seem "easy" to care for. In the early weeks, a baby who regularly sleeps for four hours or more at a time should be seen by the pediatrician to make sure he is gaining weight as expected.

One of the most accurate ways to judge your baby's intake over time is by checking her weight gain. We now recommend that babies be examined by a health-care provider at the third to fifth day of life, which provides an opportunity to check her weight, feeding, and head circumference. During the first week of life, the average weight loss is less than 8 percent of birth weight (that's about 8 ounces [226 grams] in an approximately 7½-pound [3.4 kg] full-term baby), but after that she should gain fairly steadily. By the end of her second week, she ought to be back to her birth weight. If you've breastfed other children, lactation probably will get established more quickly this time around, so the new baby may lose little weight and return to her birth weight within days.

Once your milk supply is established, your baby should gain between ½ and 1 ounce (14–28 grams) a day during his first three months. Between three and six months, his weight gain will taper off to about ½ ounce (14 grams) a day, and after six months, the amount your baby gains each day will be even less. Your pediatrician typically will weigh the baby at every visit. If you have concerns between visits, call to schedule an appointment to have the baby weighed; don't depend on a home scale, which is not very reliable for young infants.

uation is evaluated, the easier it is to address the cause. Once evaluated, if breastfeeding is going smoothly, your milk supply is well established, and the baby is gaining weight, you may decide to provide a pacifier for extra sucking. But be aware that the early introduction of pacifiers is associated with a shorter duration of breastfeeding.

What About Bottles?

It is usually best to try to breastfeed your newborn around the clock, which can be made easier by having your baby "rooming in" with you in your hospital room as much as possible. You might be tempted to have your baby sleep in the nursery for one night so you can get an uninterrupted night's sleep. But research has shown that those mothers who keep their babies with them in their hospital room twenty-four hours per day sleep just as long in total as mothers whose babies are returned to the nursery. Also, if your baby is always with you, you can avoid any unnecessary water or

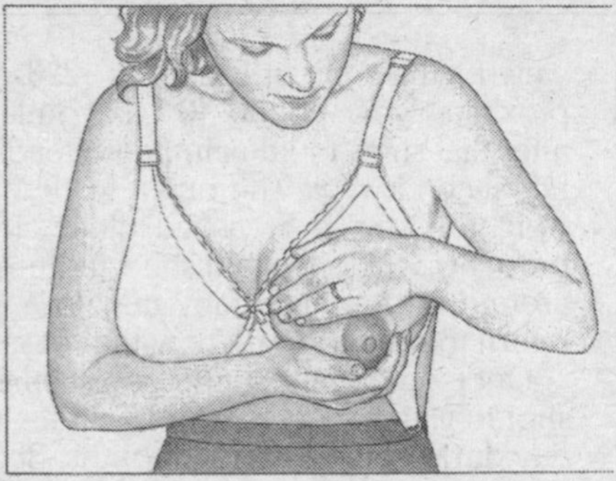

Expressing milk is easier if you stimulate the breast first by massaging it gently.

formula supplementation, which may interfere with your ability to have a successful breastfeeding experience.

If circumstances keep you away from your baby, you will need to express breastmilk, manually or mechanically, in order to stimulate continued milk production. Only rarely are there serious situations where mother's milk may not be used. If you use bottles of formula when you are away, your baby receives less breastmilk and fewer benefits of breastfeeding. Avoiding formula may be particularly important in babies from families with a history of allergy. Always check with your pediatrician or other expert before you stop giving your milk to your baby.

Once breastfeeding is going well and the milk supply is established, usually three or four weeks after delivery, you may decide to use an occasional bottle so you can be away during some feedings. But you won't need to substitute formula: If you express breastmilk in advance and store it, your baby can continue to receive the benefits of your milk by bottle. In addition, using expressed breastmilk will maintain your body's full milk production for your baby. An occasional bottle at this stage probably won't interfere with your baby's nursing habits, but it may cause another problem: Your breasts may become engorged, and they can leak milk. You can relieve the engorgement by expressing milk to drain the breasts; store this milk to replace the breastmilk that was used while you were away. Wearing nursing pads will help you manage the problem of leakage. (Some women wear

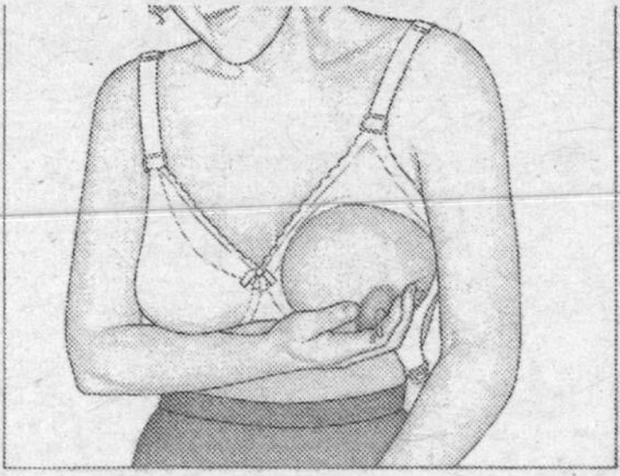

To express manually, hold the breast with the thumb and index finger at the edge of the areola on opposite sides of the breast, then press toward the chest wall with a rhythmic motion. Rotate position of fingers so all parts of the breast are emptied.

nursing pads constantly during the first month or two of lactation to avoid milk stains on their clothing.)

Milk Expression and Storage

Milk can be expressed either by hand or by pump. In either case, you must have the let-down reflex in order to get the milk out of the breast. Manual expression is easier to learn if someone shows you, rather than just reading about it. Manual expression can be quick and effective once it is learned, but it requires practice.

Initially breast pumps seem easier to use than learning hand expression, but the quality of pumps varies widely. A poor-quality breast pump will not remove milk effectively, resulting in engorgement or a gradually lower milk supply over time. Poor-quality breast pumps also may irritate the nipples or be quite painful.

If you choose to express manually, wash your hands and use a clean container to collect the milk. Place your thumb on the breast, above the areola, and your fingers underneath. Gently but firmly roll the thumb and fingers toward each other while compressing the breast tissue and pushing toward the chest wall. Do not slide your fingers toward your nipple as this can cause soreness. Transfer the milk into a clean bottle, rigid plastic container, or specially made plastic bag for storage in the freezer. (See page 121.) If your baby is hospitalized, the hospital may give you more specific and detailed information about milk collection and storage, and

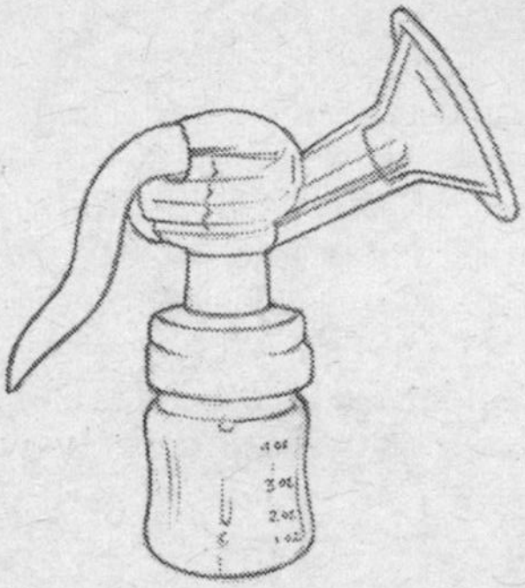

Hand pumps are available at most drug and baby stores.

may loan you a hospital-grade breast pump to express milk for your baby.

While hand pumps are available, good-quality electric pumps are a wonderful option and can stimulate the breast more effectively than manual expression. These pumps have regulated pressures and are self-cycling for efficient milk removal. They are used primarily to induce or maintain lactation when a mother is unable to feed her infant directly for several days or more, or when the mother returns to work or school. Electric pumps are efficient but can be costly—ranging in price from $150 to $300 and up. If you will need the pump for only a limited period, it's often much more economical to rent one from a medical supply store, hospital, or a lactation rental agency. If you have a hospitalized newborn or return to work shortly after your baby is born and want to continue breastfeeding, obtaining a breast pump is essential.

When shopping for an electric pump to buy or rent, make sure it creates a steady milking action with variable pressure and is not simply a suction device. You also may want to consider a pump that expresses both breasts at the same time; such a pump will increase your milk volume as well as save time. Make sure that all parts of the pump that come in contact with the skin or milk can be removed for proper cleaning. Sterilization is not required for pumps and containers for a healthy baby; simply washing them well with hot soapy water is fine, as is running them through the dishwasher. Talk to your pediatrician or a lactation consultant for advice about which type of pump may be best for you. And remember, whenever you use a pump, wash your hands immediately before pumping.

As with breastmilk that is expressed manually, milk that is pumped should be stored in clean containers, preferably glass or rigid plastic containers or special plastic bags. Baby bottle insert bags are not sufficiently strong or thick to protect the milk from contamination. If the milk is to be fed to the baby within seventy-two hours, it should be sealed and cooled immediately. If this refrigerated milk goes unused for more than seventy-two hours, it should be discarded. It may be frozen after up to twenty-four hours of refrigeration.

If you know in advance that the milk won't be used within four days, freeze it immediately. Breastmilk will safely keep in your freezer for at least one month. Store it in the back of the freezer. If you have a separate deep freeze, it can be kept for about three to six months. (Because the fats in human milk begin to break down over time, use the frozen milk as soon as possible.)

It's a good idea to place a label with the date on each container so you can use the oldest milk first. It's useful to freeze milk in quantities of about 3 to 4 ounces (90–120 ml)—the amount of a single feeding. You also can freeze some 1- to 2-ounce portions (30–60 ml); these will come in handy if the baby wants a little extra at any feeding.

When it's time to use this stored milk, keep in mind that your baby is accustomed to breastmilk at body temperature, so the baby may prefer that the milk be heated to at least room temperature (68 to 72 degrees Fahrenheit [20–22 degrees Celsius]) for feeding. Frozen milk may be thawed in the refrigerator, or the container of frozen milk may be held under warm running water, or placed in a container of warm water.

Do not heat breastmilk, formula, or bottles in a microwave oven. Microwaving overheats the milk in the center of the container. Even if the bottle feels comfortably warm to your touch, the superheated milk in the center can scald your baby's mouth. Also, the bottle itself can explode if left in the microwave too long. Bear in mind that heat also can destroy some of the anti-infectious, nutritious, and protective properties of breastmilk.

Incidentally, once milk is thawed, its fat may separate, but that does not affect its quality. You may swirl the container gently until the milk returns to a uniform consistency. Thawed milk should be used within twenty-four hours. Never refreeze it. Do not save unfinished milk from a partially consumed bottle to use at another feeding.

Not all breastfed babies react to the bottle the same way. Some accept it easily, regardless of when it is first introduced. Others are willing to take an occasional bottle, but not from the mother or when the mother is in the house.

You can increase the likelihood that your baby will accept a bottle the first few times if someone other than the mother offers it, and she is out of sight at the time. Once familiar with the bottle, he may be willing to take it in his mother's presence, possibly even from the mother herself. If your breastfed baby refuses a bottle, try using a cup or "sippie cup" instead. Even premature newborns are able to cup feed. Some breastfed babies go from breast to cup without ever using a bottle.

Possible Nursing Concerns and Questions

For some babies and mothers, nursing goes well from the start and there are never any problems. But breastfeeding can have its ups and downs, especially in the beginning. Fortunately, many of the most common difficulties can be prevented with proper positioning and latch-on, along with frequent feedings. Once problems crop up, many may resolve quickly if you seek advice right away. Don't hesitate to ask your pediatrician or his office nurse for help with the following problems.

Sore and Cracked Nipples. Breastfeeding may produce some initial mild soreness, especially with latch-on in the first week or so. But breastfeeding should not cause sustained pain, discomfort, or open cracks. Proper latch-on is the most important factor in preventing sore and cracked nipples. If your nipple or other areas of the breast are painful, you should seek advice from your lactation expert.

During your bath or shower, wash your breasts only with water, not soap. Creams, lotions, and more vigorous rubbing actually may aggravate the problem. Also, try varying the baby's position at each feeding.

In humid climates, the best treatments for cracked nipples are sunlight, heat, and keeping the area dry. Don't wear plastic breast shields or plastic-lined nursing pads, which hold in moisture; instead, expose your breasts to the air as much as possible. Also, after nursing, express a little milk from your breasts and let it dry on the nipples. This dried milk will leave a protective coating that may help the healing process. In a dry climate, you might want to apply purified hypoallergenic lanolin. If these measures do not solve the problem, consult your doctor for further advice; you might have a yeast or bacterial infection of the nipple.

Engorgement. As we've already mentioned, your breasts can become severely engorged if your baby doesn't nurse often or efficiently during the first few days after your milk comes in. While some engorgement is to be expected when you start lactation, extreme engorgement causes swelling of the milk ducts in the breasts and of blood vessels across the entire chest area. The best treatment is to feed your baby frequently; express milk between feedings, either manually or with a pump; and make sure the baby nurses at both breasts at every feeding. Since warmth encourages milk flow, standing in a warm shower as you manually express the milk may help, or use warm compresses. You also may get some relief with the use of warm compresses during nursing and cool compresses between nursing.

If you have very severe engorgement, however, warmth may aggravate the situation because it increases blood flow to the area. If this is the case, try using cool compresses between feedings. The engorgement should subside in a few days. Ibuprofen has been shown to be safe and effective in the treatment of engorgement. Use the same dose that your doctor recommends for uterine cramping.

Mastitis. Mastitis is an infection of the breast tissue caused by bacteria. Mastitis causes flulike symptoms of fever, chills, headache, nausea, dizziness, and lack of energy. These general symptoms occur along with local breast symptoms of redness, tenderness, swelling, heat, and pain. If you experience any of these symptoms, call your doctor at once. The

Supplemental Nurser (Infant Feeding Device)

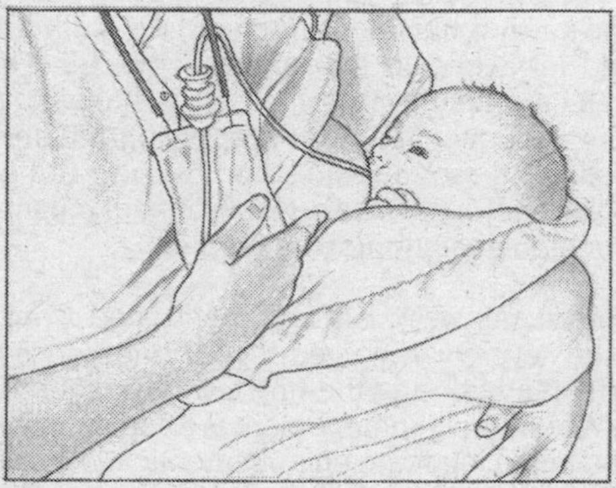

The amount of milk your breasts produce depends on the amount of milk that is removed from them. If you miss too many feedings, your body automatically will decrease milk production. This can occur even if you express milk during missed feedings, since pumps do not stimulate or empty the breasts nearly as efficiently as your baby's sucking.

If your milk supply is not meeting the needs of your baby, if you miss a number of feedings because of illness, or if your baby is unable to nurse for some reason, you may be able to reestablish your milk supply with the help of a device called a supplemental nurser (also known as a supplementer tube, infant feeding device, or nursing trainer). Unlike a bottle, which trains the baby away from the breast, this device provides supplemental formula while the infant is at the breast.

The supplemental nurser also is used for premature infants or to train babies with feeding problems. It even can help stimulate lactation in adoptive mothers, or in mothers who have stopped breastfeeding for a prolonged period and wish to start again.

The device consists of a small plastic container that holds formula or expressed breastmilk and hangs from a cord around your neck. The container has a thin flexible tube that is held or taped along the breast with its tip adjacent to the nipple and placed in the corner of the baby's mouth as she sucks. Her suction draws the formula from the container into her mouth, so that even if you aren't producing much milk, she still will be getting a full feeding. This process reinforces her desire to nurse at the breast. At the same time, her sucking stimulates your body to step up milk production.

Supplemental nursers are available from lactation specialists, medical supply stores, some pharmacies, or via mail order. If possible, purchase the device from someone who can help you use it for the first time and show you how to clean it. Most mothers and babies need a few days of practice to get comfortable with the device. Using a supplemental nurser requires commitment and dedication, as it may take weeks or months to rebuild the milk supply and the breastfeeding relationship.

infection is treated with milk removal (by feeding or pumping), rest, fluids, antibiotics, and pain medicine if needed. Your doctor will prescribe an antibiotic that is safe during breastfeeding. Be sure to take all the antibiotics even if you feel better. Do not stop nursing; doing so will worsen the mastitis and cause increased pain. The milk itself is *not* infected. Your baby will not be harmed by nursing during mastitis, and mastitis and the antibiotics will not cause changes in the composition of your milk.

Mastitis may be a sign that your body's immune defenses are down. Bed rest, sleep, and decreased activity will help you recover your stamina. Rarely, you may find that it's too painful to have the baby nurse on the infected breast; in that case, open up both sides of your bra and let the milk flow from that breast onto a towel or absorbent cloth such as a clean diaper, relieving the pressure as you feed the baby on the opposite side. Then she can finish the feeding on the infected side with less discomfort. Some women with severe pain find that it is more comfortable to pump the breast than it is to feed the baby. The pumped milk can be stored or can be fed to the baby.

A mother's return to work is a peak time for the development of mastitis. It is important to express milk regularly, approximately on the same schedule with which the baby would feed, to try to prevent the infection from occurring.

Infant Fussiness. There are a number of reasons for a breastfed baby to be unusually fussy. These range from normal variations in personality to a serious illness. Although most "fussy babies" do not have a serious medical problem, their constant crying can become extremely difficult for parents. The fussy baby wears on Mom and Dad's energy, time, and enjoyment of their young infant. Here are some general causes for excessive crying in the breastfed baby and suggestions for working with your pediatrician to pinpoint and treat the problem.

- **Hunger:** If your newborn infant feeds constantly and is never satisfied after coming off the breast, your breastfeeding needs to be evaluated by an experienced healthcare provider. He will weigh and examine your baby, examine your breast and nipples, and observe an entire breastfeeding session. The solution may be as simple as improving the baby's positioning and latch-on. It may be more complicated, however, particularly if the baby has lost too much weight or is not gaining well.

- **Growth spurt:** A rapid growth phase often happens at two to three weeks of age, again around six weeks, and once more at about three months. During these growth spurts, babies will want to nurse *constantly*. Remember, this is normal, and it is only temporary, usually lasting about four to five days. Many women are tempted to give supplemental bottles at this time, because they do not understand why the baby is eating all the time. Keep breastfeeding very often, and do not give other liquids. If the growth spurt lasts longer than five days, or if you are tempted to start your baby on bottles, call your pediatrician's office for assistance. He should see the baby, check her weight, and evaluate the feeding process (or refer you to a lactation specialist if needed).

- **Hyperalert or high-needs infants:** These babies require more of everything, except sleep. They cry seemingly around the clock. They are not very regular in their eating, sleeping, or reactions to others. They need lots of holding, carrying, and usually motion, such as rocking. Sometimes swaddling in a blanket helps them, but at other times it makes them worse. They tend to "snack" at the breast frequently and sleep in catnaps, brief fifteen- to thirty-minute naps while someone is holding or carrying them. Slings or other baby carriers, as well as swings, are good to try to help calm these babies. In spite of their fussiness, they should be gaining weight normally.
- **Colic:** Colic begins around two weeks of age. Colicky babies generally have at least one period of time each day when they appear to be in pain with their legs drawn up, crying hard, and turning red. They may act hungry during these times, but then pull back and refuse the breast. Your baby's doctor can provide suggestions for managing colic. (See Chapter 6, page 190.)
- **Oversupply or overactive let-down of breastmilk:** This could begin at almost any time in the first month. Your breasts will feel very full, and you may experience lots of leaking and spraying. Your baby will be gulping down milk very fast, sometimes pulling away to catch his breath or coughing or sputtering milk. This rapid drinking causes the baby to swallow lots of air and milk. Later, gas bubbles will form, causing plenty of discomfort and tummy rumbling. Your pediatrician may guide you to a lactation consultant to assist with this problem. (Also see *Engorgement,* page 123.)
- **Reflux (also called gastroesophageal reflux):** Most newborns spit up after feeding. When spitting up results in problems for the baby, such as pain or weight loss, he should be evaluated by your pediatrician. (See page 256.)

- **Food sensitivities:** Occasionally a particular food (including caffeinated beverages) that you're eating may cause problems in your breastfed baby. If you think this might be the case, avoid that food for one week to see if the symptoms go away. Then you may try the food again carefully to see if the symptoms return.
- **Allergies:** Although infant crying often is blamed on food allergies, such allergies are less common than some other reasons for fussiness. Allergies occur more often in babies from families where mother, father, or siblings are affected by asthma, eczema, or other allergic diseases. In the breastfed baby, the mother's diet may be the source of these allergies. It can be difficult to pinpoint the precise food, however, and allergic symptoms can linger for more than a week after the food has been removed from the mother's diet. Food allergies can be very serious, with blood in the stools, wheezing, hives, or shock (collapse). True food allergies definitely require the attention of your pediatrician.
- **Serious illness:** Other serious illnesses may not be related to feeding and may cause babies to cry endlessly, unable to be comforted. If this occurs suddenly or seems unusually severe, call your pediatrician or seek emergency care immediately.

The Cancer Question. Most studies indicate that breastfeeding offers some protection against breast cancer. If a woman has been diagnosed with cancer or has had a malignant tumor removed, but is no longer getting chemotherapy or radiation treatment, breastfeeding should be acceptable. (Check with your physician.) Most doctors feel that breastfeeding is safe after a woman has had a benign (noncancerous) lump or cyst removed.

Breastfeeding After Plastic Surgery on the Breasts. Plastic surgery to enlarge the breasts should not interfere with breastfeeding—provided that the breasts were normal to begin with and that the nipples have not been moved and no ducts have been cut. (It is a good sign if there are no surgical scars close to the nipple or areola.) Saline implants pose no risk to the baby. Women with silicone implants may worry about leakage of silicone causing problems for their baby. But most authorities recommend breastfeeding even after implant surgery and feel that it does not pose any dangers to the baby.

The course of breastfeeding after breast reduction surgery is highly individual. Plastic surgery to reduce the size of the breasts typically involves at least some disruption of normal breast tissue and often movement of the entire nipple and areola. Each mother-baby pair must be helped and followed individually. Your baby's weight should be checked at least twice a week for the first few weeks, until the baby is gaining well. Even if you don't have a full supply, you can still breastfeed and supplement with formula. This will provide your baby with some of the benefits of receiving breastmilk.

Make sure you discuss all your concerns with your doctor. Your baby's pediatrician needs to be aware of previous breast surgery that you've had so your infant can be followed closely.

For additional difficulties such as jaundice and worries about milk supply, refer to pages 173 and 116, respectively.

Bottle-Feeding

While recognizing the benefits of breastfeeding, mothers—and fathers, too—may feel that bottle-feeding gives the mother more freedom and time for duties other than those

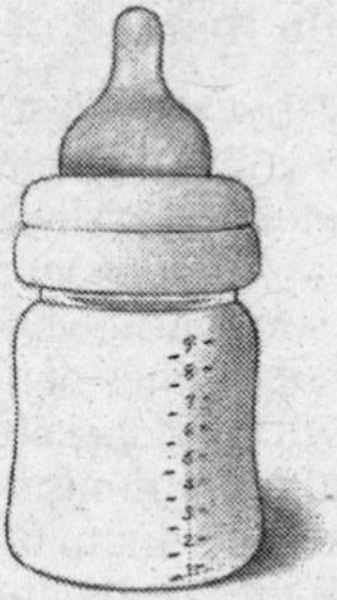

involving baby care. Dad, grandparents, sitters, and even older siblings can feed an infant breastmilk or formula in a bottle. This may give some mothers more flexibility.

There are other reasons why some parents feel more comfortable with bottle-feeding. They know exactly how much food the baby is getting, and there's no need to worry about the mother's diet or medications that might affect the milk.

Even so, formula manufacturers have not yet found a way to reproduce the components that make human milk so unique. Although formula does provide the basic nutrients an infant needs, it lacks the antibodies and many of the other components that only mother's milk contains.

Formula-feeding is also costly and may be inconvenient for some families. The formula must be bought and prepared (unless you use the more expensive, ready-to-use types). This means trips to the kitchen in the middle of the night, as well as extra bottles, nipples, and other equipment. Unintended contamination of formula also must be considered a potential risk.

If you have decided to bottle-feed your baby, you'll have to start by selecting a formula. Your pediatrician will help you pick one based on your baby's needs. The American Academy of Pediatrics does not recommend homemade baby formulas, since they tend to be deficient in vitamins and other important nutrients. Today there are several varieties and brands of commercial formulas from which to choose.

Why Formula Instead of Cow's Milk?

Many parents ask why they can't just feed their baby regular cow's milk. The answer is simple: Young infants cannot digest cow's milk as completely or easily as they digest formula. Also, cow's milk contains high concentrations of protein and minerals, which can stress a newborn's immature kidneys and cause severe illness at times of heat stress, fever, or diarrhea. In addition, cow's milk lacks the proper amounts of iron, vitamin C, and other nutrients that infants need. It may even cause iron-deficiency anemia in some babies, since cow's milk protein can irritate the lining of the stomach and intestine, leading to loss of blood into the stools. Cow's milk also does not contain the healthiest types of fat for growing babies. For these reasons, your baby should not receive any regular cow's milk for the first twelve months of life.

Choosing a Formula

To maintain safety standards for infant health in this country, an act of Congress governs the contents of infant formula, and the Food and Drug Administration monitors all formulas. When shopping for infant formula, you'll find several basic types.

Cow's milk–based formulas account for about 80 percent of the formula sold today. Although cow's milk is the basis for such formulas, the milk has been changed dramatically to make it safe for infants. It is treated by heating and other methods to make the protein more digestible. More milk sugar (lactose) is added to make the concentration equal to that of breastmilk, and the fat (butterfat) is removed and replaced with vegetable oils and other fats that infants can more easily digest and are better for infant growth.

Cow's milk formulas have additional iron added. These iron-fortified formulas have dramatically reduced the rate of iron-deficiency anemia in infancy in recent decades. Some infants do not have enough natural reserves of iron, a mineral necessary for normal human growth and development, to meet their needs. For that reason, the American Academy of Pediatrics currently recommends that iron-fortified formula be used for all infants who are not breastfed, or who are only partially breastfed, from birth to one year of age. Additional iron is available in many baby foods, especially in meats, egg yolks, and iron-fortified cereals. Low-iron formulas should not be used, since they do not provide enough iron to optimally support your baby's growth and development. Some mothers worry about the iron in infant formula causing constipation, but the amount of iron provided in infant formula does not contribute to constipation in babies. Most formulas also have docosahexaenoic acid (DHA) and arachidonic acid (ARA) added to them, which are fatty acids, believed to be important for the development of a baby's brain and eyes.

Another type of formula are *hydrolyzed formulas*. They often are called "predigested," meaning that their protein content has already been broken down into smaller proteins that can be digested more easily. In infants who have a high risk of developing allergies (because of family history, for example) and who have not been breastfed exclusively for four to six months, there is some evidence that skin conditions like eczema or atopic dermatitis can be prevented or delayed by feeding them either extensively or partially hydrolyzed (hypoallergenic) formulas. However, these hydrolyzed formulas tend to be costlier than regular formulas. Your pediatrician can advise you on whether your child is a candidate for hydrolyzed formulas.

The so-called hypoallergenic formulas will help at least 90 percent of babies who have food allergies, which can cause symptoms such as hives, a runny nose, and intestinal problems. In these types of situations, breastfeeding is particularly desirable because—when there is a strong family history of allergies—it could help avoid some infant's food allergies, especially when the child is exclusively breastfed for about six months.

Soy formulas contain a protein (soy) and carbohydrate (either glucose or sucrose) different from milk-based formulas. They are sometimes recommended for babies unable to digest lactose, the main carbohydrate in cow's milk formula, although simple lactose-free cow's milk–based formula is also available. Many infants have brief periods when they cannot digest lactose, particularly following bouts of diarrhea, which can damage the digestive enzymes in the lining of the intestines. But this is usually only a temporary problem and does not require a change in your baby's diet. It is rare for babies to have a significant problem digesting and absorbing lactose (although it tends to occur in older children and adults). If your pediatrician suggests a lactose-free formula, know that it provides your baby with everything that she needs to grow and develop just as a lactose-containing formula does.

When a true milk allergy is present, causing colic, failure to thrive, and even bloody diarrhea, the allergy is to the protein in the cow's milk formula. In this case soy formulas, with soy as the protein, might seem like a good alternative. However, as many as half the infants who have milk allergy are also sensitive to soy protein, and thus they must be given a specialized formula (like amino-based or elemental) or breastmilk.

Some strict vegetarian parents choose to use soy formula because it contains no animal products. Remember that breastfeeding is the best option for vegetarian families. Also, although some parents believe that a soy formula might prevent or ease the symptoms of colic or fussiness, there is no evidence to support its effectiveness for this purpose.

The American Academy of Pediatrics believes that there are few circumstances in which soy formula should be chosen instead of cow milk–based formula in term infants. One of these situations is in infants with a rare disorder called galactosemia; children with this condition have an intolerance to galactose, one of the two sugars that make up lactose, and they cannot tolerate breastmilk and must be fed a formula free of lactose. Most states include a test for galactosemia in routine newborn screening, which involves performing a blood test on all newborns after birth.

Specialized formulas are manufactured for infants with specific disorders or diseases. There are also formulas made specifically for premature babies. If your pediatrician recommends a specialized formula for your infant, follow his guidance about feeding requirements (amounts, scheduling, special preparations), since these may be quite different from regular formulas.

Some formulas also are fortified with probiotics, which are types of "friendly" bacteria. Others are now fortified with prebiotics, natural food substances that promote healthy intestinal lining. For more information, see page 142.

Preparing, Sterilizing, and Storing Formula

Most infant formulas are available in ready-to-feed liquid forms, concentrates, and powders. Although ready-to-feed formulas are very convenient, they are also the most expensive. Formula made from concentrate is prepared by mixing equal amounts of concentrate and water. If the entire can is not used, the remaining concentrate may be covered and left in the refrigerator for no more than forty-eight hours. Powder, the least expensive form, comes either in premeasured packets or in a can with a measuring scoop. To prepare

Preparing Formula from Concentrate (One Bottle at a Time)

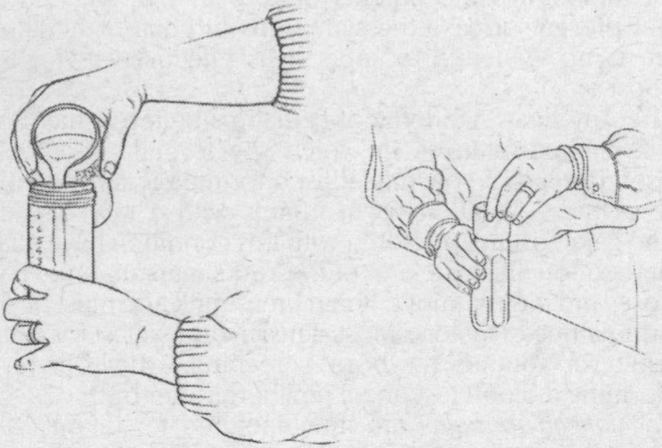

Wash hands and measure concentrate.

Pour in an equal amount of water. Shake and use promptly. If the entire can is not used, the remaining concentrate may be covered and left in the refrigerator for no more than forty-eight hours.

most formula, you'll add one level scoop of powder for every 2 ounces (60 ml) of water, and then mix thoroughly to make sure there are no clumps of undissolved powder in the bottle. The solution will mix more easily and the lumps will dissolve faster if you use room-temperature water. Always read the label to make sure you are mixing the formula properly.

Aside from the price, one advantage of the powder is its light weight and portability. The powder will not spoil, even

Preparing Formula from Powder

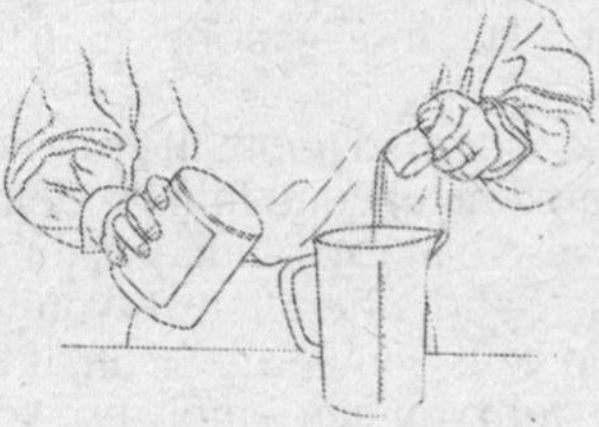

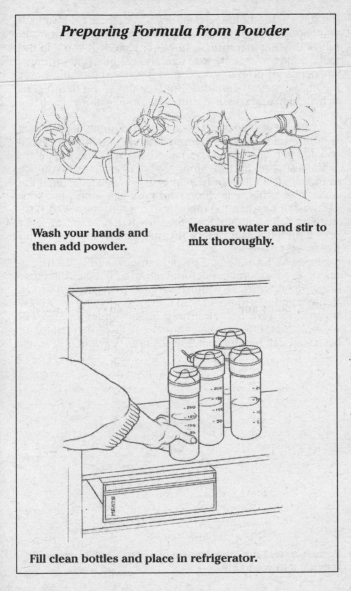

Wash your hands and then add powder.

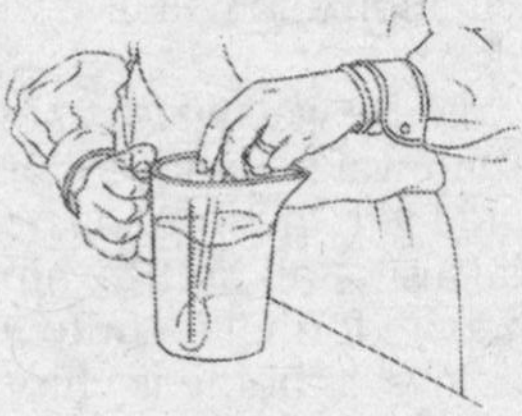

Measure water and stir to mix thoroughly.

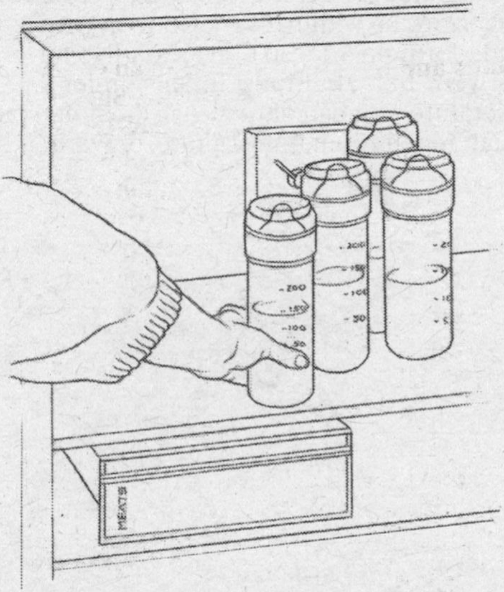

Fill clean bottles and place in refrigerator.

if it stays in the bottle several days before you add water. If you choose a formula that requires preparation, be sure to follow the manufacturer's directions exactly. If you add too much water, your baby won't get the calories and nutrients she needs for proper growth; and if you add too little water, the high concentration of formula could cause diarrhea or dehydration and will give your infant more calories than she needs.

If you use well water or are concerned about the safety of your tap water, boil it for approximately one minute before you add it to the formula. You also can use bottled water.

Make sure all bottles, nipples, and other utensils you use to prepare formula—or to feed your baby—are clean. If the water in your home is chlorinated, you can simply use your dishwasher or wash the utensils in hot tap water with dish-washing detergent and then rinse them in hot tap water. For nonchlorinated water, place the utensils in boiling water for five to ten minutes.

Store any formula you prepare in advance in the refrigerator to discourage bacterial growth. If you don't use refrigerated formula within twenty-four hours, discard it. Refrigerated formula doesn't necessarily have to be warmed for your baby, but most infants prefer it at least at room temperature. You can either leave the bottle out for an hour so it can reach room temperature, or warm it in a pan

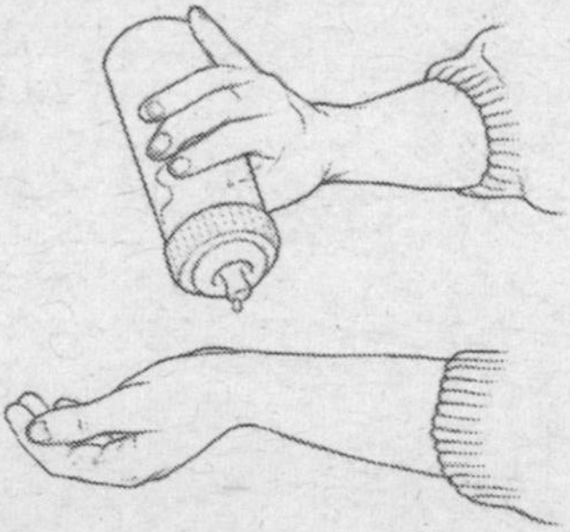

Be sure to test the temperature of warmed milk before feeding it to your child.

of hot water. (Again, do not use a microwave.) If you warm it, test it in advance to make sure it's not too hot for your child. The easiest way to test the temperature is to shake a few drops on the inside of your wrist.

The bottles you use may be glass, plastic, or plastic with a soft plastic liner. These inner liners are convenient to use and may help limit the amount of air your baby swallows when she sucks, but they are also more expensive. As your baby gets older and begins holding the bottle herself, avoid using breakable glass bottles. Also, bottles that are designed to promote self-feeding are not recommended, as they may contribute to nursing-bottle tooth decay by promoting constant feeding and exposure of the teeth to sugars throughout the day and night. When milk collects behind the teeth, bacterial growth occurs. Also, self-feeding in a supine position (lying down on the back) has been shown to contribute occasionally to ear infections. (See *Middle Ear Infections,* page 557.) Infants and older children should not receive a bottle to suck on during the night. If you give your baby a feeding at bedtime, take away the bottle before she falls asleep.

In selecting bottles, you may need to try several nipples before finding the one your baby prefers. You can choose from among the standard rubber nipples, orthodontic ones, and special designs for premature infants and babies with cleft palates. Whichever type you use, always check the size of the hole. If it's too small, your baby may suck so hard that she swallows too much air; if it's too big, the formula may flow so fast that she chokes. Ideally, formula should flow at a rate of one drop per second when you first turn the bottle upside down. (It should stop dripping after a few seconds.) Many parents find that a nipple with a single small hole is adequate for feeding water (although healthy babies under six months do not require extra water), but that they need one with a larger hole or with several holes when feeding formula.

The Feeding Process

Feeding times should be relaxing, comforting, and enjoyable for both you and your baby. They provide opportunities to show your love and to get to know each other. If you are calm

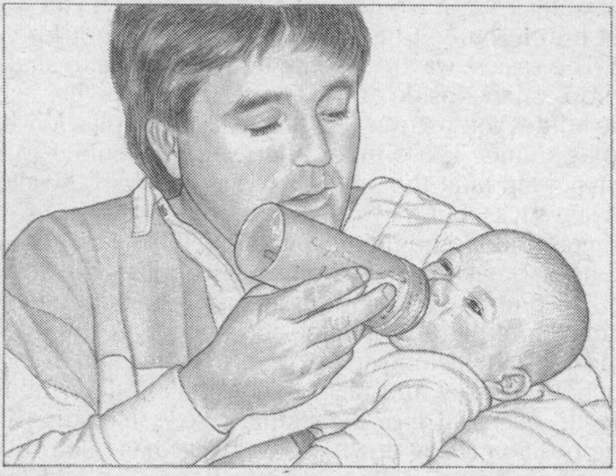

and content, your infant will respond in kind. If you are nervous or uninterested, he may pick up these negative feelings and a feeding problem can result.

You probably will be most comfortable in a chair with arms or in one with pillows that let you prop up your own arms as you feed your infant. Cradle him in a semiupright position and support his head. Don't feed him when he's lying down totally flat, because this will increase the risk of choking; it also may cause formula to flow into the middle ear, where it can lead to an infection.

Hold the bottle so that formula fills the neck of the bottle and covers the nipple. This will prevent your baby from swallowing air as he sucks. To get him to open his mouth and grasp the nipple, stimulate his rooting reflex by stroking the nipple against the lower lip or cheek. Once the nipple is in his mouth, he will begin to suck and swallow naturally.

Amount and Schedule of Formula Feedings

After the first few days, your formula-fed newborn will take from 2 to 3 ounces (60–90 ml) of formula per feeding and will eat every three to four hours on average during her first few weeks. (Breastfed infants usually take smaller, more frequent feedings than formula-fed infants.) During the first month, if your baby sleeps longer than four to five hours and

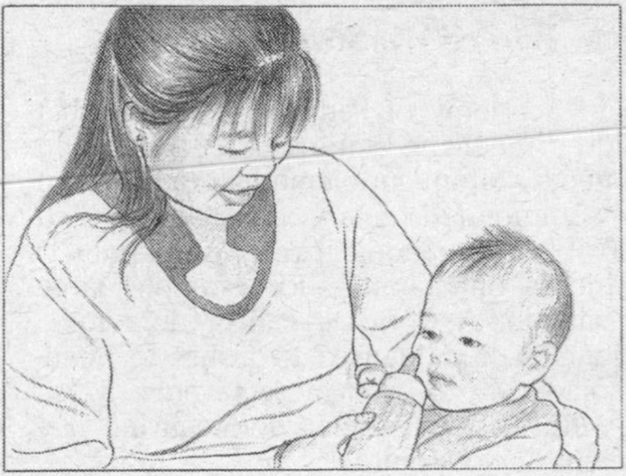

Always hold your baby closely for formula feeding.

starts missing feedings, wake her up and offer a bottle. By the end of her first month, she'll be up to at least 4 ounces (120 ml) per feeding, with a fairly predictable schedule of feedings about every four hours. By six months, your baby will consume 6 to 8 ounces (180–240 ml) at each of four or five feedings in twenty-four hours.

On average, your baby should take in about 2½ ounces (75 ml) of formula a day for every pound (453 grams) of body weight. But he probably will regulate his intake from day to day to meet his own specific needs. So instead of going by fixed amounts, let him tell you when he's had enough. If he becomes fidgety or easily distracted during a feeding, he's probably finished. If he drains the bottle and still continues smacking his lips, he might still be hungry. There are high and low limits, however. Most babies are satisfied with 3 to 4 ounces (90–120 ml) per feeding during the first month and increase that amount by 1 ounce (30 ml) per month until they reach a maximum of about 7 to 8 ounces (210–240 ml). If your baby consistently seems to want more or less than this, discuss it with your pediatrician. Your baby should drink no more than 32 ounces (960 ml) of formula in 24 hours. Some babies have higher needs for sucking and may just want to suck on a pacifier after feeding.

Initially it is best to feed your formula-fed newborn on

Where We Stand

The American Academy of Pediatrics believes that healthy children receiving a normal, well-balanced diet do not need vitamin supplementation over and above the recommended dietary allowances, which includes 400 IU (International Units) of vitamin D a day. Megadoses of vitamins—for example, large amounts of vitamins A, C, or D—can produce toxic symptoms, ranging from nausea to rashes to headaches and sometimes to even more severe adverse effects. Talk with your pediatrician before giving vitamin supplements to your child.

demand, or whenever he cries because he's hungry. As time passes, he'll begin to develop a fairly regular timetable of his own. As you become familiar with his signals and needs, you'll be able to schedule his feedings around his routine.

Between two and four months of age (or when the baby weighs more than 12 pounds [5.4 kg]), most formula-fed babies no longer need a middle-of-the-night feeding, because they're consuming more during the day and their sleeping patterns have become more regular (although this varies considerably from baby to baby). Their stomach capacity has increased, too, which means they may go longer between daytime feedings—occasionally up to four or five hours at a time. If your baby still seems to feed very frequently or consume larger amounts, try distracting him with play or with a pacifier. Sometimes patterns of obesity begin during infancy, so it is important not to overfeed your baby.

The most important thing to remember, whether you breastfeed or bottle-feed, is that your baby's feeding needs are unique. No book can tell you precisely how much or how often he needs to be fed or exactly how you should handle him during feedings. You will discover these things for yourself as you and your baby get to know each other.

SUPPLEMENTATION FOR BREASTFED AND BOTTLE-FED INFANTS

Vitamin Supplements

Human milk contains a natural balance of vitamins, especially C, E, and the B vitamins, so if you and your baby are both healthy, and you are well nourished, your child may not require any supplements of these vitamins.

Breastfed infants need supplemental vitamin D. This vitamin is naturally manufactured by the skin when it is exposed to sunlight. However, the American Academy of Pediatrics feels strongly that all children should be kept out of the direct sun as much as possible and wear sunscreen while in the sun to avoid long-term risk of sun exposure, which may contribute to skin cancer. Sunscreen keeps the skin from manufacturing vitamin D. For that reason, talk to your pediatrician about the need for supplemental vitamin D drops. The current Academy recommendation is that all infants and children should have a minimum intake of 400 IU (International Units) of vitamin D per day beginning soon after birth. Prepared formula has vitamin D added to it; so if your baby is drinking at least 32 ounces of formula, vitamin D supplementation is not needed. In addition, once your baby is one year old and on vitamin D milk, extra vitamins with vitamin D are no longer needed. Your baby also may need vitamin supplements if he was born prematurely or has certain other medical problems. Discuss the need for supplements of vitamins or minerals with your doctor.

A regular, well-balanced diet should provide all the vitamins necessary for both nursing mothers and their babies. However, pediatricians recommend that mothers continue taking a daily prenatal vitamin supplement to ensure the proper nutritional balance. If you are on a strict vegetarian diet, you need to take an extra B-complex supplement, since certain B vitamins are available only from meat, poultry, or fish products. If your baby is on infant formula, he generally will receive adequate vitamins because formula has added vitamins.

Probiotics in Formulas

Probiotics (meaning "for life") is a word that you may run across when shopping for infant formula for your baby. Some formulas are fortified with these probiotics, which are types of live bacteria. They are "good" or "friendly" bacteria that are already present at high levels in the digestive system of breastfed babies. In formula-fed babies, the introduction of probiotics to formulas is designed to promote a balance of bacteria in your baby's intestines, and offset the growth of "unfriendly" organisms that could cause infections and inflammation.

The most common types of probiotics are strains of tiny organisms called *Bifidobacterium* and *Lactobacillus*. Some research has shown that these probiotics may prevent or treat disorders such as infectious diarrhea and atopic dermatitis (eczema) in children (see pages 440 and 470). Other possible health benefits are being studied as well, including whether probiotics can lower your child's risk of food-related allergies and asthma, prevent urinary tract infections, or improve the symptoms of infant colic.

With many of these health conditions, the evidence confirming any positive effects of probiotic use is limited and more research is needed. At this time, any benefits appear to occur only as long as the probiotics are being taken. Once your baby stops consuming probiotic-fortified formula, the bacteria in the intestines will return to their previous levels.

Before giving your child infant formula that is fortified with probiotics, discuss the issue with your pediatrician. (For more information about probiotics, see page 447.)

Iron Supplements

Most babies are born with sufficient reserves of iron that will protect them from anemia. If your baby is breastfed, there is sufficient, well-absorbed iron to give her an adequate supply so that no additional supplement is necessary. When she is between four and six months old, you should be starting your breastfed infant on baby foods that contain supplemental iron (cereals, meats, green vegetables), which should further guarantee sufficient iron for proper growth.

If you are bottle-feeding your baby, it is now recommended that you use iron-fortified formula (containing from 4 to 12 mg of iron) from birth through the entire first year of life. Premature babies have fewer iron stores, so they often need additional iron beyond what they receive from breastmilk or formula.

Water and Juice

Until your baby starts eating solid foods, he'll get all the water he needs from breastmilk or formula. In the first six months, additional water or juice is generally unnecessary for breastfed or bottle-fed infants. After a bottle-fed baby is six months old, you may offer him water between feedings, but don't force it on him or worry if he rejects it. He may prefer to get the extra liquid from more frequent feedings. Breastfed infants generally do not need extra water if they are permitted adequate access to the breast for feeding.

Once your baby is eating solid foods, his need for liquid will increase. Getting your infant used to the taste of plain water is a healthy habit that will last a lifetime. Juice is not recommended; although if you do give your infant juice, make sure your child's daily juice intake does not exceed 4 to 6 ounces (120–180 ml). About 9 out of 10 of all infants consume fruit juice by the time they are one year of age. The most common fruit juices are apple juice, grape juice, and pear juice. Fruit juice can provide extra water for normal infants and young children. However, giving plain water is a much healthier option. If a child drinks too much juice, sometimes it can't be digested properly, and can result in gas or diarrhea. Some fruit juices, such as white grape juice, may be digested more easily than others because they contain a balance of carbohydrates and lack sorbitol, which can contribute to cramping and diarrhea.

In addition, most fruit juices do not contain any significant

Where We Stand

The American Academy of Pediatrics recommends that fruit juice not be given to infants under six months of age since it offers no nutritional benefit to babies in this age group. After six months of age, infants may have limited amounts of juice each day. For youngsters older than six months, fruit juice offers no nutritional benefits over whole fruit. Whole fruits also provide fiber and other nutrients. Infants should not be given fruit juice at bedtime, nor as a treatment of dehydration or management of diarrhea. For children ages one to six years old, limit fruit juice consumption to 4 to 6 ounces (120–180 ml) each day.

amount of protein, fat, minerals, or vitamins other than vitamin C. So rather than giving your child juice in excess, try giving him water with his meals. Some children who drink too much juice have an increased risk of being overweight. To help regulate the amount of fruit juice your child drinks, offer juice with food to slow down the rate at which it's absorbed, and serve a combination of one-half juice and one-half water. If you offer him extra milk, formula, or juice at mealtimes, you may curb his appetite for solid foods. In fact, infants who drink too much fruit juice may become malnourished as a result of the juice replacing formula or breastmilk. Your baby may need extra fluids when he's ill, especially when he has a fever or experiences vomiting and diarrhea. Ask your pediatrician to help you determine how much water your baby needs at these times. The best fluid for a breastfed infant who is ill is breastmilk.

Fluoride Supplements

Babies should not receive fluoride supplementation during the first six months of life, whether they are breastfed or formula-fed. After that time, breastfed and formula-fed infants need appropriate fluoride supplementation if local drinking water contains less than 0.3 parts per million (ppm) of fluoride. If your home is supplied by its own well, have the well tested to determine the amount of natural fluoride in the water. If your baby consumes bottled water instead or your home is connected to a municipal water supply, check to see if the water is fluoridated. If your family prefers to use bottled water rather than tap water, you should consider purchasing water marketed for babies with specific amounts of fluoride added; sometimes called "nursery water," it is available in the baby food aisle in grocery stores, and can be used when mixing formula.

Your pediatrician or pediatric dentist can advise you on whether there is a need for fluoride drops for your baby and prescribe the appropriate dosage. Formula-fed infants receive some fluoride from their formula if the drinking water is fluoridated in their community or if it is made with bottled or well water containing fluoride. The American Academy of Pediatrics recommends that you check with

How Do You Burp a Baby?

Here are a few tried-and-true techniques. After a little experimentation, you'll find which ones work best for your child.

1. Hold the baby upright with his head on your shoulder, supporting his head and back while you gently pat his back with your other hand.

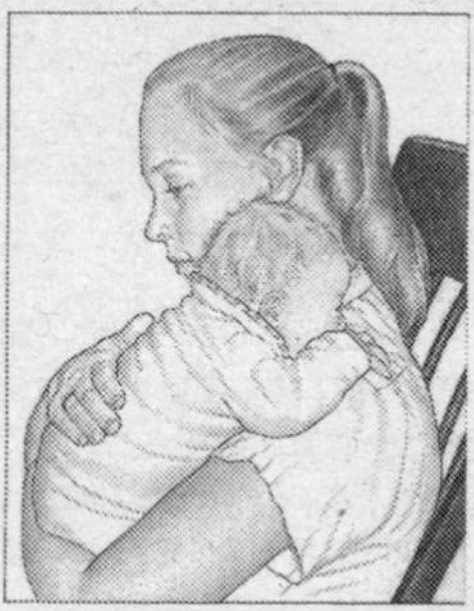

2. Sit the baby on your lap, supporting his chest and head with one hand while patting his back with your other hand.

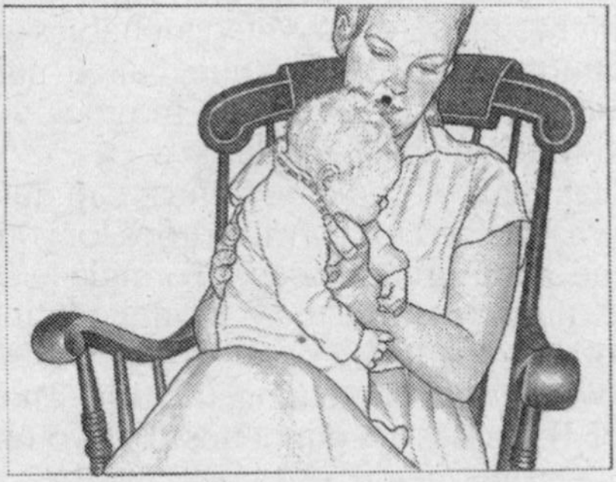

3. Lay the baby on your lap with his back up. Support his head so it is higher than his chest, and gently pat or rotate your hand on his back.

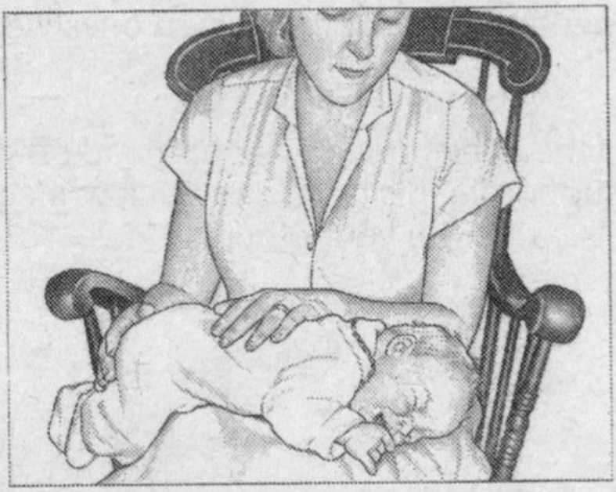

If he still hasn't burped after several minutes, continue feeding him and don't worry; no baby burps every time. When he's finished, burp him again and keep him in an upright position for ten to fifteen minutes so he doesn't spit up.

your pediatrician or pediatric dentist to find out if any additional fluoride supplements are necessary, or whether your child is already receiving the right amount.

Remember, appropriate fluoride supplementation is based on each child's unique needs. A supplement should be considered by you and your doctor until all of a child's permanent teeth are present in the mouth.

BURPING, HICCUPS, AND SPITTING UP

Burping

Young babies naturally fuss and get cranky when they swallow air during feedings. Although this occurs in both breastfed and bottle-fed infants, it's seen more often with the bottle. When it happens, it may be helpful to stop the feeding rather than letting your infant fuss and nurse at the same time. This continued fussing will cause her to swallow even more air, which will only increase her discomfort and may make her spit up.

A much better strategy is to burp her frequently, even if she shows no discomfort. The pause and the change of position alone will slow her gulping and reduce the amount of air she takes in. If she's bottle-feeding, burp her after every 2 to 3 ounces (60–90 ml). If she's nursing, burp her when she switches breasts. Some breastfed babies don't swallow very much air, and therefore they may not need to burp frequently.

Hiccups

Most babies hiccup from time to time. Usually this bothers parents more than the infant, but if hiccups occur during a feeding, change his position, try to get him to burp, or help him relax. Wait until the hiccups are gone to resume feeding. If they don't disappear on their own in five to ten minutes, try to resume feeding for a few minutes. Doing this usually stops them. If your baby gets hiccups often, try to feed him when he's calm and before he's extremely hungry. This will usually reduce the likelihood of hiccups occurring during the feeding.

Spitting Up

Spitting up is another common occurrence during infancy. Sometimes spitting up means the baby has eaten more than her stomach can hold; sometimes she spits up while burping or drooling. Although it may be a bit messy, it's usually no cause for concern. It almost never involves choking, coughing, discomfort, or danger to your child, even if it occurs while she's sleeping.

Some babies spit up more than others, but most are out of this phase by the time they are sitting. A few "heavy spitters" will continue until they start to walk or are weaned to a cup. Some may continue throughout their first year.

It is important to know the difference between normal spitting up and true vomiting. Unlike spitting up, which most babies don't even seem to notice, vomiting is forceful and usually causes great distress and discomfort for your child. It generally occurs soon after a meal and produces a much greater volume than spitting up. If your baby vomits on a regular basis (one or more times a day) or if you notice blood or a bright green color in your baby's vomit, consult your pediatrician. (See *Vomiting,* pages 227 and 458.)

While it is practically impossible to prevent all spitting up, the following steps will help you decrease the frequency of these episodes and the amount spit up.

1. Make each feeding calm, quiet, and leisurely.
2. Avoid interruptions, sudden noises, bright lights, and other distractions during feedings.
3. Burp your bottle-fed baby at least every three to five minutes during feedings.
4. Avoid feeding while your infant is lying down.
5. Hold the baby in an upright position for twenty to thirty minutes after each feeding.
6. Do not jostle or play vigorously with the baby immediately after feeding.
7. Try to feed her before she gets frantically hungry.
8. If bottle-feeding, make sure the hole in the nipple is neither too big (which lets the formula flow too fast) nor too

Developing the Right Attitude

You can do it! This should be your attitude about breastfeeding from the beginning. There's plenty of help available, and you should take advantage of the expert advice, counseling, classes, and group meetings that are available. For example, you can:

- Talk to your obstetrician and pediatrician. They can provide not only medical information but also encouragement and support when you need it most.
- Talk to your prenatal instructors and attend a breastfeeding class.
- Talk to women who have breastfed or are breastfeeding successfully and ask their advice. Sisters-in-law, cousins, office mates, yoga instructors, and fellow congregants at your place of worship are precious resources.
- Talk to members of La Leche League or other mother-to-mother support groups in your community. La Leche League is a worldwide organization dedicated to helping families learn about and enjoy the experience of breastfeeding. Information and support for parents is available at www.llli.org.
- Read about breastfeeding. A recommended book is the *American Academy of Pediatrics New Mother's Guide to Breastfeeding,* by J. Y. Meek, editor-in-chief, and S. Tippins (Bantam); and the booklet "Breastfeeding Your Baby: Answers to Common Questions" available at www.aap.org.

small (which frustrates your baby and causes her to gulp air). If the hole is the proper size, a few drops should come out when you invert the bottle, and then stop.

9. Elevate the head of the entire crib with blocks (don't use a pillow) and put her to sleep on her back. This keeps her head higher than her stomach and prevents her from choking in case she spits up while sleeping.

As you can tell from the length and detail of this chapter, feeding your baby is one of the most important and, at times, confusing challenges you'll face as a parent. The recommendations in this section apply to infants in general. Please remember that your child is unique and may have special needs. If you have questions that these pages have not answered to your satisfaction, ask your pediatrician to help you find the answers that apply specifically to you and your infant.

5

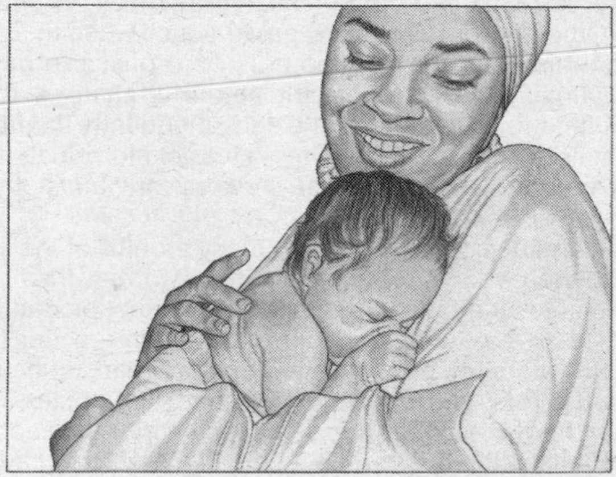

Your Baby's First Days

After all the months of pregnancy, you may believe that you already know your baby. You've felt his kicks, monitored his quiet and active periods during the day, and run your hands over your abdomen as he nestled in the womb. Although all of this does bring you closer to him, nothing can prepare you for the sight of his face and the grip of his fingers around yours.

For the first few days after his birth, you may not be able to take your eyes off him. Watching him, you may see hints of yourself or other members of the family reflected in his features. But despite any distinct resemblance, he is uniquely special—unlike anyone else. And he'll have a definite personality all his own that may start making itself known immediately. As he turns and stretches, only he knows what he wants and feels.

Some babies waste no time protesting wet or messy diapers from the day they are born and complain loudly until they are changed, fed, and rocked back to sleep. Infants who behave like this not only tend to spend more time awake than other babies, but they also may cry and eat more. Other newborns won't seem to notice when their diapers are dirty and may be more likely to object to having their bottoms exposed to the cold air during changes. These babies tend to sleep a lot and eat less frequently than their more sensitive counterparts. These kinds of individual differences are both normal and can serve as early hints of your child's future personality.

Some mothers say that after so many months of the baby being in their wombs, it becomes difficult to view their baby as a separate human being, with thoughts, emotions, and desires of his own. Making this adjustment and respecting their baby's individuality, however, are important parts of being a parent. If parents can welcome their child's uniqueness from the time he is born, they'll have a much easier time accepting the person the baby will become in the years ahead.

Your Newborn's First Days

How Your Newborn Looks

As you relax with your baby in your own room, unwrap his blankets and examine him from head to toe. You'll notice many details that may have escaped you in the first moments after birth. For instance, when your baby opens his eyes, you'll see their color. While many Caucasian newborns have blue eyes, the color may actually change over the first

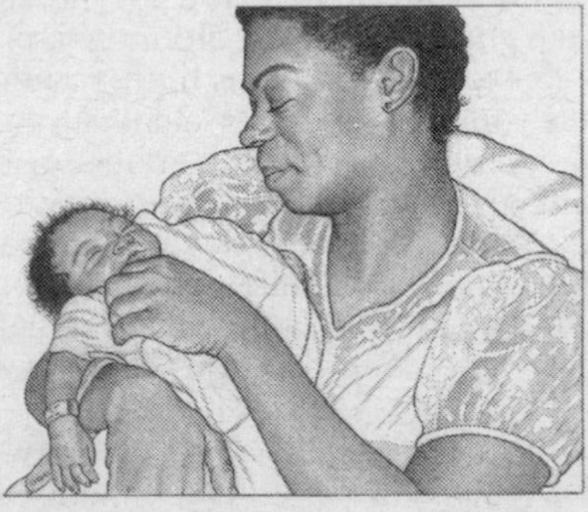

year. If a baby's eyes are going to turn brown, they'll probably become "muddy"-looking during the first six months; if they're still blue at that time, they'll probably remain so. In contrast, infants with dark-skinned heritage generally have brown eyes at birth, and they tend to remain that color throughout life.

You may notice a bloodred spot in the white area of one or both of your newborn's eyes. This spot, as well as the general puffiness of a newborn's face, are most commonly caused by pressures exerted during labor. Although you might find them a bit worrisome at first, fortunately both tend to fade in a few days. If your baby was delivered by C-section, he won't have this puffiness and the whites of his eyes should not have any red spots right from the start.

Bathed and dry, your baby's skin will seem very delicate. If he was born after his due date, it may peel and appear wrinkled as a result of having lost the vernix (a whitish, creamy substance covering the skin). If he was born on time or early, he may still peel a little as a newborn because of his skin's sudden exposure to air after the vernix is washed away. Either way, peeling skin is a normal newborn process and requires no treatment. All babies, including those with a dark-skinned heritage, have lighter-appearing skin at birth. This gradually darkens as they become older.

As you examine your baby's shoulders and back, you also may notice some fine hair, called lanugo. This hair is produced toward the end of pregnancy; however, it's usually shed before birth or soon thereafter. If your baby was born before his due date, he is more likely to still have this hair, and it may take a couple of weeks to disappear.

You also may notice a lot of pink spots and marks on your baby's skin. Some, like those that appear around the edges of his diaper, may simply be due to pressure. Mottled or blotchy-looking patches are commonly caused by exposure to cool air and will disappear quickly if you cover him again. If you find scratches, particularly on your baby's face, it serves as a good reminder that it's time to trim his fingernails. This will help prevent him from continuing to scratch himself as he randomly moves his hands and arms. For some new parents, this can seem like a monumental and nerve-racking task, so don't hesitate to ask for advice from the nurse at the hospital nursery, or at your pediatrician's office, or from anyone else with experience on how to clip an infant's nails. Your baby also may develop other newborn rashes and have some birthmarks. Most will fade or resolve on their own without treatment (although some birthmarks may be permanent).

The following are the most common newborn rashes and birthmarks:

Salmon Patches or "Stork Bites." So-called because they are distributed over the areas that a stork would supposedly carry a baby in its beak, in reality "stork bites" are simply patches, light to deep pink in color, and most commonly located on the bridge of the nose, lower forehead, upper eyelids, back of the head, and/or on the neck. They are the most common birthmark, especially in light-skinned babies. They also may be referred to as "angel kisses," and typically disappear over the first few months.

Mongolian Spots. These birthmarks can vary considerably in size but are all flat areas of skin that contain extra pigment, which causes them to appear brown, gray, or even blue (like a bruise). Most often located on the back or buttocks, Mongolian spots are very common, especially in dark-skinned babies. They usually disappear before school age and are of no medical significance.

Pustular Melanosis. Small blisters that typically appear at birth, they peel open and dry up within a couple of days. They leave dark spots like freckles that usually disappear over several weeks. Some newborns may have only the spots, indicating that they had the rash before birth. While pustular melanosis is common (particularly in babies with darker skin) and is a harmless newborn rash, it is always important to have all blisterlike rashes evaluated by your baby's doctor to make sure they aren't due to an infection.

Milia. These tiny white bumps or yellow spots are found on the cheeks, chin, or across the tip of the nose, and are caused by skin-gland secretion. This common newborn rash generally disappears on its own within the first two to three weeks of life.

Miliaria. Often referred to as a "heat rash" or "prickly heat," miliaria most often occurs in hot, humid climates or when babies are overbundled. The rash can contain tiny sweat blisters and/or small red bumps. It shows up most often in skin folds and covered areas, and usually goes away within a few days.

Erythema Toxicum. Often called "E tox" for short, this rash is very common and usually appears within the first few days after birth. It consists of multiple red splotches with yellowish-white bumps in the center, and goes away within a week or so. It generally resolves if it's left completely alone.

Capillary Hemangiomas. These raised red spots are caused by a strawberrylike collection of blood vessels in the skin. For the first week or so, they may appear white or pale, then turn red later. While they often enlarge during the first year, most shrink and almost disappear by the time a child reaches school age usually without requiring treatment.

Port Wine Stain. Large, flat, and irregularly shaped dark red or purple areas. Caused by extra blood vessels under the skin, port wine stains are usually located on the face or neck but, unlike hemangiomas, don't disappear without treatment. These birthmarks can be treated, sometimes with laser surgery by either a plastic surgeon or a pediatric dermatologist. (See also *Birthmarks and Hemangiomas,* page 696.)

If your baby was born vaginally, in addition to the elongated shape of his head, there also may be some scalp swelling in the area that was pushed out first during birth. If you press gently on this area, your finger may even leave a small indentation. This swelling (called *caput*) is not serious and should disappear in a few days.

Sometimes there may be swelling under a newborn's scalp that is present on only one side of the head, and will seem to spring right back after it is gently pressed. This type of swelling is likely to be what is called a *cephalohematoma,* and it, too, is caused by the intense pressure on the head during labor. While not serious, it typically represents some bleeding in the scalp (but outside the skull bones—not inside the brain) and usually takes six to ten weeks to disappear. Parents should be careful not to injure this area with their long nails or a sharp-toothed comb, since this swelling may get infected.

All babies have two soft spots, or *fontanelles,* on the top of the head. These are the areas where the immature bones of the skull are still growing together. The larger opening is on the top of the head toward the front; a smaller one is at the back. Parents needn't be afraid to touch these areas gently, as there is a thick, durable membrane that protects the brain.

All infants are born with hair but the amount, texture, and color vary from one newborn to another. Most, if not all, of this "baby hair" falls out during the first six months of life and is replaced by mature hair. The color and texture of the mature hair may be quite different from the hair the baby was born with.

In the weeks following their birth, babies can be affected by the large amount of their mother's hormones that they were exposed to during pregnancy. As a result, babies' breasts may be enlarged temporarily and they might even secrete a few drops of milk. It is equally likely to occur in boy and girl babies, and normally lasts less than a week, although it can last several weeks. It is best not to press on or squeeze a baby's breasts, since this won't reduce the swelling and could cause an infection. In infant girls, there could be a discharge from the vagina. Although disconcerting to some new parents, this so-called "pseudomenses" is actually quite harmless.

As you examine your baby's abdomen, it will seem prominent, and you may even notice an area that seems to bulge during crying spells. These small hernias are most commonly seen around the umbilical cord/belly button, but may also appear in a line down the center of the abdomen. (For more information, see *Umbilical Hernia* on page 177 of this chapter.)

The genitals of newborn babies can be somewhat reddish and seem quite large for bodies so small. The scrotum of a baby boy may be smooth and barely big enough to hold the testicles, or it might be large and wrinkled. The testicles can seem to move in and out of the scrotum. Sometimes they will move as far up in the scrotum as the base of the penis or even to the crease at the top of the thigh/belly. As long as a baby boy's testicles are located in the scrotum most of the time, the fact that they move around is normal.

Some boys have a buildup of fluid in a sac called a hydrocele (see page 454) inside the scrotum. This buildup will shrink gradually without treatment over several months as the fluid is reabsorbed by the body. If the scrotum swells up suddenly or gets larger when the baby cries, notify your pediatrician; this could be a sign of what is called an *inguinal* hernia, which requires treatment.

At birth, a baby boy's foreskin is attached to the head, or glans, of the penis, and it cannot be pushed back as it can in older boys and men. There is a small opening at the tip through which urine flows. If you have your son circumcised, the connections between the foreskin and the glans are artificially separated and the foreskin is removed, leaving the head of the penis visible. Without a circumcision, the foreskin will separate from the glans naturally during the first few years. (For a detailed description of circumcision, see *Should the Baby Be Circumcised?*, on page 28.)

While you're still in the hospital, the staff will watch carefully for your baby's first urination and bowel movement to make sure he has no problem with these important tasks. They may occur right after birth or up to a day later. The first bowel movement or two will be dark black-green and very slimy. It contains meconium, a substance that fills the infant's intestines before he is born. If meconium is not passed within the baby's first forty-eight hours, further evaluation is required to make sure that no problems exist in the lower bowel.

Care of the Penis

Caring for the Circumcised Penis. If you chose to have your son circumcised, the procedure probably has been performed in the hospital on the second or third day after birth, but may be done after discharge during the first week of life (see *Should the Baby Be Circumcised?*, on page 28). Ritual circumcisions for religious reasons are usually performed in the second week of life. Afterward, a light dressing such as gauze with petroleum jelly will have been placed over the head of the penis. The next time the baby urinates, this dressing usually will come off. Some pediatricians recommend keeping a clean dressing on until the penis is fully healed, while others advise leaving it off. The important thing is to keep the area as clean as possible. If particles of stool get on the penis, wipe it gently with soap and water during diaper changes.

The tip of the penis may look quite red for the first few days, and you may notice a yellow secretion. Both indicate that the area is healing normally. The redness and secretion should disappear gradually within a week. If the redness persists or there is swelling or crusted yellow sores that contain cloudy fluid, there may be an infection. This does not happen very often, but if you suspect that infection is present, consult your pediatrician.

Usually, after the circumcision has healed, the penis requires no additional care. Occasionally a small piece of the foreskin remains. You should pull back this skin gently each time the child is bathed. Examine the groove around the head of the penis and make sure it's clean.

If circumcision is not performed within the baby's first two weeks (perhaps for medical reasons), it is usually put off for several weeks or months. The follow-up care is the same whenever it is done. Should circumcision become necessary after the newborn period, general anesthesia is often used and requires a more formal surgical procedure necessitating control of bleeding and suturing of skin edges.

Caring for the Uncircumcised Penis. In the first few months, you should simply clean and bathe your baby's uncircumcised penis with soap and water, like the rest of the diaper area. Initially, the foreskin is connected by tissue to the glans, or head, of the penis, so you shouldn't try to retract it. No cleansing of the penis with cotton swabs or antiseptics is necessary, but you should watch your baby urinate occasionally to make sure that the hole in the foreskin is large enough to permit a normal stream. If the stream consistently is no more than a trickle, or if your baby seems to have some discomfort while urinating, consult your pediatrician.

The doctor will tell you when the foreskin has separated and can be retracted safely. This will not be for several months or years, and should never be forced; if you were to force the foreskin to retract before it is ready, you could cause painful bleeding and tears in the skin. After this separation occurs, retract the foreskin occasionally to gently cleanse the end of the penis underneath.

As your son gets older, you'll need to teach him what he must do in order to urinate and wash his penis. Teach him to clean his foreskin by:

- Gently pulling it back away from the head of the penis.
- Rinsing the head of the penis and inside fold of the foreskin with soap and warm water.
- Pulling the foreskin back over the head of the penis.

On occasion, newborns have a little blood in their bowel movements. Especially if it occurs during the first few days, it generally means that the infant swallowed some blood during birth or while breastfeeding. Both causes are harmless, but even so, let your pediatrician know about any signs of blood in order to make sure this is really the reason behind it, since there are other causes of blood in the stool that require further evaluation and treatment.

Your Baby's Birth Weight and Measurements

What makes a baby big or small? The following are some of the most common causes:

Large Babies: An infant can be born large when the parents are large or the mother is overweight. There is also a greater likelihood of a large newborn due to factors such as:

- The pregnancy lasting longer than forty-two weeks
- The fetus's growth overstimulated in the uterus
- Fetal chromosomal abnormalities
- Weight gain during pregnancy
- The mother's ethnicity
- The mother having diabetes before or during pregnancy
- The mother having given birth to other children
- Having a boy

Large infants may have metabolic abnormalities (such as low blood sugar and calcium), traumatic birth injuries, higher hemoglobin levels, jaundice, or various congenital abnormalities. Almost one-third of large babies initially have feeding difficulties. Your pediatrician will keep a close watch on these issues.

Small Babies: A baby may be born small for a number of reasons, including:

- Being born early (preterm)
- Being born to small parents
- The mother's ethnicity
- Fetal chromosomal abnormalities
- The mother's chronic diseases such as high blood pressure, or heart or kidney disease
- Malnutrition
- The mother's substance abuse during pregnancy

A small baby may need to have his temperature, glucose, and hemoglobin level closely monitored. After birth, the pediatrician will thoroughly evaluate a small infant and decide when he is ready to go home.

To determine how your baby's measurements compare with those of other babies born after the same length of pregnancy, your pediatrician will refer to one of the growth charts (see Appendix).

The first two growth charts examine length and weight in boys and girls, from birth to thirty-six months. They are followed by body mass index for age charts for boys and girls, ages two to twenty years. (Body mass index, or BMI, is a measure of weight in relation to height.)

As illustrated in the first two charts, eighty out of every one hundred babies born at forty weeks of pregnancy, or full term, weigh between 5 pounds 11½ ounces (2.6 kg) and 8 pounds 5¾ ounces (3.8 kg). This is a healthy average. Those above the ninetieth percentile on the chart are considered large, and those below the tenth percentile are regarded as small. Keep in mind that these early weight designations (large or small) do not predict whether a child will be above or below average when he grows up, but they do help the hospital staff determine whether he needs extra attention during the first few days after birth.

At every physical exam, beginning with the first one after birth, the pediatrician will routinely measure the baby's length, weight, and head circumference (the distance around his head) and will plot them on growth charts similar to the ones in the Appendix. In a healthy, well-nourished infant, these three important measurements should increase at a predictable rate. Any interruption in this rate can help the doctor better detect and address any feeding, developmental, or medical issues.

How Your Newborn Behaves

Lying in your arms or in the crib beside you, your newborn makes a tight little bundle. Just as he did in the womb, he'll keep his arms and legs bent up close to his body and his fingers tightly clenched, although you should be able to straighten them gently with your hands. His feet will naturally

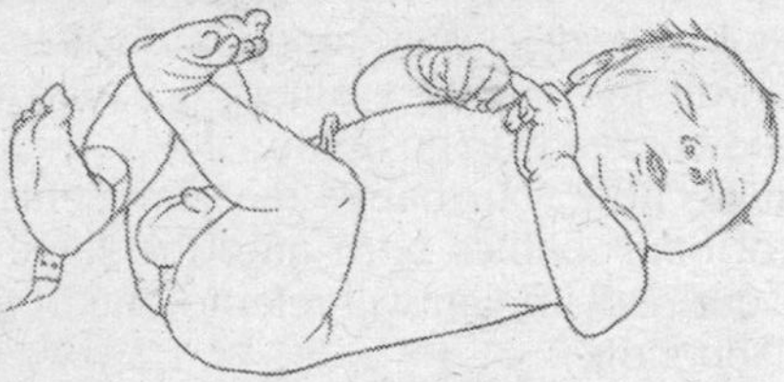

curve inward. It may take several weeks for his body to unfold from this preferred fetal position.

You'll have to wait even longer for him to make the cooing or babbling sounds we generally think of as "baby talk." However, from the beginning he'll be very noisy. Besides crying when something is wrong, he'll have a wide variety of grunts, squeaks, sighs, sneezes, and hiccups. (You may even remember the hiccups from pregnancy!) Most of these sounds, just like his sudden movements, are reactions to disturbances around him; a shrill sound or a strong odor may be all it takes for him to jump or cry.

These reactions, as well as more subtle ones, are signs of how well your baby's senses are functioning at birth. After all those months in the womb, he'll quickly recognize his mother's voice (and possibly his father's, as well). If you play soothing music, he may become quiet as he listens or he'll move gently in time with it.

By using the senses of smell and taste, your newborn is able to distinguish breastmilk from any other liquid. Born with a sweet tooth, he'll prefer sugar water to plain water and will wrinkle his nose at sour or bitter scents and tastes.

Your baby's vision will be best within an 8- to 12-inch (20.3 to 30.5 cm) range, which means he can see your face perfectly as you hold and feed him. But when you are farther away, his eyes may wander, giving him a cross-eyed appearance. During the first couple of months of his life, don't worry about this. As his eye muscles mature and his vision improves, both eyes will remain focused on the same thing at the same time. This usually occurs between two and three months of age. If it does not, bring it to the attention of your baby's pediatrician.

While your infant will be able to distinguish light from

dark at birth, he will not yet see the full range of colors. While young infants who are shown a pattern of black and white or sharply contrasting colors may study them with interest, they are not likely to respond at all when shown a picture with lots of closely related colors.

Perhaps the newborn's most important sense is touch. After months of being bathed in warm fluid in the womb, your baby will now be exposed to all sorts of new sensations—some harsh, some wonderfully comforting. While he may cringe at a sudden gust of cold air, he'll love the feel of a soft blanket and the warmth of your arms around him. Holding your baby will give him as much pleasure as it does you. It will give him a sense of security and comfort, and it will tell him he is loved. Research shows that close emotional bonding actually will promote his growth and development.

Going Home

Most hospitals will discharge you and your baby within forty-eight hours if you have delivered vaginally. However, if you undergo a Cesarean section, you may stay at the facility for four to five days. If your baby is born in an alternative birthing center, you may be able to go home within twenty-four hours. Nevertheless, just because a full-term, healthy infant *could* be discharged from the hospital in less than forty-eight hours doesn't mean it should necessarily occur. The American Academy of Pediatrics believes that the health and well-being of the mother and her child is paramount. Since every child is different, the decision to discharge a newborn should be made on a case-by-case basis. If a newborn does leave the hospital early, he or she should be seen by a doctor twenty-four to forty-eight hours after discharge.

Prior to making the decision about when to go home, you and your doctor need to weigh the advantages and disadvantages carefully. From an emotional and physical standpoint, there are arguments for both a short (one to two days) and a longer (three-plus days) stay. Some women simply dislike being in the hospital and feel more comfortable and relaxed at home; as soon as they and their baby are proclaimed healthy and able to travel, they're eager to leave. By keeping the hospital stay short, they'll certainly save themselves—or their insurance company—money. However, many new mothers often cannot get as much rest at home as in the hospital—especially if there are older children clamoring for attention. Nor are they likely to have access to the valuable support that trained nurses can offer in the hospital during the first days of breastfeeding and baby care.

If a newborn does leave the hospital early, he should have received all the appropriate newborn tests such as a hearing screen (see *Newborn Screening Tests,* page 64), and he also should be seen by the pediatrician twenty-four to forty-eight hours *after* discharge. Of course, the doctor should be called immediately whenever a newborn appears listless or is feverish, is vomiting, has difficulty feeding, or develops a yellow color to his skin (jaundice).

Before you do leave the hospital, your home and car should be equipped with at least the bare essentials. Make sure you have a federally approved car safety seat that is appropriate for your baby's size, and which you have correctly installed rear-facing in the backseat of your vehicle. It is extremely important to follow the car seat manufacturer's instructions on installation and proper use carefully,

Where We Stand

The timing of newborn discharge from the hospital should be a mutual decision between the parents and the physician caring for the infant. The American Academy of Pediatrics believes that the health and well-being of the mother and her baby should take precedence over financial considerations. Academy policy has established minimum criteria for early discharge of a mother and her baby, which include term delivery, appropriate growth, and normal physical examination, and states that it is unlikely that all of its criteria can be met in less than forty-eight hours. The Academy supports state and federal legislation based on AAP guidelines as long as physicians, in consultation with parents, have the final authority in determining when to discharge the patient.

and if possible, it is helpful to get your car seat installation checked by a certified child passenger safety technician to ensure that you've gotten it right. (For more information on the choice and proper use of car safety seats, see pages 406–418.)

At home you'll need a safe place for the baby to sleep, plenty of diapers, and enough clothing and blankets to keep him warm and protected. If you're formula-feeding, you'll also need a supply of formula.

PARENTING ISSUES

Mother's Feelings

If you find your first few days with your baby to be a mixture of delight, pain, utter exhaustion, and—especially if this is your first child—some apprehension about your capabilities as a parent—take comfort in knowing you are not alone.

If you're like many other women, you're so excited about your new arrival that you may not even notice how tired and sore you are. In spite of the fatigue, it still may be difficult to relax enough to fall asleep. Your own rooming-in arrangements may add to the problem; however, if you imagine that every crying baby you hear is your own, having your baby sleep in the nursery may not give you the peace you thought it would. You can solve these problems by letting him sleep in his hospital-supplied bassinet next to

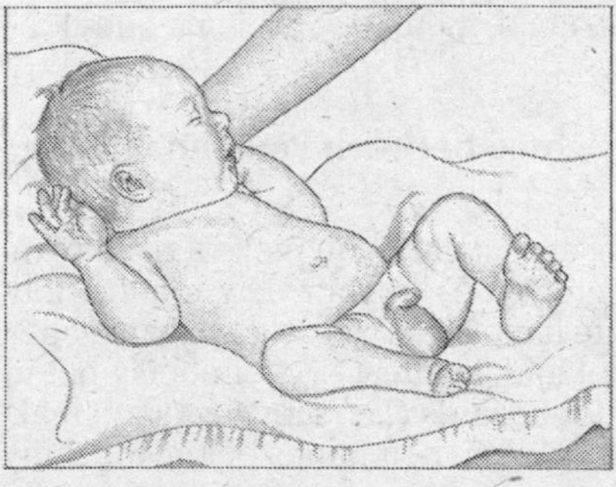

You have just given birth to a wonderful new being, but also to a new awesome responsibility.

you, so you can sleep when he does and hold him when he awakens.

On the other hand, particularly if you had a long, hard labor or a Cesarean section, you simply may not have the strength to keep the baby with you full-time, and that's understandable. After having a C-section, you may initially find it painful to lift your baby and are likely to find it more comfortable to try positions for both holding and nursing him that put less strain on your stitches. These obstacles may make you feel that you're not bonding with your baby as you imagined you would, and you may feel especially disappointed if you had planned for a problem-free, natural delivery. Fortunately, your child's major preoccupation during these first few days also will be sleeping and recuperating, and he won't much care where he does it as long as he's warm, dry, and fed when he's hungry. So for the moment, the hospital nursery will suit him fine. You will have plenty of time to form a secure bond with each other after your physical recoveries are complete.

In general, instead of worrying while in the hospital, it is best to take advantage of your time in the hospital to rest, learn from the trained professionals around you, and let your body recover. If and when your anxiety levels peak, it can admittedly be difficult to believe that you'll ever be an expert on baby care. But rest assured. Once new parents have had a few days to get used to routine baby care and get home, things start to fall into place for most of them. If they don't, be sure to enlist the help of your pediatrician, friends, and family. (For more information about postpartum blues and depression, see the description on pages 168–169.)

If this is not your first child, there may be some questions on your mind, such as:

- **Will this new baby come between you and an older child?**

  This needn't happen, especially if you make a point of including your older child(ren) in your new routine. Toddlers are usually quite happy to go retrieve a clean diaper, and older children often take great pride in being put in charge of checking for hazards (i.e., stray toys) and making sure that all visitors wash their hands before touching the new baby. As you become more comfortable with your daily routine, be sure to include special times with your older child.

- **Will you be able to give the same intensity of love to the new child?**

  In fact, each child is special and will draw out different responses and feelings from you. Even the birth order of your children may influence the way you relate to each of them. It is often helpful to keep in mind that "new" isn't "better" or "worse," but usually just . . . different. This concept is an important one for both you and your child(ren) to remember.

- **How can you avoid comparing one to another?**

  It's only natural to compare. You may even find yourself thinking that the new baby is not as beautiful or as alert as another child was right after birth, or you may worry because he's more attractive and attentive. In the beginning, these comparisons are inevitable, but as the new baby's own unique qualities begin to emerge, you'll become as proud of your children's differences as you are of their similarities.

On a more practical note, the prospect of taking care of two or more young children may worry you. This only makes sense, but as greater time demands and fears of sibling rivalry loom before you, don't let yourself get overwhelmed. Given time and patience, all of you will adjust and learn to be a family.

If the newness, fatigue, and seemingly unanswerable questions push you to tears, don't feel bad. You won't be the first new mother to cry—or the last. The hormonal changes you went through as an adolescent or experienced during your menstrual cycles are minor compared to the hormonal shifts associated with giving birth. So blame it on the hormones!

In addition to the hormonal effects, significant emotional changes are taking place. You have just given birth not only to a wonderful new human being, but also to a new and awesome responsibility. There are sure to be significant changes taking place in your family life. It is normal to think about these things and easy to attach too much importance to them.

The emotional changes of this time can sometimes lead mothers to feel sadness, fear, irritability, or anxiety—or even anger toward their baby—feelings doctors call the postpartum blues or baby blues. About three out of four new mothers experience these baby blues a few days after birth. Fortunately, these feelings tend to subside on their own as quickly as they develop, typically lasting no more than several days.

Some new mothers, however, have such severe feelings of sadness, emptiness, apathy, and even despair that doctors categorize them as having *postpartum depression*. They also may experience feelings of inadequacy, and they may begin to withdraw from family and friends. These feelings may develop a few weeks after the baby is born and affect about one out of ten new mothers. The symptoms can last for many months (or even for more than a year), worsen with time, and become so intense that these mothers may feel helpless and incapable of caring for their baby and their other children. If they don't receive care for their postpartum depression, the condition may worsen with time, and in some cases they may worry about harming themselves or their baby.

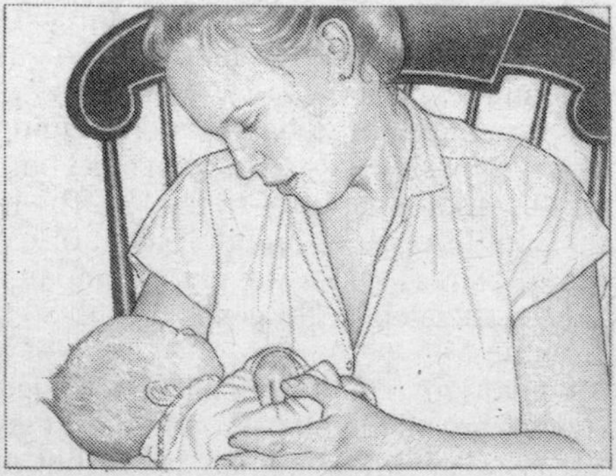

Do not be afraid to ask for help if your concerns seem too great for you to handle.

You should discuss your feelings with the baby's father, your extended family, and close friends. Allow them to give you brief breaks from being the primary caregiver, and try to reduce your stress and anxiety by getting some exercise and as much rest as possible. If this doesn't help and these feelings are severe and haven't subsided in about two weeks, talk to your obstetrician or pediatrician, or seek help from a mental health professional; counseling and/or antidepressant medications may be recommended (check in with your pediatrician if you're breastfeeding). Do not be afraid to ask for help from professionals if your concerns seem too great for you to handle, or if you feel increasingly depressed. Although a certain amount of post-delivery depression may be normal, it should not be overwhelming or last more than a few days.

Father's Feelings

As a new dad, your new role is no less complicated than the mother's. No, you didn't have to carry the baby for nine months, but you did have to make adjustments physically and emotionally as the due date approached and the preparations for the baby became all-important. On one hand, you may have felt as if you had nothing to do with this birth; but on the other, this is very much your baby, too.

When the baby finally arrived, you may have been tremendously relieved as well as excited and somewhat awed. In witnessing your baby's birth, feelings of commitment and love may have surfaced that you had worried you might never feel for this child. You also may have experienced a greater admiration and love for your wife than you ever felt before. At the same time, contemplating the responsibility of caring for this child for the next twenty years may have been more than a little unnerving.

Depending on the hospital and your own schedule, you may have been able to room in with mother and/or child until it was time to take the baby home. This helps you feel less like a bystander and more like a key participant, allowing you to get to know your baby right from the start. It also allows you to share an intense emotional experience with Mom.

If you continue to feel conflicting emotions, how should

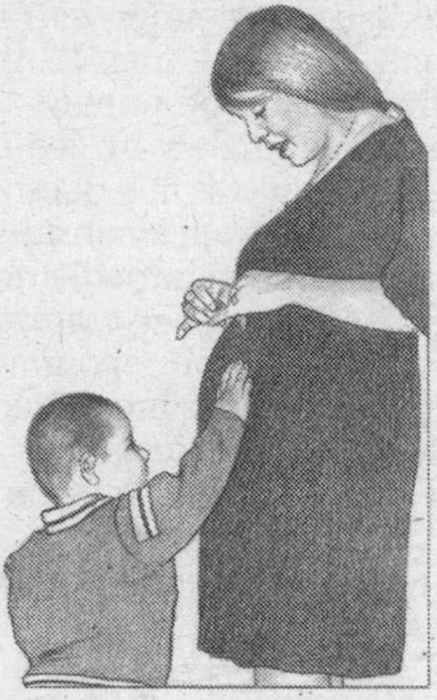

you deal with them? The best approach is to become as actively involved in fathering as possible. Once the entire family is home, you can—and should—help feed (if bottle-fed), diaper, bathe, and comfort your baby. Contrary to old-fashioned stereotypes, these jobs are not exclusively "woman's work." They are the best way for you to bond with your child, and they are wonderful opportunities for the entire family—mother, father, and even older siblings—to get to know, love, and welcome this new member home.

Sibling's Feelings

Older children may greet a new baby with either open arms or closed minds. Their reaction will depend largely on their age and developmental level. Consider a toddler, for instance. There's little you can do to prepare him in advance for the changes that will come with a new sibling. To begin with, he may have been confused by the sudden disappearance of his parents when the baby was born. Upon visiting the hospital, he may have been frightened by the sight of his mother in bed, perhaps attached to intravenous tubing.

He also may be jealous that his parents are holding someone else instead of him, and he may misbehave or begin acting younger—for example, by insisting on wearing diapers or suddenly having accidents several months after being toilet trained. These are normal responses to stress and change, and don't deserve discipline. Instead of punishing him or insisting that he share your love for the new baby, give him extra love and reassurance. Also, try very hard to catch him "being good," so he'll get lots of attention for appropriate behaviors. Praise him for acting "like the big brother," letting him know that he, too, has an important new role to play. Tell him that there's plenty of room in your heart to love both him and the new baby. Over time, his attachment to the baby will build, gradually and naturally.

If your older child is a preschooler, he'll be better able to understand what's happening. If you prepared him during the pregnancy, you may have helped ease his confusion, if not his jealousy. He would have been able to understand the basic facts of the situation ("The baby is in Mommy's tummy"; "The baby will sleep in your old crib"), and he probably became very curious about this mysterious person.

If your older child is of school age, he'll still need to adapt to a new role. At the same time, he was probably fascinated by the process of pregnancy and childbirth and eager to meet the new baby. Once the infant arrived, he may have become very proud and protective. Let him help take care of the little one at times, but don't forget that he still needs time and attention himself.

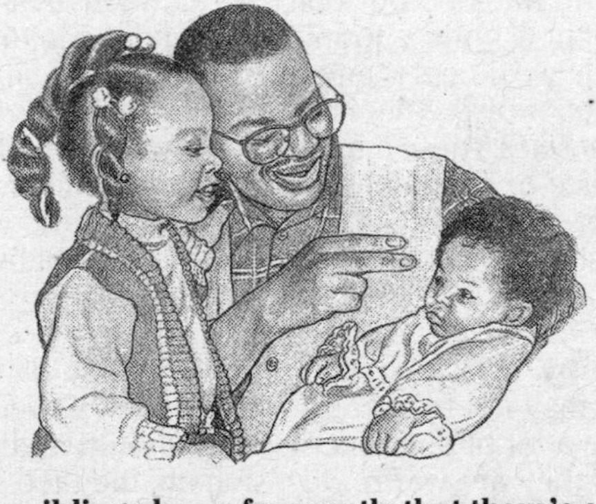

Let the older siblings know frequently that there's enough room and love in your heart for both children.

(If you're the grandparent of a newborn, see pages 217–220 for some thoughts about your new role now that your new grandson or granddaughter has arrived.)

Health Watch

Some physical conditions are especially common during the first couple of weeks after birth. If you notice any of the following in your baby, contact your pediatrician.

Abdominal Distension. Most babies' bellies normally stick out, especially after a large feeding. Between feedings, however, they should feel quite soft. If your child's abdomen feels swollen and hard, and if he has not had a bowel movement for more than one or two days or is vomiting, call your pediatrician. Most likely the problem is due to gas or constipation, but it also could signal a more serious intestinal problem.

Birth Injuries. It is possible for babies to be injured during birth, especially if labor is particularly long or difficult, or when babies are very large. While newborns recover quickly from some of these injuries, others persist longer term. Quite often the injury is a broken collarbone, which will heal quickly if the arm on that side is kept relatively motionless. Incidentally, after a few weeks a small lump may form at the site of the fracture, but don't be alarmed; this is a positive sign that new bone is forming to mend the injury.

Muscle weakness is another common birth injury, caused during labor by pressure or stretching of the nerves attached to the muscles. These muscles, usually weakened on one side of the face or one shoulder or arm, generally return to normal after several weeks. In the meantime, ask your pediatrician to show you how to nurse and hold the baby to promote healing.

Blue Baby. Babies may have mildly blue hands and feet, but this may not be a cause for concern. If their hands and feet turn a bit blue from cold, they should return to pink as soon as they are warm. Occasionally, the face, tongue, and lips may turn a little blue when the newborn is crying hard, but once he becomes calm, his color in these parts of the body should quickly return to normal. However, persistently blue skin coloring, especially with breathing difficulties and feeding difficulties, is a sign that the heart or lungs are not operating properly, and the baby is not getting enough oxygen in the blood. Immediate medical attention is essential.

Coughing. If the baby drinks very fast or tries to drink water for the first time, he may cough and sputter a bit; but this type of coughing should stop as soon as he adjusts to a familiar feeding routine. This may also be related to how strong or fast a breastfeeding mom's milk comes down. If he coughs persistently or routinely gags during feedings, consult the pediatrician. These symptoms could indicate an underlying problem in the lungs or digestive tract.

Excessive Crying. All newborns cry, often for no apparent reason. If you've made sure that your baby is fed, burped, warm, and dressed in a clean diaper, the best tactic is probably to hold him and talk or sing to him until he stops. You cannot "spoil" a baby this age by giving him too much attention. If this doesn't work, wrap him snugly in a blanket or try some of the approaches listed on pages 190–191 and 193.

You'll become accustomed to your baby's normal pattern of crying. If it ever sounds peculiar—for example, like shrieks of pain—or if it persists for an unusual length of time, it could mean a medical problem. Call the pediatrician and ask for advice.

Forceps Marks. When forceps are used to help during a delivery, they can leave red marks or even superficial scrapes on a newborn's face and head where the metal pressed against the skin. These generally disappear within a few days. Sometimes a firm, flat lump develops in one of these areas because of minor damage to the tissue under the skin, but this, too, usually will go away within two months.

Jaundice. Many normal, healthy newborns have a yellowish tinge to their skin, which is known as jaundice. It is caused by a buildup of a chemical called bilirubin in the child's blood. This occurs most often when the immature liver has not yet begun to efficiently do its job of removing bilirubin from the bloodstream (bilirubin is formed from the

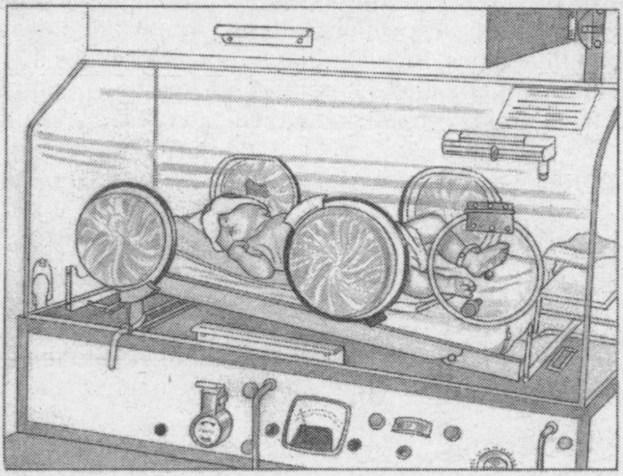

Phototherapy—or light treatment—can be delivered through different light sources or by a blanket that has a special lighting source.

body's normal breakdown of red blood cells). While babies often have a mild case of jaundice, which is harmless, it can become a serious condition when bilirubin reaches what the pediatrician considers to be a very high level. Although jaundice is quite treatable, if the bilirubin level is very high and is not treated effectively, it can even lead to nervous system or brain damage in some cases, which is why the condition must be checked for and appropriately treated. Jaundice tends to be more common in newborns who are breastfeeding, most often in those who are not nursing well; breastfeeding mothers should nurse at least eight to twelve times per day, which will help produce enough milk and help keep bilirubin levels low.

Jaundice appears first on the face, then on the chest and abdomen, and finally on the arms and legs in some instances. The whites of the eyes may also be yellow. The pediatrician will examine the baby for jaundice, and if she suspects that it may be present—based not only on the amount of yellow in the skin, but also on the baby's age and other factors—she may order a skin or blood test to definitively diagnose the condition. If jaundice develops before the baby is twenty-four hours old, a bilirubin test is *always* needed to make an accurate diagnosis. At three to five days old, newborns should be checked by a doctor or nurse, since this is the time when the bilirubin level is highest; for that reason, if an infant is discharged before he is seventy-two hours old, he should be seen by the pediatrician within two days of that discharge. Some newborns need to be seen even sooner, including:

- Those with a high bilirubin level before leaving the hospital
- Those born early (more than two weeks before the due date)
- Those whose jaundice is present in the first twenty-four hours after birth
- Those who are not breastfeeding well
- Those with considerable bruising and bleeding under the scalp, associated with labor and delivery
- Those who have a parent or sibling who had high bilirubin levels and underwent treatment for it

When the doctor determines that jaundice is present and needs to be treated, the bilirubin level can be reduced by placing the infant under special lights when he is undressed—either in the hospital or at home. His eyes will be covered to protect them during the light therapy. This kind of treatment can prevent the harmful effects of jaundice. In infants who are breastfed, jaundice may last for more than two to three weeks; in those who are formula-fed, most cases of jaundice go away by two weeks of age.

Lethargy and Sleepiness. Every newborn spends most of his time sleeping. As long as he wakes up every few hours, eats well, seems content, and is alert part of the day, it's perfectly normal for him to sleep the rest of the time. But if he's rarely alert, does not wake up on his own for feedings, or seems too tired or uninterested to eat, you should consult your pediatrician. This lethargy—especially if it's a sudden change in his usual pattern—may be a symptom of a serious illness.

Respiratory Distress. It may take your baby a few hours after birth to form a normal pattern of breathing, but then he should have no further difficulties. If he seems to be breathing in an unusual manner, it is most often from blockage of the nasal passages. The use of saline nasal drops, followed by the use of a bulb syringe, are what may be needed to fix the problem; both are available over the counter at all pharmacies.

However, if your newborn shows any of the following warning signs, notify your pediatrician immediately:

- Fast breathing (more than sixty breaths in one minute), although keep in mind that babies normally breathe more rapidly than adults.
- Retractions (sucking in the muscles between the ribs with each breath, so that her ribs stick out)
- Flaring of her nose
- Grunting while breathing
- Persistent blue skin coloring

Umbilical Cord. You'll need to keep the stump of the umbilical cord clean and dry as it shrivels and eventually falls off. To keep the cord dry, sponge bathe your baby rather than submersing him in a tub of water. Also keep the diaper folded below the cord to keep urine from soaking it. You may notice a few drops of blood on the diaper around the time the stump falls off; this is normal. But if the cord does actively bleed, call your baby's doctor immediately. If the stump becomes infected, however, it will require medical treatment. Although an infection is quite uncommon, contact your doctor if any of these signs is present:

- Foul-smelling yellowish discharge from the cord
- Red skin around the base of the cord
- Crying when you touch the cord or the skin next to it

The umbilical cord stump should dry up and fall off by the time your baby is eight weeks old. If it remains beyond that time, there may be other issues at play. See the baby's doctor if the cord has not dried up and fallen off by the time the baby is two months old.

Umbilical Granuloma. Sometimes instead of completely drying, the cord will form a granuloma or a small reddened mass of scar tissue that stays on the belly button after the umbilical cord has fallen off. This granuloma will drain a light-yellowish fluid. This condition will usually go away in about a week, but if not, your pediatrician may need to burn off (cauterize) the granulamatous tissue.

Umbilical Hernia. If your baby's umbilical cord area seems to push outward when he cries, he may have an umbilical hernia—a small hole in the muscular part of the abdominal wall that allows tissue to bulge out when there's pressure inside the abdomen (e.g., when the baby cries). This is not a serious condition, and it usually heals by itself in the first twelve to eighteen months. (For unknown reasons it takes longer to heal in African American babies.) In the unlikely event that it doesn't heal, the hole may need to be surgically closed. Taping this area or putting a "taped coin" over this area may be harmful.

Your Newborn's First Physical Exams

Your baby should have one thorough physical examination within his first twenty-four hours and a follow-up at some point before you and the baby leave the hospital. If you take your baby home early (less than twenty-four hours after delivery), your pediatrician should see the baby again in her office twenty-four to forty-eight hours after discharge for follow-up. The purpose of this visit is to assess your baby's general health, such as weight; discuss important topics such as your baby's stool and urine patterns, and sleep habits; review feeding techniques, including those associated with breastfeeding (adequate position, latch-on, and swallowing); and evaluate for jaundice, besides identifying any new questions or concerns you may have. The American Academy of Pediatrics also recommends that you and your baby schedule a doctor's visit when he's age two to four weeks. As we described in Chapter 3 on pages 90–93, your doctor will physically examine your baby and take measurements such as his length, weight, and head circumference. She'll listen to your baby's heart and lungs to ensure that they are normal; look into his eyes, ears, and mouth; feel his abdomen for tenderness; evaluate how his belly button is healing and check a baby boy's circumcision; check his reflexes; and examine other parts of the body from head to toe, including the hips. If there is a persistent "clunking" sound of the hip, especially in a girl born breech, your pediatrician may request that an orthopedist do an ultrasound and/or a repeat physical exam at four to eight weeks of age.

These early visits to the pediatrician are also opportunities to ask questions about baby care and relieve any worries you may have. Don't hesitate to ask questions; the goal is for you to get valuable information and leave confident and reassured.

6

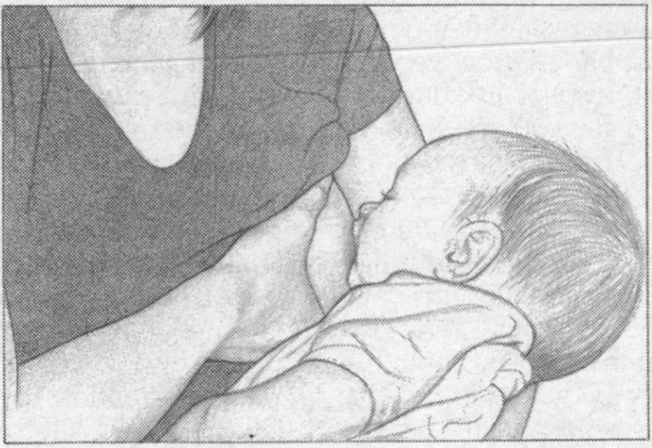

THE FIRST MONTH

GROWTH AND DEVELOPMENT

In the very beginning, it may seem that your baby does nothing but eat, sleep, cry, and fill her diapers. By the end of the first month, she'll be much more alert and responsive. Gradually she'll begin moving her body more smoothly and with much greater coordination—especially in getting her hand to her mouth. You'll realize that she listens when you speak, watches you as you hold her, and occasionally moves her own body to respond to you or attract your attention. But before we explore her expanding capabilities, let's look at the changes in her physical appearance during the first month.

Physical Appearance and Growth

When your baby was born, her birth weight included excess body fluid, which she lost during her first few days. Most babies lose about one-tenth of their birth weight during the first five days, then regain it over the next five, so that by about day ten they usually are back to their original birth weight. You can plot your own infant's growth on the charts in the Appendix.

Most babies grow very rapidly after regaining their birth weight, especially during growth spurts, which occur around seven to ten days and again between three and six weeks. The average newborn gains weight at a rate of ⅔ of an ounce (20–30 grams) per day and by one month weighs about ten pounds (4.5 kg). She grows between 1½ and 2 inches (4.5 to 5 cm) during this month. Boys tend to weigh slightly more than girls (by less than 1 pound, or approximately 350 grams). They also tend to be slightly longer than girls at this age (by about ½ inch, or 1.25 cm).

Your pediatrician will pay particular attention to your child's head growth, because it reflects the growth of her brain. The bones in your baby's skull are still growing together, and the skull is growing faster during the first four months than at any other time in her life. The average newborn's head circumference measures about 13¾ inches (35 cm), growing to about 15 inches (38 cm) by one month. Because boys tend to be slightly larger than girls, their heads are larger, though the average difference is less than ½ inch (1 cm).

During these first weeks your baby's body gradually will straighten from the tightly curled position she held inside the uterus during the final months of pregnancy. She'll begin to stretch her arms and legs and may arch her back from time to time. Her legs and feet may continue to rotate inward, giving her a bowlegged look. This condition usually will correct itself gradually over the first year of life. If the bowlegged appearance is particularly severe or associated with pronounced curving of the front part of the foot, your pediatrician may suggest a splint or a cast to correct it, but in most instances these circumstances are extremely unusual. (See *Bowlegs and Knock-Knees,* page 689; *Pigeon Toes* [*Intoeing*], page 693.)

If your baby was born vaginally and her skull appeared misshapen at birth, it soon should resume its normal shape. Any bruising of the scalp or swelling of the eyelids that occurred during birth will be gone by the end of the first week or two. Any red spots in the eyes will disappear in about three weeks.

To your dismay, you may discover that the fine hair that covered your child's head when she was born soon begins falling out. If she rubs the back of her head on her sleep surface, she may develop a temporary bald spot there, even if the rest of her hair remains. This loss is not medically significant. The bare spots will be covered with new hair in a few months.

Another normal development is baby acne—pimples that break out on the face, usually during the fourth or fifth week of life. They are thought to be due to stimulation of oil glands in the skin by hormones passed across the placenta during pregnancy. This condition may be made worse if the baby lies in sheets laundered in harsh detergents or soiled by milk that she's spit up. If your baby does have baby acne, place a soft, clean receiving blanket under her head while she's awake and wash her face gently once a day with a mild baby soap to remove milk or detergent residue.

Your newborn's skin also may look blotchy, ranging in color from pink to blue. Her hands and feet in particular may be colder and bluer than the rest of her body. The blood vessels leading to these areas are more sensitive to temperature changes and tend to shrink in response to cold. As a result, less blood gets to the exposed skin, causing it to look pale or bluish. If you move her arms and legs, however, you should notice that they quickly turn pink again.

Your baby's internal "thermostat," which causes her to sweat when she's too hot or shiver when she's too cold, won't be working properly for some time. Also, in these early weeks, she'll lack the insulating layer of fat that will protect her from sudden temperature shifts later on. For these reasons, it's important for you to dress her properly—warmly in cool weather and lightly when it's hot. A general rule of thumb is to dress her in one more layer of clothing than *you* would wear in the same weather conditions. Don't automatically bundle her up just because she's a baby.

Between ten days and three weeks after birth, the stump from the umbilical cord should have dried and fallen off, leaving behind a clean, well-healed area. Occasionally a raw spot is left after the stump is gone. It may even ooze a little blood-tinged fluid. Just keep it dry and clean (using a cotton ball dipped in rubbing alcohol) and it will heal by itself. If it is not completely healed and dry in two weeks, consult your pediatrician.

Reflexes

Much of your baby's activity in her first weeks of life is reflexive. For instance, when you put your finger in her mouth, she doesn't think about what to do, but sucks by reflex. When confronted by a bright light, she will tightly shut her eyes, because that's what her reflexes make her do. She's born with many of these automatic responses, some of which remain with her for months, while others vanish in weeks.

In some cases, reflexes change into voluntary behavior. For example, your baby is born with a "rooting" reflex that prompts her to turn her head toward your hand if you stroke her cheek or mouth. This helps her find the nipple at feeding time. At first she'll root from side to side, turning her head toward the nipple and then away in decreasing arcs. But by about three weeks she'll simply turn her head and move her mouth into position to suck.

Sucking is another survival reflex present even before birth. If you had an ultrasound test done during pregnancy, you may have seen your baby sucking her thumb. After birth, when a nipple (either breast or bottle) is placed in your baby's mouth and touches the roof of her mouth, she automatically begins to suck. This motion actually takes place in two stages: First, she places her lips around the areola (the circular area of pigmented skin surrounding the nipple) and squeezes the nipple between her tongue and palate. (Called "expression," this action forces out the milk.) Then comes the second phase, or the milking action, in which the tongue moves from the areola to the nipple. This whole process is helped by the negative pressure, or suction, that secures the breast in the baby's mouth.

Coordinating these rhythmic sucking movements with breathing and swallowing is a relatively complicated task for a newborn. So even though this is a reflexive action, not all babies suck efficiently at first. With practice, however, the reflex becomes a skill that they all manage well.

As rooting, sucking, and bringing her hand to her mouth

Newborn Reflexes

The following are some of the normal inborn reflexes you will see your baby perform during her first weeks. Not all infants acquire and lose these reflexes at exactly the same time, but this table will give you a general idea of what to expect.

Reflex	*Age When Reflex Appears*	*Age When Reflex Disappears*
Moro reflex	Birth	2 months
Walking/Stepping	Birth	2 months
Rooting	Birth	4 months
Tonic neck reflex	Birth	5–7 months
Palmar grasp	Birth	5–6 months
Plantar grasp	Birth	9–12 months

become less reflexive and more directed, your infant will start to use these movements to console herself. She also may be comforted when you give her a pacifier or when you help her find her thumb or her fingers.

Another, more dramatic reflex during these first few

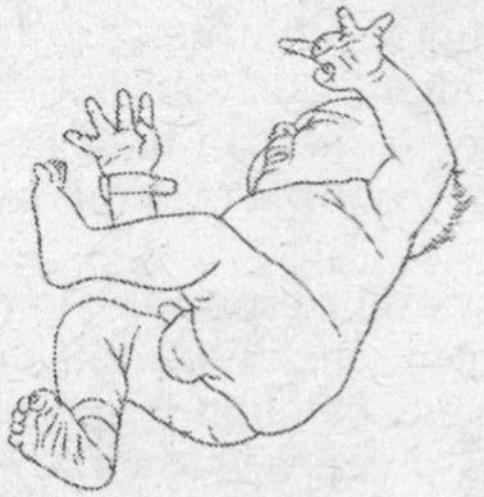

Moro reflex

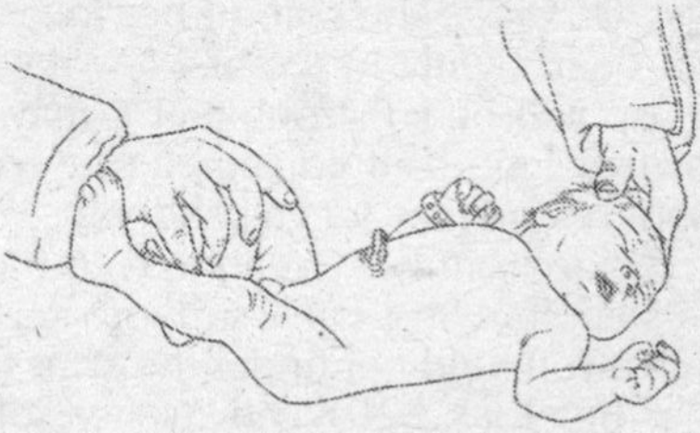

Tonic neck reflex

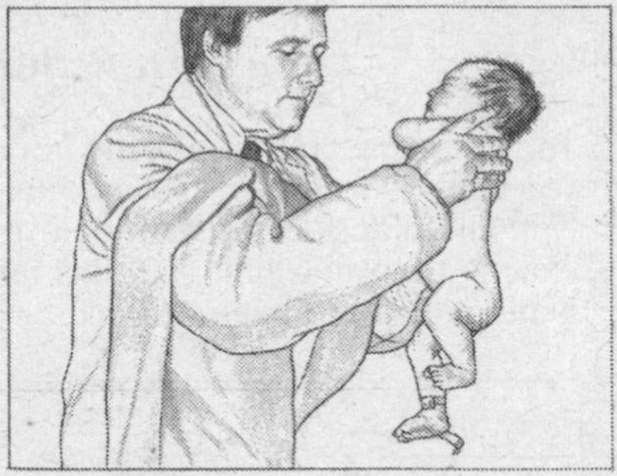

Walking/stepping reflex

weeks is called the Moro reflex. If your baby's head shifts positions abruptly or falls backward, or she is startled by something loud or abrupt, she will react by throwing out her arms and legs and extending her neck, then rapidly bringing her arms together and she may cry loudly. The Moro reflex, which may be present in varying degrees in different babies, peaks during the first month and then disappears after two months.

One of the more interesting automatic responses is the tonic neck reflex, otherwise known as the fencing posture. You may notice that when your baby's head turns to one side, her arm on that side will straighten, with the opposite arm bent as if she's fencing. Do not be surprised if you don't see this response, however. It is subtle, and if your baby is disturbed or crying, she may not perform it. It disappears at five to seven months of age.

You'll see still another reflex when you stroke the palm of your baby's hand and watch her immediately grip your finger. Or stroke the sole of her foot, and watch it flex as the toes curl tightly. In the first few days after birth, your baby's grasp will be so strong that it may seem she can hold her own weight—but don't try it. She has no control over this response and may let go suddenly.

Aside from her strength, your baby's other special talent is stepping. She can't support her own weight, of course, but if you hold her under the arms (being careful to support her head, as well) and let her soles touch a flat surface, she'll place one foot in front of the other and "walk." This reflex will disappear after two months, then recur as the learned voluntary behavior of walking toward the end of the first year.

Although you may think of babies as utterly defenseless, they actually have several protective reflexes. For instance, if an object comes straight toward her, she'll turn her head and try to squirm out of its way. (Amazingly, if the object is on a path that would make it a near miss instead of a collision, she will calmly watch it approach without flinching.) Yes, she's very dependent on her mother and father at this age, but she's not totally defenseless.

Early Brain Development

As a parent, you know that your actions affect your child. You laugh, she laughs. You praise her, she gloats. You frown at her misbehavior, she saddens. You are at the center of your child's universe.

Research shows that during the first three years of a baby's life, the brain grows and develops significantly and patterns of thinking and responding are established. What does this mean for you as a parent? It means that you have a very special opportunity to help your baby develop appropriately and thrive socially, physically, and cognitively throughout her life. The first years last forever.

For years, people have mistakenly believed that the baby's brain is an exact replica of the genetic codes of her parents. For example, if the mother is a good artist, then the baby has more potential to possess the same artistic skills when she grows up. While genetics does play a role in determining your child's skills and abilities, new research highlights the equally significant role that environment plays. Recently, neuroscientists realized that the experiences that fill a baby's first days, months, and years have a great impact on how the brain develops. Both nature and nurture work hand in hand in the development of young children.

Studies have shown that children need certain

elements in the early stages of life to grow and develop to their full potential:

- A child needs to feel special, loved, and valued.
- She needs to feel safe.
- She needs to feel confident about what to expect from her environment.
- She needs guidance.
- She needs a balanced experience of freedom and limits.
- She needs to be exposed to a diverse environment filled with language, play, exploration, books, music, and appropriate toys.

While it may seem that what goes on in a baby's brain would be relatively simple compared to an adult's, in fact, a baby's brain is twice as active as an adult's brain. Neuroscientists are focusing especially on the first three years of a baby's life because they have identified these as times of special importance. During these years, the human brain has the greatest potential for learning. Not only is learning occurring rapidly, but basic ways of thinking, responding, and solving problems are established. For example, notice how easy it is for a child to pick up words from a foreign language. How difficult is that same task for an adult?

What does this mean for you as a parent? It means that you and the environment that you create for your baby will influence the way she deals with her emotions, the way she interacts with people, the way she thinks, and the way she grows physically. By creating an appropriate environment for your child, you are allowing normal brain development to take place. You may wonder what is considered an "appropriate" environment. It's one that is "child-centered" and provides opportunities for learning that are geared to your child's development, interests, and personality. Fortunately, the components of a good environment include basic things that many parents want to provide for their children: proper nutrition; a warm, responsive, and loving family as well as other providers; fun playtime; consistent positive reinforcement; engaging conversation; good books to read and to listen to; music to stimulate brain activities; and the freedom to explore and learn from their surroundings.

Review the following elements of children's health and how each one contributes to a child's brain development:

- *Language.* Direct face-to-face communication between parents and other caregivers and their young children supports language development, as does reading to them beginning in early infancy.
- *Early identification of developmental problems.* Many developmental and medical problems can be treated if detected early. Children with disabilities and other special healthcare needs also can greatly benefit from close monitoring of early brain development.
- *Positive parenting.* Raising a child in a loving, supportive, and respectful environment enhances self-esteem and self-confidence, and has a great impact on the child's development. Your parental nurturing and your responsiveness to your infant will play a critical role in shaping your baby's future.
- *Stimulating environment.* Exploring and problem solving in a variety of safe places promotes learning.

More and more behavioral researchers are discovering how much the environment plays a role in shaping a baby's life. This new science helps us understand exactly how significant our role is in the development of the child's brain.

To build a positive environment for your baby in your home and in your community, follow these suggestions:

- **Get good prenatal care.** Since brain development begins in the womb, good prenatal care can help ensure the healthy development of your child's brain. Start prenatal care early, see your doctor regularly, and be sure to follow her instructions. Eating a balanced, healthy diet and avoiding drugs, alcohol, and tobacco are just a few steps you can take to contribute to your child's future health.
- **Try to create a "village" around you.** Since it's hard to raise a child on your own, seek support from your family, friends, and community. Talk to your pediatrician about parent-support groups and activities.
- **Interact with your child as much as possible.** Talk with your child, read, listen to music, draw pictures, and play together. These kinds of activities allow you to spend time focused on your child's thoughts and interests. This, in turn, can make your child feel special and important. You also can teach the language of communication that your child will use to form healthy relationships over a lifetime.
- **Give your child plenty of love and attention.** A warm and loving environment helps children feel safe, competent, and cared for, as well as helping them feel concern for others. Such attention cannot "spoil" a child.
- **Provide consistent guidelines and rules.** Be sure you and other care providers are working with the same rules. Also, be sure your own rules and guidelines are consistent while taking into account your child's growing competency. Consistency helps children feel confident about what to expect from their environment.

States of Consciousness

As you get to know your baby, you'll soon realize that there are times when she's very alert and active, times when she's watchful but rather passive, and times when she's tired and irritable. You may even try to schedule your daily activities to capitalize on her "up" times and avoid overextending her during the "down" periods. Don't count on this schedule, however. These so-called states of consciousness will change dramatically in this first month.

There are actually six states of consciousness through which your baby cycles several times a day. Two are sleep states; the others are waking states.

State 1 is deep sleep, when the baby lies quietly without moving and is relatively unresponsive. If you shake a rattle loudly in her ear, she may stir a little, but not much. During lighter, more active sleep (State 2), the same noise will startle her and may awaken her. During this light sleep, you also can see the rapid movements of her eyes beneath her closed eyelids. She will alternate between these two sleep states, cycling through both of them within a given hour. Sometimes she'll retreat into these sleep states when she's overstimulated, as well as when she's physically tired.

Your Baby's States of Consciousness

State	Description	What Your Baby Does
State 1	Deep sleep	Lies quietly without moving
State 2	Light sleep	Moves while sleeping; startles at noises
State 3	Drowsiness	Eyes start to close; may doze
State 4	Quiet alert	Eyes open wide, face is bright; body is quiet
State 5	Active alert	Face and body move actively
State 6	Crying	Cries, perhaps screams; body moves in very disorganized ways

As your baby wakes up or starts to fall asleep, she'll go through State 3. Her eyes will roll back under drooping eyelids and she may stretch, yawn, or jerk her arms and legs. Once awake, she'll move into one of the three remaining states. She may be wide awake, happy, and alert but relatively motionless (State 4). Or she may be alert, happy, and very active (State 5). Or she may cry and flail about (State 6).

If you shake a rattle by your baby's ear when she's happy and alert (States 4 and 5), she'll probably become quiet and turn her face to look for the source of this strange sound. This is the time when she'll appear most responsive to you and the activity around her, and be most attentive and involved in play.

In general, it's a mistake to expect much attention from a baby who is crying. At these times, she's not receptive to new information or sensations; what she wants instead is to be comforted. The same rattle that enchanted her when she was happy five minutes earlier will only irritate her and make her more upset when she's crying. As she gets older, sometimes you may be able to distract her with an attractive object or sound so that she stops crying, but at this young age, the best way to comfort her usually is to pick her up and hold her. (See *Responding to Your Baby's Cries,* page 67.)

As your baby's nervous system becomes more developed, she'll begin to settle into a pattern of crying, sleeping, eating, and playing that matches your own daily schedule. She still may need to eat every three to four hours, but by the end of the month she'll be awake for longer periods during the day and be more alert and responsive at those times.

Colic

Does your infant have a regular fussy period each day when it seems you can do nothing to comfort her? This is quite common, particularly between 6:00 p.m. and midnight—just when you, too, are feeling tired from the day's trials and tribulations. These periods of crankiness may feel like torture, especially if you have other demanding children or work to do, but fortunately they don't last long. The length of this fussing usually peaks at about three hours a day by six weeks and then declines to one or two hours a day by three to four months. As long as the baby calms within a few hours and is relatively peaceful the rest of the day, there's no reason for alarm.

If the crying does not stop, but intensifies and persists throughout the day or night, it may be caused by colic. About one-fifth of all babies develop colic, usually between the second and fourth weeks. They cry inconsolably, often screaming, extending or pulling up their legs, and passing gas. Their stomachs may be enlarged or distended with gas. The crying spells can occur around the clock, although they often become worse in the early evening.

Unfortunately, there is no definite explanation for why this happens. Most often, colic means simply that the child is unusually sensitive to stimulation or cannot "self-console" or regulate her nervous system. (Also known as an immature nervous system.) As she matures, this inability to self-console—marked by constant crying—will improve. Generally this "colicky crying" will stop by three to four months, but it can last until six months of age. Sometimes, in breastfeeding babies, colic is a sign of sensitivity to a food in the mother's diet. The discomfort is caused only rarely by sensitivity to milk protein in formula. Colicky behavior also may signal a medical problem, such as a hernia or some type of illness.

Although you simply may have to wait it out, several things might be worth trying. First, of course, consult your pediatrician to make sure that the crying is not related to any serious medical condition that may require treatment. Then ask him which of the following would be most helpful.

- **If you're nursing,** you can try to eliminate milk products, caffeine, onions, cabbage, and any other potentially irritating foods from your own diet. If you're feeding formula to your baby, talk with your pediatrician about a protein hydrolysate formula. If food sensitivity is causing the discomfort, the colic should decrease within a few days of these changes.

- **Do not overfeed** your baby, which could make her uncomfortable. In general, try to wait at least two to two and a half hours from the start of one feeding to the start of the next one.

Abusive Head Trauma: Shaken Baby Syndrome

Shaking a baby is a serious form of child abuse that occurs mostly in infants in the first year of life. The act of severely or violently shaking a baby—which may also include striking the baby's head—is often the result of a parent's or caregiver's frustration or anger in response to a baby's or toddler's constant crying or irritability. Shaking or striking a baby's head can cause serious physical and mental damage, even death.

Serious injuries associated with abusive head trauma may include blindness or eye injuries, brain damage, damage to the spinal cord, and delay in normal development. Signs and symptoms may include irritability, lethargy (difficulty staying awake), tremors (shakiness), vomiting, seizures, difficulty breathing, and coma.

The American Academy of Pediatrics feels strongly that it is *never* okay to shake your baby. If you suspect that a care provider has shaken or hurt your baby—or if you or your spouse have done so in a moment of frustration—take your baby to the pediatrician or an emergency room immediately. Any brain damage that might have occurred will only get worse without treatment. Don't let embarrassment or fear keep you from getting treatment for your baby.

If you feel as if you might lose control when caring for your baby:

- Take a deep breath and count to ten.
- Put your baby in her crib or another safe place, leave the room, and let her cry alone.
- Call a friend or relative for emotional support.
- Give your pediatrician a call. Perhaps there's a medical reason why your baby is crying.

- **Walk your baby** in a baby carrier to soothe her. The motion and body contact will reassure her, even if her discomfort persists.
- **Rock her,** run the vacuum in the next room, or place her where she can hear the clothes dryer, a fan or a white-noise machine. Steady rhythmic motion and a calming sound may help her fall asleep. However, be sure to never place your child *on top* of the washer/dryer.
- **Introduce a pacifier.** While some breastfed babies will actively refuse it, it will provide instant relief for others. (See page 206.)
- **Lay your baby** tummy-down across your knees and gently rub her back. The pressure against her belly may help comfort her.
- **Swaddle her** in a large, thin blanket so that she feels secure and warm.
- **When you're feeling** tense and anxious, have a family member or a friend look after the baby—and get out of the house. Even an hour or two away will help you maintain a positive attitude. No matter how impatient or angry you become, a baby should *never* be shaken. Shaking an infant hard can cause blindness, brain damage, or even death (see sidebar *Abusive Head Trauma: Shaken Baby Syndrome*, page 192). Let your own doctor know if you are depressed or are having trouble dealing with your emotions, as she can recommend ways to help.

The First Smile

A few of the most important developments during this month are your baby's first smiles and giggles. These start during sleep, for reasons that are not understood. They may be a signal that the baby feels aroused in some way or is responding to some internal impulse. While it's great fun to watch a newborn smile her way through a nap, the real joy comes near the end of this month when she begins to grin back at you during her alert periods.

Those first loving smiles will help you tune in even more closely to each other, and you'll soon discover that you can predict when your baby will smile, look at you, make sounds, and, equally important, pause for time-out from play. Gradually you'll recognize each other's patterns of responsiveness so that your play together becomes a kind of dance in which you take turns leading and following. By identifying and responding to your child's subtle signals, even at this young age, you are telling her that her thoughts and feelings are important and that she can affect the world around her. These messages are vital to her developing self-esteem and sense of fun.

Movement

For the first week or two, your baby's movements will be very jerky. Her chin may quiver and her hands may tremble. She'll startle easily when moved suddenly or when she hears a loud sound, and the startling may lead to crying. If she appears overly sensitive to stimulation, she may be comforted if you hold her close to your body or swaddle her tightly in a blanket. There are even special blankets for swaddling small babies who are particularly difficult to console. But by the end of the first month, as her nervous system matures and her muscle control improves, these shakes and quivers will give way to much smoother arm and leg movements that look almost as if she's riding a bicycle. Lay her on her stomach now and she will make crawling motions with her legs and may even push up on her arms.

Your baby's neck muscles also will develop rapidly, giving her much more control over her head movements by the

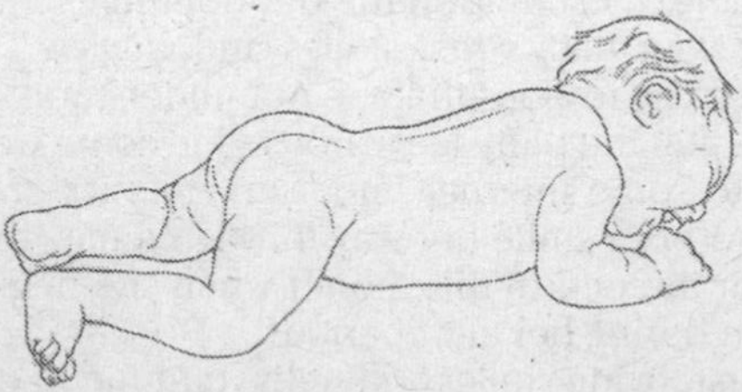

Movement Milestones by the End of This Period

- Makes jerky, quivering arm thrusts
- Brings hands within range of eyes and mouth
- Moves head from side to side while lying on stomach
- Head flops backward if unsupported
- Keeps hands in tight fists
- Strong reflex movements

end of this month. Lying on her stomach, she may lift her head and turn it from one side to the other. However, she won't be able to hold her head independently until about three months, so make sure you support it whenever you're holding her.

Your baby's hands, a source of endless fascination throughout much of this first year, will probably catch her eyes during these weeks. Her finger movements are limited, since her hands are likely to be clenched in tight fists most of the time. But she can flex her arms and bring her hands to her mouth and into her line of vision. While she can't control her hands precisely, she'll watch them closely as long as they're in view.

Vision

Your baby's vision will go through many changes this first month. She was born with peripheral vision (the ability to see to the sides), and she'll gradually acquire the ability to focus closely on a single point in the center of her visual field. She likes to look at objects held about 8 to 15 inches (20.3 to 38.1 cm) in front of her, but by one month she'll focus briefly on things as far away as 3 feet (91.4 cm).

At the same time, she'll learn to follow, or track, moving objects. To help her practice this skill, you can play tracking

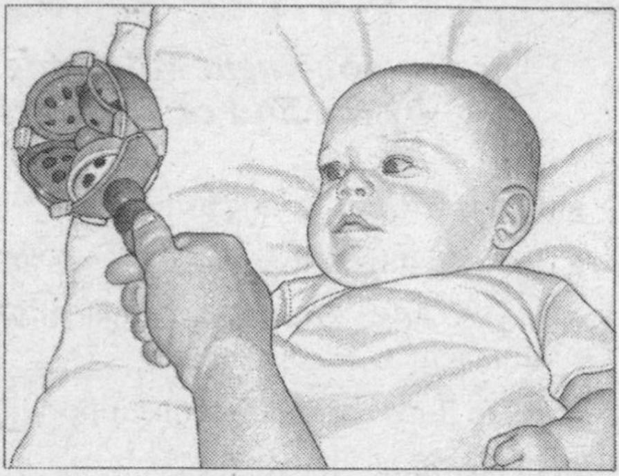

Your baby likes to look at objects held about 8 to 15 inches (20.3 to 38.1 cm) in front of him.

games with her. For example, move your head slowly from side to side as you hold her facing you; or pass a patterned object up and down or side to side in front of her (making sure it's within her range of focus). At first she may only be able to follow large objects moving slowly through an extremely limited range, but soon she'll be tracking even small, speedy movements.

At birth your baby was extremely sensitive to bright light, and her pupils were constricted (small) to limit the amount of light that entered her eyes. At two weeks of age, her pupils will begin to enlarge, allowing her to experience a broader range of shades of light and dark. As her retina (the light-sensitive tissue inside the eyeball) develops, her ability to see and recognize patterns also will improve.

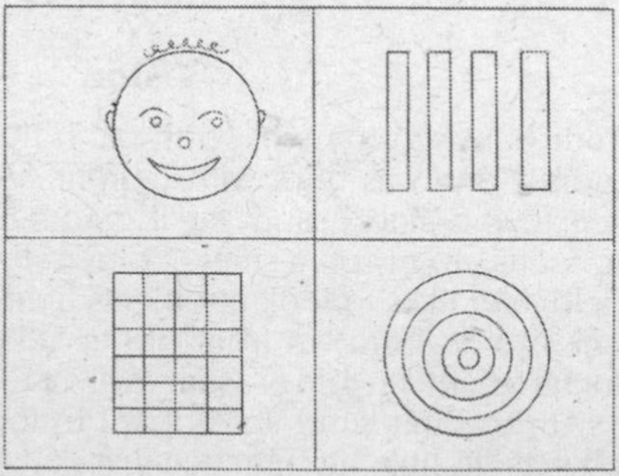

He is most attentive to black-and-white pictures or high contrast patterns, such as sharply contrasting stripes, bull's-eyes, checks, and very simple faces.

Visual Milestones by the End of This Period

- Focuses 8 to 12 inches (20.3 to 30.4 cm) away
- Eyes wander and occasionally cross
- Prefers black-and-white or high-contrast patterns
- Prefers the human face to all other patterns

The more contrast there is in a pattern, the more it will attract her attention, which is why she is most attentive to black-and-white pictures or high-contrast patterns, such as sharply contrasting stripes, bull's-eyes, checks, and very simple faces.

If you show your infant three identical toys—one blue, one yellow, one red—she probably will look longest at the red one, although no one yet understands why. Is it the color red itself? Or is it the brightness of this color that attracts newborn babies? We do know that color vision doesn't fully mature before about four months, so if you show your baby two related colors, such as green and turquoise, she probably can't tell the difference at this age.

Hearing

Your baby may have had a hearing test shortly after birth; in fact, the American Academy of Pediatrics recommends that newborn hearing screenings occur prior to every baby's discharge from the hospital, and parents should ask their pediatrician for the results. (See *Hearing Loss*, pages 549–553.)

Infants born with normal hearing abilities will pay close attention to human voices during the first month, especially high-pitched ones speaking "baby talk." When you talk to her, she'll turn her head to search for you and listen closely as you sound out different syllables and words. Watch carefully

Hearing Milestones by the End of This Period

- Hearing is fully mature
- Recognizes some sounds
- May turn toward familiar sounds and voices

and you may even see her make subtle movements of her arms and legs in time with your speech.

Your infant also will be sensitive to noise levels. If you make a loud clicking sound in her ear or bring her into a noisy, crowded room, she may "shut down," becoming as unresponsive as if she had heard nothing. Or she may be so sensitive that she startles, erupts into crying, and turns her entire body away from the noise. (Extremely sensitive babies also will cry when exposed to a very bright light.) Substitute the sound of a soft rattle or quiet music and she'll become alert and turn her head and eyes to locate the source of this interesting sound.

Not only does your baby hear well, but even at this age, she'll remember some of the sounds she hears. Some mothers who repeatedly read a story aloud late in their pregnancy have found—and some research supports—that their babies seemed to recognize the story when it was read to them again after birth—the babies became quiet and looked more attentive. Try reading your favorite children's story aloud for several days in a row at times when your baby is alert and attentive. Then wait a day or two and read it again. Does she seem to recognize it?

Smell and Touch

Just as babies prefer certain patterns and sounds, they are typically very particular about tastes and smells. They will breathe deeply to catch a whiff of milk, vanilla, banana, or sugar, but will turn up their nose at the smell of alcohol or vinegar. By the end of their first week, if they're nursing, they'll turn toward their mother's breast pad but will ignore

Smell and Touch Milestones by the End of This Period

- Prefers sweet smells
- Avoids bitter or acidic smells
- Recognizes the scent of her own mother's breastmilk
- Prefers soft to coarse sensations
- Dislikes rough or abrupt handling

the pads of other nursing mothers. This radarlike system helps direct them at feeding times and warn them away from substances that could harm them.

Babies are equally sensitive to touch and the way you handle them. They'll nestle into a soft piece of flannel or satin, but pull away from scratchy burlap or coarse sandpaper. When they are stroked gently with a palm, they'll relax and become quiet. If they're picked up roughly, they'll probably take offense and start to cry. If they're picked up gently and rocked slowly, they'll become quiet and attentive. Holding, stroking, rocking, and cuddling will calm them when they're upset and make them more alert when they're drowsy. It also sends a clear message of a parent's love and affection. Long before they understand a word that parents say, they'll understand parental moods and feelings from the way they are touched.

Temperament

Consider these two babies, both from the same family, both girls:

- **The first infant** is calm and quiet, happy to play by herself. She watches everything that happens around her, but rarely demands attention herself. Left on her own, she sleeps for long periods and eats infrequently.

- **The second baby** is fussy and startles easily. She thrashes her arms and legs, moving almost constantly whether awake or asleep. While most newborns sleep fourteen hours a day, she sleeps only ten, and wakens whenever there's the slightest activity nearby. She seems in a hurry to do everything at once and even eats in a rush, gulping her feedings and swallowing so much air that she needs frequent burping.

Both these babies are absolutely normal and healthy. One is no "better" than the other, but because their personalities are so far apart, the two will be treated very differently, right from birth.

Like these babies, your infant will demonstrate many unique personality traits from the earliest weeks of life. Discovering these traits is one of the most exciting parts of having a new baby. Is she very active and intense, or relatively slow-going? Is she timid when faced with a new situation, such as the first bath, or does she enjoy it? You'll find clues to

Developmental Health Watch

If during the second, third, or fourth weeks of your baby's life she shows any of the following signs of developmental delay, notify your pediatrician.

- Sucks poorly and feeds slowly
- Doesn't blink when shown a bright light
- Doesn't focus and follow a nearby object moving side to side
- Rarely moves arms and legs; seems stiff
- Seems excessively loose in the limbs or floppy
- Lower jaw trembles constantly, even when not crying or excited
- Doesn't respond to loud sounds

Toys Appropriate for Your Baby's First Month

- Mobile with highly contrasting colors and patterns
- Unbreakable mirror attached securely to inside of crib
- Music players with soft music
- Soft, brightly colored and patterned toys that make gentle sounds

her personality in everything she does, from falling asleep to crying. The more you pay attention to these signals and learn to respond appropriately to her unique personality, the calmer and more predictable your life will be in the months to come.

While most of these early character traits are built into the newborn's hereditary makeup, their appearance may be delayed if your baby is born quite prematurely. Premature babies don't express their needs—such as hunger, fatigue, or discomfort—as clearly as other newborns. They may be extra sensitive to light, sound, and touch for several months. Even playful conversation may be too intense for them and cause them to become fussy and look away. When this happens, it's up to the parent to stop and wait until the baby is alert and ready for more attention. Eventually most of these early reactions will fade away, and the baby's own natural character traits will become more evident.

Babies who are less than 5.5 pounds or 2.5 kg at birth (low birth weight), even if they're full term, also may be less responsive than other newborns. At first they may be very sleepy and not seem very alert. After a few weeks they seem to wake up, eating eagerly but still remaining irritable and hypersensitive to stimulation between feedings. This irritability may last until they grow and mature further.

From the very beginning, your baby's temperamental traits will influence the way you treat her and feel about her. If you had specific ideas about child rearing before she was born, reevaluate them now to see if they're really in tune with her character. The same goes for expert advice—from books, articles, and especially from well-meaning relatives and friends—about the "right way" to raise a child. The truth is, there is no right way that works for every child. You have to create your own guidelines based on your child's unique personality, your own beliefs, and the circumstances of your family life. The important thing is to remain responsive to your baby's individuality. Don't try to box her into some previously set mold or pattern. Your baby's uniqueness is her strength, and respecting that strength from the start will help lay the best possible foundation for her high self-esteem and for loving relationships with others.

BASIC CARE

Feeding and Nutrition

(See Chapter 4 for additional information)

Breastmilk or formula should be your child's sole nutritional source for the first four to six months, and the major source of nutrition throughout the first twelve months. During this time, you and your pediatrician will need to pay attention to her pattern of feedings and make sure that she's getting enough for growth. Regular checkups and monitoring of growth is the best way to ensure this.

Here are some important points to keep in mind about feeding:

- **Establishing a pattern** of feedings does not mean setting a rigid timetable and insisting that your baby breastfeed for a set amount of time or eat a full 4 ounces (120 ml) at each feeding. It's much more important to pay attention to your baby's signals and work around her needs. If she is bottle-fed, she probably will cry at the end of her feeding if she is not getting enough. On the other hand, if she is getting an adequate amount in the first ten minutes, she may stop and fall asleep.
- **During the first** month, breastfed babies indicate interest in feeding when they begin to root (reflexively turn

Vitamin D and Your Baby

With the nutrition of infants and other children in mind, pediatricians are now giving more attention to the importance of vitamin D in the overall well-being of children. The American Academy of Pediatrics recommends that all infants and children should have a daily intake of vitamin D of at least 400 IU, starting soon after birth. This recommendation is based on recent research that this level of vitamin D can be given safely in babies, strengthening their immune system and preventing diseases such as diabetes and cancer.

Talk to your pediatrician about the importance of giving vitamin D to your own baby, and the optimal way to administer it.

Signs of Feeding Difficulties

The following are some possible warning signs of feeding problems, and should be discussed with your pediatrician.

Too Much Feeding:

- If bottle-fed, the baby is consuming more than 4 to 6 ounces (120 to 180 ml) per feeding.
- She vomits most or all the food after a complete feeding.
- Her stools are loose and very watery, eight or more times a day. (Keep in mind that breastfed babies normally tend to have much more frequent and looser stools.)

Too Little Feeding:

- If breastfed, the baby stops feeding after ten minutes or less.

- She wets fewer than four diapers per day; particularly if she has begun sleeping through the night, she may be feeding inadequately (since most babies feed at least once during the night), and may urinate less often and become mildly dehydrated.
- She has infrequent or very hard stools in the first month.
- She appears hungry, searching for something to suck shortly after feedings.
- She becomes more yellow, instead of less, during the first week.

Feeding Allergy or Digestive Disturbance:

- Your baby vomits most or all food after a complete feeding.
- She produces loose and very watery stools eight or more times a day or has blood in the stools.
- She has a severe skin rash.

toward the breast) or place their fist in their mouth and start sucking. Crying is a late sign of hunger. It is easier to get the baby to latch on and feed when she is showing the early signs of rooting or lip smacking.

- **Your baby should** be fed at least every two to three hours on demand, with attempts to feed eight to twelve times a day. During the first month, your baby should be feeding through the day and night. In fact, it may be troubling if your baby is sleeping contentedly through the night; she may not be getting enough to eat.
- **Generally, your baby** will feed adequately in about fifteen to twenty minutes. By this time, she will frequently begin to look drowsy or fall asleep. If she still acts hungry after feeding well on the first breast or wakes up during a diaper change, offer the other breast. Very long feedings may indicate that the baby is not latched on well or ingesting enough milk to become full or satiated.

Growth spurts can occur at different times for different babies. At the beginning of the second week and again between three and six weeks, your baby may go through growth spurts that may make her hungrier than usual. Even if you don't notice any outward growth, her body is changing in important ways and needs extra calories during these times. Be prepared to feed her more often if she's breastfed; more frequent breastfeeding will stimulate more milk production by the mother's body. If your baby is bottle-fed, try giving her slightly more at each feeding.

If your baby has a nutritional problem, she's likely to start losing weight or not gain adequately. There are some signals that may help you detect such a problem. Your breasts will typically become quite full from two to five days after giving birth. After this time, you should notice that your breasts feel full and somewhat firm before feeding and soften after feeding. While your baby nurses on one breast, you may notice some milk dripping or spraying from the other breast.

If you fail to notice fullness in your breasts after five days or you don't see milk dripping from your breast at the start of each feeding, you may not have an adequate milk supply or the baby may not be providing enough stimulation when she sucks. These also may be signs of medical problems that are unrelated to your baby's nutrition, so call your pediatrician if they persist. Every infant should have a checkup within three to five days after birth and forty-eight to seventy-two hours after hospital discharge to help detect any problems.

Most babies this age begin to spit up occasionally after feedings. That's because the muscular valve between the esophagus (the passage between throat and stomach) and the stomach is immature. Instead of closing tightly, it remains open enough to allow the contents of the stomach to come back up and gently spill out of the mouth. This could be normal, may not harm your baby, and will resolve as your baby grows, usually by one year of age. If your baby is gaining weight appropriately and does not have any other problems, it should reassure you. But if spitting up occurs frequently or is associated with diarrhea, rash, or failure to gain weight, this may indicate a food allergy or problem with the gastrointestinal tract and your physician should be contacted.

You also do not necessarily need to be concerned if your newborn has a bowel movement every time she feeds—or only once a week. If your infant is otherwise feeding normally, there is a wide range of acceptable bowel patterns. (Other warning signs of feeding problems appear in the box *Signs of Feeding Difficulties* on pages 203–204.)

Carrying Your Baby

A newborn or very young infant who has not developed head control needs to be carried in a way that keeps her head from flopping from side to side or snapping from front to back. This is done by cradling the head when carrying the baby in a lying position and supporting the head and neck with your hand when carrying the baby upright.

Pacifiers

Many babies soothe themselves by sucking. If your baby wants to suck beyond nursing or bottle-feeding, a pacifier can satisfy that need.

A pacifier is meant to satisfy your baby's noneating sucking needs, not to replace or delay meals. So offer a pacifier to your baby only after or between feedings, when you are

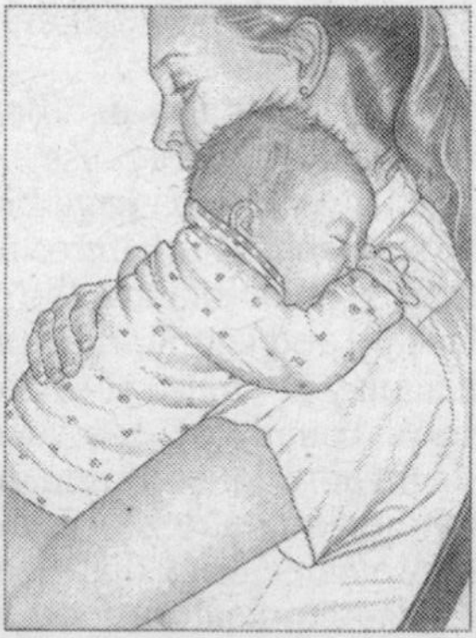

A very young infant who has not developed head control needs to be carried in a way that keeps her head from flopping from side to side or snapping from front to back.

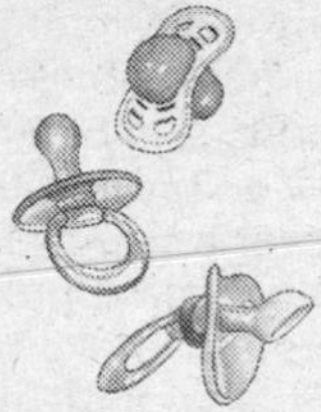

sure she is not hungry. If she is hungry, and you offer a pacifier as a substitute, she may become so angry that it interferes with feeding or she may not get enough to eat. Remember, the pacifier is for your baby's benefit, not your convenience, so let her decide whether and when to use it.

Still, offering a pacifier when your baby is going to sleep may help reduce the risk of SIDS (sudden infant death syndrome), although doctors do not know the reason for this. If you are breastfeeding, wait until your baby is one month old before using a pacifier. However, if your baby doesn't want it or if it falls out of her mouth, don't force it because it may interfere with breastfeeding.

If your baby does use a pacifier to fall asleep, she may wake up when it falls out of her mouth. When she's younger, she may cry for you to put it back for her. Babies who suck their fingers or hands have a real advantage here, because their hands are always readily available. Once your baby is older and has the hand coordination to find and replace it, there should be no problem.

When shopping for a pacifier, look for a one-piece model that has a soft nipple. (Some models can break into two pieces and become a choking hazard.) It should be dishwasher-safe so you can either boil it or run it through the dishwasher before your baby uses it. Until she's six months old, you should clean the pacifier this way frequently, so she's not exposed to any increased risk of infection, as her immune system is still maturing. After that, the likelihood of her picking up an infection in that way is minimal, so you can just wash it with soap and rinse it in clear water.

Pacifiers are available in a variety of shapes and sizes. Once you decide which your baby prefers, buy some extras. Pacifiers have a way of disappearing or falling on the floor or street when you need them most. However, never try to solve this problem by fastening the pacifier with a cord around your baby's neck. Babies can choke or strangle on the cords, strings, ribbons, and fasteners attached to pacifiers, whether or not they go around the child's neck. Also, for safety reasons, it's never a good idea to make pacifiers out of a bottle nipple. Babies have pulled the nipple out of such homemade pacifiers and choked on them. Babies also can choke on a pacifier that's not the right size for their age, so be sure to follow the recommended age range for each pacifier.

Going Outside

Fresh air and a change of surroundings are good for both you and your baby, even in her first month, so take her out for walks when the weather is nice. Be sure to dress her properly for these outings, however. Her internal temperature control isn't fully mature until the end of her first year. This makes it difficult for her to regulate her body temperature when she's exposed to excessive heat or cold. Her clothing must do some of this work for her by keeping heat in when she is in a cold location and letting heat escape when she's in a very warm place. In general, she should wear one more layer than you do.

Here are a few suggestions for those outings with your baby:

- **Your infant's skin** also is extremely susceptible to sunburn during the first six months, so it's important to keep her out of direct and reflected sunlight (e.g., off of water, sand, or concrete) as much as possible. If you must take her out in the sun, dress her in lightweight and light-colored clothing, with a bonnet or hat to shade her face. If she is lying or sitting in one place, make sure it is shady, and adjust her position to keep her in the shade as the sun moves. Sunscreen can be used in infants under six months of age if protective clothing, hats, and shade are not available, but apply it only on small areas of the body such as the face and the backs of the hands. Test it out ahead of time on a small patch on her back to make sure she isn't sensitive to it. (When your child is a little older—over six months of age—sunscreen can be applied to all areas of the body, while being careful to avoid the eyes.)

- **Another warning for** the hot-weather months: Do not let baby equipment (such as car safety seats and strollers) sit in the sun for a long period of time. When that happens, the plastic and metal parts can get hot enough to burn your child. Check the surface temperature of any such equipment before you allow your baby to come in contact with it.
- **In uncomfortably cold** or rainy weather, keep your baby inside as much as possible. If you have to go out, bundle her up and use a warm hat to cover her head and ears. You can shield her face from the cold with a blanket when you're outside.
- **To check whether** she's clothed appropriately, feel her hands and feet and the skin on her chest. Her hands and feet should be slightly cooler than her body, but not cold. Her chest should feel warm. If her hands, feet, and chest feel cold, take her to a warm room, unwrap her, and feed her something warm or hold her close so the heat from your body warms her. Until her temperature is back to normal, extra layers of clothing will just trap the cold, so use these other methods to warm her body before wrapping her in additional blankets or clothing.

Finding Help at Home

Most families need some in-house help when they bring a new baby home. If your partner is able to take a few days off from work during the first week or two, this will help a lot. If this isn't an option, the next best choice is to ask a close relative or friend. If relatives are not available, hiring a baby nurse is sometimes a good option. If you think you'll need the extra help, especially if it is going to be a baby nurse, it is wise to make these arrangements in advance rather than waiting until after the delivery to seek it.

Some communities have a visiting nurse or homemaking service. This will not solve your middle-of-the-night problems, but it will provide an hour or two during the day to catch up on work or simply rest a little. These arrangements, too, should be made in advance.

Be selective about the help you seek. Look for assistance from those who will really support you. Your goal is to reduce the stress level in your home, not add to it.

Before you start interviewing or asking friends or family for assistance, decide exactly what kind of help will work best for you. Ask yourself the following questions:

- Do you want someone who can help you tend to the baby, or do the housework, or cook meals—or a little bit of everything?
- During what hours do you want help?
- Do you need someone who can drive (to pick up other children at school, shop for groceries, run errands, and the like)?

Once you know what you need, make sure the person you choose to help out understands and agrees to meet those needs. Explain your expectations clearly to her, and if this is an employment situation, put those expectations in writing. She should be someone you trust. If employing help, be certain that a background check has been performed and the person has basic life-support training. If she will be driving, her driving record should be checked. Regardless if this is a relative, friend, or employee, ask her to notify you if she is ill so she doesn't pass any infections to your baby.

Your Baby's First Sitter. Sometime in the first month or two, you may need to leave your baby for the first time, often to take a break or run an errand. The more confidence you have in your babysitter, the easier this experience will be for you. Therefore, you may want to have your first sitter be someone very close and trusted—a grandparent, close friend, or relative who's familiar with both you and the child.

After your first separation, you may want to look for a regular babysitter. You can ask your friends, neighbors, and coworkers for recommendations, or see if your pediatrician or nurse practitioner can refer you to someone. Local child care agencies or referral services are great resources and should be one of the first places to look. If that still doesn't yield any names, contact the placement services at local colleges for a listing of child development or early education students who babysit. You also can find the names of sitters in community newspapers, telephone directories, and church and grocery store bulletin boards, but remember that no one screens the people in these listings. *It is absolutely essential that you check references—inquiring about the sitter's responsibility, maturity, and ability to adhere to instructions—particularly for someone you've only recently met or don't know well.*

Interview every candidate in person and with your baby present. You should be looking for someone who is affectionate, capable, and supports your views about child care. If you feel comfortable with the individual after you've talked awhile, let her hold the baby so you can see how she handles the infant. Ask if she's had experience caring for babies. Although experience, references, and good health are very important, the best way to judge a babysitter is by giving her a trial run while you're home. It will give your baby and the babysitter a chance to get to know each other before they're alone together, and it will give you an opportunity to make sure you feel comfortable with the sitter.

Whenever you leave your child with a sitter, give her a list of all emergency phone numbers, including those where you or other close family members can be contacted if problems arise; she should know where you'll be and how to reach you at all times. Establish clear guidelines about what to do in an emergency, and remind her about calling 911 for emergency help. Show her where all exits from your home are located, as well as smoke detectors and fire extinguishers. Make sure your sitter has taken an approved CPR class (from the American Red Cross, for example), and has learned how to respond when a child is choking or not breathing. (See *Cardiopulmonary Resuscitation and Mouth-to-Mouth Resuscitation,* page 575; *Choking,* page 576); in fact, some local YMCAs or American Red Cross chapters can provide a list of babysitters who have taken CPR or babysitting safety courses. Give your sitter any other guidelines that you feel are important (e.g., she should never open the door to strangers, including delivery people). Ask the sitter to jot down any notes or questions she has about your child. Let friends and neighbors know about your arrangement so they can help if there's an emergency, and ask them to tell you if they suspect any problems in your absence.

Traveling with Your Baby

The key to traveling with your baby during this time is to maintain her normal patterns as much as possible. Long trips involving a change of time zones can disturb your baby's sleep schedule. So do your best to plan your activities according to the schedule your child is on and allow several days for her to adjust to a time change if possible. If she awakens very early in the morning, plan to start your own activities earlier. Be ready to stop earlier, too, because your little one might be getting tired and cranky long before the clock says it's time to go to bed. Always remember to perform a safety inspection of any cribs when checking into a hotel. (See *Cribs,* page 388.)

If you're going to remain in a new time zone for more than two or three days, your baby's internal time clock gradually will shift to coincide with the time zone you're in. You'll have to adjust mealtimes to match the times when her body is telling her she's hungry. Mom and Dad—and even older children—may be able to postpone meals to fit the new time zone, but a baby isn't able to make those adjustments as easily.

Here are some other suggestions when traveling:

- **Your baby will** adapt to her new environment more quickly if you bring some familiar things from home. A favorite rattle and toy will provide some comfort and reassurance. Use her regular soap, a familiar towel, and bring along one of her tub toys to make her more at ease during baths.
- **When packing for** a trip with your baby, it's usually best to use a separate bag for her things. This makes it easier to find items quickly when you want them and reduces the chance that you'll forget an important one. You'll also need a large diaper bag for bottles, formula if formula-feeding, pacifier, a changing pad, diapers, diaper ointment, and baby wipes. Keep this bag with you at all times.

- **When traveling by** car, make sure your child is safely strapped into her safety seat. For more information on car safety seats, see page 406. The backseat is the safest place for children to ride. Rear-facing seats should never be placed in the front seat of a car with a passenger-side airbag. At this age a baby always should ride in the rear-facing position. The same car seat safety rules apply in rental cars, taxis, and any vehicle your baby rides in.
- **Always use a** car safety seat on planes and trains. If you're not sure how to secure your baby safely on a plane or train, ask a flight attendant or a conductor to help you. Unless you buy a ticket for the baby, you'll be expected to carry her on your lap, which the AAP and numerous other safety advocates strongly discourage. All children should travel with proper restraints on an aircraft. This would mean that your baby needs her own seat on the plane. When there is extra room on board, you may be able to get a separate seat for the baby without paying for it. Talk with your travel agent or an airline ticketing representative about how to increase the chances that an empty seat will be available, but the only way to ensure that your baby has her own seat is to purchase one for her ahead of time.
- **If your baby** is bottle-fed, bring not only enough formula for the expected travel time, but plenty extra in case any unexpected delays occur. If you're nursing and are concerned about privacy on a plane or train, bring a nursing cover or ask for some blankets you can use as a screen.
- **A bottle (or pacifier)** may have other benefits when traveling with a baby by plane. The rapid changes in air pressure associated with air travel can cause discomfort in the baby's middle ear. Babies cannot intentionally "pop" their ears as adults can (by swallowing or yawning), but this relief within the ear may occur when they suck on a bottle or pacifier. To reduce the risk of pain, feed your baby during takeoff and landing.

The Family

A Special Message to Mothers

One reason why this first month can be especially difficult is that you are still recovering physically from the stress of pregnancy and delivery. It may take weeks before your body is back to normal, your incisions (if you had an episiotomy or C-section) have healed, and you're able to resume everyday activities. You also may experience strong mood swings due to changes in the amount of hormones in your body. These changes can prompt sudden crying episodes for no apparent reason or feelings of mild depression for the first few weeks. These emotions may be intensified by the exhaustion that comes with waking up every two or three hours at night to feed and change the baby.

If you experience these so-called postpartum blues, they may make you feel a little "crazy," embarrassed, or even that you're a "bad mother." Difficult as it may be, try to keep these emotions in perspective by reminding yourself that they're normal after pregnancy and delivery. Even fathers sometimes feel sad and unusually emotional after a new baby arrives (possibly a response to the psychological intensity of the experience). To keep the blues from dominating your life—and your enjoyment of your new baby—avoid isolating yourself in these early weeks. Try to nap when your baby does, so you don't get overtired. If these feelings persist past a few weeks or become severe, consult your pediatrician or your own physician about getting extra help. (For more information about the postpartum blues, see also Chapter 5, pages 168–169.)

Visitors often can help you combat the blues by celebrating the baby's arrival with you. They may bring welcome gifts for the baby or—even better during these early weeks—offer food or household help. But they also can be exhausting for you and overwhelming for the baby, and may expose her to infection. It is wise to strictly limit the number of visitors during the first couple of weeks, and keep anyone with a cough, cold, or contagious disease away from your newborn. Ask all visitors to call in advance, wash their hands before holding the baby, and keep their visits brief until you're back to a regular schedule. If the baby seems unsettled by all the attention, don't let anyone outside the family hold or come close to her.

If you become overwhelmed with phone calls, consider leaving a message on your voice mail with information you may want to share about your new baby such as sex, name, birth date, time, weight, and length. State that you are spending time with your family and you will return the call when you have a moment. Then turn off your ringer. This way you can return the calls on your schedule without feeling stressed or guilty every time the phone rings. With a new baby, constant visitors, an aching body, unpredictable mood swings, and, in some cases, other siblings demanding attention, it's no wonder many routine activities in your home will get neglected. Resign yourself ahead of time to knowing that this will happen. What's important is to concentrate on recuperating and enjoying your new baby. If need be, allow extended family and friends to lend a hand with all the other tasks now and then. This is not a sign of weakness; it shows that your priorities are in the right place. And it also allows loved ones to both care for you and feel like they, too, are a part of this new child's life.

A Special Message to Fathers

While this time can be challenging for new fathers, it can also be uniquely rewarding. Just as mothers occasionally need to readjust their priorities, fathers now have a golden opportunity to show more of their nurturing side by caring for Mom, the baby, and possibly other siblings. Although not all fathers have the option of paternity leave from work, those who do and take advantage of it may find it priceless. If Mom was the center of a sibling's universe and Dad was only an afterthought, Dad may suddenly be more "cool" once a newborn comes home. By adjusting his priorities (at home and at work) and "rising to the occasion," Dad can strengthen an already strong bond with Mom as well as with the new child. By working as a team, parenting couples may be amazed at how well they can adapt to their new, stressful circumstances.

Of course, balancing the seemingly constant demands of the baby, the needs of other children, and the household

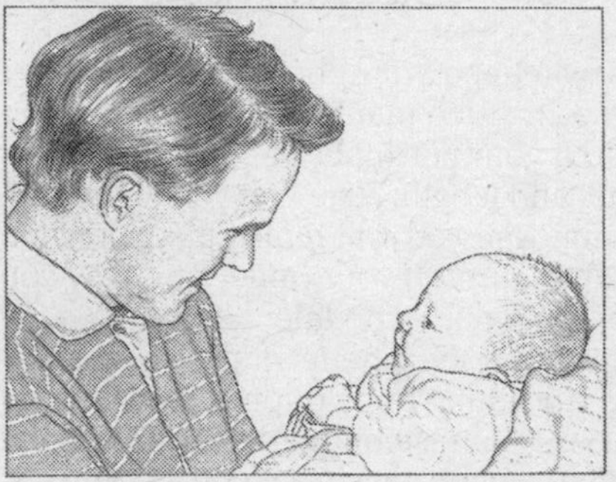

Become as involved as possible in caring for and playing with the new baby. You'll get just as emotionally attached to her as her mother will.

chores is not always easy. Nights spent feeding, diapering, and walking the floor with a crying baby can quickly take their toll in fatigue for both parents. But by working as a team to relieve each other for naps, for exercise, and for "downtime," parenting couples might find that even though they share less "quality time" together, they may actually feel closer than ever. Sometimes there may be conflict and jealous feelings. These are normal, and thankfully, temporary. Life soon settles into a fairly regular routine that will once again give you some time to yourselves and restore your sex life and social activities to normal. Meanwhile, make an effort for just the two of you to spend some time together each day enjoying each other's company while the baby is sleeping or somebody else is caring for her.

Remember, you're entitled to hold, hug, cuddle, and kiss each other as well as the baby.

A positive way for men to deal with these issues is to become as involved as possible in caring for and playing with the new baby. When you spend this extra time with your child, you'll get just as emotionally attached to her as her mother will.

This is not to say that moms and dads play with babies the same way. In general, fathers play to arouse and excite their babies, while mothers generally concentrate on more low-key stimulation such as gentle rocking, quiet interactive

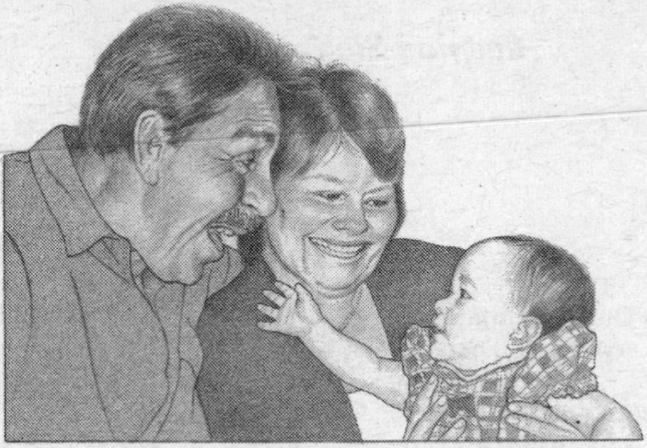

games, singing, and soothing activities. From the baby's viewpoint, both play styles are equally valuable and complement each other beautifully, which is another reason why it's so important to have both of you involved in the care of the baby.

A Special Message to Grandparents

The first time you gaze into the eyes of your new grandchild, you probably will be overwhelmed by many feelings: love, wonder, amazement, and joy, among many other emotions. You might find yourself reflecting back on when your own children were born and feel enormous pride now that your own adult child is raising a family of her own.

Depending on your other responsibilities and how close you live to your grandchild, you can and should play as active a role as possible in the life of the new baby. Research shows that children who have grandparents participating in their lives fare better throughout childhood and later in life. You have plenty of love and lots of hugs to give, and they can make a difference. As you spend time with your grandchild, you'll form and strengthen a lasting bond and become an invaluable source of nurturing and guidance.

If you live in the same city as your new grandchild, make frequent visits at times deemed appropriate by your

Keeping Siblings Happy

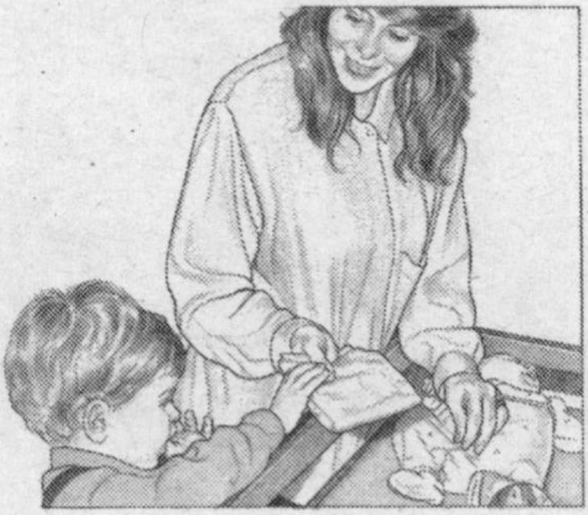

Once the infant arrives, you can expect your older child to be very proud and protective.

With all the excitement over the new baby's arrival, siblings might feel somewhat neglected. They still may be a little upset over their mother's hospitalization, especially if this was their first prolonged separation from her. Even after Mom returns home, they may have trouble understanding that she's tired and cannot play with them as much as they're used to. Compound this with the attention she's now devoting to the baby—attention that just a couple of weeks ago belonged to them!—and it's no wonder that they may feel jealous and left out. It's up to both parents to find ways to reassure the siblings that they're still very much loved and valued, and to help them come to terms with their new "competition."

Here are some suggestions to help soothe your older children and make them feel more involved during the first month home with your new baby.

1. If possible, have the siblings visit mother and baby in the hospital.

2. When Mom comes home from the hospital, bring each sibling a special gift to celebrate.

3. Set aside a special time to spend alone with each sibling every day. Make sure that both Mom and Dad have time with each child, individually and together.

4. While you're taking pictures of the new baby, take some of the older children—alone and with the baby.

5. Ask the grandparents or other close relatives to take the older children on a special outing—to the zoo, a movie, or just dinner. This special attention may help them through moments when they feel abandoned.

6. Have some small gifts for the older child and present them when friends come with gifts for the baby.

7. Especially during the first month, when the baby needs to eat so often, older children can get very jealous of the intimacy you have with the baby during feedings. Show them that you can share this intimacy by turning feeding times into story times. Reading stories that specifically deal with issues of jealousy encourages a toddler or preschooler to voice her feelings so that you can help her become more accepting.

adult child. (Don't show up uninvited on the doorstep, and of course know when to leave.) At the same time, also encourage their family to visit you at your home. (Make sure that your home is childproofed in the ways recommended in this book.) Minimize the advice and certainly the criticism you offer the new parents; instead, give them support, respect their opinions, and be patient. They may have approaches to child rearing that are somewhat different from yours, but remember that they're the parents now. If they should ask, "Mom, what do you think I should do about . . . ?", then of course provide some input. Share your point of view, but don't try to impose your beliefs on them.

Remember, it's been a while since you were raising your

own babies, and although much may be the same, much has changed, as well. Ask how you can support the new parents in the child-rearing process, and take your lead from them on how, when, and how often to get involved. For example, you might focus on basic baby care, including feeding and changing diapers, but don't try to take over. Also, offer them a break from time to time by giving them a night out (or, at some point, perhaps a weekend away). No matter how often you visit, however, make regular phone calls, not only during your grandchild's infancy, but also in the upcoming years when you're actually able to have a conversation with her.

Later, as your grandchild grows, tell her stories of what her own mother or father was like during childhood. (Sharing the family history and teaching family values are important contributions you can make as your grandchild becomes older.) In the meantime, consider keeping your own scrapbook of photos and other mementos of your grandchild that you can share with her someday; as part of that scrapbook, create a family tree that the entire family can contribute to. Make it a priority to get together on holidays, attend birthday parties, and, later on, go to as many soccer matches and Little League games as possible.

If you live hundreds of miles away, and thus can't be as much of a presence in your grandchild's life as you'd like, you still can be an excellent long-distance grandparent. One option: E-mail is a wonderful way to stay in touch. If the new parents have a digital camera, ask them to e-mail photographs of your grandchild to you that you can view on your computer or on a digital photo frame. Maybe they can make and share videotapes of your grandchild, as well. Make some videos of you and your spouse that your children can share with your grandchild when she is older.

Health Watch

The following medical problems are of particular concern to parents during the first month. (For problems that occur generally throughout childhood, check the listings in Part II.)

Breathing Difficulties. Normally, your baby should take from twenty to forty breaths per minute. This pattern is most regular when she is asleep and healthy. When awake, occasionally she may breathe rapidly for a short period, then take a brief pause (less than ten seconds) before returning to normal breathing. This is called periodic breathing. A runny nose may interfere with breathing because your baby's nasal passages are narrow and fill easily. This condition can be eased by using a cool-mist humidifier and gently suctioning the nose with a rubber aspirating bulb (ordinarily given to you by the hospital; for its use, see page 260). Occasionally, mild salt-solution nose drops are used to help thin the mucus and clear the nasal passages. If she has a fever, notify your pediatrician right away. Her breathing may become faster, increasing by about two breaths per minute for each degree of temperature elevation. When the number of breaths exceeds sixty per minute, or the baby's chest muscles are retracting, her nose is flaring, or she is coughing a lot, be sure to contact your pediatrician. A fever with a temperature higher than 100.4 degrees Fahrenheit (38 degrees Celsius) in a one-month-old baby may be serious and you should call the doctor.

Diarrhea. A baby has diarrhea if she produces loose, very watery stools more than six to eight times a day. Diarrhea usually is caused by a viral infection. The danger, especially at this young age, is of losing too much fluid and becoming dehydrated. The first signs of dehydration are a dry mouth and a significant decrease in the number of wet diapers. But don't wait for dehydration to occur. Call your pediatrician if the stools are very loose or occur more often than after each feeding (six to eight per day).

Constipation. The first week a baby should be producing a stool at least once a day. If not, call your pediatrician as your infant may have a condition that makes it difficult for the stool to pass. Or it may be a sign that your baby isn't getting enough to eat. Once your baby has demonstrated that he is eating and pooping well, at a few weeks of age his pattern will become more predictable.

Excessive Sleepiness. Since each infant requires a different amount of sleep, it's difficult to tell when a baby is excessively drowsy. If your infant starts sleeping much more than usual, it might indicate the presence of an infection, so notify your pediatrician. Also, if you are nursing and your baby sleeps more than five hours without a feeding in the first month, you must consider the possibility that she is not getting enough milk or perhaps is being affected, through the breastmilk, by a medication that you are taking. Bottle-fed babies may also be sleepy from inadequate feeding or any herbal medication administered by parents.

Eye Infections/Tear-Production Problems. Some babies are born with one or both tear ducts partially or totally blocked. They typically open by about two weeks, when tear production begins. If they don't, the blockage may cause a watery or mucous tearing. In this case, the tears will back up and flow over the eyelids instead of draining through the nose. This is not harmful, and the ducts generally will open without treatment, usually by nine months of age. You also may help open them by gently massaging the inner corner of the eye and down the side of the nose. However, do this only at the direction of your pediatrician.

If the ducts remain blocked, it will keep the tears from draining properly. Although this will produce pus, it does not mean your baby has an infection, or "pinkeye" (see page 225). You may see a greenish-yellow or white discharge in the corner of the eye, and the eyelashes may become sticky and may dry together at night so the eyelid can't open when your baby wakes up in the morning. But since this discharge does not indicate an infection, it usually is not treated with an antibiotic (see *Tear Production Problems,* page 622).

On the other hand, if your doctor believes that this *does* represent a true infection, it will usually be treated with special drops or an ointment that he will prescribe after examining the eye. But in many cases, all that's needed is a gentle cleansing with sterile water. When the lashes are sticky, dip a cotton ball in sterile water, and use it to gently wipe from the part of the lid nearest the nose to the outside. Use each cotton ball just once, moving in one clean motion from inside to outside (avoid going back and forth), then discard it. Use as many cotton balls as you need to clean the eye thoroughly.

Sudden Infant Death Syndrome (SIDS)

Approximately one newborn out of every two thousand dies in her sleep, for no apparent reason, usually between three and six months. These babies generally are well cared for and show no obvious symptoms of illness. Their autopsies turn up no identifiable cause of death, so the term *sudden infant death syndrome (SIDS)* is used.

The risk factor most clearly associated with SIDS is stomach-sleeping. Therefore, unless your pediatrician has advised otherwise, *your baby should be placed down for sleep on her back.* Babies of mothers who smoke and those who sleep in adult beds with other family members also appear to be at increased risk. Soft or loose bedding, pillows, and stuffed toys are also risk factors and should be kept out of the baby's sleeping environment. Babies who sleep in their own bassinet or crib, particularly when the crib is in the parents' room and those who use a pacifier when going to sleep, have a lower incidence of SIDS.

There are many theories about the cause of SIDS, but none has been proven. Infection, milk allergy, pneumonia, and immunizations all have been disproven as causes. The most plausible theory at this time is that there is a delay in the maturation of the arousal centers in the brains of certain babies, which predisposes them to stop breathing under certain conditions.

If your baby occasionally stops breathing or turns blue, your pediatrician probably will want to hospitalize her to look for treatable causes for the episodes and to assess the severity of the condition. If the spells are severe, you may be advised to learn cardiopulmonary resuscitation (CPR) and use a home monitor while the baby sleeps. This device measures her respiration and heart rate, and sounds an alarm if they go too low. If your baby was born prematurely, the pediatrician may choose to control the condition with medications such as caffeine or theophylline, which stimulate breathing.

Along with the normal feelings of grief and depression, many parents who lose a child to SIDS feel guilty and become extremely protective of older siblings or any babies born afterward. Help for parents is available through local groups or through the national First Candle organization (www.firstcandle.org; 1-800-221-7437). Ask your pediatrician about other resources in your area.

At this time, the best preventive measure that parents can take is to place their baby to sleep on her back. Since 1992, the American Academy of Pediatrics has recommended that babies always be placed in this sleep position. Before this recommendation was made, more than 5,000 babies died from SIDS every year in the United States. But today, with the decrease in the number of babies sleeping on their stomach, the deaths from SIDS have declined to less than 2,500 per year. Each of these deaths is tragic, and campaigns are continuing to promote a back-to-sleep message to parents and others who care for young children. Between the ages of four and seven months, however, you may notice that your infant begins rolling over when placed to sleep on her back. Fortunately, SIDS decreases markedly after an infant is over six months of age and rolling over is a sign that she has some head and neck control. So while it is important to continue to place your infant to sleep on her back, you should not stay up all night constantly flipping her onto her back. Still, this situation has not been scientifically studied so a definitive answer on how best to handle it cannot be given.

Although this type of mild discharge may recur several times during your baby's first months, it will not damage the eye and she probably will outgrow it, even without more intensive treatment. Only rarely does this tear-duct blockage require surgical care.

If the eye itself is bloodshot or pinkish, your infant could have conjunctivitis or "pinkeye," and you should notify your pediatrician (see *Eye Infections,* page 616).

Fever. Whenever your child is unusually cranky or feels warm, take her temperature. (See *Taking a Rectal Temperature,* page 87.) If her rectal temperature reads 100.4 degrees Fahrenheit (38 degrees Celsius) or higher on two separate readings, and she's not overly bundled up, call your pediatrician at once. Fever in these first few weeks can signal an infection, and babies this age can become seriously ill quickly.

Floppiness.. Newborn infants all seem somewhat floppy because their muscles are still developing, but if your baby feels exceptionally loose or floppy, it could be a sign of a more serious problem, such as an infection. Consult your pediatrician immediately.

Hearing. Pay attention to the way your baby responds to sounds even if she passed her newborn hearing screening. Does she startle at loud or sudden noises? Does she become quiet or turn toward you when you talk to her? If she does not respond normally to sounds around her, ask your pediatrician about formal hearing testing. (See *Hearing Loss,* pages 549–553.) This testing might be particularly appropriate if your infant was extremely premature, if she was deprived of oxygen or had a severe infection at birth, or if your family has a history of hearing loss in early childhood. If there is any suspicion of hearing loss, your infant should be tested as early as possible, as a delay in diagnosis and treatment is likely to interfere with normal language development.

Jaundice. Jaundice, the yellow color that often appears in the skin shortly after birth, sometimes lasts for more than two to three weeks in a baby who is breastfed. In formula-fed babies, most jaundice goes away within two weeks. If your baby is jaundiced for more than three weeks or the jaundice seems to be increasing, see your pediatrician. If you are having trouble breastfeeding, ask your pediatrician or nurse or lactation specialist for help, as breastmilk is the ideal food for your baby. For additional information about jaundice, see Chapter 5, page 173.

Jitters. Many newborns have quivery chins and shaky hands, but if your baby's whole body seems to be shaking, it could be a sign of low blood sugar or calcium levels, or some type of seizure disorder. Notify your pediatrician so he can determine the cause.

Rashes and Infections. Common newborn rashes include the following:

- **Cradle cap** (**seborrheic dermatitis**) appears as scaly patches on the scalp. Washing the hair and brushing out the scales daily helps control this condition. It usually disappears on its own within the first few months, but may have to be treated with a special shampoo. (See *Cradle Cap and Seborrheic Dermatitis*, page 701.)
- **Fingernail or toenail infections** will appear as redness around the edge of the toenail or fingernail, which may seem to hurt when touched. These infections may respond to warm compresses, but at this age they should be taken seriously and be examined by a doctor, as they may require medication.
- **Umbilical infections** are rare, but if one occurs it often appears as redness around the umbilical stump. There's usually pus and often tenderness. These infections should be examined by your pediatrician. If your baby is also running a fever, see your pediatrician right away as she may need antibiotics or hospitalization. It is normal, though, to have a small amount of clear oozing, drops of blood, and a scab around the umbilical stump without any redness or fever. If this is the case, watch it for a few days and if it doesn't heal on its own, see your pediatrician.

- **Diaper rash.** See instructions for handling this problem on pages 77–78.

Thrush. White patches in the mouth may indicate that your baby has thrush, a common yeast infection. This condition is treated with an oral antifungal medication prescribed by your pediatrician.

Vision. Watch how your baby looks at you when she is alert. When you're about 8 to 15 inches (20.3 to 38.1 cm) from her face, do her eyes follow you? Will she follow a light or small toy passing before her at the same distance? At this age, the eyes may appear crossed, or one eye occasionally may drift inward or outward. This is because the muscles controlling eye movement are still developing. Both eyes should be able to move equally and together in all directions, however, and she should be able to track slowly moving objects at close range. If she can't, or if she was born premature (less than thirty-two weeks into the pregnancy), or if she needed oxygen as a newborn, your pediatrician may refer you to an eye specialist for further examination.

Vomiting. If your baby starts forcefully vomiting (shooting out several inches rather than dribbling from the mouth), contact your pediatrician at once to make sure she does not have an obstruction of the valve between the stomach and the small intestine (hypertrophic pyloric stenosis; see pages 256–257). Any vomiting that persists for more than twelve hours or is accompanied by diarrhea or fever also should be evaluated by your pediatrician.

Weight Gain. Your baby should be gaining weight rapidly (½ to 1 ounce per day [14 to 28 grams]) by the middle of this month. If she isn't, your pediatrician will want to make sure that she's getting adequate calories in her feedings and that she is absorbing them properly. Be prepared to answer these questions.

- How often does the baby eat?
- How much does she eat at a feeding, if bottle-feeding? How long does she nurse, if breastfeeding?

- How many bowel movements does the baby have each day?
- What is the amount and thinness or thickness of the stools?
- How often does the baby urinate?

If your baby is eating well and the contents of her diapers are normal in amount and consistency, there is probably no cause for alarm. Your baby may just be getting off to a slow start, or her weight could even have been inaccurately measured. Your pediatrician may want to schedule another office visit in two or three days to reevaluate the situation.

SAFETY CHECK

Car Safety Seats

- Your baby should ride in a properly installed, federally approved car safety seat *every time* she is in the car. At this age, she should ride in the rear-facing position, in the backseat. Never place a baby in the front seat of a car with a passenger-side air bag.

Bathing

- If you are bathing your baby in the sink, seat her on a washcloth or bath mat to prevent slipping, and hold her under the arms. Never run the dishwasher at the same time that your baby is being bathed in the sink; otherwise, you may risk scald burns from the dishwasher's hot water. Also, don't run the faucet while your baby is in the sink; instead, fill it first, test the temperature, and then put the baby in the water.
- Adjust the maximum temperature of your water heater to 120 degrees Fahrenheit (48.9 degrees Celsius) or lower so hot water can't scald her.

Changing Table

- Never leave your baby unattended on any surface above the floor. Even at this young age, she can suddenly extend her body and flip over the edge.

Suffocation Prevention

- Do not use baby or talcum powders on the baby. If inhaled, talc-containing powders can cause severe lung damage and breathing problems in babies.
- Keep the crib free of all small objects (safety pins, small parts of toys, etc.) that she could swallow.
- Never leave plastic bags or wrappings where your baby can reach them.
- Don't have your baby sleep in your own bed next to you. Keep her in her crib.
- Instead of using loose blankets that your baby could get tangled in, dress her in appropriate-weight sleepwear (like a wearable blanket or sleep sack).
- Don't allow your baby to sleep on her stomach, nor should she sleep on a soft comforter or pillow. Put her down to sleep only on her back.

Fire Prevention

- Dress your baby in flame-resistant clothing.
- Install smoke detectors in the proper places throughout your home.

Supervision

- Never leave your baby unattended in the house, yard, or car.

Necklaces and Cords

- Don't let strings or cords dangle in the crib.

- Don't attach pacifiers, medallions, or other objects to the crib or body with a cord.
- Don't place a string or necklace around the baby's neck.
- Don't use clothing with drawstrings.

Jiggling

- Be careful not to jiggle or shake the baby's head too vigorously.
- Always support the baby's head and neck when moving her body.

7

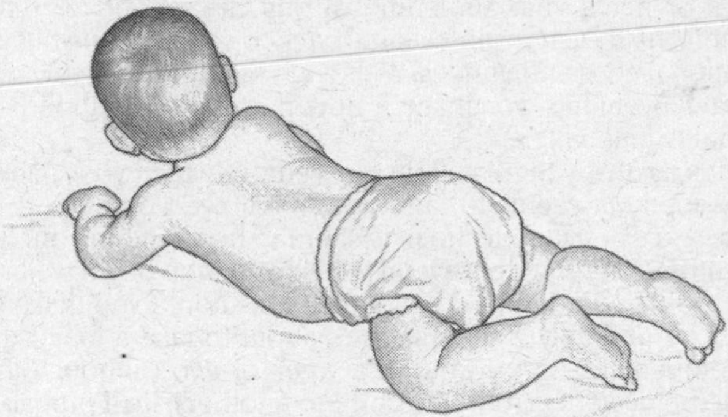

AGE ONE MONTH THROUGH THREE MONTHS

By the beginning of your baby's second month, much of the awe, exhaustion, and uncertainty that you may have felt immediately after his birth is likely to give way to self-confidence. You hopefully have settled into a fairly routine (if still demanding) schedule around his feedings and naps. You've adjusted to having a new member of the family and are beginning to understand his general temperament. And you probably already have received the crowning reward that makes all the sacrifice worthwhile: his first true smile. This smile is just a glimmer of the delights in store over the next three months.

Between one and four months, your baby will undergo a dramatic transformation from a totally dependent newborn to an active and responsive infant. He'll lose many of his newborn reflexes while acquiring more voluntary control of his body. You'll find him inspecting his hands and watching their movements. He'll also become increasingly interested in his surroundings, especially the people close to him. He'll often smile when he sees or hears you. Sometime during his second or third month, he'll even begin "talking" back to you in gentle but intentional coos and gurgles. With each of his new discoveries or achievements, you'll see a new part of your child's personality emerging.

Occasionally there will be moments in which your baby's development seems to lag, usually followed by a spurt in progress. For example, he may seem to be stretching out his nighttime feedings for several weeks and then begin waking up again to feed more frequently. What should you make of this? It's probably a sign that he's about to take a major developmental leap forward. In a week or two (although the time frame varies from one child to another), he'll probably be sleeping longer stretches at night again and maybe take fewer naps, although each nap may be for a longer period of time. In addition, he'll have longer periods during the day where he will be considerably more alert and responsive to people and events around him. Many other types of developmental progress, including physical growth, may occur in spurts and pauses, with periods where there even seems to be a slight setback or lag. As challenging as this may be at first, you'll soon learn to read the signals, anticipate, and appreciate these periods of change.

Growth and Development

Physical Appearance and Growth

From months one through four, your baby will continue growing at the same rate he established during his first few weeks of life. In general, babies gain between 1½ and 2 pounds (0.7 to 0.9 kg) and grow 1 to 1½ inches (2.5 to 4 cm). Their head size will increase in circumference by about ½ inch (1.25 cm) each month. These figures are only averages, however, so keep track of your child's development to see if it matches one of the normal curves on the growth charts in the Appendix on pages 736–739.

At two months, the soft spots on your baby's head should still be open and flat, but by two to three months, the soft spot at the back should be closed. Also, his head is more likely to be proportionately larger as compared to his body because it is growing faster. This is quite normal; his body will soon catch up.

At two months, your baby will look round and chubby, but as he starts using his arms and legs more actively, muscles will develop. His bones also will grow rapidly, and as his arms and legs loosen up, his body and limbs will seem to stretch out, making him appear taller and leaner.

Movement

Many of your baby's movements still will be reflexive at the beginning of this period. For example, he may assume a "fencing" position every time his head turns (tonic neck reflex; see page 183) and throw out his arms if he hears a loud noise or feels that he's falling (Moro reflex, pages 183–184). But as we've mentioned, most of these common newborn reflexes will begin to fade by the second or third month. He may temporarily seem less active after the reflexes have diminished, but now his movements, however subtle, are intentional ones and will build steadily toward mature activity.

One of the most important developments of these early months will be your baby's increasing neck strength. Try placing him on his stomach and see what happens. Before two months, he'll struggle to raise his head to look around. Even if he succeeds for only a second or two, that will allow him to turn for a slightly different view of the world. These momentary exercises also will strengthen the muscles in the back of his neck so that, by sometime around his four-month birthday, he'll be able to hold up his head and chest as he supports himself on his elbows. This is a major accomplishment, giving him the freedom and control to look all around at will, instead of just staring at his crib or the mobile directly overhead.

For you, it's also a welcome development because you no longer have to support his head quite so much when carrying him (although sudden movements or force will still require some head support). If you use a front or back carrier, he'll now be able to hold his own head up and look around as you walk.

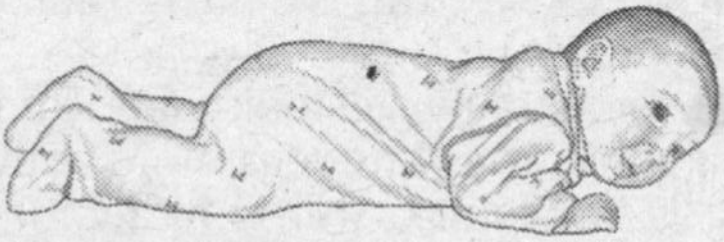

A baby's control over the front neck muscles and abdominal muscles develops more gradually, so it will take a little longer for your baby to be able to raise his head when lying on his back. At one month, if you gently pull your baby by the arms to a sitting position, his head will flop backward; by four months, however, he'll be able to hold it steady in all directions.

Your child's legs also will become stronger and more active. During the second month, they'll start to straighten from their inward-curving newborn position. Although his kicks will remain mostly reflexive for some time, they'll quickly gather force, and by the end of the third month, he might even kick himself over from front to back. (He probably won't roll from back to front until he's about six months old.) Since you cannot predict when he'll begin rolling over, you'll need to be especially careful and pay close attention whenever he's on the changing table or any other surface above floor level.

Another newborn reflex—the stepping reflex (described in Chapter 6, page 184)—will allow him to take steps

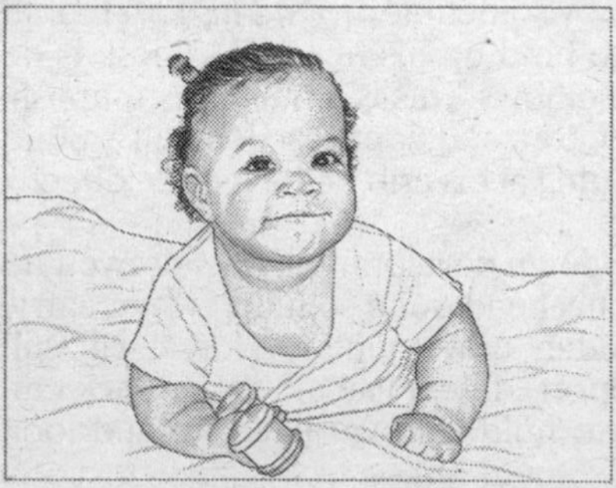

By her four-month birthday, your baby will be able to hold up her head and chest as she supports herself on her elbows.

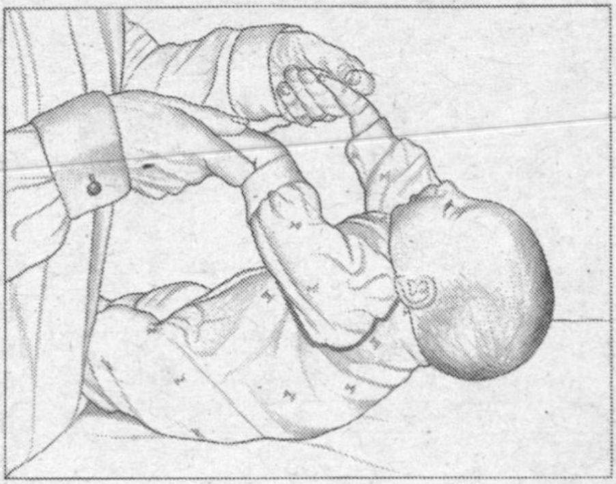

At one month, your baby's head will flop backward if you gently pull her to a sitting position (so always support your baby's head when picking her up).

when you hold him under his arms, while his feet touch the floor. But this reflex will disappear at about six weeks, and you may not see your baby step again until he's ready to walk. By three or four months, however, he'll be able to flex and straighten his legs at will. Lift him upright with his feet on the floor and he'll push down and straighten his legs so that he's virtually standing by himself (except for the balance you're providing). Then he'll try bending his knees and discover that he can bounce himself. Although parents are often concerned about whether this kind of bouncing is harmful to the baby's legs, it is perfectly healthy and safe.

Your baby's hand and arm movements also will develop rapidly during these three months. In the beginning, his hands will be tightly clenched with his thumb curled inside his fingers; if you uncoil the fingers and place a rattle in his palm, he'll grasp it automatically, yet he won't be able to shake it or bring it to his mouth. He'll gaze at his hands with interest when they come into view by chance or because of reflexive movements, but he probably won't be able to bring them to his face on his own.

However, many changes will occur within just a month or two. Suddenly your baby's hands will seem to relax and his arms will open outward. During the third month, his hands will be half-open most of the time, and you'll notice him carefully opening and shutting them. Try placing a rattle in

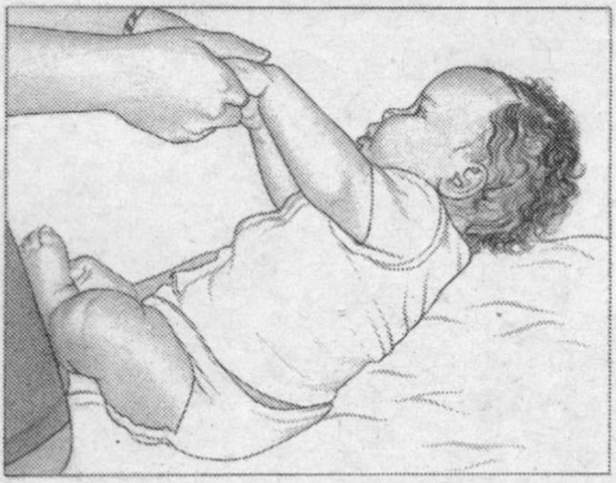

By four months, however, she will be able to hold her head steady in all directions.

his palm and he'll grip it, perhaps bring it to his mouth, and then drop it only after he's explored it fully. (The more lightweight the toy, the better he'll be able to control it.) He'll never seem to grow bored with his hands themselves; just staring at his fingers will amuse him for long stretches of time.

Your baby's attempts to bring his hands to his mouth will be persistent, but mostly in vain at first. Even if his fingers occasionally reach their destination, they'll quickly fall away. By four months, however, he'll probably have finally mastered this game (which is also an important developmental skill) and be able to get his thumb to his mouth and keep it there whenever he wishes. Put a rattle in his palm now and he'll clench it tightly, shake it, mouth it, and maybe even transfer it from hand to hand.

Your baby also will be able to reach accurately and quickly—not only with both hands but with his entire body. Hang a toy overhead and he'll reach up eagerly with arms and legs to bat at it and grab for it. His face will tense in concentration, and he may even lift his head toward his target. It's as if every part of his body shares in his excitement as he masters these new skills.

Vision

At one month your baby still can't see very clearly beyond 12 inches (30.4 cm) or so, but he'll closely study anything

Movement Milestones by the End of This Period

- Raises head and chest when lying on stomach
- Supports upper body with arms when lying on stomach
- Stretches legs out and kicks when lying on stomach or back
- Opens and shuts hands
- Pushes down on legs when feet are placed on a firm surface
- Brings hands to mouth
- Takes swipes at dangling objects with hands
- Grasps and shakes hand toys

within this range: the corner of his crib, toys attached to the side rail, or the shapes of his mobile dangling above the crib. The human face is his favorite image, however. As you hold him in your arms, his attention is drawn automatically to your face, particularly your eyes. Often the mere sight of your eyes will make him smile. Gradually his visual span will broaden so that he can take in your whole face instead of just a single feature like your eyes. As this happens he'll be much more responsive to facial expressions involving your mouth, jaw, and cheeks. He'll also love flirting with himself in the mirror. Buy an unbreakable mirror that's specially made to attach inside cribs and playpens, so he can entertain himself when you're not nearby.

In his early weeks, your baby will have a hard time following

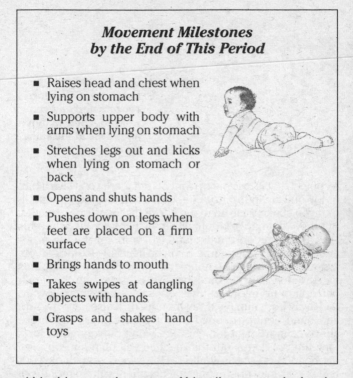

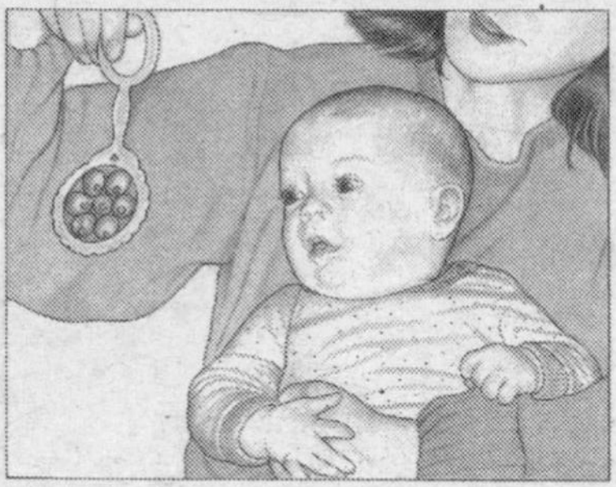

By two months your baby's eyes are more coordinated and can work together to move and focus at the same time.

an object that is moving in front of his face. If you wave a ball or toy quickly in front of him, he'll seem to stare through it, or if you shake your head, he'll lose his focus on your eyes. But this will change dramatically by two months, when his eyes are more coordinated and can work together to move and focus at the same time. Soon he'll be able to track an object moving through an entire half-circle in front of him. This increased visual coordination also will give him the depth perception he needs to track objects as they move toward and away from him. By three months, he'll also have the arm and hand control needed to bat at objects as they move above or in front of him; his aim won't be very good for a long time to come, but the practice will help him develop his hand-to-eye coordination. However, if you think your baby's eyes may not be tracking together by three months of age, talk with your pediatrician.

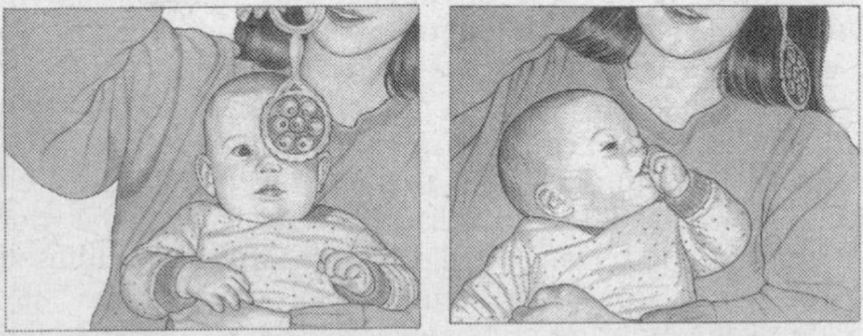

Soon he'll be able to track an object moving through an entire half-circle in front of him.

Your baby's distance vision also is developing at this time. You may notice at three months that he's smiling at you halfway across the room, or studying a toy several feet away. By four months, you'll catch him staring at the distant wall hanging or looking out the window. These are clues that his distance vision is developing properly.

Your infant's color vision will mature at about the same rate. At one month, he'll be quite sensitive to the brightness or intensity of color; consequently, he'll prefer to look at bold patterns in sharply contrasting colors or in black-and-white. Young infants do not appreciate the soothing pastels we usually associate with a newborn's nursery because of the babies' limited color vision. By about four months, your

Visual Milestones by the End of This Period

- Watches faces intently
- Follows moving objects
- Recognizes familiar objects and people at a distance
- Starts using hands and eyes in coordination

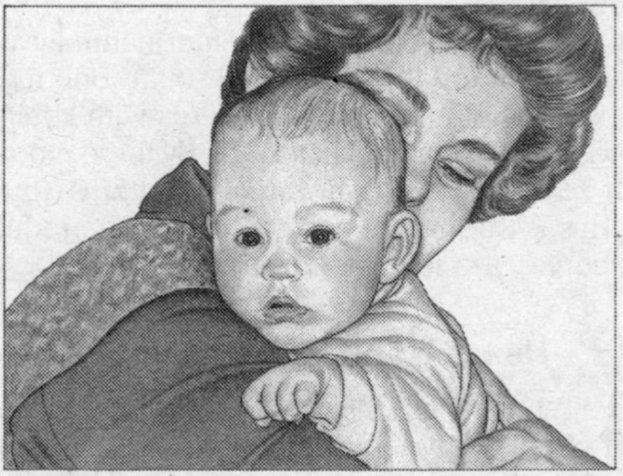

Hearing and Speech Milestones by the End of This Period

- Smiles at the sound of your voice
- Begins to babble
- Begins to imitate some sounds
- Turns head toward direction of sound

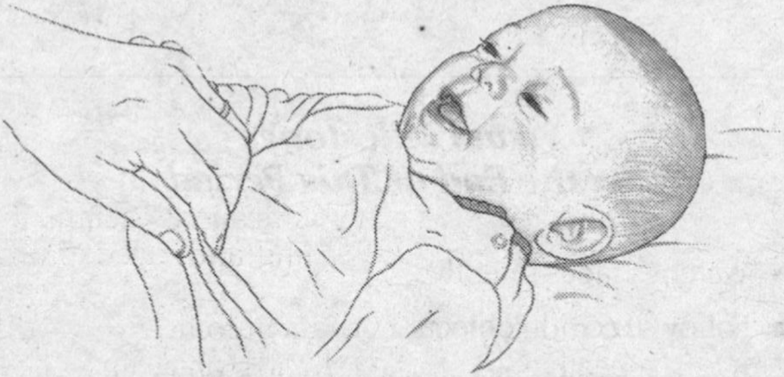

baby finally will be responsive to the full range of colors and their many shades.

As his eyesight develops, your infant naturally will seek out more stimulating things to see. Around one month, his favorite patterns will be simple patterns with straight lines such as big stripes or a checkerboard. By three months, he'll be much more interested in circular patterns (bull's-eyes, spirals). This is one reason why faces, which are full of circles and curves, are so appealing to him.

Hearing and Making Sounds

Just as your baby naturally prefers the human face over any other visual pattern, he also prefers the human voice to other sounds. His mother's voice is his absolute favorite, because he associates it with warmth, food, and comfort. Babies like the high-pitched voices of women in general—a fact that most adults seem to understand intuitively and respond to accordingly, without even realizing it.

Just listen to yourself the next time you talk to your baby. You'll probably notice that you raise the pitch of your voice, slow your rate of speech, exaggerate certain syllables, and widen your eyes and mouth more than normal. This dramatic approach is guaranteed to capture almost any baby's attention—and usually make him smile.

By listening to you and others talk to him, your baby will discover the importance of speech long before he understands or repeats any specific words himself. By one month, he'll be able to identify you by voice, even if you're in another room, and as you talk to him, he'll be reassured, comforted, and entertained. When he smiles and gurgles back at you, he'll see the delight on your face and realize that talk is a two-way process. These first conversations will teach him many of the subtle rules of communication, such as turn-taking, vocal tone, imitation and pacing, and speed of verbal interaction.

At about two months, you may begin to hear your infant cooing and repeating some vowel sounds (ah-ah-ah, ooh-ooh-ooh). Go ahead and imitate his cooing, while also adding simple words and phrases to your "conversations" over the first four to six months. Along the way, it's easy to fall into a habit of baby talk, but you should try to mix your conversations with adult language and eventually phase out the baby talk. During early infancy, you also should read to your baby, even though you may not think he comprehends what you're reading.

By four months, your infant will babble routinely, often amusing himself for long periods by producing strange new sounds (muh-muh, bah-bah). He'll also be more sensitive to your tone of voice and the emphasis you put on certain words or phrases. As you move through each day together, he'll learn from your voice when you're going to feed him, change his diapers, go out for a walk, or put him down to sleep. The way you talk will tell him a great deal about your mood and personality, and the way he responds will tell you a lot about him. If you speak in an upbeat or comforting way, he may smile or coo. Yell or talk angrily, and he'll probably startle or cry.

Emotional and Social Development

By the second month, your baby will spend much of each day watching and listening to the people around him. He learns that they will entertain and soothe him, feed him, and make him comfortable. He feels good when they smile at him, and he seems to know instinctively that he can smile, too. Even during his first month, he'll experiment with primitive grins and grimaces. Then, during the second month, these movements will turn to genuine signals of pleasure and friendliness.

Have you experienced his first true smile yet? It's a major turning point for both you and your infant. In case there was any doubt in your mind, all the sleepless nights and erratic days of these first weeks suddenly seem worthwhile at the sight of that first grin, and you'll do everything in your power to keep those smiles coming. For his part, your baby suddenly will discover that just by moving his lips he can have two-way "conversations" with you, as his grins bring him even more attention than usual and make him feel good. Smiling also will give him another way besides crying to express his needs and exert some control over what happens to him. The more engaged he is with you and your smiles, and eventually with the rest of this great big world around him, not only will his brain development advance, but the more he'll be distracted from internal sensations (hunger, gas, fatigue) that once strongly influenced much of his behavior. His increasing socialization is further proof that he enjoys and appreciates these new experiences. Expanding his world with these experiences is not only fun for both of you but also important to his overall development.

At first your baby actually may seem to smile past you without meeting your gaze, but don't let this disturb you. Looking away from you gives him some control and protects him from being overwhelmed by you. It's his way of taking in the total picture without being "caught" by your eyes. In this way, he can pay equal attention to your facial expressions, the sound of your voice, the warmth of your body, and the way you're holding him. As you get to know each other,

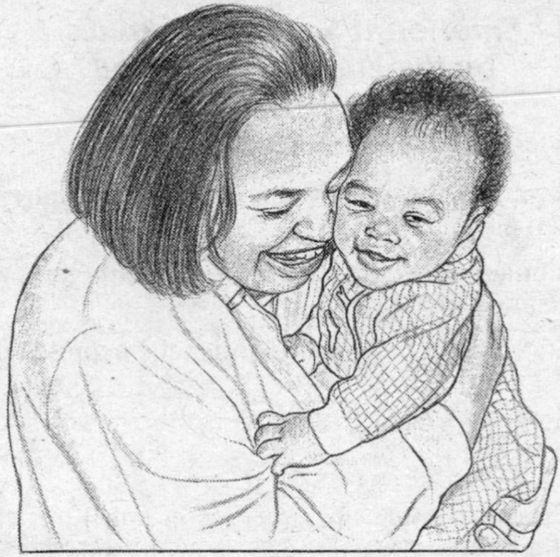

he'll gradually hold your gaze for longer and longer periods, and you'll find ways to increase his "tolerance"—perhaps by holding him at a certain distance, adjusting the level of your voice, or modifying your expressions.

By three months, your baby will be a master of "smile talk." Sometimes he'll start a "conversation" by aiming a broad smile at you and gurgling to catch your attention. At other times he'll lie in wait, watching your face until you give the first smile and then beaming back his enthusiastic response. His whole body will participate in these dialogues. His hands will open wide, one or both arms will lift up, and his arms and legs will move in time with the rhythms of your speech. His facial movements also may mirror yours. As you talk he may open his mouth and widen his eyes, and if you stick out your tongue, he may do the same!

Of course, your baby probably won't act this friendly with everyone. Like adults, your infant will prefer certain people to others. And his favorites, naturally, will be his parents. Then, at about three or four months, he'll become intrigued by other children. If he has brothers or sisters, you'll see him beaming as soon as they start talking to him. If he hears

Emotional/Social Milestones by the End of This Period

- Begins to develop a social smile
- Enjoys playing with other people and may cry when playing stops
- Becomes more communicative and expressive with face and body
- Imitates some movements and facial expressions

children's voices down the street or on television, he may turn to find them. This fascination with children will increase as he gets older.

Grandparents or familiar sitters may receive a hesitant smile at first, followed by coos and body talk once they've played with your baby awhile. By contrast, strangers may receive no more than a curious stare or a fleeting smile. This selective behavior tells you that even at this young age, he's starting to sort out who's who in his life. Although the signals are subtle, there's no doubt that he's becoming very attached to the people closest to him.

This unspoken give-and-take may seem like no more than a game, but these early exchanges play an important part in his social and emotional development. By responding quickly and enthusiastically to his smiles and engaging him often in these "conversations," you'll let him know that he's important to you, that he can trust you, and that he has a certain amount of control in his life. By recognizing his cues and not interrupting or looking away when he's "talking," you'll also show him that you are interested in him and value him. This contributes to his developing self-esteem.

As your baby grows, the way the two of you communicate will vary with his needs and desires. On a day-to-day basis you'll find that he has three general levels of need, each of which shows a different side of his personality:

Developmental Health Watch

Although each baby develops in his own individual way and at his own rate, failure to reach certain milestones may signal medical or developmental problems requiring special attention. If you notice any of the following warning signs in your infant at this age, discuss them with your pediatrician.

- Still has Moro reflex after four months
- Doesn't seem to respond to loud sounds
- Doesn't notice his hands by two months
- Doesn't smile at the sound of your voice by two months
- Doesn't follow moving objects with his eyes by two to three months
- Doesn't grasp and hold objects by three months
- Doesn't smile at people by three months
- Cannot support his head well at three months
- Doesn't reach for and grasp toys by three to four months
- Doesn't babble by three to four months
- Doesn't bring objects to his mouth by four months
- Begins babbling, but doesn't try to imitate any of your sounds by four months
- Doesn't push down with his legs when his feet are placed on a firm surface by four months
- Has trouble moving one or both eyes in all directions
- Crosses his eyes most of the time (Occasional crossing of the eyes is normal in these first months.)

- Doesn't pay attention to new faces, or seems very frightened by new faces or surroundings
- Still has the tonic neck reflex at four to five months

1. When his needs are urgent—when he's very hungry or in pain, for instance—he'll let you know in his own special way, perhaps by screaming, whimpering, or using desperate body language. In time you'll learn to recognize these signals so quickly that you usually can satisfy him almost before he himself knows what he wants.

2. While your baby is peacefully asleep, or when he's alert and entertaining himself, you'll feel reassured that you've met all his needs for the moment. This will give you a welcome opportunity to rest or take care of other business. The times when he's playing by himself provide you with wonderful opportunities to observe—from a distance—how he is developing important new skills such as learning to play by himself, reaching, tracking objects, or manipulating his hands. These activities set the stage for learning to self-soothe, which will help him settle down and ultimately sleep through the night. These are especially important skills for more colicky or difficult-to-console babies to learn.

3. Each day there will be periods when your baby's obvious needs are met but he's still fussy or fitful. He may let you know this with a whine, agitated movements, or spurts of aimless activity between moments of calm. He probably won't even know what he wants, and any of several responses might help calm him. Playing, talking, singing, rocking, and walking may work sometimes; on other occasions, simply repositioning him or letting him "fuss it out" may be the most successful strategy. You also may find that while a particular response calms him down momentarily, he'll soon become even fussier and demand more attention. This cycle may not break until you either let him cry a few minutes or distract him by doing something different—for example, taking him outside or feeding him. As

For the Grandparents

As a grandparent, your role can be especially important in the lives of not only your newborn grandchild and his parents, but also the other children in the family. Make sure you pay plenty of attention to the older youngsters, who might feel a little neglected with all the attention showered on the baby. You can serve as a "pinch hitter" when the new parents are adjusting to their infant by planning some special activities just for you and the baby's older brother(s) or sister(s). For example, make time for the sibling(s) with:

- Trips to the store or other activities
- Car rides
- Appropriate stimulating times with music or reading stories
- Sleepovers at Grandma's house

As we've suggested elsewhere in the book (see pages 217, 345, and 429), you can play other important roles to help your daughter or son adjust to the new addition to their family. Help them with cleaning, shopping, and other errands. At the same time, without being overly intrusive, pass along some of your own wisdom and reassurances about baby care—perhaps explaining the "normalness" of crying, the color of bowel movements, the little rashes or other changes in skin color, and a host of other occurrences in the early months. For example, there will be times of frustration for the new parents, such as when the baby is crying excessively and is difficult to console. Provide support and encouragement for the parents—and give them a breather, if possible, by taking the baby out for a stroll in the carriage. The insights and assistance of both grandfathers and grandmothers can have a calming and "life-saving" effect on new parents.

trying as these spells can be, you'll both learn a lot about each other because of them. You'll discover how your baby likes to be rocked, what funny faces or voices he most enjoys, and what he most likes to look at. He'll find out what he has to do to get you to respond, how hard you'll try to please him, and where your limits of tolerance lie.

Over time your baby's periods of acute need will decrease, and he'll be able to entertain himself for longer stretches. In part, this is because you're learning to anticipate and care for many of his problems before he's uncomfortable. But also, his nervous system will be maturing, and, as a result, he'll be better able to cope with everyday stresses by himself. With greater control over his body, he'll be able to do more things to amuse and console himself and he'll experience fewer frustrations. The periods when he seems most difficult to satisfy probably won't disappear entirely for a few years, but as he becomes more active, it will be easier to distract him. Ultimately he should learn to overcome these spells on his own.

During these early months, don't worry about spoiling your baby with too much attention. Observe him closely and respond promptly when he needs you. You may not be able to calm him down every time, but it never hurts to show him how much you care. In fact, the more promptly and consistently you comfort your baby's fussing in the first six months, the less demanding he's likely to be when he's older. At this age, he needs frequent reassurance in order to feel secure about himself and about you. By helping him establish this sense of security now, you're laying a foundation for the confidence and trust that will allow him gradually to separate from you and become a strong, independent person.

Basic Care

Feeding

Ideally, your baby will continue on his exclusive diet of breastmilk or formula until four to six months. The best way to monitor whether your baby is getting enough is by making sure his growth is appropriate. Your doctor will measure his weight, length, and head at each visit. Most breastfed

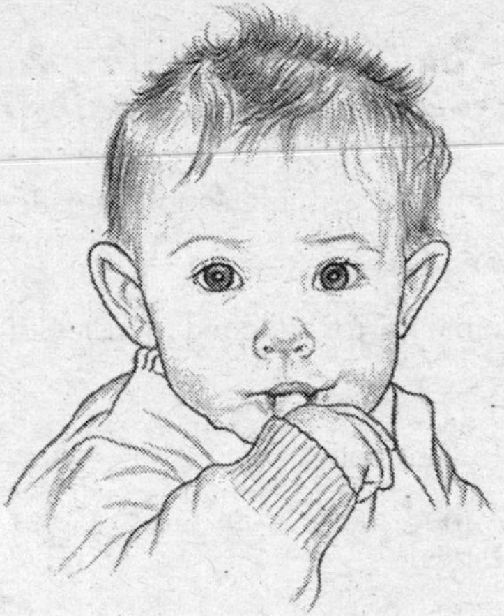

babies will continue to request feedings on demand throughout the day and night. The average amount he consumes at a feeding will increase gradually from about 4 or 5 ounces (120 to 150 ml) during the second month, to 5 or 6 ounces (150 to 180 ml) by four months, but these amounts vary from baby to baby and from feeding to feeding. His daily intake should range from about 25 to 30 ounces (750 to 900 ml) by four months. Ordinarily, this amount will supply all his nutritional needs at this age.

But if your baby seems persistently hungry after what you think are adequate feedings, consult your pediatrician for advice. When a breastfeeding infant is not gaining weight, your milk supply may have decreased. If the milk supply had once been adequate but has recently declined, this decrease could be associated with Mom's return to work without adequate pumping, or increased stress for the mother, longer sleep intervals in the baby, or a variety of other factors. Several techniques can be used to increase the milk supply and the baby's intake of it. Try increasing the frequency or the length of feedings, and use a breast pump to increase milk production. If you continue to be concerned about your milk supply, however, mention it again to your doctor, and/or see a certified lactation consultant.

Toys and Activities Appropriate for a One- to Three-Month-Old

- Images or books with high-contrast patterns
- Bright, varied mobile
- Unbreakable mirror attached to inside of crib
- Rattles
- Singing to your baby
- Playing varied music from music boxes, CDs, records, or tapes

Generally, you should avoid introducing solid foods before four to six months of age. When you do give him solids, feed him from a spoon. However, placing a spoon in the baby's mouth before four months will cause the baby to thrust out his tongue, which is normal at this stage, even though parents or care providers may mistake this behavior for refusing or disliking the food. At four to five months old, this tongue thrusting will go away and the baby will be able to move a small amount of pureed solid food from the front of the mouth to the back of the mouth and swallow it. But if your baby seems resistant to solid foods, talk to your pediatrician to ensure that his resistance is not the sign of any

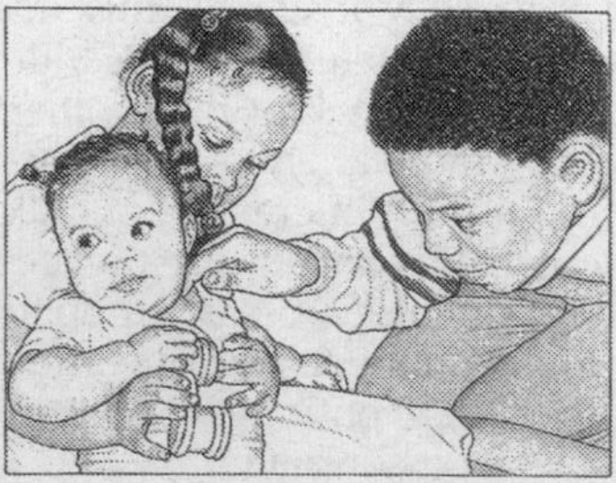

Invite older siblings to play with the baby.

problem. (For more information about introducing solids, see pages 280–285 in Chapter 8.)

Even if you don't make any additions to your baby's diet, you'll probably notice a change in his bowel movements during these months. His intestines can hold more now and absorb a greater amount of nutrients from the milk, so his stools may be more solid. The gastrocolic reflex (see *Bowel Movements,* page 79) is also diminishing, so he should no longer have a bowel movement after each feeding. In fact, between two and three months, the frequency of stools in both breastfed and formula-fed babies may decrease dramatically; some breastfed babies have only one bowel movement every three or four days, and a few perfectly healthy breastfed infants have just one a week. As long as your baby is eating well, gaining weight, and his stools are not too hard or dry, there's no reason to be alarmed by this drop in frequency.

Sleeping

By two months, your baby will be more alert and social and will spend more time awake during the day. Meanwhile, his stomach capacity will be growing, so that he'll need less frequent feedings; as a result, he may start skipping one middle-of-the-night feeding. Around three months, most (but not all) infants consistently sleep through the night (six to eight hours without disruption).

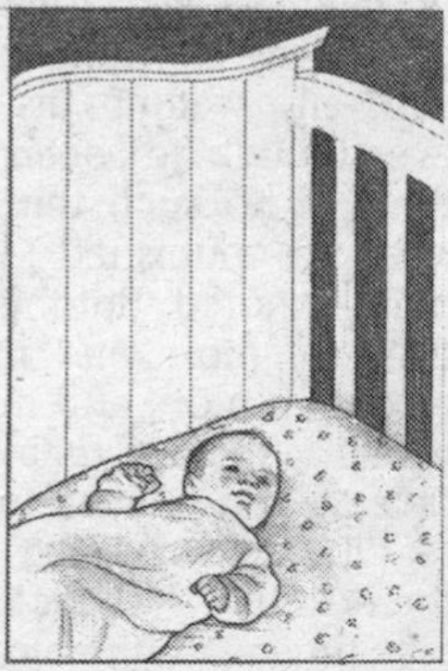

After three months, most (but not all) infants consistently sleep through the night.

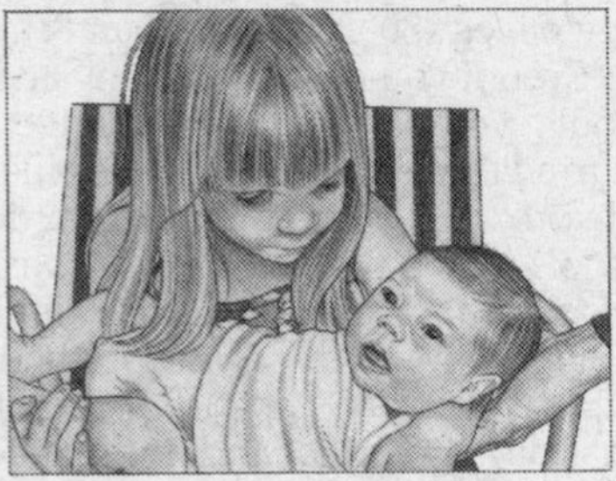

Set clear and consistent rules, such as never picking up the baby without permission.

Remember, at this age, children should be put to sleep on their back (but be sure to give him some "tummy time" during his waking hours, which is good for his normal physical development). See Chapter 30 (pages 715–728) for detailed information on sleep.

Siblings

By the second month, although you may be used to having a new baby in the house, your older children still may be having a hard time adjusting. Especially if the baby is your second child, your first probably may be saddened by not being the primary focus of the family.

Sometimes your older child might display his frustration by talking back, doing something he knows is forbidden, or literally shouting for attention. He also might regress, suddenly wetting his bed or having daytime accidents even though he's been toilet-trained for months. Remember, there is no such thing as "negative" attention. He would rather be punished for bad behavior than feel like he is being ignored. But this can quickly escalate into a vicious cycle of more and more inappropriate behavior associated with more and more attention. One important way to reverse this frustrating cycle is to actively "catch him being good." Giving him praise for playing by himself or reading a book makes those activities more likely to occur the next time he's looking for attention. Having each parent take time with him alone each day may also help. Also, you

Stimulating Infant Brain Growth: Age One Month Through Three Months

- Provide healthful nutrition as your baby grows; have periodic checkups and timely immunizations from a regular source of medical care.
- Give consistent, warm, physical contact—hugging, skin-to-skin, body-to-body contact—to establish your infant's sense of security and well-being. Talk or sing to your baby during dressing, bathing, feeding, playing, walking, and driving. Use simple, lively phrases and address your baby by name. Respond to his gestures, as well as to the faces and the sounds he makes.
- Be attentive to your baby's rhythms and moods. Learn to read his cues and respond to him when he is upset as well as when he is happy. Babies cannot be spoiled.
- Provide colorful objects of different shapes, sizes, and textures that he can play with. Show him children's picture books and family photographs.
- Your face is by far the most interesting visual object at this age. Play peekaboo with your baby.
- Place a child-safe mirror in your infant's crib so he can look at his own face.
- If you speak a foreign language, use it at home.
- Avoid subjecting your baby to stressful or traumatic experiences, physical or psychological.
- Make sure other people who provide care and supervision for your baby understand the importance of forming a loving and comforting relationship with your child and also provide consistent care.

may need to pick your battles. If you suspect that your child is doing something to get your attention that is not harmful or dangerous (whining, for example), if you ignore that behavior, he will likely find some other way to get your attention.

However, if your older child takes out his frustration on the baby—pulling away his bottle or even hitting him—you'll need to take more direct action. Sit down and talk with him, and be prepared to hear things such as "I wish that baby had never come here." Try to keep these and his other feelings in mind as you confront him. Reassure him that you still love him very much, but explain firmly that he must not hurt the baby. Make an extra effort to include him in all family activities, and encourage him to interact with the newborn. Make him feel like an important "big kid" by giving him specific baby-related jobs, such as carrying the diaper bag, putting away toys, helping dress the baby, or being the one in charge of making sure that visitors and other people wash their hands before they get to hold "his" baby. At the same time, set clear and consistent rules, such as never picking up the baby without permission.

Health Watch

A newborn can get very sick very quickly, so if your infant is under three months of age and has a temperature of 100.4 degrees Fahrenheit or higher, call your pediatrician. The following medical problems are common between the ages of two and four months. If you are concerned that your baby has any of these conditions while younger than two months of age, contact your pediatrician. Check Part II of this book for other illnesses and conditions that occur throughout childhood.

Diarrhea (see also *Diarrhea,* page 440). If your baby has a vomiting spell followed a day or two later by diarrhea, he probably has a viral infection in his intestinal tract. If you're breastfeeding, your pediatrician probably will suggest that you continue nursing him as usual. If you're formula-feeding, in most cases you can continue to do so. You may be advised to use a "reduced" lactose formula for a few days before returning to the original formula if diarrhea persists. In some instances your pediatrician may advise you to limit your baby's intake to a special solution containing electrolytes (i.e., salt and potassium) and sugar. This is because diarrhea can sometimes "wash out" the enzymes needed to properly and effectively digest the sugar in cow's milk–based formulas.

Ear Infections (see also *Middle Ear Infections,* page 557). Although ear infections are more common in older babies, occasionally they occur in infants under three months. Babies are prone to ear infections because the tube that connects the nasal passages to the middle ear is very short, making it easy for a virus that causes a cold in the nasal passages to spread to the ear. The virus infection in the middle ear can then have an added bacterial infection. When this occurs, your pediatrician will examine your baby and diagnose a true middle ear infection.

The first sign of an ear infection is usually irritability, especially at night. The infection may also produce a fever. If your pediatrician's ear examination confirms that an infection is present, the doctor may recommend giving liquid acetaminophen to your baby in an appropriate dose. (Do *not* give him aspirin; it can cause a serious brain disorder called Reye syndrome.) Your pediatrician also may prescribe a course of antibiotics, although if your child does not have a fever or is not severely ill, antibiotics may not be necessary. While ear infections can be caused by bacteria or viruses, antibiotics treat only bacterial infections, and thus your pediatrician may not recommend them if he isn't convinced that a bacterial infection is present.

Eye Infections. In infants, conjunctivitis, or "pinkeye," usually is caused by a viral or bacterial infection. In babies, the infection is occasionally associated with chlamydia or gonorrhea, acquired as the newborn moves through the birth canal. The eyedrops or ointments that all babies receive in the delivery room may not clear this infection in the eyes, nor do they prevent it from spreading to the nose and throat and from there to the lungs, causing pneumonia. Because of this danger, babies who have been exposed to bacteria such as chlamydia during the birthing process are treated with an oral antibiotic such as azithromycin.

Any signs of eye infection such as eye swelling, redness, or discharge during the first few weeks of life can be potentially serious, but that's certainly not always the case. For example, there can be discharge and tearing—but generally without redness—if a tear duct is blocked, which can set the stage for a subsequent eye infection. If you suspect any kind of eye problem, even if it seems rather routine, report it to your pediatrician. (For more information, see *Eye Infections*, page 616.)

Spitting (Gastroesophageal Reflux). This condition occurs when contents from the stomach make their way back into the esophagus (the tube through which food and liquids are transported from the throat to the stomach). This so-called reflux takes place when the sphincter (the muscle responsible for keeping the stomach contents from coming back up into the esophagus) relaxes at the wrong time or, less commonly, is too weak, allowing food and/or liquid to flow upward in the direction from which it came. Because of this immaturity of the sphincter, all babies reflux to some degree, although the level decreases over time with most children. In some cases, however, it becomes a problem that may require the advice of your pediatrician.

Recent research shows that chronic gastroesophageal reflux is more common in children than was once believed, and can begin as early as infancy. Not long after eating, an infant with this condition may vomit, have periods of coughing, become irritable, have difficulty swallowing, arch his back, and may be underweight. Spitting/vomiting in infancy is common in about half of the infants less than six months of age who vomit and about 5 percent of infants at twelve months of age. To minimize the problem, stop to burp your baby several times during a feed, as well as afterward. Because the condition can worsen when your infant is lying flat, try keeping him in an upright position for about half an hour following each feeding. Because of concerns about SIDS (sudden infant death syndrome) when babies sleep, do not place them in a prone position (on stomach) for sleep or to help their reflux symptoms, unless recommended by a specialist for babies with very severe reflux. The safest way for your baby to sleep is always on his back. Remember . . . "back to sleep."

A baby with gastroesophageal reflux should be evaluated by a pediatrician or pediatric gastroenterologist. In some cases, your doctor may recommend thickening your baby's formula or breastmilk to help reduce the amount of reflux. In some cases, he might suggest switching to a protein hydrolysate formula (ask your doctor what kind to buy), and then see if symptoms improve in the next week or two. If your infant has an allergy to cow's milk, this switch in formulas may help. In cases where your baby isn't keeping enough down to gain weight properly, or if she is very uncomfortable, medications may be prescribed as well.

Some cases of vomiting in the first few months of age may be caused by *pyloric stenosis*, a condition in which there is a narrowing of the opening connecting the stomach to the small intestine, causing forceful vomiting and a change in bowel movement patterns. If your pediatrician is concerned that your baby may have pyloric stenosis he will order an ultrasound and, if needed, refer you for further treatment. (See also *Vomiting,* pages 458–462.)

Rashes and Skin Conditions. Many of the rashes seen in the first month may persist through the second or third month of life. In addition, eczema may occur anytime after one month. Eczema, or atopic dermatitis (see also *Eczema,* page 470), is a skin condition that can result in dry, scaly skin, and often red patches, usually on the face, in the bends of the elbows, and behind the knees. In young infants, elbows and knees are the most common locations. The patches can range from small and mild to extremely itchy, which may make a baby irritable. Ask your pediatrician to recommend treatment, which may vary depending on the severity of the condition, and could include either over-the-counter or prescription lotions or creams (only use the OTC products if your doctor specifically recommends them, since he can guide you toward those products that are most effective). For babies who have only occasional and mild eczema (small patches), he may feel no treatment is necessary.

To prevent a recurrence of this condition, make sure you use only the mildest soaps to wash your baby and his clothes, and dress him only in soft clothing (no wool or rough weaves). Bathe him no more than three times a week, since frequent baths may further dry his skin. (If your doctor believes that certain foods may be triggering your child's eczema, particularly once he's feeding on solid foods, he may recommend avoiding these foods.) For more information about eczema, see pages 470–473.

Respiratory Syncytial Virus (RSV) Infections. RSV is the most common cause of lower respiratory tract infections in infants and young children, and is one of many viruses that causes colds in children. Infecting the lungs and breathing passages, it is frequently responsible for bronchiolitis and pneumonia in children under age one. In fact, the highest incidence of RSV illness occurs in infants from two months to eight months of age. RSV is also the most common reason that infants under one year of age are hospitalized.

RSV is a highly contagious infection, occurring most often during the months from fall through spring. It causes symptoms such as a runny or stuffy nose with or without an accompanying sore throat, a mild cough, and sometimes a fever. The infection can remain in the nose or involve the ears and it can spread to the lower respiratory tract causing bronchiolitis. The symptoms of bronchiolitis include abnormally rapid breathing and wheezing.

If your baby was born prematurely, or has chronic lung disease, he has a higher risk of having a serious RSV infection. Premature babies frequently have underdeveloped lungs, and may not have received enough antibodies from their mother to help them combat RSV if they encounter it.

You can reduce your infant's chances of developing a more serious RSV infection by:

- Having people wash their hands with warm water and soap before picking up and holding your baby
- Reducing close contact with people who have runny noses or other sicknesses. Continue to breastfeed when you have a cold, however, since doing so will supply the baby with nourishment and protective antibodies

- As much as possible, limiting your baby's siblings from spending time with your infant when they have a cold (and make sure they wash their hands frequently)
- Keeping your baby away from crowded areas, such as shopping malls and elevators, where he'll have close contact with people who may be sick
- Avoiding smoking around your baby, since secondhand smoke could increase his susceptibility to a serious RSV infection

If your pediatrician determines that your baby has developed bronchiolitis or another RSV infection, she may recommend symptomatic treatment, such as easing nasal stuffiness with a nasal aspirator or mild salt-solution nasal drops. Severe pneumonia or bronchiolitis may require hospitalization in order to administer humidified oxygen and medications to help your child breathe more easily. (For more information about RSV infections, see *Bronchiolitis,* page 494.)

Upper Respiratory Infections (URI) (see also *Colds/ Upper Respiratory Infection,* page 554). Many babies have their first cold during these months. Breastfeeding provides some immunity, but it is not complete protection by any means, especially if another member of the family has a respiratory illness. The infection can spread easily through respiratory droplets in the air or by hand contact. (Exposure to cold temperatures or drafts, on the other hand—contrary to popular opinion—does not cause colds.) Washing hands, covering mouths while sneezing or coughing, and refraining from kissing when you have a cold will decrease spreading viruses to others; at the same time, keep in mind that you won't be able to avoid the spread of all colds, since people can spread most viruses even before they develop symptoms.

Most respiratory infections in young babies are mild, producing a cough, runny nose, and slightly elevated temperature, but rarely a high fever. A runny nose, however, can be troublesome for an infant. He cannot blow his nose, so the mucus blocks the nasal passages. Before three or four months of age, an infant doesn't breathe well through his mouth, so this blockage of his nose causes more discomfort for him than for older children. A congested nose also often disturbs sleep and causes babies to wake up when they're not able to breathe well. It can interfere with feeding, too, since infants must interrupt sucking in order to breathe through their mouth.

If congestion does occur and is interfering with your baby's ability to drink and breathe comfortably, try using a bulb syringe to suction the mucus from his nose, especially before feedings and when it's obviously blocked. Put a few drops of normal saline (prescribed by your pediatrician) into his nose first to thin the mucus, making it easier to suction. Squeeze the bulb first; then insert the tip **gently** into the nostril and slowly release the bulb. (Caution: Too vigorous or frequent suctioning may cause increased swelling of delicate nasal tissues.) Although acetaminophen will lower an elevated temperature and calm him if he's irritable, you should give it to a baby in this young age group *only* on your pediatrician's advice. *Do not use aspirin.* (See *Medication,* page 647.) Fortunately, in the case of most common colds and upper respiratory infections, babies don't need to see the doctor. You should call, however, if any of the following occurs:

- A persistent cough
- Loss of appetite and refuses several feedings
- Fever: *Contact your pediatrician anytime a baby under three months of age has a rectal temperature of 100.4 degrees Fahrenheit (38.0 degrees Celsius) or higher*
- Excessive irritability
- Unusual sleepiness or hard to awaken

Immunization Update

Your baby should receive the hepatitis B vaccine soon after birth and before he is discharged from the hospital, and again at least four weeks after the first dose.

At two months, and again at four months, your baby should receive:

- DTaP vaccine
- Inactivated polio vaccine
- Hib vaccine
- Pneumococcal vaccine
- Rotavirus vaccine

(For detailed information, see page 93 and Chapter 27, *Immunizations.*)

Safety Check

Falls

- Never place the baby in an infant seat on a table, chair, or any other surface above floor level.
- Never leave your baby unattended on a bed, couch, changing table, or chair. When purchasing a changing table, look for one with two-inch (or higher) guardrails. To avoid a serious fall, don't place it near a window. (For more information about changing tables, see page 391.)
- On all kinds of gear, always use their safety straps or bars.

Burns

- Never hold your baby while smoking, drinking a hot liquid, or cooking by a hot stove or oven.
- Never allow anyone to smoke around your baby.
- Before placing your baby in the bath, always test the water temperature with the inside of your wrist or forearm. Also, fill up the bathing tub (or sink) with water—and then test its temperature—before placing your baby in the water. To prevent scalding, the hottest temperature at the faucet should be no more than 120 degrees Fahrenheit (48.9 degrees Celsius).
- Never heat your baby's milk (or, later on, food) in a microwave oven. Mix it well and test the temperature before serving.

Choking

- Routinely check all toys for small parts that could be pulled or broken off. Also look for sharp edges, which can pose a danger, too.
- If you attach a toy to the crib, make sure it is fastened securely and tightly so the baby cannot pull it down or entangle himself in it.

8

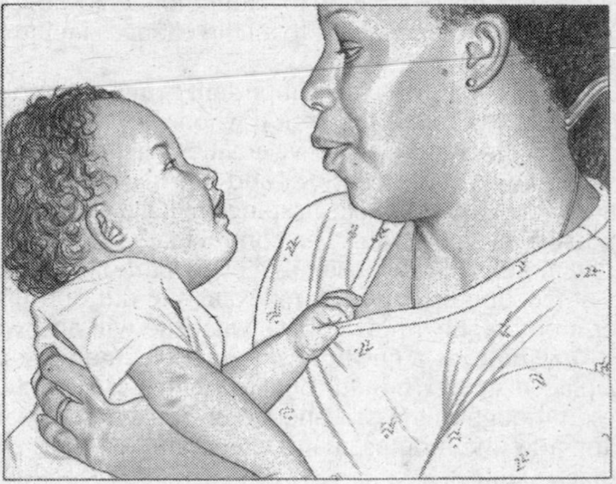

Age Four Months Through Seven Months

These months are glorious ones for you and your baby. As his personality emerges, his laughter, giggles, and joy of being with you and all he sees are a wonder every day. For him each day has new surprises, new accomplishments, and for you there is a growing sense of just how special the experience is.

By your infant's four-month birthday, you'll probably have a daily routine for his feeding, napping, bathing, and going to sleep at night. This routine will provide a predictability that will help your baby feel secure while allowing you to budget your time and activities. The schedule should be flexible, however, to allow for spur-of-the-moment fun. Short strolls when the sun finally appears on a dreary day, an unexpected lunch visit from grandparents, or a family excursion to the zoo or park are all wonderful excuses to break the routine. Being open to impulse will make your life together more enjoyable and help your baby learn to adapt to all the changes facing him in his life ahead.

For the time being, the most important changes are taking place within her. This is the period when she'll learn to coordinate her emerging perceptive abilities (the use of senses like vision, touch, and hearing) and her increasing motor abilities to develop skills like grasping, rolling over, sitting up, and possibly even crawling. The control that's evident in her budding motor skills will extend to every part of her life. Instead of reacting primarily by reflex, as she did during her earlier months, she'll now choose what she will and won't do. For example, as a newborn, she sucked on almost anything placed in her mouth, but now she has definite favorites. Although in the past she merely looked at a strange new toy, now she mouths, manipulates, and explores every one of its qualities.

Your baby will be better able to communicate her emotions and desires now, and she'll voice them frequently. For example, she'll cry not only when she's hungry or uncomfortable, but also when she wants a different toy or a change in activity.

You may find that your five- or six-month-old also occasionally cries when you leave the room or when she's suddenly confronted by a stranger. This is because she's developing a strong attachment for you and the other people who regularly care for her. She now associates you with her own well-being and can distinguish you from other people. Even if she doesn't cry out for you, she will signal this new awareness by curiously and carefully studying a stranger's face. By eight or nine months, she may openly object to strangers who come too close. This signals the start of a normal developmental stage known as stranger anxiety.

During these months before stranger anxiety hits full force, however, your child probably will go through a period of delightful showmanship, smiling and playing with everyone she meets. Her personality will be coming out in full bloom, and even people meeting her for the first time will notice many of her unique character traits. Take advantage of her sociability to acquaint her with people who will help care for her in the future, such as babysitters, relatives, or child care workers. This won't guarantee clear sailing through the stranger-anxiety period, but it may help smooth the waters.

You'll also learn during these months, if you haven't before, that there is no formula for raising an ideal child. You and your baby are each unique, and the relationship between the two of you is unique, as well. So what works for one baby may not for another. You have to discover what succeeds for you through trial and error. While your neighbor's child may fall asleep easily and sleep through the night, your baby may need some extra holding and cuddling to settle her down at bedtime and again in the middle of the night. While your first child might have needed a great deal of hugging and comforting, your second might prefer more time alone. These individual differences don't necessarily indicate that your parenting is "right" or "wrong"; they just mean that each baby is unique.

Over these first months and years, you will get to know your child's individual traits and you'll develop patterns of activity and interaction that are designed especially for her. If you remain flexible and open to her special traits, she'll help steer your actions as a parent in the right direction. (Also see the discussion of *temperament* on page 277 of this chapter.)

GROWTH AND DEVELOPMENT

Physical Appearance and Growth

Between four and seven months, your baby will continue to gain approximately 1 to 1¼ pounds (0.45 to 0.56 kg) a month. By the time she reaches her eight-month birthday, she probably will weigh about two and a half times what she did at birth. Her bones also will continue to grow at a rapid rate. As a result, during these months her length will increase by about 2 inches (5 cm) and her head circumference by about 1 inch (2.5 cm).

Your child's specific weight and height are not as important as her rate of growth. By now you should have established her position on the growth curve in the Appendix. Continue to plot her measurements at regular intervals to

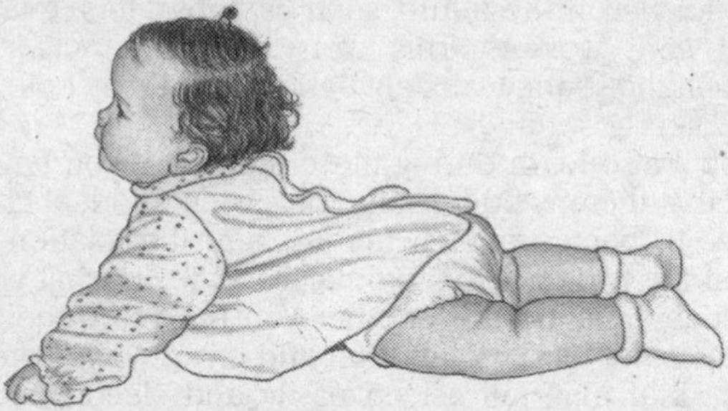

make sure she keeps growing at the same rate. If you find that she's beginning to follow a different curve or gaining weight or height unusually slowly, discuss it with your pediatrician.

Movement

In her first four months, your baby established the muscle control she needed to move both her eyes and her head so

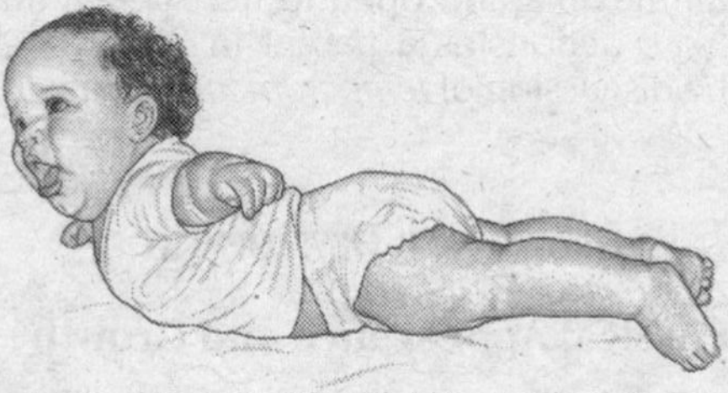

she could follow interesting objects. Now she'll take on an even greater challenge: sitting up. She'll accomplish this in small steps as her back and neck muscles gradually strengthen and she develops better balance in her trunk, head, and neck. First she'll learn to raise her head and hold it up while lying on her stomach. You can encourage this by placing her on her stomach and extending her arms forward; then hold a rattle or other attractive toy in front of her to get her attention and coax her to hold her head up and look at you. This also is a good way to check her hearing and vision.

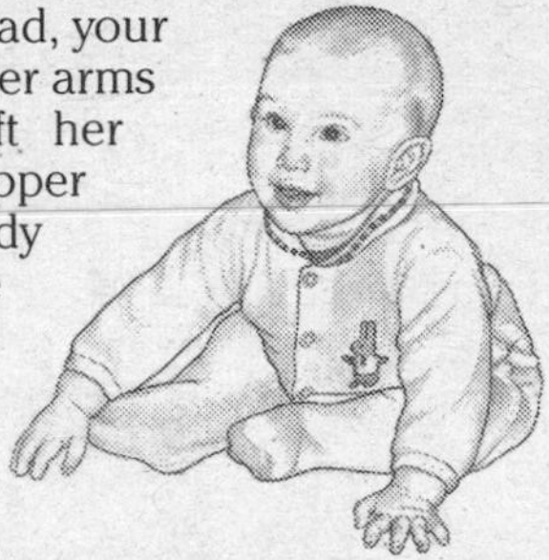

Once she's able to lift her head, your baby will start pushing up on her arms and arching her back to lift her chest. This strengthens her upper body so she can remain steady and upright when sitting. At the same time she may rock on her stomach, kick her legs, and "swim" with her arms. These abilities, which usually appear at about five months, are necessary for rolling over and crawling. By the end of this period, she'll probably be able to roll over in both directions, although babies normally vary in the age when they're able to do so. Most children roll first from the stomach to the back and later in the opposite direction, although doing it in the opposite sequence is perfectly normal.

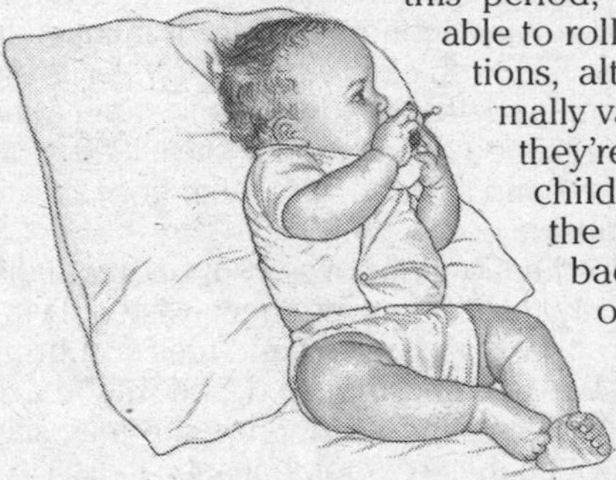

Once your baby is strong enough to raise her chest, you can help her practice sitting up. Hold her up or support her back with pillows or a couch corner as she learns to balance herself. Soon she'll learn to "tripod," leaning forward as she extends her arms to balance her upper body. Bright, interesting toys placed in front of her will give her something to focus on as she gains her balance. It will be some time before she can maneuver herself into a sitting posture without your assistance, but by six to eight months, if you position her upright, she'll be able to remain sitting without leaning forward on her arms. Then she can discover all the wonderful things that can be done with her hands as she views the world from this new vantage point.

By the fourth month, your baby can easily bring interesting objects to her mouth. During her next four months,

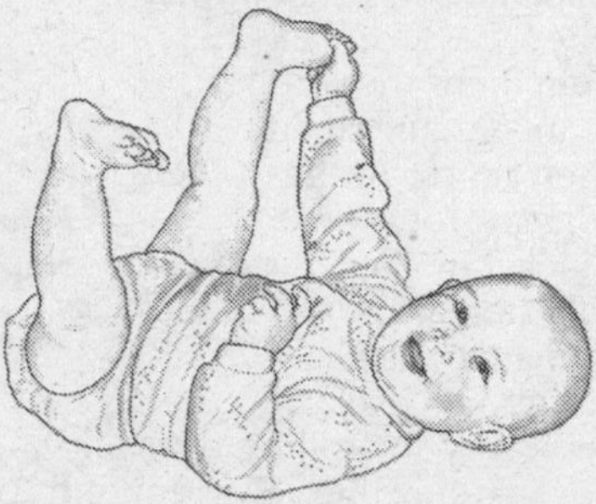

she'll begin to use her fingers and thumbs together in a mitten or clawlike grip or raking motion, and she'll manage to pick up many things. She won't develop the pincer grasp using her index finger and thumb until she's about nine months old, but by the sixth to eighth month, she'll learn how to transfer objects from hand to hand, turn them from side to side, and twist them upside down.

As her physical coordination improves, your baby will discover parts of her body that she never knew existed. Lying on her back, she can now grab her feet and toes and bring them to her mouth. While being diapered, she may reach down to touch her genitals. When sitting up, she may slap her knee or thigh. Through these explorations she'll discover many new and interesting sensations. She'll also start to understand the function of each body part. For example, when you place her newly found feet on the floor, she may first curl her toes and stroke the carpet or wood surface, but soon she'll discover she can use her feet and legs to practice "walking" or just to bounce up and down. Watch out! These are all preparations for the next major milestones: crawling and standing.

Vision

As your baby works on her important motor skills, have you noticed how closely she watches everything she's doing? The concentration with which she reaches for a toy may remind you of a scientist engrossed in research. It's obvious that her good vision is playing a key role in her early motor

Movement Milestones by the End of This Period

- Rolls both ways (front to back, back to front)
- Sits with, and then without, support of her hands
- Supports her whole weight on her legs
- Reaches with one hand
- Transfers object from hand to hand
- Uses raking grasp (not pincer)

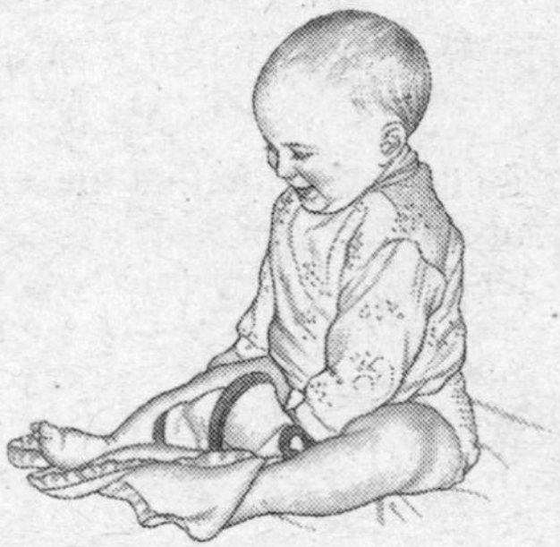

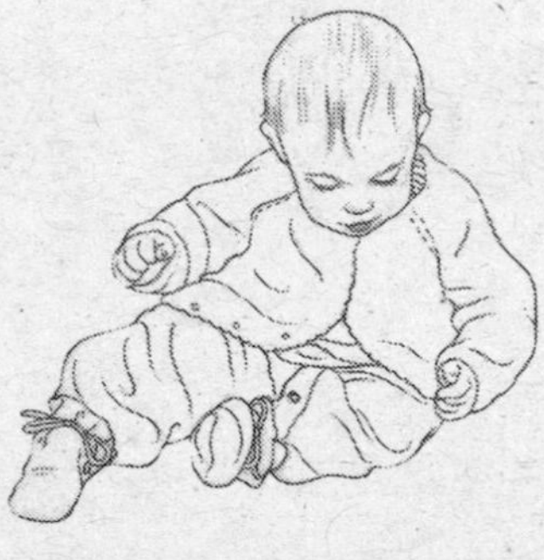

and cognitive development. Conveniently, her eyes become fully functional just when she needs them most.

Although your baby was able to see at birth, her total visual ability has taken months to develop fully. Only now can she distinguish subtle shades of reds, blues, and yellows. Don't be surprised if you notice that she prefers red or blue to other colors; these seem to be favorites among many infants this age. Most babies also like increasingly complex patterns and shapes as they get older—something to keep in

Toys Appropriate for a Four- to Seven-Month-Old

- Unbreakable mirror attached to inside of crib or playpen
- Soft balls, including some that make soft, pleasant sounds

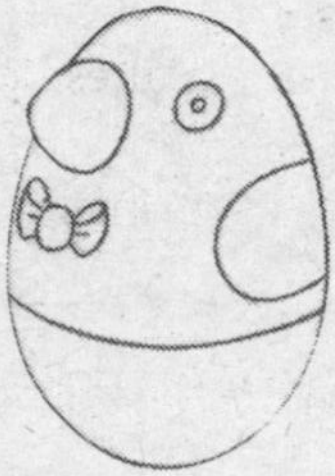

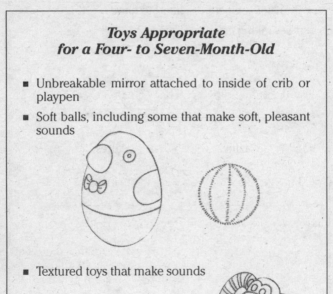

- Textured toys that make sounds

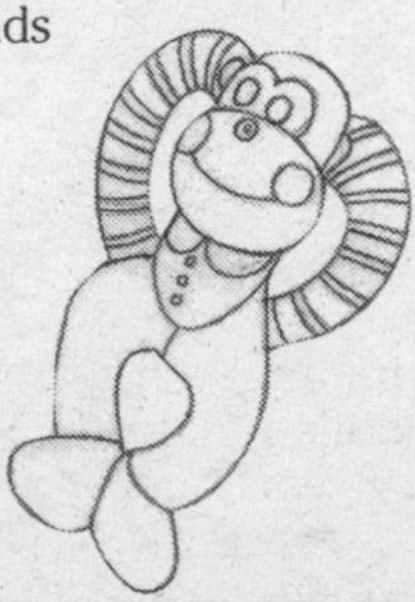

- Toys that have fingerholds

- Musical toys, such as bells, maracas, tambourines (Make sure none of the parts can become loose.)
- See-through rattles that show the pieces making the noise
- Old magazines with bright pictures for you to show her
- Baby books with board, cloth, or vinyl pages

mind when you're shopping for picture books or posters for your child's nursery.

By four months, your baby's range of vision has increased to several feet (meters) or more, and it will continue to expand until, at about seven months, her eyesight will be more nearly mature. At the same time, she'll learn to follow faster and faster movements with her eyes. In the early months, when you rolled a ball across the room, she couldn't coordinate her eyes well enough to track it, but now she'll follow the path of moving objects easily. As her hand-to-eye coordination improves, she'll be able to grab these objects as well.

A mobile hung over the crib or in front of an infant's "bouncy" seat is an ideal way to stimulate a young baby's vision. However, by about five months, your baby will quickly get bored and search for other things to watch. Also by this

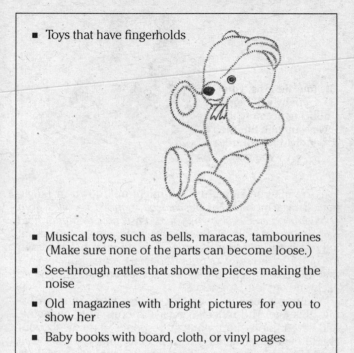

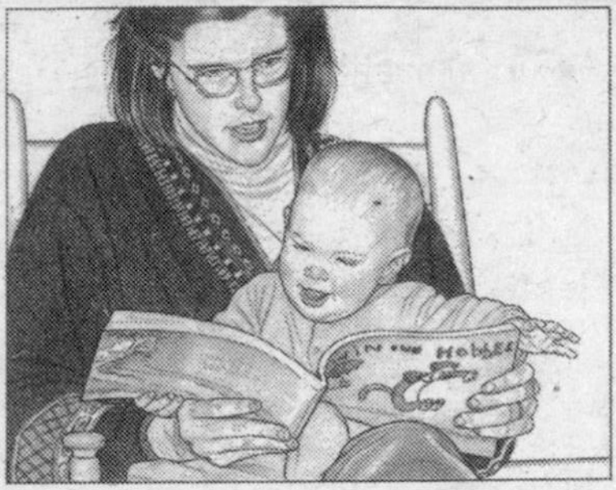

By four months, your baby will begin noticing not only the way you talk but the individual sounds you make.

age, she may be sitting up and might pull down or tangle herself in a mobile. *For this reason, remove mobiles from cribs or playpens as soon as your baby is able to pull or hold herself upright.* Still another way to hold your baby's visual interest is to keep her moving—around your home, down the block, to the store, or out on special excursions. Help her find things to look at that she's never seen before, and name each one out loud for her.

A mirror is another source of endless fascination for babies this age. The reflected image is constantly changing, and, even more important, it responds directly to your child's own movements. This is her clue that the person in the mirror is actually herself. It may take your baby a while to come to this realization, but it probably will register during this period.

In general, then, your child's visual awareness should clearly increase during these four months. Watch how she responds as you introduce her to new shapes, colors, and objects. If she doesn't seem to be interested in looking at new things, or if one or both eyes turn in or out, inform your pediatrician. (See also Chapter 21, *Eyes.*)

Language Development

Your baby learns language in stages. From birth, she receives information about language by hearing people make sounds and watching how they communicate with one another. At first she is most interested in the pitch and level of your voice. When you talk to her in a soothing way, she'll stop crying be-

Vision Milestones by the End of This Period

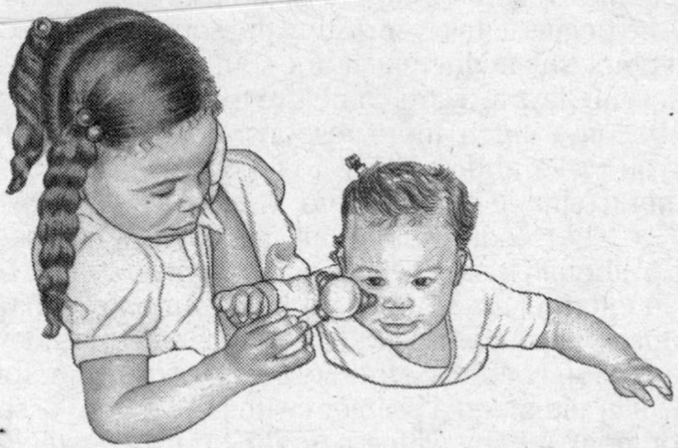

- Develops full color vision
- Distance vision matures
- Ability to track moving objects improves

cause she hears that you want to comfort her. By contrast, if you shout out in anger, she probably will cry, because your voice is telling her something is wrong. By four months, she'll begin noticing not only the way you talk but the individual sounds you make. She'll listen to the vowels and consonants and begin to notice the way these combine into syllables, words, and sentences.

Besides receiving sounds, your baby also has been producing them from the very beginning, first in the form of cries and then as coos. At about four months, she'll start to babble, using many of the rhythms and characteristics of her native language. Although it may sound like gibberish, if you listen closely, you'll hear her raise and drop her voice as if she were making a statement or asking a question. Encourage her by talking to her throughout the day. When she says a recognizable syllable, repeat it back to her and then say some simple words that contain that sound. For example, if her sound of the day is "bah," introduce her to "bottle," "box," "bonnet," and "Baa, Baa, Black Sheep."

Your participation in your child's language development will become even more important after six or seven months, when she begins actively imitating the sounds of speech. Up to that point, she might repeat one sound for a whole day or even several days at a stretch before trying another. But now she'll become much more responsive to the sounds she hears you make, and she'll try to follow your lead. So introduce her to simple syllables and words such as "baby," "cat," "dog," "go," "hot," "cold," and "walk," as well as "Mama" and "Dada." Although it may be as much as a year or more before you can interpret any of her babbling, your baby can understand many of your words well before her first birthday.

If she doesn't babble or imitate any sounds by her seventh month, it could mean a problem with her hearing or speech development. A baby with a partial hearing loss still can be startled by loud noises or will turn her head in their direction, and she may even respond to your voice. But she will have difficulty imitating speech. If your child does not babble or produce a variety of sounds, alert your pediatrician. If she has had frequent ear infections, she might have some fluid remaining in her inner ear, and this could interfere with her hearing.

Special equipment is used to check a very young baby's

Language Milestones by the End of This Period

- Responds to own name
- Begins to respond to "no"
- Distinguishes emotions by tone of voice
- Responds to sound by making sounds
- Uses voice to express joy and displeasure
- Babbles chains of consonants

hearing. All newborns should be tested for hearing loss. Your observations are the early warning system that tells whether further testing is needed. If you suspect a problem, you might ask your pediatrician for a referral to a children's hearing specialist.

Cognitive Development

During your baby's first four months, did you have doubts that she really understood much that was happening around her? This parental reaction is not surprising. After all, although you knew when she was comfortable and uncomfortable, she probably showed few signs of actually thinking. But studies show that from the minute your baby is born, she is learning about the world around her, even though it may not be apparent to you or others. Now, as her memory and attention span increase, you'll start to see evidence that she's not only absorbing information but also applying it to her day-to-day activities.

During this period, one of the most important concepts she'll refine is the principle of cause and effect. She'll probably stumble on this notion by accident somewhere between four and five months. Perhaps while kicking her mattress, she'll notice the crib shaking. Or maybe she'll realize that her rattle makes a noise when she hits or waves it. Once she understands that she can cause these interesting reactions, she'll continue to experiment with other ways to make things happen.

Your baby will quickly discover that some things, such as bells and keys, make interesting sounds when moved or shaken. When she bangs certain things on the table or drops them on the floor, she'll start a chain of responses from her audience, including funny faces, groans, and other reactions that may lead to the reappearance—or disappearance—of the object. Before long, she'll begin dropping things intentionally to see you pick them up. As annoying as this may be at times, it's one important way for her to learn about cause and effect and her personal ability to influence her environment.

It's important that you give your child the objects she needs for these experiments and encourage her to test her "theories." But make sure that everything you give her to play

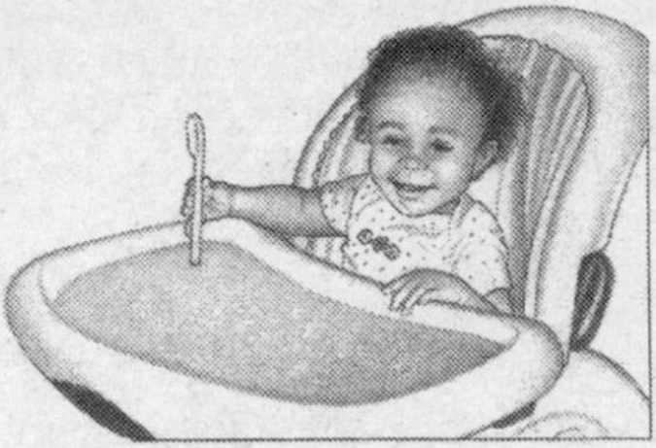

When she bangs certain things on the table or drops them on the floor, she'll start a chain of responses from her audience.

with is unbreakable, lightweight, and large enough that she can't possibly swallow it. If you run out of the usual toys or she loses interest in them, plastic or wooden spoons, unbreakable cups, and jar or bowl lids and boxes are endlessly entertaining and inexpensive.

Another major discovery that your baby will make toward the end of this period is that objects continue to exist when they're out of her sight—a principle called object permanence. During her first few months, she assumed that the world consisted only of things that she could see. When you left her room, she assumed you vanished; when you returned, you were a whole new person to her. In much the same way, when you hid a toy under a cloth or a box, she thought it was gone for good and wouldn't bother looking for it. But sometime after four months, she'll begin to realize that the world is more permanent than she thought. You're the same person who greets her every morning. Her teddy bear on the floor is the same one that was in bed with her the night before. The block that you hid under the can did

Cognitive Milestones by the End of This Period

- Finds partially hidden objects
- Explores with hands and mouth
- Struggles to get objects that are out of reach

not actually vanish after all. By playing hiding games like peekaboo and observing the comings and goings of people and things around her, your baby will continue to learn about object permanence for many months to come.

Emotional Development

Between four and seven months, your baby may undergo a dramatic change in personality. At the beginning of this period, she may seem relatively passive and preoccupied with getting enough food, sleep, and affection. But as she learns to sit up, use her hands, and move about, she's likely to become increasingly assertive and more attentive to the world outside. She'll be eager to reach out and touch everything she sees, and if she can't manage on her own, she'll demand your help by yelling, banging, or dropping the nearest object at hand. Once you've come to her rescue, she'll probably forget what she was doing and concentrate on you—smiling, laughing, babbling, and imitating you for many minutes at a stretch. While she'll quickly get bored with even the most engaging toy, she'll never tire of your attention.

The more subtle aspects of your baby's personality are determined largely by her constitutional makeup or temperament. Is she rambunctious or gentle? Easygoing or easily upset? Headstrong or compliant? To a large extent, these are inborn character traits. Just as infants come in different sizes and shapes, their temperaments differ as well. Their unique character traits include their activity levels, their persistence, and their adaptability to the world around them—and these traits will become increasingly apparent during these months. You won't necessarily find all of their personal characteristics enjoyable all the time—especially not when your determined six-month-old is screaming in frustration as she lunges for the family cat. But in the long run, adapting to her natural personality is best for both of you. And because your baby's temperament is real and directly affects you and the rest of the family, it's important to understand her as completely as possible.

Your child's "behavioral style" even affects how you parent and how you feel about yourself. An agreeable, even-tempered child, for example, is more likely to make you feel competent as a parent than one who is constantly irritable.

Developmental Health Watch

Because each baby develops in her own particular manner, it's impossible to tell exactly when or how your child will perfect a given skill. The developmental milestones listed in this book will give you a general idea of the changes you can expect, but don't be alarmed if your own baby's development takes a slightly different course. Alert your pediatrician, however, if your baby displays any of the following signs of possible developmental delay for this age range.

- Seems very stiff, with tight muscles
- Seems very floppy, like a rag doll
- Head still flops back when body is pulled up to a sitting position
- Reaches with one hand only
- Refuses to cuddle
- Shows no affection for the person who cares for her
- Doesn't seem to enjoy being around people
- One or both eyes consistently turn in or out
- Persistent tearing, eye drainage, or sensitivity to light
- Does not respond to sounds around her
- Has difficulty getting objects to her mouth
- Does not turn her head to locate sounds by four months
- Doesn't roll over in either direction (front to back or back to front) by five to seven months
- Seems inconsolable at night after five months
- Doesn't smile spontaneously by five months
- Cannot sit with help by six months

- Does not laugh or make squealing sounds by six months
- Does not actively reach for objects by six to seven months
- Doesn't follow objects with both eyes at near (1 foot [30 cm]) and far (6 feet [180 cm]) ranges by seven months
- Does not bear some weight on legs by seven months
- Does not try to attract attention through actions by seven months
- Does not babble by eight months
- Shows no interest in games of peekaboo by eight months

As you've probably discovered already, some infants of this age are "easy," calm and predictable, while others are much more difficult. Strong-willed and high-strung babies require an extra dose of patience and gentle guidance. They often don't adapt to changing surroundings as easily as calmer babies, and will become increasingly upset if pushed to move or perform before they're ready. To a large degree, you'll fare better not by trying to change your child's temperament, but by accommodating it. You can reduce the stresses of rearing an infant by recognizing and acknowledging her temperament rather than resisting or working against it.

Language and cuddling sometimes will do wonders to calm the nerves of an irritable child. Distracting her can help refocus her energy. For instance, if she screams because you won't retrieve the toy she dropped for the tenth time, move her to the floor so she can reach the toy herself.

The shy or "sensitive" child also requires special attention, particularly if you have more boisterous children in the household who overshadow her. When a baby is quiet and undemanding, it's easy to assume she's content, or if she

> ### *Social/Emotional Milestones by the End of This Period*
>
> - Enjoys social play
> - Interested in mirror images
> - Responds to other people's expressions of emotion and appears joyful often

doesn't laugh or smile a lot, you may lose interest in playing with her. But a baby like this often needs personal contact even more than other children. She may be overwhelmed easily and needs you to show her how to be assertive and become involved in the activities around her. How should you do this? Give her plenty of time to warm up to any situation, and make sure that other people approach her slowly. Let her sit on the sidelines before attempting to involve her directly with other children. Once she feels secure, gradually she'll become more responsive to the people around her.

Also let your pediatrician know if you have any concerns about your baby's emotional development. Your pediatrician can help if she knows there are problems, but such concerns can often be difficult to detect in a routine office visit. That's why it's important for you to call the doctor's attention to your concerns and describe your day-to-day observations. Write them down so you don't forget them. And take comfort in the fact that with time and patience, some of her personality traits that you wish you could change will evolve. In the meantime, enjoy her as she is.

BASIC CARE

Introducing Solid Foods

At four months, your baby's diet should consist of breastmilk and/or formula (with iron), but by four to six months, you can begin adding solid foods. Babies are born with a tongue thrust reflex. Because of this reflex, the young infant will push her tongue against a spoon or anything else inserted into her mouth, including food. Most babies lose this reflex at about four months, enabling them to begin taking solid food. Talk with your pediatrician at the four-month checkup to see when she feels your infant should begin eating solid food.

Once you decide to begin, you may start solid food at whichever feedings during the day are most acceptable to you and your baby. However, remember that as she gets older, she will want to eat with the other family members. To minimize the chances of choking, make sure your baby is sitting upright when you introduce solids. If she cries or turns away when you try to feed her, don't force the issue. It's more important that you both enjoy her mealtimes than for her to start these foods by a specific date. Go back to nursing or bottle-feeding exclusively for a week or two, then try again.

Always use a spoon to feed your baby solids unless, at your pediatrician's recommendation, you are thickening the formula because your infant has gastro-esophageal reflux (spitting up stomach contents). Some parents try putting solid foods in a bottle or infant feeder with a nipple, but feeding a baby this way can drastically increase the amount of food she takes in at each feeding and lead to excessive weight gain. Besides, it's important for your baby to get used to the process of eating—sitting up, taking bites from a spoon, resting between bites, and stopping when she's full. This early experience will help lay the foundation for good eating habits throughout her life.

Even standard baby spoons may be too wide for a child this young, but a small coffee spoon will work well; use of a rubber-coated baby spoon is also a good choice and can avoid injury. Start with half a spoonful or less, and talk your baby through the process ("Mmm, see how good this is"). She probably won't know what to do the first time or two. She may look confused, wrinkle her nose, and roll the food around her mouth or reject it entirely. This is an understandable reaction, considering how different her feedings have been up to this point.

One way to ease the transition to solids is to give your infant a little breastmilk or formula first, then switch to very small half-spoonfuls of food, and finally finish off with more breastmilk or formula. This will prevent her from being overly frustrated when she's very hungry, and it will link the

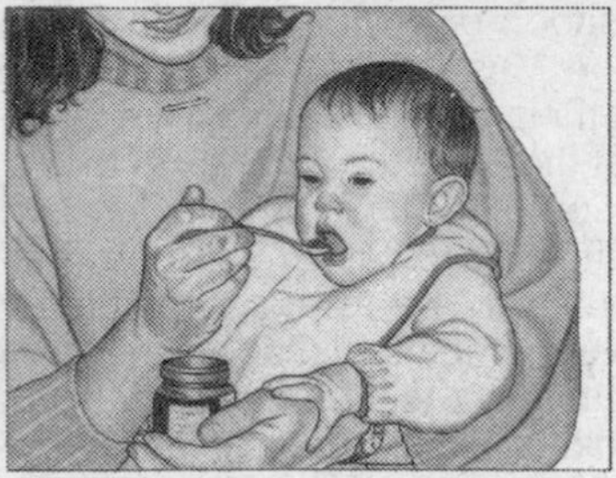

It is important for your baby to get used to the process of eating while sitting up.

satisfaction of nursing with this new experience of spoon-feeding.

No matter what you do, most of the first few solid-food feedings are sure to wind up outside her mouth on her face and bib, so increase the size of her feedings very gradually, starting with just a teaspoonful or two, until she gets the idea of swallowing solids.

What foods should you feed her? By tradition, single grain cereals have usually been introduced first. However, there is no medical evidence that introducing solid foods in any particular order has an advantage for your infant. Though many pediatricians recommend starting vegetables before fruits, there is no research indicating that your infant will develop a dislike for vegetables or an allergy if vegetables follow the introduction of fruit.

Many babies enjoy eating cereals. You may use premixed baby cereals in a jar or dry varieties to which you add formula, breastmilk, or water. The prepared cereals are convenient, but the dry ones are richer in iron and can be varied in consistency to suit your baby. Whichever you choose, make sure that it's made for babies. This assures you that it contains the extra nutrients your child needs at this age and not additional salt, etc.

If your infant has been mostly breastfeeding, she may benefit from baby meats, which contain iron and zinc. These nutrients are more easily absorbed, and are needed by four to six months of age.

Give your baby just one new food at a time, and wait at least four days before starting another. After each new food, watch for responses such as diarrhea, rash, or vomiting. If any of these occur, eliminate the suspect food from her diet until you've consulted your pediatrician. Within two or three months, your baby's daily diet should include breastmilk or formula, cereal, vegetables, meats, and fruits, distributed among three meals.

Talk with your pediatrician about the best time to start eggs and fish. Although many pediatricians previously recommended against giving these foods in the first year of life because of allergic reactions, there is no evidence that introducing these nutrient-dense foods after four to six months of age determines whether or not your baby will become allergic to them. It's also important to note that because canned adult-type foods generally contain added salt and preservatives, they should not be fed to babies.

Once your baby sits up independently, you can begin to give her finger foods to help her learn to feed herself. Most infants can begin learning to self-feed around eight months of age. Make sure anything you give her is soft, easy to swallow, and breaks down into small pieces that she can't possibly choke on. Well-cooked cut-up yams, sweet potatoes, green beans, peas, and small pieces of bread, wafer-type cookies, or crackers are good examples. Don't give her any food that requires chewing at this age, even if she already has teeth.

When feeding your baby solid foods, do not feed directly from the jar but rather from a small dish into which a portion of the jar of food has been placed. This will prevent the jar of food from becoming contaminated from the introduction of bacteria from the baby's mouth. The portion in the dish also should be discarded, not saved.

What if you want your baby to have fresh food instead of canned or dehydrated? In that case, use a blender or food processor, or just mash softer foods with a fork. Everything should be soft, unsalted, well cooked, and unseasoned. Cooked fresh vegetables and stewed fruits are the easiest to prepare. Although you can feed your baby mashed raw bananas, all other fruits should be cooked until soft. Refrigerate any food you don't use immediately, and then inspect it carefully for signs of spoilage before giving it to your baby. Unlike commercial foods, your own are not bacteria-free, so they will spoil more quickly.

Although water is a healthier drinking option, if you must

give your infant fruit juice, wait until your baby is at least six months old. Because of the nonabsorbed carbohydrates in juices, large amounts of fruit juice can increase the frequency of stools and make them looser. These more frequent loose stools can cause diaper rash that is bright red and painful when the baby is wiped during her diaper change. Contact with air and the application of a heavy, protective diaper ointment usually will heal the rash. Fruit juice also gets children used to drinking sweet beverages and can lead to excessive weight gain.

Bear in mind that babies do not need juice. If you choose to give her juice (after six months of age), offer it only in a cup, not in a bottle. Limit this juice intake to no more than four ounces a day and offer it only with a meal or snack; any more than four ounces will reduce her appetite for other, more nutritious foods, including breastmilk or formula.

If your infant seems to be thirsty between feedings, put her to the breast or offer her extra formula. After six months, you can offer her small sips of extra water if she seems to be thirsty between feedings. Getting a child used to the taste of plain water is a healthy habit for life. During the hot months when your child is losing fluid through sweat, offer water two or more times a day. If you live in an area where the water is fluoridated, these feedings also will help prevent future tooth decay.

By the time your baby is six or seven months old, she'll probably sit up well enough to use a high chair during mealtime. To ensure her comfort, the seat of the chair should be covered with a pad that's removable and washable, so you can clean out the food that probably will accumulate there. Also, when shopping for a high chair, look for one with a detachable tray with raised rims. (See page 398 for safety recommendations.) The rims will help keep dishes and food from sliding off during your baby's more rambunctious feeding sessions. The detachable tray can be carried straight to the sink for cleaning, a feature you're bound to appreciate in the months to come. (There still may be days when the only solution is to put the entire chair in the shower for a complete wipe-down!)

As your child's diet expands and she begins feeding herself more regularly, discuss her personal nutritional needs with your pediatrician. Poor eating habits established in infancy can lead to health problems later on.

Your pediatrician will help you determine whether your baby is overfed, not eating enough, or eating too many of the wrong kinds of foods. By familiarizing yourself with the caloric and nutritional contents of what she eats, you can make sure she's eating a proper diet. Be aware of the food habits of others in your family. As your baby eats more and more "table foods" (this usually starts at eight to ten months in quantities similar to those used for baby foods), she'll imitate the way you eat—including using the saltshaker and nibbling on salty snacks and processed foods. For her sake as well as your own, cut your salt use to a minimum.

What if you're concerned that your baby is *already* overweight? Even when infants are young, some parents are already worried that their babies are gaining too much weight. On one hand, there *is* a rise in childhood obesity and all of its potential complications (such as diabetes), and thus it's wise to be sensitive to the problem, no matter what age your child is. Some evidence indicates that bottle-fed infants gain weight more rapidly than breastfed babies, perhaps because some parents encourage their infant to finish a bottle feeding. **However, *don't let any anxiety over obesity lead you to underfeed your infant during the first year.*** Get your pediatrician's advice before making any dietary adjustments. During these months of rapid growth, your infant needs the proper balance of fat, carbohydrates, and protein. As soon as you start giving your child solid foods, her stools will become more solid and variable in color. Due to the added sugars and fats, they'll also have a much stronger odor. Peas and other green vegetables may turn the stool deep green; beets may make it red. (Beets sometimes make urine red, as well.) If her meals aren't strained, her stools may contain undigested particles of food, especially hulls of peas or corn, and the skin of tomatoes or other vegetables. All of this is perfectly normal. If the stools are extremely loose, watery, or full of mucus, however, it may mean her digestive tract is irritated. In this case, consult your pediatrician to determine if your infant or child has a digestive problem.

Dietary Supplements

Although the American Academy of Pediatrics recommends breastfeeding your baby for the first twelve months of her life, human milk does not contain sufficient vitamin D to prevent a deficiency of this vitamin, which can produce diseases such as rickets (the severe form of vitamin D deficiency characterized by the softening of bones). Even though sunlight stimulates the skin to manufacture vitamin D, all children should wear sunscreen when they're outdoors, and sunscreen prevents the skin from making vitamin D.

As a result, the Academy recommends that if you are breastfeeding your baby, you need to provide her with supplemental vitamin D, beginning soon after birth. Vitamin D supplements of 400 IU (International Units) (contained in a 1 ml combination multivitamin or a vitamin that contains vitamins A, C, and D) per day are recommended for breastfed babies unless they are weaned to at least 32 ounces (1,000 ml) of vitamin D–fortified formula, and for all nonbreastfed infants who are consuming less than 32 ounces (1,000 ml) per day of vitamin D–fortified formula. You should discuss this issue with your pediatrician. Vitamin D has already been added to infant formula, so no additional supplementation of vitamin D is necessary.

What about iron? For the first four to six months, your breastfed baby needs no additional iron. The iron she had in her body at birth was enough to see her through her initial growth. But now the reserves will be running low and her need for iron will increase as her growth speeds up. The Academy believes that babies who are not breastfed or are only partially breastfed should receive an iron-fortified formula (containing between 4 and 12 mg of iron) from birth through twelve months of age. We discourage the use of low-iron infant formulas as they do not contain enough iron to support an infant's proper growth and development. Fortunately, once you start your baby on solid foods, she'll also receive iron from meats, iron-fortified baby cereals, and green vegetables. For example, four level tablespoons of fortified cereal, diluted with breastmilk or formula, provides 7 mg of iron; meat is another very good source of iron. (See also *Supplementation for Breastfed and Bottle-Fed Infants,* page 141.)

Sleeping

Most babies this age still need at least two naps a day, one at midmorning and the other midday. Some babies may nap a third time later in the afternoon. In general, it's best to let your baby sleep as long as she wants, unless she has trouble falling asleep at her normal nightly bedtime. If this becomes a problem, wake her up earlier from her afternoon nap.

Because your child is more alert and active now, she may have trouble winding down at the end of the day. A consistent bedtime routine will help. Experiment to see what works best, taking into consideration both the activities in the rest of the household and your baby's temperament. A warm bath, a massage, rocking, a story or lullaby, and a breast- or bottle-feeding will all help relax her and put her in a bedtime mood. *Remember to begin these activities before your baby becomes overtired.* Eventually she'll associate these activities with going to sleep, and that will help relax and soothe her.

Settle your baby in her crib while she's still awake so she learns to fall asleep on her own. Gently put her down, whisper your good night, and leave the room. If she cries, check on her and offer a few comforting words and then leave the room. As the days pass, gradually give her less attention at night.

If parents are consistent, most babies will cry less each night and will be more likely to learn self-soothing. See Chapter 30 for more information on sleep.

Teething

Teething usually starts during these months. The two front teeth (central incisors), either upper or lower, usually appear first, followed by the opposite front teeth. The first molars come in next, followed by the canines or eyeteeth.

There is great variability in the timing of teething. If your child doesn't show any teeth until later than this age period, don't worry. The timing may be determined by heredity, and it doesn't mean that anything is wrong.

Teething *occasionally* may cause mild irritability, crying, a low-grade temperature (but not over 101 degrees Fahrenheit or 38.3 degrees Celsius), excessive drooling, and a desire to chew on something hard. More often, the gums around the new teeth will swell and be tender. To ease your baby's discomfort, try gently rubbing or massaging the gums with one of your fingers. Teething rings are helpful, too, but they should be made of firm rubber. (The teethers that you freeze tend to get too hard and can cause more harm than good.) Pain relievers and medications that you rub on the gums are not necessary or useful since they wash out of the baby's mouth within minutes. Some medication you rub on your child's gums can even be harmful if too much is used and the child swallows an excessive amount. If your child seems particularly miserable or has a fever higher than 101 degrees Fahrenheit (38.3 degrees Celsius), it's probably not because she's teething, and you should consult your pediatrician.

How should you clean the new teeth? Simply brush them with a soft child's toothbrush when you first start seeing her teeth. To prevent cavities, never let your baby fall asleep with a bottle, either at nap time or at night. By avoiding this situation, you'll keep milk from pooling around the teeth and creating a breeding ground for decay.

Swings and Playpens

Many parents find that mechanical swings, especially those with cradle attachments, can calm a crying baby when noth-

Stimulating Infant Brain Growth: Age Four Months Through Seven Months

Many connections are being made in your baby's brain during this time in her young life, reflected in her behaviors, such as showing strong attachments to you and others who regularly take care of her, crying when you leave the room or when she is approached suddenly by a stranger, or crying when she wants a particular toy or a change in activity. She is becoming more interested in the world around her and is better able to communicate her emotions and desires—all the while developing new skills such as grasping, rolling over, and sitting up.

Without overstimulating your baby, try these activities to help strengthen the connections in her developing brain:

- Provide a stimulating, safe environment where your baby can begin to explore and roam freely.
- Give consistent, warm, physical contact—hugging, skin-to-skin, body-to-body contact—to establish your infant's sense of security and well-being.
- Be attentive to your baby's rhythms and moods. Respond to her when she is upset as well as when she is happy.
- Talk and sing to your baby during dressing, bathing, feeding, playing, walking, and driving. She may not yet understand the language, but as she hears it all the time, her language skills will develop. Check with your pediatrician if your baby doesn't seem to hear sounds or doesn't imitate your words.
- Engage your child in face-to-face talk. Mimic her sounds to show interest.
- Read books to your baby every day. She'll love the sound of your voice, and before long she'll enjoy looking at the pictures and "reading" on her own.
- If you speak a foreign language, use it at home.
- Engage in rhythmic movement with your child, such as dancing together with music.
- Avoid subjecting your baby to stressful or traumatic experiences, physical or psychological.
- Introduce your child to other children and parents; this is a very special period for infants. Be sensitive to cues indicating that she is ready to meet new people.

- Encourage your child to reach for toys. Give her baby blocks and soft toys that can stimulate her eye-hand coordination and her fine motor skills.
- Make sure other people who provide care and supervision for your baby understand the importance of forming a loving and comforting relationship with your child.
- Encourage your child to begin to sleep for extended periods at night; if you need advice about this important step in your infant's development, ask your pediatrician.
- Spend time on the floor playing with your child every day.
- Choose quality child care that is affectionate, responsive, educational, and safe. Visit your child care provider frequently and share your ideas about positive caregiving.

ing else seems to work. If you use one of these devices, don't put your baby in the seat of the swing until she can sit on her own. Use only swings that stand firmly on the floor, not the ones that hang suspended from door frames. Also, don't use a swing more than half an hour twice a day; while it may quiet your baby, it is no substitute for your attention. Secure your baby properly with a safety strap at all times.

Once your baby starts to move about, you may need to start using a playpen (also called a portable play yard). But even before she crawls or walks, a playpen offers a protected place where she can lie or sit outdoors as well as in rooms where you have no crib or bassinet. (See *Playpens,* page 400, for specific recommendations.) Remember never to leave the side of the playpen down. If the baby gets used to a playpen now, she may be more willing to stay in it as she gets older. Don't count on this, though; while some babies don't mind being enclosed, others resist it vigorously.

Be sure the playpen or swing that you're considering buying has not been recalled. Check the Consumer Product Safety Commission website (www.cpsc.gov) for recalled products.

BEHAVIOR

Discipline

As your baby becomes more mobile and inquisitive, she'll naturally become more assertive, as well. This is wonderful for her self-esteem and should be encouraged as much as possible. When she wants to do something that's dangerous or disrupts the rest of the family, however, you'll need to take charge.

For the first six months or so, the best way to deal with such conflicts is to distract her with an alternative toy or activity. Standard discipline won't work until her memory span increases around the end of her seventh month. Only then can you use a variety of techniques to discourage undesired behavior.

When you finally begin to discipline your child, it should never be harsh. Remember that discipline means to teach or instruct, not necessarily to punish. Often the most successful approach is simply to reward desired behavior and withhold rewards when she does not behave as desired. For example, if she cries for no apparent reason, make sure there's nothing wrong physically; then when she stops, reward her with extra attention, kind words, and hugs. If she starts up again, wait a little longer before turning your attention to her, and use a firm tone of voice as you talk to her. This time, don't reward her with extra attention or hugs.

The main goal of discipline is to teach limits to the child, so try to help her understand exactly what she's doing wrong when she breaks a rule. If you notice her doing something that's not allowed, such as pulling your hair, let her know that it's wrong by calmly saying "no," stopping her, and redirecting her attention to an acceptable activity.

If your child is touching or trying to put something in her mouth that she shouldn't, gently pull her hand away as you tell her this particular object is off-limits. But since you do want to encourage her to touch *other* things, avoid saying

"Don't touch." More pointed phrases, such as "Don't eat the flowers" or "No eating leaves" will convey the message without confusing her.

Because it's still relatively easy to modify her behavior at this age, this is a good time to establish your authority and a sense of consistency. Be careful not to overreact, however. She's still not old enough to misbehave intentionally and won't understand if you punish her or raise your voice. She may be confused and even become startled when told that she shouldn't be doing or touching something. Instead, remain calm, firm, consistent, and loving in your approach. If she learns now that you have the final word, it may make life much more comfortable for both of you later on, when she naturally becomes more headstrong.

Siblings

If your baby has a big brother or sister, you may start to see increasing signs of rivalry at about this time, particularly if

A Word for Grandparents

As a grandparent, you thoroughly love watching your grandchild develop. During this time of her life (ages four to seven months), she's continuing to discover the world around her and has more physical skills and cognitive abilities to engage and enjoy her environment.

As sights and sounds take on more meaning for your grandchild, and as laughter abounds, these are great months for both of you. Smiles, interactive play, and recognition of familiar objects, sounds, people, and names will become part of these discovery months. Her vision is better, her hand transfer is more efficient, and her curiosity is unstoppable. Be sure to reinforce these early learning milestones that are occurring along the way.

Your grandchild also is beginning to move during this time. Although it is a wondrous period of life, you need to be particularly vigilant as she begins to sit.

While she will be upright more frequently, she is also likely to tip over.

You have an important role to play as a grandparent, and can make the most of it—enjoying your time with her and stimulating her parents' development—by taking these steps:

- Follow your own child's lead with respect to activities to do with your grandchild, adding some special things of your own when appropriate. Special names you share ("Nana,""Grandpa Stan"), places that the two of you go, and books or music that you share can be unique to her experiences with you. Also consider inviting other grandparents and their grandchildren to join you from time to time, which can be a special treat for your own grandchild.
- When buying gifts for your grandchild, choose age-appropriate books, as well as toys that encourage creative play.
- Make yourself available as a babysitter as often as possible when your son or daughter requests it. These times spent alone with your grandchild will be special moments that you'll always treasure. Take her on field trips (to the park or the zoo), and as the years pass, help her develop hobbies that you can do together.
- You will get a better idea of your grandchild's temperament as she moves through this time of life. Inevitably, you will make comparisons as to who she really resembles in the family. Some of her own likes and dislikes will start to emerge, and it is best to respect them. If your grandchild is particularly boisterous and active, you may need extra patience at times to fully enjoy her company. Give her some space, let her be the person she is—but rein her in if she gets too far out of bounds. The same with a shy child; don't expect her to break free of

her bashfulness the moment you show up. Enjoy her for who she is.

- Diaper changing is often an exercise in controlling the "wiggly worm," and you may need all of your strength just to keep the baby from rolling onto the floor. Switching from the changing table to the bed or floor is often a good idea; remember to keep all of the diapering paraphernalia close by and within reach.
- When it comes to discipline, discuss it with the baby's parents, and make sure your own approach is consistent with their wishes.
- Consider investing in a grandchild-appropriate crib and other furniture for your home. A high chair certainly will come in handy if she occasionally (or frequently) eats meals at your home. A stroller and a car safety seat may be very useful, as well. And keep some everyday medications at your home (for a fever, diaper rash, etc.), and a few toys that she can enjoy.
- Your grandchild's eating has become more regular, and by the end of this time period, she will be on solid foods (i.e., infant cereal and pureed vegetables, fruits, and meats). When you're caring for your grandchild, again follow the guidance of her parents on what and when to feed her. If they're on her menu, let her explore your own versions of "junior foods," such as fruit, pureed vegetables, and meats. Stay away from adult-type canned foods. Avoid giving her food chunks that are too large and could cause choking. If your grandchild is still breastfeeding, keep some frozen breastmilk in your freezer.
- Your grandchild should be sleeping through the night, so "overnighters" will be more enjoyable and less disruptive of your own schedule. When she spends the night at your home, you and your spouse can take turns on who's going to take the

early morning shift if the baby awakens before you normally would.

- Make your home a safe environment for your grandchild. Follow the guidelines in Chapter 11 to baby-proof your home, from placing protective covers on unused electrical outlets, to ensuring that matches are nowhere where the baby can reach them.
- At times, having your grandchild and her siblings staying at your home at the same time may be too much for you to handle. Try caring for one youngster at a time, especially at first. Doing this will allow you to tailor-make the activities you do, while still providing much-needed relief to your own daughter or daughter-in-law, who can then focus her energies on the child(ren) she has remaining at her home. Your continued, valued role in assisting your child to become the most effective parent possible remains the core purpose for all that you do.
- You can promote your grandchild's development now and in the future by taking family pictures and movies, creating photo albums, and putting family stories down on paper (accompanied by old and new photos).

there are less than two years separating their ages. Earlier, the baby was more dependent, slept a lot, and didn't require your constant attention. But now that she's becoming more demanding, you'll need to ration your time and energy so you have enough for each child individually as well as all of them together. This rationing is even more important—and more difficult—if you go back to work.

Your older child may still be experiencing jealousy over having to share your attention with the baby. One way to give some extra attention to your older child is to set aside special "big brother" or "big sister" chores that don't involve the baby. Doing this allows you to spend some time together and get the housework done. Be sure to show the child how much you appreciate this help.

You also might help sibling relations by including the older child in activities with the baby. If the two of you sing a song or read a story, the baby will enjoy listening. The older child also can help take care of the baby to some extent, assisting you at bathtime or changing time. But unless the child is at least twelve years old, don't leave him alone with the baby, even if he's trying to be helpful. Younger children can easily drop or injure an infant without realizing what they're doing.

For more information, see the section entitled *Siblings* in Chapter 7 (*Age One Month Through Three Months*). Many of the same issues and guidelines described there also apply to children ages four through seven months.

Health Watch

Don't be surprised if your baby catches her first cold or ear infection soon after her four-month birthday. Now that she can actively reach for objects, she'll come into physical contact with many more things and people, so she'll be much more likely to contract contagious diseases.

The first line of defense is to keep your child away from anyone you know is sick. Be especially careful of infectious diseases such as influenza (the flu), chickenpox, or measles (see *Chickenpox,* page 699; *Measles,* page 703). If someone in your playgroup has caught one of these diseases, keep your child out of the group until you're sure no one else is infected. But remember that children and adults are contagious a day or so before they have symptoms, so it is impossible to prevent some exposures.

No matter how you try to protect your baby, of course, there will be times when she gets sick. This is an inevitable part of growing up, and will happen more frequently as she has more direct contact with other children. It's not always easy to tell when a baby is ill, but there are some signs that will tip you off. Does she look pale or have dark circles under her eyes? Is she acting less energetic or more irritable than usual? If she has an infectious disease, she'll probably have a fever (see Chapter 23, *Fever*), and she may be losing weight due to loss of appetite, diarrhea, or vomiting. Some difficult-to-detect infections of the kidneys or lungs also can prevent weight gain in babies. At this age, weight loss could mean that the baby has some digestive problem, such as an allergy to wheat or milk protein (see *Milk Allergy*, page 485)

Your Child and Antibiotics

Antibiotics are among the most powerful and important medicines known; there are several types of antibiotics: antivirals, antibacterials, and antifungals. When used properly, they can save lives, but when used improperly, antibiotics actually can harm your child.

Two main types of germs—viruses and bacteria—cause most infections. Viruses cause all colds and most coughs. There are some antiviral medications, but so far, none for the common cold. Antibacterials never cure common viral infections. Your child recovers from these common viral infections when the illness has run its course. *Antibacterial antibiotics should not be used to treat viral infections.*

Antibacterials can be used to treat bacterial infections, but some strains of bacteria have become resistant to certain antibiotics. If your child is infected with resistant bacteria, she might need a different antibiotic or even need to be treated in the hospital with more powerful medicines given by vein (intravenously [by IV]). A few new strains of bacteria are already untreatable. To protect your child from antibiotic-resistant bacteria, use antibiotics only when your pediatrician has determined that they might be effective, since repeated or improper use of antibiotics contributes to the increase in resistant bacteria and viruses.

- When are antibiotics needed? When are they not needed?

These complicated questions are best answered by your pediatrician, as the answer depends on the specific diagnosis. If you think your child might need treatment, contact your pediatrician.

- *Ear infections:* Some types need antibacterial antibiotics and some do not.
- *Sinus infections:* These are very uncommon at this age, in large part because the sinuses themselves are so small. Just because your child's mucus is yellow or green does not mean that she has a bacterial infection. It is normal for the mucus to get thick and change color during a viral cold.
- *Bronchitis:* Children rarely need antibiotics for bronchitis.
- *Colds:* Colds are caused by viruses and sometimes can last for two weeks or more. Antibacterial antibiotics have no effect on colds. Your pediatrician may have suggestions for comfort measures while the cold runs its course.
- *Influenza:* There are antiviral medications for this infection but they cannot be used in children under a year of age.

Viral infections sometimes may lead to bacterial infections. But treating viral infections with antibacterials that prevent bacterial infections does not work and may lead to infection with resistant bacteria. Keep your pediatrician informed if the illness gets worse or lasts a long time, so that proper treatment can be given as needed.

If an antibiotic is prescribed, make sure your child takes the entire course, even if she's feeling better before all of the pills or liquid are gone. Never save antibiotics for later use or let other family members use a prescription that wasn't intended for them.

or lacks the digestive enzymes needed to digest certain solid foods. If you suspect that your child may be ill but can't identify the exact problem, or if you have any concerns about what is happening, call your pediatrician and describe the symptoms that worry you.

The following illnesses are the most common ones that occur at this age. (All are described in Part II of this book.)

Bronchiolitis	Diarrhea	Viral Infections
Colds (URIs)	Earache/	Vomiting
Conjunctivitis (pinkeye)	Ear Infection	
Croup	Fever	
	Pneumonia	

IMMUNIZATION UPDATE

At four months, your baby should receive:

- Second DTaP vaccine
- Second polio vaccine
- Second Hib (*Haemophilus influenzae* type b) vaccine
- Second pneumococcal vaccine
- Second hepatitis B vaccine (may be given between one and four months)
- Second rotavirus vaccine (may be given as early as four weeks after the first dose)

And at six months:

- First dose of influenza vaccine if during flu season; second dose given one month later
- Third DTaP vaccine
- Third polio vaccine (which can be given between six and eighteen months)
- Third pneumococcal vaccine
- Third Hib vaccine (depending on vaccine type given for doses one and two)
- Third hepatitis B vaccine, given between six and eighteen months

- Third rotavirus vaccine (depending on vaccine type; one requires two doses and the other three)

Safety Check

Car Safety Seats

- Buckle your baby into an approved, properly installed infant car safety seat before you start the car. It should be equipped with a five-point harness. When your child reaches the top weight or height allowed by her infant-only car safety seat (check the labels or instructions to find these limits), she will need to use a convertible car safety seat, which is bigger and heavier than an infant-only seat and can accommodate larger children rear-facing. You may choose to use a convertible car safety seat rear-facing from birth; this is safe as long as the seat fits your baby properly.
- The backseat is the safest place for all children to ride. Never place a rear-facing car seat in the front seat of a car that has a passenger-side air bag.

Drowning

- Never leave a baby alone even for a moment in a bath or near a pool of water, no matter how shallow it is. Infants can drown in just a few inches of water. Baby bath seats or supporting rings are not a substitute for adult supervision. Practice touch supervision by staying within arm's reach anytime your baby is in or near water.

Falls

- Never leave the baby unattended in high places, such as on a tabletop, changing table, or in a crib with the sides down. If she does fall and seems to be acting abnormally in any way, call the pediatrician immediately.

Burns

- Never smoke or eat, drink, or carry anything hot while holding a baby.
- Keep all hot liquids, like coffee and tea, out of baby's reach.
- Prevent scalding by making sure the hottest temperature at the faucet is no more than 120 degrees Fahrenheit (48.9 degrees Celsius).

Choking

- Never give a baby any food or small object that could cause choking. All foods should be mashed, ground, or soft enough to swallow without chewing.

9

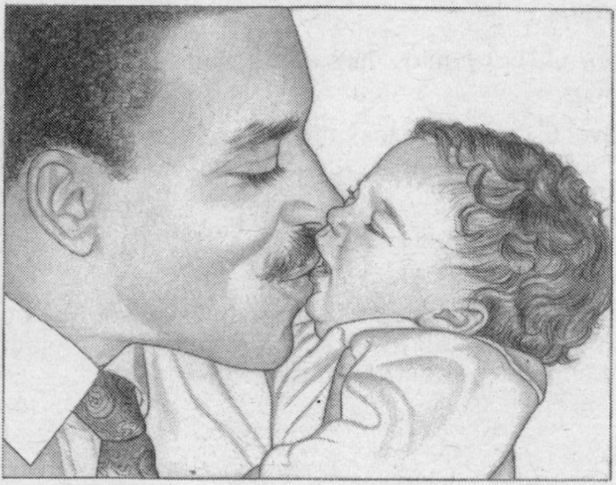

Age Eight Months Through Twelve Months

During these months, your baby is becoming increasingly mobile, a development that will thrill and challenge both of you. Being able to move from place to place gives your baby a delicious sense of power and control—her first real taste of physical independence. And while this is quite exhilarating for her, it's also frightening, since it comes at the time when she may be upset by separation from you. So as eager as she is to move out on her own and explore the farthest reaches of her domain, she may wail if she wanders out of your sight or you move too far from her.

From your point of view, your baby's mobility is a source of considerable concern as well as great pride. Crawling and walking are signals that she's developing right on target, but these achievements also mean that you'll have your hands full keeping her safe. If you haven't already fully childproofed your home, do it now. (See Chapter 11, on safety.) At this age, your baby has no concept of danger and only a limited memory for your warnings. The only way to protect her from the hundreds of hazards in your home is to secure cupboards and drawers, place dangerous and precious objects out of her reach, and make perilous rooms such as the bathroom inaccessible unless she's supervised.

By childproofing your home, you'll also give your baby a greater sense of freedom. After all, fewer areas will be off-limits, and thus you can let her make her own discoveries without your intervention or assistance. These personal accomplishments will promote her emerging self-esteem; you might even think of ways of facilitating them—for example:

1. Fill a low kitchen cupboard with safe objects and let your baby discover it herself.
2. Pad edges of a coffee table or sofa and allow her to learn to pull up and cruise.
3. Equip your home with cushions of assorted shapes and sizes and let her experiment with the different ways she can move over and around them.

Knowing when to guide a child and when to let her do things for herself is part of the art of parenting. At this age, your baby is extremely expressive and will give you the cues you need to decide when to intervene. When she's acting frustrated rather than challenged, for instance, don't let her struggle alone. If she's crying because her ball is wedged under the sofa out of her reach, if she's pulled to a standing position and can't get down, she needs your help. At other times, however, it's important to let her solve her own problems. Don't let your own impatience cause you to intervene any more than absolutely necessary. You may be tempted to feed your nine-month-old, for instance, because it's faster and less messy than letting her feed herself. However, that also deprives her of a chance to learn a valuable new skill. The more opportunities you can give her to discover, test, and strengthen her new capabilities, the more confident and adventurous she'll be.

Growth and Development

Physical Appearance and Growth

Your baby will continue to grow rapidly during these months. The typical eight-month-old boy weighs between 17.5 and 22 pounds (8 to 10 kg). Girls tend to weigh half a pound less. By his first birthday, the average child has tripled his birth weight and is 28 to 32 inches (71 to 81 cm) tall. Head growth between eight and twelve months slows down a bit from the first six months. Typical head size at eight months is 17½ inches (44.5 cm) in circumference; by one year, it's 18 inches (46 cm). Each baby grows at his own rate, however, so you should check your infant's height and weight curves on the growth charts in the Appendix to make sure he's following the pattern established in his first eight months.

When your child first stands, you may be surprised by his posture. His belly will protrude, his rear end will stick out, and his back will have a forward sway to it. It may look unusual, but this stance is perfectly normal from the time he starts to stand until he develops a confident sense of balance sometime in the second year.

Your child's feet also may look a little odd to you. When he lies on his back, his toes may turn inward so that he appears pigeon-toed. This common condition usually disappears by eighteen months. If it persists, your pediatrician may show you some foot or leg exercises to do with your baby. If the problem is severe, your pediatrician may refer you to a pediatric orthopedist. (See *Pigeon Toes,* page 693.)

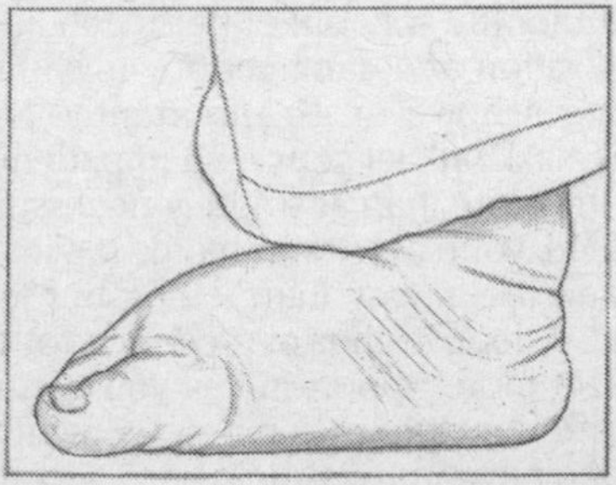

At this age your child's feet will seem flat because the arch is hidden by a pad of fat. But in two to three years this fat will disappear and his arch will be evident.

When your child takes his first teetering steps, you may notice quite a different appearance—his feet may turn outward. This occurs because the ligaments of his hips are still so loose that his legs naturally rotate outward. During the first six months of his second year, the ligaments will tighten and then his feet should point nearly straight.

At this age, your child's feet will seem flat because the arch is hidden by a pad of fat. In two to three years, this fat will disappear and his arch will be evident.

Movement

At eight months, your baby probably will be sitting without support. Although she may topple over from time to time, she'll usually catch herself with her arms. As the muscles in her trunk grow stronger, she'll also start leaning over to pick up toys. Eventually she'll figure out how to roll down onto her stomach and get back up to a sitting position.

When she's lying on a flat surface, your baby is now in constant motion. When on her stomach, she'll arch her neck so she can look around, and when on her back, she'll grab her feet (or anything else nearby) and pull them to her mouth. But she won't be content to stay on her back for long. She can turn over at will now and flip without a moment's notice. This can be especially dangerous during diaper changes, so you may want to retire her changing table, using

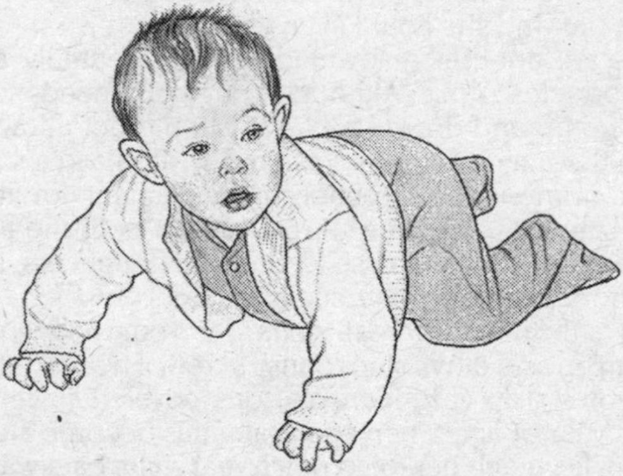

instead the floor or a bed from which she's less likely to fall. Never leave her alone for an instant at any time.

All this activity strengthens muscles for crawling, a skill that usually is mastered between seven and ten months. For a while she simply may rock on her hands and knees. Since her arm muscles are better developed than her legs, she may even push herself backward instead of forward. But with time and practice she'll discover that, by digging with her knees and pushing off, she can propel herself forward across the room toward the target of her choice.

A few children never do crawl. Instead, they use alternative movement methods, such as scooting on their bottoms or slithering on their stomachs. As long as your baby is learning to coordinate each side of her body and is using each arm and leg equally, there's no cause for concern. The important thing is that she's able to explore her surroundings on her own and is strengthening her body in preparation for walking. If you feel your baby is not moving normally, discuss your concern with the pediatrician.

How can you encourage your baby to crawl? Try presenting her with intriguing objects placed just beyond her reach. As she becomes more agile, create miniature obstacle courses using pillows, boxes, and sofa cushions for her to crawl over and between. Join in the game by hiding behind one of the obstacles and surprising her with a "peekaboo!" Don't ever leave your baby unsupervised among these props, though. If she falls between pillows or under a box, she might not be able to pull herself out. This is bound to frighten her, and she could even smother.

Stairs are another ready-made—but potentially dangerous—obstacle course. Although your baby needs to learn how to go up and down stairs, you should not allow her to play on them alone during this time. If you have a staircase in your home, she'll probably head straight for it every chance she gets, so place sturdy gates at both the top and the bottom of your staircase to close off her access. (To see a safe, horizontal-type gate, see page 398.)

As a substitute for real stairs, let your baby practice climbing up and down steps constructed of heavy-duty foam blocks or sturdy cardboard cartons covered in fabric. At about a year of age, when your baby has become a competent crawler, teach her to go down real stairs backward. She may take a few tumbles before she understands the logic of going feet first instead of headfirst, so practice on carpeted steps and let her climb only the first few. If your home doesn't have carpeted stairs, let her perfect this skill when you visit a home that does.

Although crawling makes a huge difference in how your baby sees the world and what she can do in it, don't expect her to be content with that for long. She'll see everyone else around her walking, and that's what she'll want to do, too. In preparation for this big step, she'll pull herself to a standing position every chance she gets—although when she first starts, she may not know how to get down. If she cries for your help, physically show her how to bend her knees so she can lower herself to the floor without falling. Teaching her this skill will save you many extra trips to her room at night when she's standing in her crib and crying because she doesn't know how to sit down.

Once your baby feels secure standing, she'll try some tentative steps while holding on to a support. For instance, when your hands aren't available, she'll "cruise" alongside furniture. Just make sure that whatever she uses for support has no sharp edges and is properly weighted or securely attached to the floor so it won't fall on her.

As her balance improves, occasionally she may let go, only to grab for support when she feels herself totter. The first time she continues forth on her own, her steps will be shaky. At first, she may take only one step before dropping, either in surprise or relief. Soon, however, she'll manage to keep herself up and moving until you catch her several steps later. As miraculous as it may seem, most children advance from these first steps to quite confident walking in a matter of days.

Although both of you will feel excited over this dramatic development, you'll also find yourself unnerved at times, especially when she stumbles and falls. But even if you take pains to provide a safe and soft environment, it's almost impossible to avoid bumps and bruises. Just be matter-of-fact about these accidents. Offer a quick hug or a reassuring word and send your little one on her way again. She won't be unduly upset by these falls if you're not.

At this stage, or even earlier, many parents start using a baby walker. Contrary to what the name suggests, these

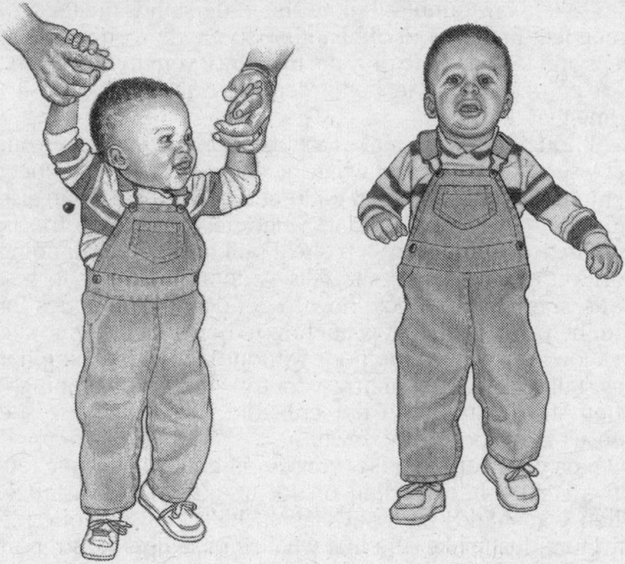

Soon he'll manage to keep himself up and moving until you catch him several steps later.

devices do not help the process of learning to walk. They actually eliminate the desire to walk. To make matters worse, they present a serious safety hazard because they can tip over easily when the child bumps into an obstacle, such as a small toy or a throw rug. Children in walkers also are more likely to fall down stairs and get into dangerous places that would otherwise be beyond their reach. For these reasons, ***the American Academy of Pediatrics strongly urges parents not to use baby walkers.***

A stationary walker or activity center is a better choice. These do not have wheels, but seats that rotate and bounce. You may also want to consider a sturdy wagon or a "kiddie push car." Be sure the toy has a bar she can push and that it's weighted so it won't tip over when she pulls herself up on it.

As your baby begins to walk outside, she'll need shoes to protect her feet. They should be comfortable and flexible

Movement Milestones by the End of This Period

- Gets to sitting position without assistance
- Crawls forward on belly by pulling with arms and pushing with legs
- Assumes hands-and-knees position
- Creeps on hands and knees supporting trunk on hands and knees
- Gets from sitting to crawling or prone (lying on stomach) position
- Pulls self up to stand
- Walks holding on to furniture
- Stands momentarily without support
- May walk two or three steps without support

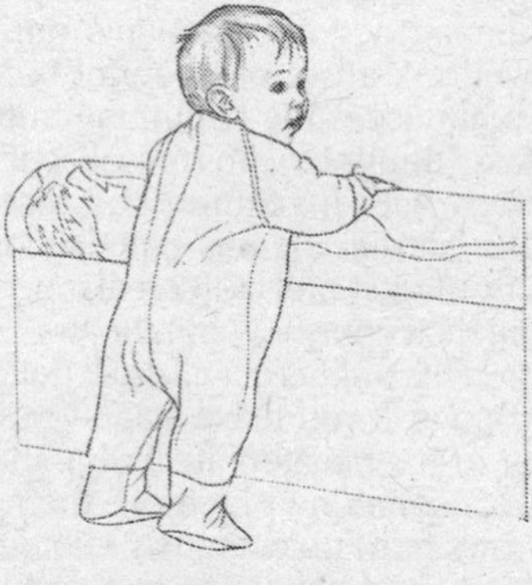

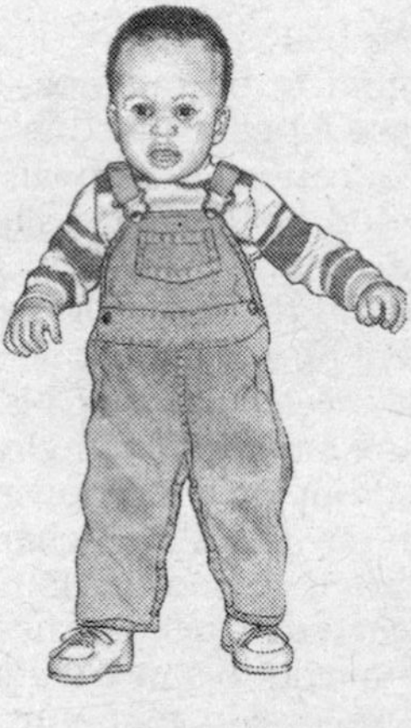

with nonskid soles to avoid slips and provide room to grow; sneakers are fine. She does not need wedges, inserts, high backs, reinforced heels, special arches, and other features designed to shape and support the feet as they have no proven benefit for the average child. Her feet will grow rapidly during these months, and her shoes will have to keep pace. Her first pair of shoes probably will last two to three months, but you should check the fit of her shoes as often as monthly during this formative period. It's often best to have your infant's shoes fit by a professional trained in a child's specific foot needs.

Many babies' first steps are taken around their first birthday, although it's perfectly normal for children to start walking a little earlier or later. At first, your baby will walk with her feet wide apart to improve her shaky sense of balance. During those initial days and weeks, she accidentally may get going too fast and fall when she tries to stop. As she becomes more confident, she'll learn how to stop and change directions. Before long, she'll be able to squat to pick something up and then stand again. When she reaches this level of accomplishment, she'll get enormous pleasure from push-pull toys—the noisier the better.

Hand and Finger Skills

Your baby's mastery of crawling, standing, and walking are bound to be his most dramatic accomplishments during these months, but don't overlook all the wonderful things he's learning to do with his hands. At the beginning of this period, he'll still clumsily "rake" things toward himself, but by the end, he'll grasp accurately with his thumb and first or second finger. You'll find him practicing this pincer movement on any small object, from dust balls to cereal, and he may even try to snap his fingers if you show him how.

As your baby learns to open his fingers at will, he'll delight in dropping and throwing things. If you leave small toys on the tray of his high chair or in his playpen, he'll fling them down and then call loudly for someone to retrieve them so he can do it again. If he throws hard objects such as blocks, he might do some damage and probably will increase the noise level in your household considerably. Your life will be a little calmer if you redirect him toward softer objects, such

Milestones in Hand and Finger Skills by the End of This Period

- Uses pincer grasp
- Bangs two cubes together
- Puts objects into container
- Takes objects out of container
- Lets objects go voluntarily
- Pokes with index finger
- Tries to imitate scribbling

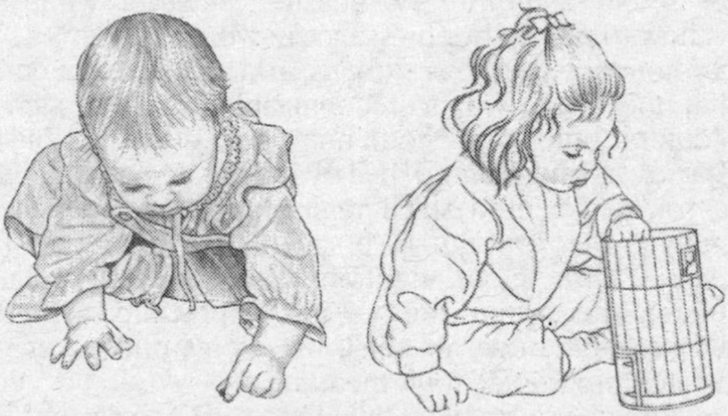

as balls of various sizes, colors, and textures. (Include some with beads or chimes inside so they make a sound as they roll.) One activity that not only is fun but allows you to observe your child's developing skills is to sit on the floor and roll a large ball toward him. At first, he'll slap randomly at it, but eventually he'll learn to swat it so it rolls back in your direction.

With his improved coordination, your baby can now investigate the objects he encounters more thoroughly. He'll pick them up, shake them, bang them, and pass them from hand to hand. He'll be particularly intrigued by toys with moving parts—wheels that spin, levers that can be moved, hinges that open and close. Holes also are fascinating because he can poke his fingers in them and, when he becomes a little more skilled, drop things through them.

Blocks are another favorite toy at this age. In fact, nothing motivates a baby to crawl quite as much as a tower waiting to be toppled. Toward the end of this period, your child may even start to build towers of his own by stacking one block on top of another.

Language Development

Toward the end of the first year, your baby will begin to communicate what she wants by pointing, crawling, or gesturing toward her target. She'll also imitate many of the gestures she sees adults make as they talk. This nonverbal communication is only a temporary measure, however, while she learns how to phrase her messages in words.

Do you notice the coos, gurgles, and screeches of earlier months now giving way to recognizable syllables, such as "ba," "da," "ga," and "ma"? Your baby may even stumble on words such as "mama" and "bye-bye" quite accidentally, and when you get excited she'll realize she's said something meaningful. Before long she'll start using "mama" to summon you or attract your attention. At this age, she may also say "mama" throughout the day just to practice saying the word. Ultimately, however, she'll use words only when she wants to communicate their meanings.

Even though you've been talking to your baby from birth, she now understands more language, and thus your conversations will take on new significance. Before she can say many, if any, words, she'll probably be comprehending more than you suspect. For example, watch how she responds when you mention a favorite toy across the room. If she looks toward it, she's telling you she understands. To help her increase her understanding, keep talking to her as much as possible. Tell her what's happening around her, particularly as you bathe, change, and feed her. Make your language simple and specific: "I'm drying you with the big blue towel. How soft it feels!" Verbally label familiar toys and objects for her, and try to be as consistent as possible—that is, if you call the family pet a cat today, don't call it a kitty tomorrow.

Picture books can enhance this entire process by reinforcing her budding understanding that everything has a name. Choose books with large board, cloth, or vinyl pages that she can turn herself. Also look for simple but colorful illustrations of things your child will recognize.

Whether you're reading or talking to her, give her plenty of opportunities to join in. Ask questions and wait for a response. Or let her take the lead. If she says "Gaagaagaa," repeat it back and see what she does. Yes, these exchanges may seem meaningless, but they tell your baby that communication is two-way and that she's a welcome participant.

Language Milestones by the End of This Period

- Pays increasing attention to speech
- Responds to simple verbal requests
- Responds to "no"
- Uses simple gestures, such as shaking head for "no"
- Babbles with inflection
- Says "dada" and "mama"
- Uses exclamations, such as "oh-oh!"
- Tries to imitate words

Paying attention to what she says also will help you identify the words she understands and make it more likely that you'll recognize her first spoken words.

These first words, incidentally, often aren't proper English. For your baby, a "word" is any sound that consistently refers to the same person, object, or event. So if she says "mog" every time she wants milk, you should treat "mog" with all the respect of a legitimate word. When you speak back to her, however, use "milk," and eventually she'll make the correction herself.

There's a tremendous variance in the age at which children

Bilingual Babies

If you speak a second language in your home, don't be concerned that your baby is going to become confused by hearing two languages. Millions of American families speak not only English but also another language in their daily lives. Research and parental experience show that when children are exposed to two (or even more) languages at a very young age, particularly when they hear both of them consistently, they are able to learn both languages simultaneously. Yes, during the child's normal language development, he may be more proficient in one or the other language, and at times he may interject words from one language when speaking the other. But with time, the two languages will become distinct and separate, and he should be able to communicate in both. (Some studies suggest that while he may be able to understand both languages, he will speak one of them better than the other for a time.)

Certainly you should encourage your child to become bilingual. It's an asset and a skill that will benefit him for the rest of his life. In general, the younger he is when both languages are introduced, the more proficiently he'll learn them; by contrast, he may have a little more difficulty learning the second language if he is introduced to it during the preschool years only after learning and speaking the first language exclusively.

begin to say recognizable words. Some have a vocabulary of two to three words by their first birthday. More likely, your baby's speech at twelve months will consist of a sort of gibberish that has the tones and variations of intelligible speech. As long as she's experimenting with sounds that vary in intensity, pitch, and quality, she's getting ready to talk. The more you respond to her as if she were speaking, the more you'll stimulate her urge to communicate.

Cognitive Development

An eight-month-old is curious about everything, but he also has a very short attention span and will move rapidly from one activity to the next. Two to three minutes is the most he'll spend with a single toy, and then he'll turn to something new. By twelve months, he may be willing to sit for as long as fifteen minutes with a particularly interesting plaything, but most of the time he'll still be a body in motion, and you shouldn't expect him to be any different.

Ironically, although toy stores are brimming with one expensive plaything after another, the toys that fascinate children most at this age are ordinary household objects such as wooden spoons, egg cartons, and plastic containers of all shapes and sizes. Your baby will be especially interested in things that differ just a bit from what he already knows, so if he's bored with the oatmeal box he's been playing with, you can renew his interest by putting a ball inside or turning it into a pull toy by tying a short string to it. These small changes will help him learn to detect small differences between the familiar and the unfamiliar. Also, when you choose playthings, remember that objects too much like what he's seen before will be given a quick once-over and dismissed, while things that are too foreign may be confusing or frightening. Look instead for objects and toys that gradually help him expand his horizons.

Often your baby won't need your help to discover objects that fall into this middle ground of newness. In fact, as soon as he can crawl, he'll be off in search of new things to conquer. He'll rummage through your drawers, empty out wastebaskets, ransack kitchen cabinets, and conduct elaborate experiments on everything he finds. (Make sure there's nothing that can hurt him in those containers, and keep an eye on him whenever he's into these things.) He'll never tire of dropping, rolling, throwing, submerging, or waving objects to find out how they behave. This may look like random play to you, but it's your baby's way of finding out how the world works. Like any good scientist, he's observing the properties of objects, and from his observations, he'll develop ideas about shapes (some things roll and others don't), textures (things can be scratchy, soft, or smooth), and sizes (some things fit inside each other). He'll even begin to understand

Variations of Peekaboo

The possible variations of peekaboo are almost endless. As your baby becomes more mobile and alert, create games that let her take the lead. Here are some suggestions.

1. Drape a soft cloth over her head and ask, "Where's the baby?" Once she understands the game, she'll pull the cloth away and pop up grinning.

2. With baby on her back facing toward you, lift both her legs together—"Up, up, up"—until they conceal your face from her. Then open them wide: "Peekaboo!" As she gets the idea, she'll move her legs herself. (This is a great game at diaper-changing time.)

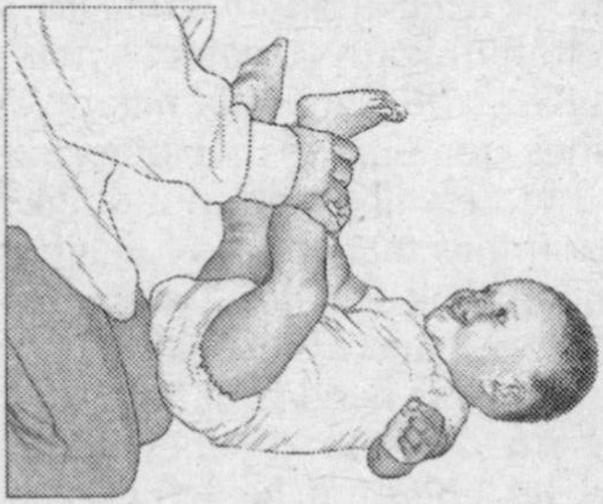

3. Hide behind a door or a piece of furniture, leaving a foot or arm in her view as a clue. She'll be delighted to come find you.

4. Take turns with your baby "hiding" your head under a large towel and letting her pull the towel off and then putting it over her head and pulling it off.

that some things are edible and others aren't, although he'll still put everything into his mouth just to be sure. (Again, make sure there's nothing dangerous lying around that he can put in his mouth.)

Cognitive Milestones by the End of This Period

- Explores objects in many different ways (shaking, banging, throwing, dropping)
- Finds hidden objects easily
- Looks at correct picture when the image is named
- Imitates gestures
- Begins to use objects correctly (drinking from cup, brushing hair, dialing phone, listening to receiver)

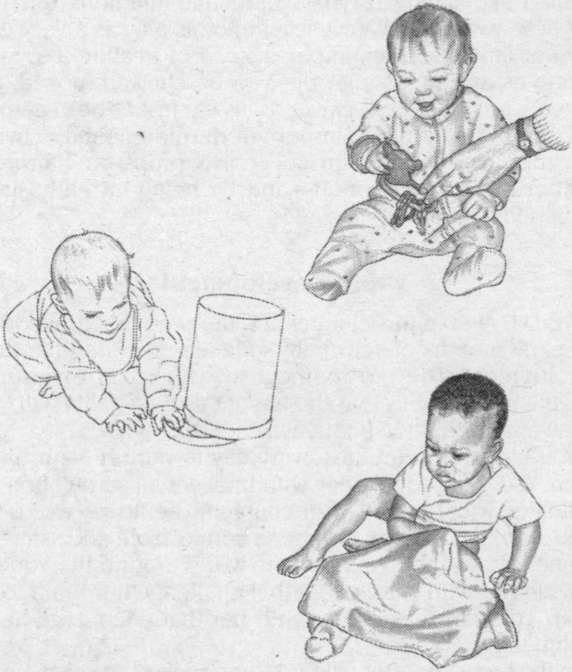

His continuing observations during these months also will help him understand that objects exist even when they're out of his sight. This concept is called object permanence. At eight months, when you hide a toy under a scarf, he'll pick up the scarf and search for the toy underneath—a response that wouldn't have occurred three months earlier. Try hiding the toy under the scarf and then removing it when he's not looking, however, and your eight-month-old will be puzzled. By ten months, he'll be so certain that the toy still exists that he'll continue looking for it. To help your baby learn object permanence, play peekaboo with him. By switching from one variation of this game to another, you'll maintain his interest almost indefinitely.

As he approaches his first birthday, your baby will become increasingly conscious that things not only have names but that they also have particular functions. You'll see this new awareness weave itself into his play as a very early form of fantasy. For example, instead of treating a toy telephone as an interesting object to be chewed, poked, and banged, he'll put the receiver to his ear just as he's seen you do. You can encourage important developmental activities like this by offering him suggestive props—a hairbrush, toothbrush, cup, or spoon—and by being an enthusiastic audience for his performances.

Brain Development

As you've read in this chapter and the ones that preceded it, the early months of your baby's life are crucial to her brain development. The environment to which you expose her and the experiences that she has at this time in life will have a powerful influence on the way her brain grows.

You have opportunities every day to nurture your baby's brain. You can provide her with intellectual stimulation just by talking with her and by encouraging her to say words that she's learning. You can give her a comfortable and safe environment in which to explore the world around her. You can provide her with simple toys that challenge her brain to develop. You can play games with her that encourage her to stretch her memory.

In the box at right, you'll find some suggestions that can be used day by day as your baby progresses from ages eight to

Stimulating Infant Brain Growth: Age Eight Months Through Twelve Months

- Talk to your baby during dressing, bathing, feeding, playing, walking, and driving, using adult talk; check with your pediatrician if your baby does not seem to respond to sound or if syllables and words are not developing.
- Be attentive to your baby's rhythms and moods. Respond to her when she is upset as well as when she is happy.
- Encourage your baby to play with blocks and soft toys, which helps her develop hand-to-eye coordination, fine motor skills, and a sense of competence.
- Provide a stimulating, safe environment where your baby can begin to explore and roam.
- Give consistent warm, physical contact—hugging, skin-to-skin, body-to-body contact—to establish your baby's sense of security and well-being.
- Read to your baby every day.
- If you speak a foreign language, use it at home.
- Avoid subjecting your baby to stressful or traumatic experiences, physical or psychological.
- Play games like peekaboo and pattycake to stimulate your baby's memory skills.
- Introduce your baby to other children and parents.
- Provide age- and developmentally appropriate toys that are safe and inexpensive. Toys do not need to be costly—ordinary household objects will do just fine. Remember, it's much more important to give your baby more attention than more toys.

- Teach your baby to wave "bye-bye" and to shake her head "yes" and "no."
- Make sure other people who provide care and supervision for your baby understand the importance of forming a loving and comforting relationship with her.
- Respect your baby's periodic discomfort around people who may not be her primary caregivers.
- Spend time on the floor playing with your child every day.
- Choose quality child care that is affectionate, responsive, educational, and safe. Visit your child care provider frequently and share your ideas about positive caregiving.

twelve months. They really can make a difference in your child's life, and not only now—they'll build a foundation for brain growth for years to come.

Emotional Development

During these months, your baby sometimes may seem like two separate babies. First there's the one who's open, affectionate, and outgoing with you. But then there's another who's anxious, clinging, and easily frightened around unfamiliar people or objects. Some people may tell you that your baby is fearful or shy because you're "spoiling" her, but don't believe it. Her widely diverse behavior patterns aren't caused by you or your parenting style; they occur because she's now, for the first time, able to tell the difference between familiar and unfamiliar situations. If anything, the predictable anxieties of this period are evidence of her healthy relationship with you.

Anxiety around strangers is usually one of the first emotional milestones your baby will reach. You may think something is wrong when this baby of yours who, at the age of three months, interacted calmly with people she didn't know is now beginning to tense up when strangers come too close. This is normal for this age, and you need not worry. Even relatives and frequent babysitters with whom your baby was once comfortable may prompt her to hide or cry now, especially if they approach her hastily.

At about the same time, she'll become much more "clutchy" about leaving you. This is the start of separation anxiety. Just as she's starting to realize that each object is unique and permanent, she'll also discover that there's only one of you. When you're out of her sight, she'll know you're somewhere, but not with her, and this will cause her great distress. She'll have so little sense of time that she won't know when—or even whether—you'll be coming back. Once she gets a little older, her memory of past experiences with you will comfort her when you're gone, and she'll be able to anticipate a reunion. But for now she's only aware of the present, so every time you leave her sight—even to go to the next room—she'll fuss and cry. When you leave her with someone else, she may scream as though her heart will break. At bedtime, she'll refuse to leave you to go to sleep, and then she may wake up searching for you in the middle of the night.

How long should you expect this separation anxiety to last? It usually peaks between ten and eighteen months and then fades during the last half of the second year. In some ways, this phase of your baby's emotional development will be especially tender for both of you, while in others, it will be painful. After all, her desire to be with you is a sign of her attachment to her first and greatest love—namely you. The intensity of her feeling as she hurtles into your arms is

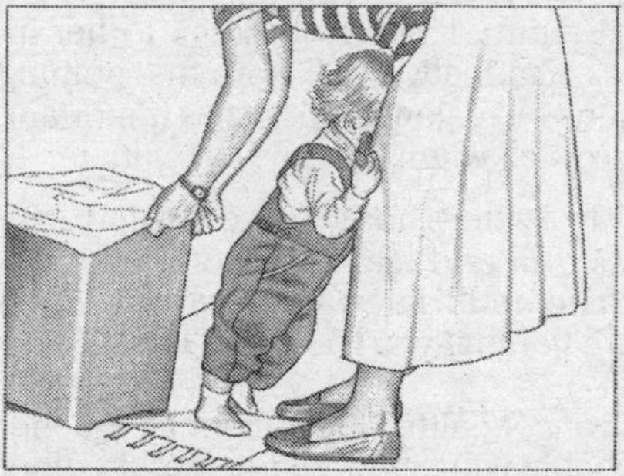

The predictable anxieties of this period are evidence of your baby's healthy relationship with you.

irresistible, especially when you realize that no one—including your child herself—will ever again think you are quite as perfect as she does at this age. On the other hand, you may feel suffocated by her constant clinging, while experiencing guilt whenever you leave her crying for you. Fortunately, this emotional roller coaster eventually will subside along with her separation anxiety. But in the meantime, try to downplay your leave-taking as much as possible. Here are some suggestions that may help.

1. Your baby is more susceptible to separation anxiety when she's tired, hungry, or sick. If you know you're going to go out, schedule your departure so that it occurs after she's napped and eaten. And try to stay with her as much as possible when she's sick.
2. Don't make a fuss over your leaving. Instead, have the person staying with her create a distraction (a new toy, a visit to the mirror, a bath). Then say good-bye and slip away quickly.
3. Remember that her tears will subside within minutes of your departure. Her outbursts are for your benefit, to persuade you to stay. With you out of sight, she'll soon turn her attention to the person staying with her.
4. Help her learn to cope with separation through short practice sessions at home. Separation will be easier on her when she initiates it, so when she crawls to another room (one that's babyproofed), don't follow her right away; wait for one or two minutes. When you have to go to another room for a few seconds, tell her where you're going and that you'll return. If she fusses, call to her instead of running back. Gradually she'll learn that nothing terrible happens when you're gone and, just as important, that you always come back when you say you will.
5. If you take your baby to a sitter's home or a child care center, don't just drop her off and leave. Spend a few extra minutes playing with her in this new environment. When you do leave, reassure her that you'll be back later.

If your baby has a strong, healthy attachment to you, her separation anxiety probably will occur earlier than in other

Social/Emotional Milestones by the End of This Period

- Shy or anxious with strangers
- Cries when mother or father leaves
- Enjoys imitating people in play
- Shows specific preferences for certain people and toys
- Tests parental responses to his actions during feedings (What do you do when he refuses a food?)
- Tests parental responses to his behavior (What do you do if he cries after you leave the room?)
- May be fearful in some situations
- Prefers mother and/or regular caregiver over all others
- Repeats sounds or gestures for attention
- Finger-feeds himself
- Extends arm or leg to help when being dressed

babies, and she'll pass through it more quickly. Instead of resenting her possessiveness during these months, maintain as much warmth and good humor as you can. Through your actions, you're showing her how to express and return love. This is the emotional base she'll rely on in years to come.

From the beginning, you've considered your baby to be a unique person with specific character traits and preferences. She, however, has had only a dim notion of herself as a person separate from you. Now her sense of identity is coming into bloom. As she develops a growing sense of herself as an individual, she'll also become increasingly conscious of you as a separate person.

One of the clearest signs of her own self-awareness is the way your baby watches herself in the mirror at this age. Up to

Acquainting Your Baby with a Sitter

Is your baby about to have a new babysitter for a few hours? Whenever possible, let your infant get to know this new person while you're there. Ideally, have the sitter spend time with him on several successive days before you leave them alone. If this isn't possible, allow yourself an extra hour or two for this get-acquainted period before you have to go out.

During this first meeting, the sitter and your baby should get to know each other very gradually, using the following steps.

1. Hold the baby on your lap while you and the sitter talk. Watch for clues that your infant is at ease before you have the sitter make eye contact with him. Wait until the baby is looking at her or playing contentedly by himself.

2. Have the sitter talk to the baby while he stays on your lap. She should not reach toward the infant or try to touch him yet.

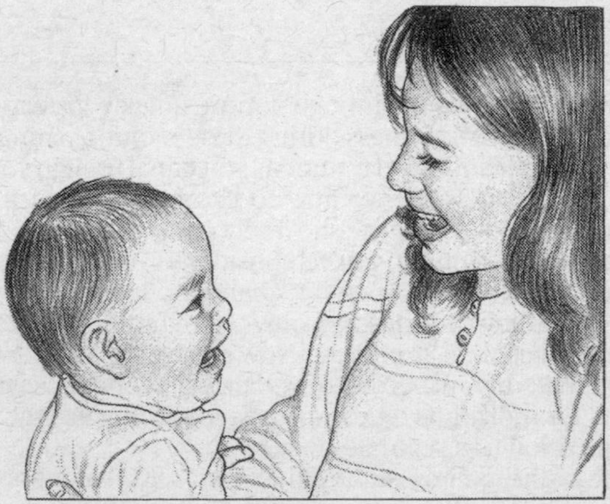

3. Once the baby seems comfortable with the conversation, put him on the floor with a favorite toy, across from the sitter. Invite the sitter to slowly come closer and play with the toy. As the baby warms up to her, you can move back gradually.

4. See what happens when you leave the room. If your baby doesn't notice you're missing, the introduction has gone well.

You can use leisurely introduction with anyone who hasn't seen the baby in the past few days, including relatives and friends. Adults often overwhelm babies of this age by coming close and making funny noises or, worse yet, trying to take them from their mothers. You have to intervene when this occurs. Explain to these well-meaning people that your baby needs time to warm up to strangers and that he's more likely to respond well if they go slowly.

about eight months, she treated the mirror as just another fascinating object. Perhaps, she thought, the reflection was another baby, or maybe it was a magical surface of lights and shadows. But now her responses will change, indicating she understands that one of the images belongs to her. While watching the mirror, for example, she may touch a smudge on her own nose or pull on a stray lock of her hair. You can reinforce her sense of identity by playing mirror games. When you're looking in the mirror together, touch different body parts: "This is Jenny's nose. This is Mommy's nose." Or move in and out of the mirror, playing peekaboo with the reflections. Or make faces and verbally label the emotions you are conveying.

As the months pass and your baby's self-concept becomes more secure, she'll have less trouble meeting strangers and separating from you. She'll also become more assertive. Before, you could count on her to be relatively compliant as long as she was comfortable. But now, more often than not, she'll want things her own particular way. For instance, don't be surprised if she turns up her nose at certain foods or

Toys Appropriate for an Eight- to Twelve-Month-Old

- Stacking toys in different sizes, shapes, colors
- Cups, pails, and other unbreakable containers
- Unbreakable mirrors of various sizes
- Bath toys that float, squirt, or hold water
- Large building blocks
- "Busy boxes" that push, open, squeak, and move
- Squeeze toys
- Large dolls and puppets
- Cars, trucks, and other vehicle toys made of flexible plastic, with no sharp edges or removable parts
- Balls of all sizes (but not small enough to fit in the mouth)
- Cardboard books with large pictures
- CDs, tapes, music boxes, and musical toys
- Push-pull toys
- Toy telephones
- Paper tubes, empty boxes, old magazines, egg cartons, empty plastic soda/juice/milk bottles (well rinsed)

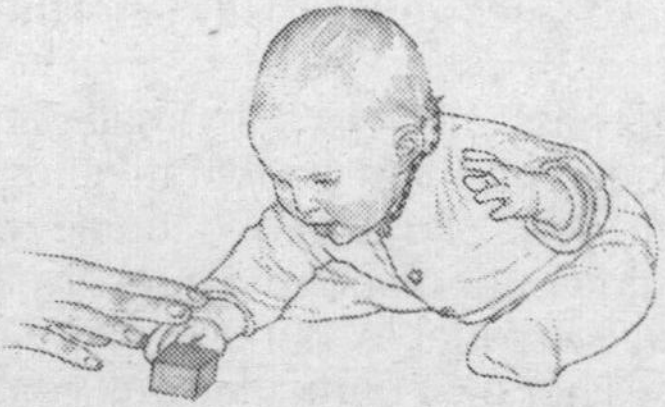

Developmental Health Watch

Each baby develops in his own manner, so it's impossible to tell exactly when your infant will perfect a given skill. Although the developmental milestones listed in this book will give you a general idea of the changes you can expect as your child gets older, don't be alarmed if his development takes a slightly different course. Alert your pediatrician if your baby displays any of the following signs of *possible* developmental delay in the eight- to twelve-month age range.

- Does not crawl
- Drags one side of body while crawling (for over one month)
- Cannot stand when supported
- Does not search for objects that are hidden while he watches
- Says no single words ("mama" or "dada")
- Does not learn to use gestures, such as waving or shaking head
- Does not point to objects or pictures

objects when you place them in front of her. Also, as she becomes more mobile, you'll find yourself frequently saying "no," to warn her away from things she shouldn't touch. But even after she understands the word, she may touch anyway. Just wait—this is only a forerunner of power struggles to come.

Your baby also may become afraid of objects and situations that she used to take in stride. At this age, fears of the dark, thunder, and loud appliances such as vacuum cleaners are common. Later you'll be able to subdue these fears by talking about them, but for now, the only solution is to eliminate the source of the fears as much as possible: Put a night-light in her room, or vacuum when she's not around.

Transitional Objects

Almost everyone knows about the Charles Schulz character Linus and his blanket. He drags it around wherever he goes, nibbling on its corner or curling up with it when the going gets tough. Security objects such as blankets are part of the emotional support system every child needs in his early years.

Your baby may not choose a blanket, of course. He may prefer a soft toy or even the satin trim on Mom's bathrobe. Chances are, he'll make his choice between months eight and twelve, and he'll keep it with him for years to come. When he's tired, it will help him get to sleep. When he's separated from you, it will reassure him. When he's frightened or upset, it will comfort him. When he's in a strange place, it will help him feel at home.

These special comforts are called transitional objects, because they help children make the emotional transition from dependence to independence. They work, in part, because they feel good: They're soft, cuddly, and nice to touch. They're also effective because of their familiarity. This so-called lovey has your child's scent on it, and it reminds him of the comfort and security of his own room. It makes him feel that everything is going to be okay.

Despite myths to the contrary, transitional objects are not a sign of weakness or insecurity, and there's no reason to keep your baby from using one. In fact, a transitional object can be so helpful that you may want to help him choose one and build it into his nighttime ritual.

You also can make things easier for yourself by having two identical security objects. Doing this will allow you to wash one while the other is being used, thus sparing your baby (and yourself) a potential emotional crisis and a very bedraggled lovey. If your baby chooses a large blanket for his security object, you can easily turn it into two by cutting it in half. He has little sense of size and won't notice the change. If he's chosen a toy instead, try to find a duplicate as soon as possible. If you don't start rotating them early, your baby may refuse the second one because it feels too new and foreign.

Parents often worry that transitional objects promote thumb sucking, and in fact they sometimes (but not always) do. But it's important to remember that thumb or finger sucking is a normal, natural way for a young child to comfort himself. He'll gradually give up both the transitional object and the sucking as he matures and finds other ways to cope with stress.

And when you can't shield her from something that frightens her, try to anticipate her reaction and be close by so she can turn to you. Comfort her, but stay calm so she understands that you are not afraid. If you reassure her every time she hears a clap of thunder or the roar of a jet overhead, her fear gradually will subside until all she has to do is look at you to feel safe.

Basic Care

Feeding

At this age, your baby needs between 750 and 900 calories each day, about 400 to 500 of which should come from breastmilk or formula (approximately 24 ounces [720 ml] a day). But don't be surprised if her appetite is less robust now than it was during the first eight months. This is because her rate of growth is slowing, and she also has so many new and interesting activities to distract her.

At about eight months, you may want to introduce "junior" foods. These are slightly coarser than strained foods and are packaged in larger jars—usually 6 to 8 ounces (180 to 240 ml). They require more chewing than baby foods. You also can expand your baby's diet to include soft foods such as puddings, mashed potatoes, yogurt, and gelatin. Eggs are an excellent source of protein, but feed her only the yolks at

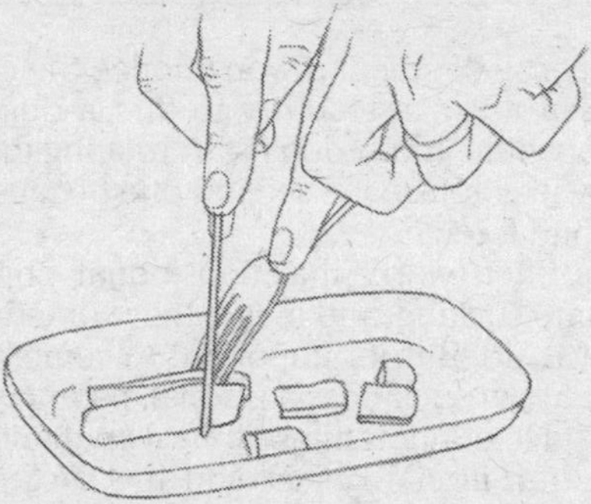

first, since their nutritional value is higher and they're less likely to cause allergies than the whites. In one or two months you can give her the whole egg. As always, introduce one food at a time, then wait two or three days before trying something else to be sure your baby doesn't develop an allergic reaction.

At about eight to nine months, as your baby's ability to use her hands improves, give her a spoon of her own and let her play with it at mealtimes. Once she's figured out how to hold it, dip it in her food and let her try to feed herself. But don't expect much in the beginning, when more food is bound to go on the floor and high chair than into her mouth. A plastic

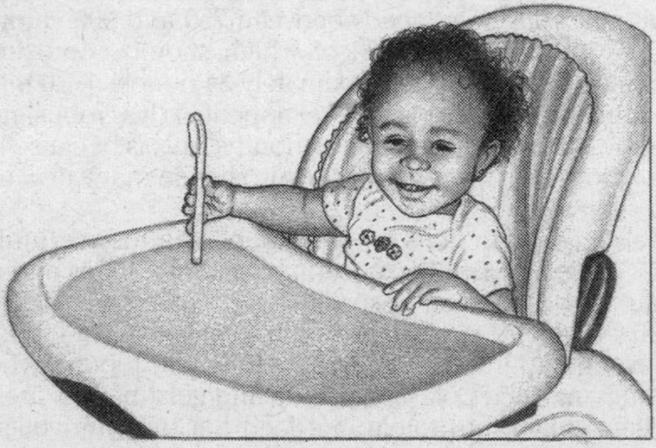

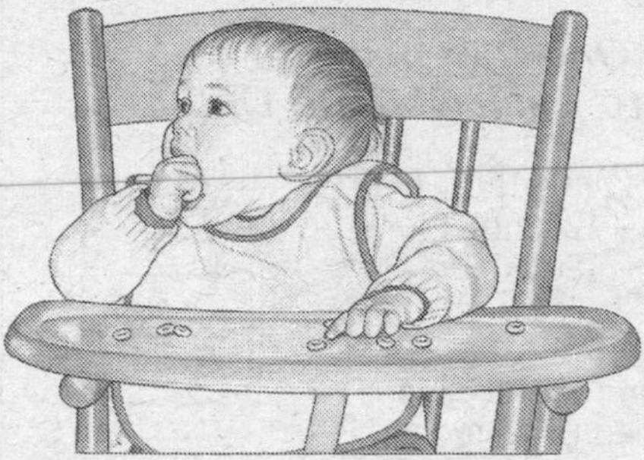

In the early weeks of self-feeding, things may go more smoothly when she's really hungry and is more interested in eating than playing.

cloth under her chair will help minimize some of the cleanup.

Be patient, and resist the temptation to grab the spoon away from her. She needs not only the practice but also the knowledge that you have confidence in her ability to feed herself. For a while you may want to alternate bites from her spoon with bites from a spoon that you hold. Once she consistently gets her own spoon to her mouth (which might not be until after her first birthday), you may keep filling her spoon for her to decrease the mess and waste, but leave the actual feeding to her.

In the early weeks of self-feeding, things may go more smoothly when she's really hungry and is more interested in eating than playing. Although your baby now eats three meals, just like the rest of the family, you may not want to impose her somewhat disorderly eating behavior on everyone else's dinnertime. Many families compromise by feeding the baby most of her meal in advance and then letting her occupy herself with finger foods while the others eat their meal.

Finger foods for babies include small pieces of steamed veggies, or soft fruit such as banana, well-cooked pasta, small pieces of bread, chicken, scrambled eggs, or cereals. Try to offer a selection of flavors, shapes, colors, and textures, but always watch her for choking in case she bites off a piece too big to swallow. (See *Choking,* page 576.) Also, because she's likely to swallow without chewing, never offer a young child

Sample One-Day Menu for an Eight- to Twelve-Month-Old

1 cup = 8 ounces [240 ml]
4 ounces = 120 ml
6 ounces = 180 ml

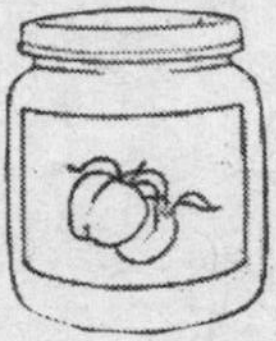

Breakfast
¼–½ cup cereal or mashed egg
¼–½ cup fruit, diced (if your child is self-feeding)
4–6 oz. formula/breastmilk

Snack
4–6 oz. breastmilk/formula or water
¼ cup diced cheese or cooked vegetables

Lunch
¼–½ cup yogurt or cottage cheese or meat
¼–½ cup yellow or orange vegetables
4–6 oz. formula/breastmilk

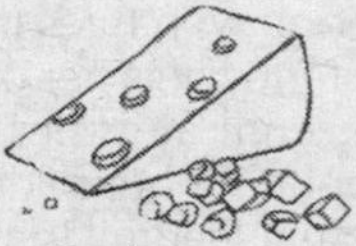

Snack
1 teething biscuit or cracker
¼ cup yogurt or diced (if child is self-feeding) fruit
water

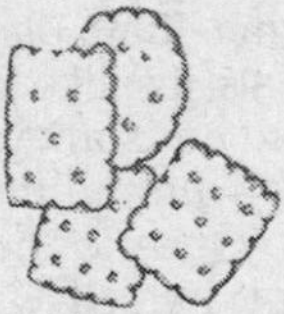

Dinner
¼ cup diced poultry, meat, or tofu
¼–½ cup green vegetables
¼ cup noodles, pasta, rice, or potato
¼ cup fruit
4–6 oz. formula/breastmilk

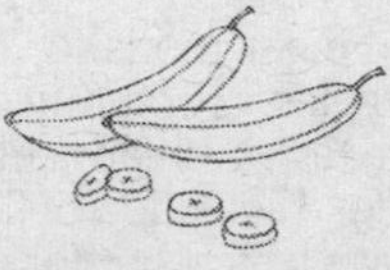

Before Bedtime
6–8 oz. formula/breastmilk or water (If formula or breastmilk, follow with water or brush teeth afterward.)

Sample One-Day Menu for a One-Year-Old

This menu is planned for a one-year-old child who weighs approximately 21 pounds (9.5 kg).
1 teaspoon = ⅓ tablespoon (5 ml)
1 tablespoon = ½ ounce (15 ml)
1 cup = 8 ounces (240 ml)
1 oz = 30 ml

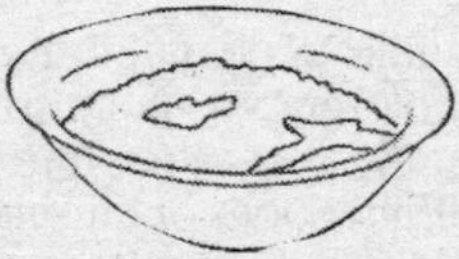

Breakfast
½ cup iron-fortified breakfast cereal or 1 cooked egg
¼–½ cup whole milk (with cereal or without)
Fruit can be added to cereal or on its own
½ banana, sliced
2–3 large sliced strawberries

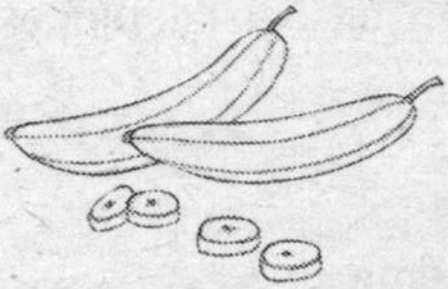

Snack
1 slice toast or whole wheat muffin with 1–2 tablespoons cream cheese or peanut butter, or yogurt with cut-up fruit
½ cup whole milk

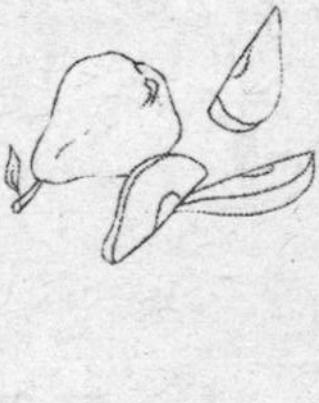

Lunch
½ sandwich sliced turkey or chicken, tuna, egg salad, or peanut butter
½ cup cooked green vegetables
½ cup whole milk

Snack
1–2 ounces cubed or string cheese, or 2–3 tablespoons fruit or berries
1 cup whole milk

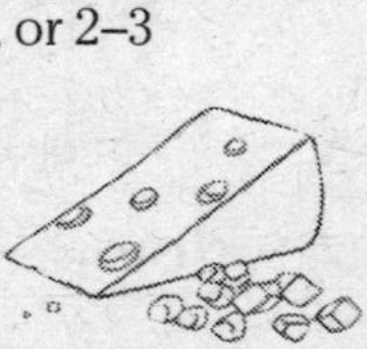

Dinner
2–3 ounces cooked meat, ground or diced
½ cup cooked yellow or orange vegetables
½ cup pasta, rice, or potato
½ cup whole milk

chunks of peanut butter, large pieces of raw vegetables, nuts, whole grapes, popcorn, uncooked peas, celery, gum, hard candies, or other hard round foods. Choking can happen with hot dogs or chunks of cheese or meat sticks (baby-food "hot dogs"), so these always should be cut lengthwise and then into smaller pieces before being fed to a baby of this age.

SOURCES OF IRON

		Excellent	
Red meats		Blackstrap molasses	
Fortified bran cereal			
		Good	
Hamburger	Shrimp	Potato, baked in skin	Dried apricots
Lean beef	Frankfurter	Navy beans	Raisins
Chicken	Egg, egg yolks	Kidney beans	Prunes, prune juice
Tuna	Spinach, mustard greens	Soybeans	Strawberries
Ham	Asparagus	Split peas	Tomato juice
		Adequate	
Enriched rice	Avocado	Broccoli	Green peas
Enriched pasta, noodles	Cranberry juice	Tomato	Bacon
Enriched bread	Orange	Carrots	Peanut butter
Banana	Apple	Green beans	

Where We Stand

Childhood overweight and obesity is becoming an increasingly common problem. In fact, over the past two decades it has doubled in children and tripled among adolescents in the United States. Throughout a child's lifetime, chronic obesity can lead to potentially serious health problems, including diabetes and high blood pressure. It also can cause psychological stresses associated with feeling different from his peers, leading to depression and low self-esteem.

The American Academy of Pediatrics believes that both parents and pediatricians need to take steps to prevent the development of overweight problems in children. Your pediatrician can monitor annually your child's weight gain from age one and help make sure that it remains within normal guidelines as he grows. When your child turns two years old, your doctor will calculate his body mass index (BMI). This is the weight in pounds divided by the height in inches squared, and then multiplied by 703 (or, weight in kilograms divided by height in meters squared). A child with a BMI greater than the 85th percentile for age and sex is considered overweight; when the BMI is at or above the 95th percentile, he is considered obese. (See *Growth Charts*, in Appendix.)

Weaning from Breast to Bottle

Mothers wean their babies for a variety of reasons. The weaning process begins when the baby first receives anything in the diet besides breastmilk or formula.

In any event, you should continue to breastfeed or provide infant formula until your baby is one year old. After that, whole cow's milk can be given. Many breastfed babies never use a bottle, but wean directly to a cup. If you plan to introduce bottle-feedings of formula or expressed milk, don't expect smooth sailing if your baby has never been given a bottle before. She probably will object to it the first few

Discontinuing the Bottle

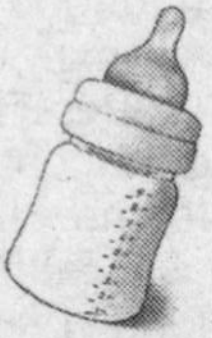

Infants who sleep with a bottle containing milk, juice, soda, or other sweetened liquids are at a high risk of developing tooth decay. It is recommended that the bottle be given up entirely at around age one and almost certainly by eighteen months. As long as your baby is drinking from a cup, he doesn't need to take liquids from a bottle. If you must give him a bottle, limit the contents to plain water. Unfortunately, weaning your baby from the bottle may not be as easy as it sounds. To help things along, eliminate the midday bottle first, then the evening and morning ones; save the bedtime bottle for last, but remember to limit the contents to plain water. If your baby will not take a bottle with plain water initially, slowly over a short period of time dilute the formula or other contents with water so that after a week or two the bottle contains *only* water.

It's easy to get into the habit of using a bottle to comfort a child or help him sleep. But at this age, he no longer needs anything to eat or drink during the night. If you are still feeding him at that time, you should stop. Even if he demands a bottle and drinks thirstily, nighttime feedings are a comfort rather than a nutritional necessity. The bottle soon turns into a crutch and prevents his learning to fall back to sleep on his own. If he cries for only a short time, try letting him cry back to sleep. After a few nights he'll probably forget all about the bottle. If this doesn't happen, consult your pediatrician and read the other sections on sleep in this book. (See, for example, pages 71 and 287.)

Incidentally, giving your toddler a drink or other snack *before bedtime* is acceptable—provided you brush his teeth afterward. In fact, it may help him fall asleep. A short breastfeeding, a drink of cow's milk or other liquid, or even some fruit or another nutritious food will do. If the snack is a bottle, gradually phase it out by substituting a cup.

Whatever the snack, have your child finish it and then clean his teeth, using a soft cloth, gauze, or brush. This can even be done while the child is sleeping on your lap. Not removing the food or liquid from your baby's teeth after he eats will allow it to remain on the teeth all night and can result in tooth decay. If he needs some comfort to get to sleep, let him use a cuddly toy, blanket, or his thumb—but never a bottle containing anything else but plain water.

times, especially if her mother tries to give it to her. By this age, she associates her mother with nursing, so it's understandable if she's confused and annoyed when there's a sudden change in the routine. Things may go more smoothly if her father or another family member feeds her—and Mom stays out of the room. After she's gotten used to the idea, then Mom can take over, but the baby should get lots of cuddling, stroking, and encouragement to make up for the lost skin-to-skin contact.

Once your baby has learned to take an occasional bottle, it should be relatively easy to wean her from the breast if you desire to do so. The time needed to wean her, however, will vary, depending on the emotional and physical needs of both child and mother. If your baby adapts well to change and you're ready for the transition, you can make a total switch in one or two weeks. For the first two days, substitute one bottle of formula for one breastfeeding per day. (Don't express milk during this time.) On the third day, use a bottle for two feedings. By the fifth day, you can jump to three or four bottle-feedings.

Once you've stopped breastfeeding entirely, breastmilk production will cease very quickly. In the meantime, if your breasts should become engorged, you may need to express milk for the first two or three days to relieve the discomfort. Gradual weaning by eliminating one feeding at a time will help to minimize engorgement. Within a week, the discomfort should subside.

Many women prefer to wean more slowly, even when their babies cooperate fully. Breastfeeding provides a closeness between mother and child that's hard to duplicate any other way, and, understandably, you may be reluctant to give up such intimacy. In this case, you can continue to offer a combination of the breast and the bottle for up to one year, or beyond. Some babies lose interest between nine and twelve months, or when they learn to drink from a cup. It's important for you to remember that this is not a personal rejection, but a sign of your child's growing independence. However, breastfeeding can continue as part of the routine feeding beyond the first year of life.

Weaning to a Cup

Once your baby is feeding himself more often, it's a natural time to introduce him to drinking from a cup. To get started, give him a trainer cup that has two handles and a snap-on lid with a spout, or a straw cup. Either option will minimize spillage as he experiments with different ways to hold (and most likely to throw) the cup.

In the beginning, fill the cup with water and offer it to him at just one meal a day. Show him how to maneuver it to his mouth and tip it so he can drink. Don't become dismayed, however, if he treats the cup as a plaything for several weeks; most babies do. Just be patient until he's finally able to get most of the liquid down his throat or suck out of the straw

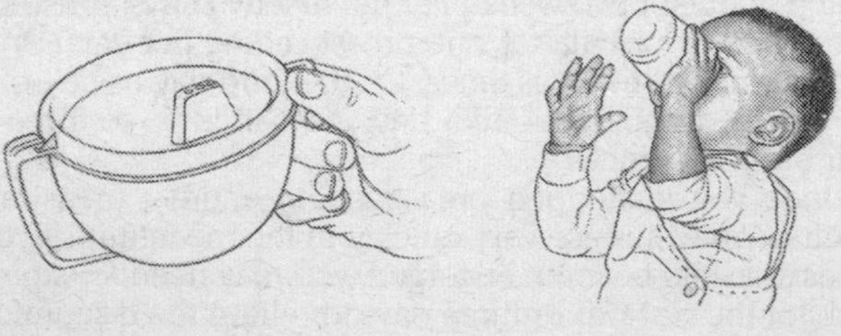

Six months may pass before your baby is willing to take all his liquid from a cup.

without the liquid dribbling down his chin or the cup flying around the room.

There are advantages to drinking from a cup: It will improve your baby's hand-to-mouth coordination, and it will begin to prepare him for the weaning process, which frequently occurs around this age. Remember, the American Academy of Pediatrics believes that breastfeeding is the best source of nutrition for babies through at least their first birthday. But as you gradually transition him to receiving other types of liquids, your baby's readiness for drinking from a cup will be signaled by his:

1. Looking around while nursing or taking the bottle

2. Mouthing the nipple without sucking

3. Trying to slide off your lap before the feeding is finished

Even under the best of circumstances, weaning may not take place overnight. Six months may pass before your baby is willing to take all his liquid from a cup. Even so, you can start the process and proceed gradually, letting his interest and willingness guide you. You'll probably find it easiest at first to substitute a cup for the bottle or breast at the midday feeding. Once he's adjusted to this change, try doing the same in the morning. The bedtime feeding probably will be the last one abandoned, and for good reason: Your baby has become accustomed to this source of nighttime comfort and calming, and it will take him some time to give it up. If he's sleeping through the night and not waking up hungry, he doesn't physically need the extra nourishment from bedtime breast- or bottle-feeding. In this case, you might break the habit in stages, first by substituting a bedtime bottle with water instead of milk and then by switching to a drink of water from a cup.

During this process, you may be tempted to put milk in his bottle to help him go to sleep, but don't do it. If he falls asleep while feeding, the milk will pool around his teeth, and this can cause his incoming teeth to decay—a condition known as baby bottle tooth decay or early childhood caries. To make matters worse, drinking while lying flat on his back can contribute to middle ear infections, since the liquid may flow through the eustachian tube into the middle ear.

There's still one more disadvantage to prolonged bottle-feeding: The bottle can become a security object, particularly if your baby keeps it beyond about age one. To avoid this, don't let him carry or drink from a bottle while playing. Restrict the use of a bottle to feedings when he's sitting down or being held. At all other times, give him a cup. If you never allow him to take the bottle with him, he won't realize that bringing it along is even an option. Don't relent once this decision has been made, or it could prompt him to demand a bottle again long after he has "officially" been weaned.

Sleeping

At eight months, your baby probably still takes two regular naps, one midmorning and the other midafternoon. She's also likely to sleep as much as ten to twelve hours at night without needing a middle-of-the-night feeding. But be aware of some possible problems ahead: As her separation anxieties intensify in the next few months, she may start to resist going to bed, and she may wake up more often looking for you.

During this difficult period, you may need to experiment with several strategies to find those that help your baby sleep. For example, some children go to sleep more easily with the door open (so they can hear you); others develop consoling habits, such as sucking their thumbs or rocking. As previously mentioned, your baby also might adopt a special blanket or stuffed animal as a transitional object, which comforts her when you're not nearby. Anything that's safe, soft and huggable, and can be stroked or sucked will serve this purpose. You can encourage your child to use a transitional object by providing her with a lightweight blanket or soft toy.

Here are some additional suggestions to help this stage pass more quickly. First of all, don't do anything that will reward your baby for calling you in the middle of the night. Go to her side to make sure she's all right, and tell her that you're nearby if she really needs you; but don't turn on the light, rock her, or walk with her. You might offer her a drink of water, but don't feed her, and certainly don't take her to your bed. If she's suffering from separation anxiety, taking her to your bed will only make it harder for her to return to her own crib.

When you do check on her, try to make her as comfortable as possible. Also make sure she isn't sick. Some problems, such as ear infections or the croup, can come on suddenly in the night. Once you're sure there's no sign of illness, then check her diaper, changing her only if she's had a bowel movement or if her diaper is uncomfortably wet. Do the change as quickly as possible in dim light and then settle her back in her crib—and on her back. Before leaving the room, whisper a few comforting words about how it's time to sleep. If she continues to cry, wait a few minutes, then go back in and comfort her for a short time. This period can be extremely difficult for parents. After all, it's emotionally and physically exhausting to listen to your baby cry, and you'll probably respond with a combination of emotions. But remember, her behavior is not deliberate. Instead, she's reacting to anxieties and stresses that are natural at her age. If you stay calm and follow a consistent pattern from one night to the next, she'll soon be putting herself to sleep. Keep this objective in sight as you struggle through the "training" nights. Doing so ultimately will make life much easier for both of you. See Chapter 30 for more information on sleep.

Behavior

Discipline

Your baby's desire to explore is almost impossible to satisfy. As a result, he'll want to touch, taste, and manipulate everything he can get into his hands. In the process, he's bound to find his way into places and situations that are off-limits. Although his curiosity is vital to his overall development and shouldn't be discouraged unnecessarily, he can't be allowed to jeopardize his own safety or to damage valuable objects. Whether he's investigating the burners on your stove or pulling up plants in your flower bed, you need to help him stop these activities.

Keep in mind that the way you handle these early incidents will lay the foundation for future discipline. Learning not to do something that he very much wants to do is a major first step toward self-control. The better he learns this lesson now, the less you'll have to intervene in years to come.

What's your best strategy? As we suggested earlier, distraction usually can deal effectively with undesirable behavior. Your baby's memory is still short, and thus you can shift his focus with minimal resistance. If he's headed for something he shouldn't get into, you don't necessarily have to say "no." Overusing that word will blunt its effect in the long run. Instead, pick him up and direct him toward something he can play with. Look for a compromise that will keep him interested and active without squelching his natural curiosity.

You should reserve your serious discipline for those situations where your baby's activities can expose him to real danger—for example, playing with electric cords. This is the time to say "no" firmly and remove him from the situation. But don't expect him to learn from just one or two incidents. Because of his short memory, you'll have to repeat the scene over and over before he finally recognizes and responds to your directions.

To improve the effectiveness of your discipline, consistency is absolutely critical. Make sure that everyone responsible for caring for your baby understands what the infant is and isn't allowed to do. Keep the rules to a minimum, preferably limited to situations that are potentially dangerous to the baby. Then make sure he hears "no" every time he strays into forbidden territory.

Immediacy is another important component of good discipline. React as soon as you see your baby heading into trouble, not five minutes later. If you delay your reprimand, he won't understand the reason you're angry and the lesson will be lost. Likewise, don't be too quick to comfort him after he's been scolded. Yes, he may cry, sometimes as much in surprise as distress; but wait a minute or two before you reassure him. Otherwise, he won't know whether he really did something wrong.

Keep in mind the importance of refraining from spanking or striking your baby in any way when disciplining him. No matter what your child's age, or what his behavior has been, physical punishment is always an inappropriate way for you to respond. Spanking only teaches a child to act aggressively when he's upset. Yes, it may relieve your own frustration temporarily, and for the moment you actually might believe that it will do some good. But this is ***not*** an effective way of disciplining your infant, and it certainly doesn't teach him any alternative way to act. It also undermines effective communication between the two of you, as well as weakening his own sense of security.

What's the alternative? The American Academy of Pediatrics recommends using "time-outs" instead of spankings—putting a baby who has misbehaved in a quiet place for a few minutes, away from other people, TV, or books. When the time-out is over, explain to him exactly why his behavior was unacceptable. (For more information about spanking and more appropriate ways to discipline, see page 291.)

As you refine your own disciplinary skills, don't overlook the importance of responding in a positive way to your baby's *good* behavior. This kind of reaction is equally important in helping him learn self-control. If he hesitates before reaching for the stove, notice his restraint and tell him how pleased you are. And give him a hug when he does something nice for another person. As he grows older, his good behavior will depend, in large part, on his desire to please you. If you make him aware now of how much you appreciate the good things he does, he'll be less likely to misbehave just to get your attention.

Some parents worry about spoiling an infant this age by giving him too much attention, but you needn't be concerned about that. At eight to twelve months, your baby still has a limited ability to be manipulative. You should assume that when he cries, it's not for effect but because he has real needs that aren't being met.

These needs gradually will become more complex, and as they do, you'll notice more variation in your baby's cries—and in the way you react to them. For example, you'll come running when you hear the shattering wail that means something is seriously wrong. By contrast, you may finish what you're doing before you answer the shrill come-here-I-want-you cry. You'll also probably soon recognize a whiny, muffled cry that means something like "I could fall asleep now if everyone would leave me alone." By responding appropriately to the hidden message behind your baby's cries, you'll let him know that his needs are important, but you'll respond only to deserving calls for attention.

Incidentally, there probably will be times when you won't

be able to figure out exactly why your baby is crying. In these cases, he himself may not even know what's bothering him. The best response is some comfort from you, combined with consoling techniques that he chooses for himself. For instance, try holding him while he cuddles his favorite stuffed animal or special blanket, or take time to play a game or read a story with him. Both of you will feel better when he's cheered up. Remember that his need for attention and affection is just as real as his need for food and clean diapers.

Siblings

As your baby becomes more mobile, she'll be better able to play with her siblings, and those brothers and sisters usually will be glad to cooperate. Older children, particularly six- to ten-year-olds, often love to build towers for an eight-month-old to destroy. Or they'll lend a finger to an eleven-month-old just learning to walk. A baby this age can be a wonderful playmate to her siblings.

However, while the baby's mobility can turn her into a more active participant in games with her brothers and sisters, it also will make her more likely to invade their private territory. This may violate their budding sense of ownership and privacy, and it can present a serious safety hazard for the baby, since the toys of older children often contain small, easily swallowed pieces. You can ensure that everyone is protected by giving older siblings an enclosed place where they can keep and play with their belongings without fear of a "baby invasion."

Also, now that the baby can reach and grab just about

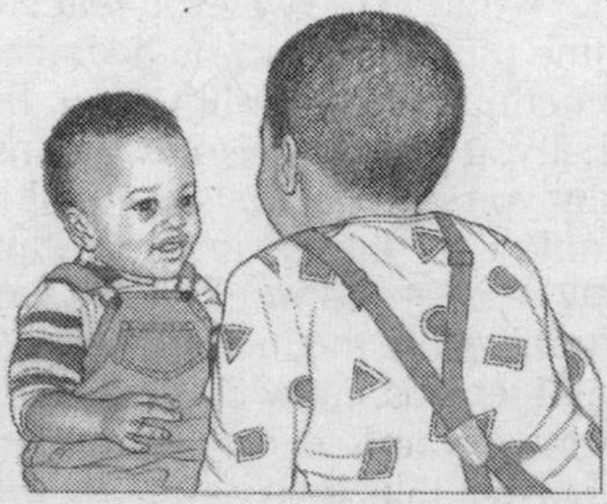

A baby this age can be a wonderful playmate to his siblings.

everything in sight, sharing is another issue that must be dealt with. Children under three just aren't capable of sharing without lots of adult prodding and, in most cases, direct intervention. As much as possible, try to sidestep the issue by encouraging both children to play with their own toys, even if they're doing so side by side. When they do play together, suggest looking at books or listening to music, rolling a ball back and forth, or playing hide-and-seek games—in other words, activities requiring limited cooperation.

Grandparents

This childhood age (eight to twelve months) is a wonderful time to enjoy your grandchild. She is now much more physically active and has more language expressions and emotional enthusiasm. However, babies of this age also may experience stranger anxiety, and could be reluctant to go to Grandma and Grandpa with much eagerness. Don't take this personally; it's part of normal development. Simply hang in there, and continue to provide all of the love and attention that you always have, but don't feel you must overdo it in the midst of these pulling-back episodes by the baby. Be patient, and the apparent standoffishness will resolve over time.

In your activities with your grandchild, you can take advantage of her developmental progress in the following areas.

Crawling. Get down on the floor with your grandchild as much as you physically can. This "floor time" is both fun and reassuring for the baby. She'll show delight if you use yourself as her crawling target or object of exploration. Remember, though, to check the floor carefully for possible hazards, since babies will pick up every object within reach and put it in their mouth.

Fine Motor Skills. Develop your own set of fine motor "games" with your grandchild—for example, opening and closing items, dumping out and putting back games and toys, and operating latches. Expect plenty of repetition since babies seem tireless doing the same activity over and over.

Language. Read books, and listen to music, tapes, and CDs with your grandchild. All the while, keep the language interactive. If you speak a language that's different from the one in which your grandchild is becoming proficient, don't be afraid to speak it to her. (Be sure her parents agree.) For more information on bilingual babies, see page 314.

Basic Care. When it comes to feeding and sleeping, consistency of routines is important in this age group. Keep "junior foods" in your home. You also can establish "Grandma's Special Menus" that your grandchild can come to expect. When the baby is staying at your home, nap times and nighttime sleep schedules should be maintained as close as possible to those at her own home. Changes of routine sometimes can create confusion for babies.

Safety. Follow the safety check items in your own home that are described at the end of this chapter to ensure your grandchild's well-being. Keep gates on the top and the bottom of stairways. Place soft, protective coverings around sharp or round edges. Don't use walkers. Also, since babies of this age can have a strong nature and are wiggly, changing diapers should be a two-person operation if possible; change the diapers on carpeted floors or sofas to minimize the risk that your grandchild will twist off the changing table. While you're changing the baby, try distracting her with something she can manipulate.

Immunization Update

At one year of age (or in the months immediately after your baby's first birthday), she should receive the measles, mumps, rubella (MMR) vaccine. This vaccine will protect your baby from three serious diseases that can cause fever, rash, and other symptoms, and potentially lead to serious complications (pneumonia in children with measles, and hearing impairment in children with mumps). The current recommendation is to have your child receive the first MMR vaccine between twelve and fifteen months of age.

The varicella vaccine, which protects your child against chickenpox, should be given at or after twelve months of age if she is susceptible to the disease—that is, if she has not already had the chickenpox.

The third hepatitis B vaccine will also be given between six and eighteen months of age, and the first hepatitis A vaccine will be given on or after one year of age.

Safety Check

Car Safety Seats

- Buckle the baby into an approved, properly installed car safety seat before you start the car. The American Academy of Pediatrics recommends that children ride rear-facing as long as possible, preferably to the maximum weight or height allowed by the seat (as long as the top of the child's head is below the top of the seat back), often around 15 to 18 months of age. At a very minimum, keep him rear-facing until he weighs at least 20 pounds (9 kg) *and* is at least one year of age.

Falls

- Use gates at the top and bottom of stairways, and in doorways to rooms with furniture or other objects that the baby might climb on or that have sharp or hard edges against which he might fall.

- Do not allow an infant to climb on a narrow-based ladder-back chair, since the child will try to climb the ladder and the chair will tip over, resulting in head injury and possible leg or arm fractures.

- Do not use a baby walker. A stationary activity center is a much safer choice.

Burns

- Never smoke or carry hot liquids or foods near your baby or while you're holding him. When you must handle hot liquids or foods, put your baby in a safe place such as a crib, play yard, or high chair.

- Never leave containers of hot liquids or foods near the edges of tables or counters.
- Do not allow your baby to crawl around hot stoves, floor heaters, or furnace vents.

Drowning

- Never leave your baby alone in a bath or around containers of water, such as buckets, wading pools, swimming pools, sinks, or open toilets. Remove all water from containers immediately after use. If you have a swimming pool, install a four-sided fence of at least 4 feet in height that completely separates the house from the pool.

Poisoning and Choking

- Never leave small objects in your baby's crawling area.
- Do not give your baby hard pieces of food, or any soft foods that could become lodged in his airway, such as hot dogs and grapes.
- Store all medicines and household cleaning products high and out of his reach.
- Use safety latches on drawers and cupboards that contain objects that might be dangerous to him.

10

Early Education and Child Care

Who will care for your baby during the hours when you are away? Sooner or later you're bound to face this question. Whether you need someone to care for your infant a few hours a week or nine hours a day, you'll want to feel confident about the person who does it. But finding the right caregiver or team of caregivers to care for your child can be a big challenge. Your top priority should be to ensure the well-being of your baby, and that should be the overriding consideration when selecting child care. This chapter provides suggestions to make your search easier. It also contains guidelines for preventing, recognizing, and resolving problems once you have made your choice.

The most important aspect of finding good child care is judging the quality of the child care program and the character and abilities of the caregiver involved with your baby. Nearly six of every ten families use in-home or out-of-home care. Parents also may choose to share care between themselves or have relatives and nonrelatives provide that service. Some children participate in more than one type of child care arrangement at different times of the day or week. If your child's caregiver is not a member of your family, chances are you'll meet this person only a few times before entrusting your child to her. (Many, though not all, caregivers are women.) Even so, you'll want to feel as confident about your choice as if she were a member of your family. While it's impossible to be absolutely sure about anyone under these circumstances, you can tell a great deal about caregivers by observing them at work for a day or two and carefully checking references. Entrust your baby to someone only after you have taken time to watch her with your child and

Never entrust your child to anyone until you've taken time to watch her with your child and other children.

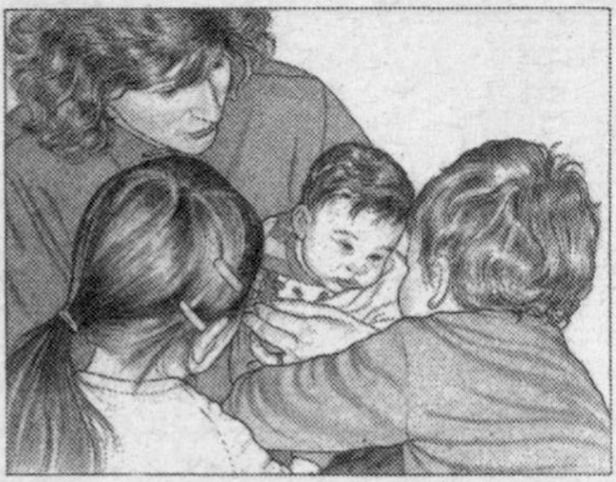

other children, and you feel confident in her abilities and dedication.

In addition to this chapter's guidance on seeking, evaluating, and selecting child care, you'll find a checklist titled *Is This the Right Place for My Child?* on page 740 of the Appendix. It will help you choose high-quality, nurturing care.

What to Look For in a Care Provider

(See also Chapter 6, page 209.)

Children thrive when they're cared for in a safe, healthy environment by supportive adults who are warmly affectionate and who help children learn, interact, and work out solutions while protecting them from making choices that could lead to harm. The following list describes several things you should look for when you are observing someone who might take care of your child. More specific suggestions appear throughout this chapter, but remember that they are general guidelines. They do apply to all out-of-home and in-home care, including babysitters and nannies. Also, keep these same criteria in mind as you play with your own child or supervise small groups of children.

A good caregiver will:

- Listen carefully to children and observe their behavior.
- Set reasonable limits for children and maintain those limits consistently.

- Tell children why certain things are not allowed, and offer acceptable alternatives.
- Deal with difficult situations as they arise and before they get out of control.
- Anticipate trouble and intervene early to prevent it.
- Live up to promises made to the children.
- Join children at play without disrupting their activity.
- Ease transitions that can be stressful to children.
- Reward children's efforts and relieve their "hurts" with an affectionate physical gesture, such as a hug or a pat.
- Talk naturally and conversationally with the children about what they are doing.
- Limit adult conversations in the children's presence.
- Show respect for the children's ideas and decisions.
- Avoid offering children choices when there is no choice.
- Allow children to make mistakes and learn from them (as long as there is no danger involved in doing so).

CHOICES IN CARE

You will want to identify your specific needs and desires. Before you meet and interview potential caregivers, the list of questions you need to answer should include:

- **Where do I** want my baby to be during the day: At home? In someone else's home? In a child care center? If out-of-home care, how far away? What other family members or friends will my child be near?
- **What days and** hours do I need or want care each week?
- **How will I** handle my infant's transportation to and from the program? If the caregiver needs transportation during the day or evening, how will it be handled?
- **What backup arrangements** can I make? How will I handle days when my baby is sick or when my baby's

caregiver is unavailable because of illness or personal business? What are the arrangements for holidays, summertime, and vacations?

- **What can I** realistically afford?
- **What size program** do I want for my baby? How much group interaction do I want for her?
- **How much structure** and stimulation do I want for my baby?
- **What qualifications do** I want the caregiver(s) to have?
- **How do I** want my baby disciplined?
- **What other basic** conditions would make me feel comfortable about leaving my infant with someone else?

While a majority of young children in the United States are in some form of child care, nearly a quarter of this care is provided by relatives, mostly grandmothers. Not only are many grandparents caring for children for part of the day, but more and more of them are involved in taking children to and from other child care arrangements.

If you have family members or friends who you would like to care for your baby and who live nearby, ask yourself if you would be comfortable with their care and whether they would be willing to provide part-time care (perhaps for a few hours a day or for two to three days a week), either on a regular basis or as a backup if other arrangements fail. Consider also, when possible, that offering payment for these services makes the arrangement fairer and creates an additional incentive for the person you depend on for child care to help you.

Other options include bringing someone into your own home or taking your baby to another person's home or a child care center. Your financial resources, the age and needs of your baby, and your own preferences about child rearing will help you decide which choice is best.

Remember that your baby will grow and develop quickly and the choice that is correct today may not be the best choice in the future. Keep reevaluating your infant's needs

A Message for Grandparents

As a grandparent, you may become the person providing part-time care for your grandchild at times, perhaps on a scheduled day or two during the week or for a few hours here and there. Therefore, many of the guidelines in this chapter would apply to your caregiving. The recommendations about the best environment for the baby, safety issues, special needs, and the size of the group (if you care for more than one baby) should be considered.

As a grandparent, your role is unique and important. You are not just "another babysitter." You have a fundamental connection, providing the continuity between generations that your grandchild will come to understand and respect. Take advantage of this irreplaceable role. Your involvement with your grandchild, introducing her to your own world, is especially valuable. Treasure it. Make the most of those special days when you are the babysitter, and offer to do it regularly if you're able.

At times, you may not be the actual caregiver for your grandchild, but rather you'll take him to and from a child care center or babysitter. You can make sure he is transported safely in an appropriate restraint, and provide another set of eyes to evaluate the quality of the center or sitter, which will help your grandchild's parents feel secure in their own choice of a child care setting.

As you know, times have changed, although caring love is still the universal and timeless ingredient to helping children to thrive. Educate yourself on the new medical discoveries since you raised your own children by asking your grandchild's parents to share information. The medical profession has learned a lot about having infants sleep safely on their backs and on safer over-the-counter medications for illnesses, as well as many other things. It keeps us young to learn new things.

By the way, if you've accepted the responsibility of picking up or dropping off your grandchild at regular times, introduce yourself to the responsible person at that site and provide them with your telephone number as a contact person. And remember, when driving with your grandchild, be sure he is properly buckled in a car safety seat at all times. At your home, make sure that you secure any of your personal medications so that your grandchild can't accidentally ingest them.

and how good a fit your current child care arrangement is over time.

Here are some suggestions to keep in mind when deciding among in-home care, family child care, or a child care center:

In-Home Care/Nanny

If you are returning to work while your child is still an infant, one choice for child care (often a more expensive one) may be to have someone come into your home on a live-in or live-out basis. Since this person will not be required to be licensed, there are some important considerations that should be part of your evaluation and the hiring process.

- Check references
- Perform a background check, if possible
- Ask for documented work experience (preferably back as far as five years)
- Ask for the caregiver's approach to discipline, scheduling, feeding, comforting, and providing appropriate activities. Determine if her approach matches your style of child rearing and is right for your child. Make sure this individual shares your philosophy about how to react to excessive crying by your child, how to respond when he has an accident, or what to do when he doesn't sleep. (Sharing

this kind of information is applicable no matter in what type of setting your child is cared for.)

HOW DO I FIND AN IN-HOME CAREGIVER?

- Ask friends for recommendations
- Scan or place ads in the paper (especially local publications for parents)
- Go through a service

AFTER CHOOSING AN IN-HOME CAREGIVER

- Arrange a trial period of at least a week when you can be home to watch the caregiver work under your supervision.
- In the days and weeks ahead, carefully monitor the performance of the person you hire.

ADVANTAGES OF IN-HOME CARE

1. Your baby will stay in familiar surroundings and receive individualized care and attention.
2. He will not be exposed to the illnesses and negative behaviors of other children.
3. When your infant is sick, you won't have to stay home from work or make different arrangements to take care of him.
4. Your caregiver may do some light housework and prepare family meals. If this is one of your expectations, make this clear from the start.
5. You will not need to worry about transportation for your baby unless you want the caregiver to take him on outings.

DISADVANTAGES OF IN-HOME CARE

1. You may have difficulty finding someone who is willing to accept the wages, benefits, and confinement of working

in your home, or you may find the costs of qualified in-home care prohibitive.

2. Since you will be considered an employer, you must meet minimum-wage, Social Security, and tax-reporting requirements. You also should provide health insurance for your employee, if she is not otherwise covered.
3. The presence of a caregiver may infringe on your family's privacy, especially if she lives in your home.
4. Because your caregiver will be alone with your baby most of the time, you have no way of knowing exactly how she will perform her job.
5. Your caregiver may not always have back-up help available for times when she isn't feeling well, has a family crisis, or wants to take a vacation. You will be responsible for securing a replacement.
6. Your caregiver will likely have less initial or ongoing training in child development and health and safety issues such as CPR, first aid, and medication administration. CPR and first aid are skills that she *has* to learn.

Family Child Care

Many people provide informal care in their homes for small groups of children, including babies, often looking after their own children or grandchildren at the same time. Some offer evening care, sick care, or care for children with special needs. Family child care is generally less expensive and more flexible than that offered by child care centers. A small family child care home typically has fewer than six children and one caregiver. Large family child care homes may have up to twelve children and one caregiver and an assistant.

Family child care may be licensed, registered, or unregulated. It is always best to seek out a setting that is licensed. (Licensing regulations vary from state to state and they can be found at places like the National Resource Center for Safe and Healthy Child Care, www.nrckids.org.)

IN CHOOSING A FAMILY CHILD CARE HOME

- Observe the caregiver's work.
- Look for signs of good quality care, such as hygienic diaper changing and safety measures.
- Ask for references.
- Check certification and licensing compliance.
- Look over the home to ensure its safety.
- Find out how many children the provider has enrolled and during what hours.
- Inquire about substitute arrangements in case the caregiver is sick or cannot provide care.
- Request information on the caregiver's plans for emergency situations.
- Ask the provider what training he or she has.
- Ask if the provider's program is accredited by the National Association for Family Child Care.

HOW DO I FIND A FAMILY CHILD CARE PROVIDER?

- Ask friends for recommendations.
- Scan or place ads in the paper (especially local publications for parents).
- Contact a local resource and referral agency: www.naccrra.org or Child Care Aware at 1-800-424-2246.

AFTER CHOOSING A FAMILY CHILD CARE PROVIDER

- Monitor your baby's adjustment and carefully observe interactions between the caregiver and your infant.
- Keep the lines of communication open to address any issues that arise.

ADVANTAGES OF FAMILY CHILD CARE

1. In good family child care settings, there is a favorable child-to-adult ratio. In general, the total number of chil-

dren to adults should be no more than about three children for one adult if some of the children are under the age of twenty-four months.

2. Your baby will have the comforts of being in a home and can be involved in many of the same household activities he'd find at home.
3. Your baby will have social stimulation that comes from having playmates (when other children are present).
4. Family child care has the potential to be relatively flexible, so special arrangements can often be made to meet your baby's individual interests and needs.
5. Your baby may have more individualized attention and quiet time.
6. Your baby may be exposed to fewer infectious diseases or negative behavior from other children.

DISADVANTAGES OF FAMILY CHILD CARE

1. You cannot observe what happens to your baby in your absence. While many providers carefully organize activities that are appropriate for children, others use the TV set as a babysitter—even letting children watch shows that are inappropriate for them.
2. Many family child care providers work without supervision or advice from other adults.
3. The caregiver might share the care of your baby with relatives, boyfriends, or other people who might not give high-quality care.

Child Care Centers

Child care centers also may be called day care, child development centers, nursery schools, preschools, and other similar names. These facilities typically provide care for children in a nonresidential building with classrooms of children in different age groups. Most centers are licensed, caring for children from birth to six years old. Of the approximately 12 million children in child care in the U.S., about 9 million of them are in licensed facilities, and thus about 25 percent of children are cared for in unlicensed/unregulated facilities and settings. Centers demonstrate a higher commitment to quality by participating in the accreditation process.

There are several types of child care centers, most notably the following:

- *Chain centers* offer a wide variety of activities and programs and very appealing activities for children. Because they are chains and run under central management, some do not offer any variation and room for individual creativity in their operations.
- *Independent for-profit centers* depend on enrollment fees to pay their overhead, and they typically earn a narrow profit for their owners. Because many of these programs are built around one or two dedicated people, they can be excellent—as long as those individuals remain actively involved in the daily operations.
- *Nonprofit centers* are sometimes linked to religious institutions, community centers, universities, or social service agencies, or they may be independently incorporated facilities. Some may have access to additional public funding, permitting discounted fees for lower-income families. Any income earned above expenses is put back into the program, directly benefiting the children.
- *Head Start* is a national child development program for children from birth to age five that provides services to promote academic, social, and emotional development, as well as providing social, health, and nutrition services for income-eligible families.

HOW DO I FIND A CHILD CARE CENTER?

- **Child care centers** are often listed on the Internet or in the phone book.
- **Ask your pediatrician** or other parents with children in child care to recommend a center.

- **Contact your community's** health or welfare agency, or a local or national resource and referral organization, such as www.childcareaware.org or Child Care Aware at 1-800-424-2246.

ADVANTAGES OF CHILD CARE CENTERS

1. More information is generally available about them since the majority of centers are regulated by licensing agencies.
2. Many centers have structured programs designed to meet children's developmental needs.
3. Most centers have several caregivers, so you are not dependent on the availability of just one person.
4. Workers in these centers have higher educational requirements and tend to be better supervised than caregivers in other settings.
5. Some centers may allow you to arrange shorter hours or fewer days of care if you work only part-time.
6. Many centers encourage parental involvement so you can help make the center better while your baby is enrolled.

DISADVANTAGES OF CHILD CARE CENTERS

1. Regulations for child care centers vary widely based on the type of center.
2. Good programs may have waiting lists for admission because they are in such demand.
3. Due to the number of children cared for in this type of program, your baby may receive less personalized attention than in a smaller program.

MAKING A FINAL SELECTION

When considering a particular child care setting, you need to know all of the rules and practices that would affect your baby. If the program is formal enough to have a printed handbook, this may answer many of your questions. Otherwise, ask the program director about the following (some of which apply to in-home or family child care as well). Also see *Is This the Right Place for My Child?* in the Appendix to help you choose high-quality, nurturing care.

1. What are the hiring requirements for staff members? (Regulations vary from state to state.) In many good programs, caregivers must have at least two years of college, pass minimum health requirements, and receive basic immunizations. Ideally, they will have some background in early child development and perhaps have children themselves. Directors generally must have a college degree or many years of experience qualifying them as experts in both child development and administration. Staff members should also have training in CPR and first aid.

2. How many staff members are available per child? Although some children need highly personalized attention and others do well with less direct supervision, the general rule to follow is: The younger the child, the more adults there should be in each group. Each baby should be assigned to one caregiver as the primary person responsible for that baby's care, and that caregiver should provide most of the baby's one-on-one care (e.g., feeding, diapering, putting the child to sleep).

How many children are in each group? Generally, smaller groups offer babies a better chance to interact with and learn from one another.

While fewer children per adult is usually better, there is a desirable maximum ratio and group size for each age category. The designated ratios vary from state to state, though, and some good facilities do not reach the ideal child/staff ratios. (Again, the chart *Is This the Right Place for My Child?* on page 740 of the Appendix provides these details.)

3. Is there a problem with frequent staff changes? If so, this may suggest that there are problems with the facility's operations. Ideally, most caregivers should have been with the program for several years, since consistency is desirable. Unfortunately, staff turnover in this profession is an issue for a variety of reasons, including low wages.

4. Are caregivers prohibited from smoking, even outside? This is important for your baby's health.

5. Are caregivers required to have updated immunizations?

6. What are the goals of the program? Some are very organized and try to teach children new skills, or attempt to change or mold their behavior and beliefs. Others are very relaxed, with an emphasis on helping children develop at their own pace. Still others fall somewhere in between. Decide what you want for your baby, and make sure the program you choose meets your desires. Avoid those that offer no personalized attention or support for your baby.

7. What are the admission procedures? Quality child care programs require relevant background information on each baby. Be prepared for very specific questions about your baby's individual needs, developmental level, and health status. You also may be asked about your own child-rearing desires and any other children in your family.

8. Does the child care provider have a valid license and recent health certificate, and does the provider enforce health and immunization requirements for children in the program? Standard immunizations and regular checkups should be required for all children and staff members.

9. How are illnesses handled? Parents should be notified if a staff member or child contracts a significant communicable disease (not just a cold, but problems like chickenpox or hepatitis). The program also should have a clear policy regarding sick children. You should know when to keep your baby home and how the center will respond if he becomes ill during the day.

10. What are the costs? How much will you have to pay to start, and how often will you make installment payments? What do the payments cover specifically? Will you need to pay when your baby is absent for illness or vacations with the family?

11. What happens on a typical day? Ideally, there should be a mix of physical activity and quiet times. Some activities should be group-oriented and others individualized. Times for meals and snacks should be set aside. While a certain amount of structure is desirable, there also should be room for free play and special events.

12. How much parental involvement is expected? Some programs rely heavily on parent participation, while others request very little. At the least, quality programs should welcome your opinions and allow you to visit your baby during the day. If the school maintains a closed-door policy for part or all of the day—typically for educational reasons—be sure that you are comfortable with this practice.

13. What are the general procedures? A well-organized program should have clearly defined rules and regulations regarding:

- Hours of operation
- Transportation of children
- Field trips
- Meals and snacks, whether they are provided by parents or are prepared on-site
- Administration of medication and first aid
- Emergency evacuations
- Notification of child's absence
- Weather cancellations
- Withdrawal of children from the program
- Supplies or equipment that parents must provide
- Sleep arrangements, especially for infants
- Special celebrations
- How parents may contact the staff during the day and at night
- Exclusion of children with certain illnesses
- Security to ensure that everyone who enters the facility, including outdoor play areas, is screened by child care personnel, that strangers cannot enter the building, and that familiar adults who are acting oddly cannot get into any child care area, indoors or out

Once you've received this kind of basic information, you should take a tour of the building and grounds during operating hours to see how the caregivers interact with the children. Your first impressions are especially important, since they'll influence all your future dealings with the program. If you sense warmth and a loving approach to the children, you'll probably feel comfortable placing your own baby there. If you see a worker spank or restrain one of the youngsters too forcefully, you should reconsider sending your own baby, even if that's the only sign of abusive behavior you've noticed.

Try to observe the daily routine, paying attention to how the day is organized and what activities are planned for the children. Watch how food is prepared, and find out how often the children are fed. Check how frequently the babies are diapered. While touring the child care home or center, also check to see if the following basic health and safety standards are being met:

- The premises are clean and reasonably neat (without discouraging play by the children).
- There is plenty of play equipment, and it is in good repair.
- The equipment is appropriate for the developmental skills of the children in the program.
- Babies are closely supervised when climbing on playthings, roughhousing, or playing with blocks (which are sometimes thrown) and other potentially dangerous toys.
- Food is stored in an appropriate manner and if the child care site is preparing the food, that it is nutritious.
- Areas where food is handled are clearly separate from toilets and diaper-changing areas.
- Diaper-changing areas are cleaned and sanitized before and after being used for each infant.
- Hand-washing sinks are available where they are needed and are used not only by the children, but also by the staff members to wash their hands:
    - Upon arrival for the day
    - When moving from one child care group to another
    - Before and after eating or touching food or food preparation surfaces

  - Before and after giving medication
  - Before and after playing in water that is used by more than one person
  - After diapering
  - After using the toilet or helping children use the toilet
  - After handling any body fluid, such as nasal discharge, blood, vomit, drool, or sores
  - After playing in sandboxes
  - After handling garbage
- Potty (or training) chairs are avoided in order to decrease the risk of spreading germs that cause diarrhea.
- Children are supervised by sight and sound at all times, even when napping.

Once you're satisfied that a particular program will provide your baby with a safe, loving, healthy environment, let him test it out while you're present. Watch how the caregivers and your baby interact, and make sure that all of you are comfortable with the situation.

Building a Relationship with Your Baby's Care Providers

For your baby's sake, you need to develop a good relationship with the person or people who care for him in your absence. The better you get along with his caregiver, the more comfortable your baby will feel as he interacts with both of you. The better you communicate with the caregiver about your infant, the more continuity there will be in his care throughout the day.

One way to build this relationship is by talking with the caregiver—even briefly—each time you leave or return for your baby. If something exciting or upsetting happened during the early morning, it might affect your baby's behavior during the rest of the day, so the caregiver should know about it. Share family stresses, both good and bad, like expecting the birth of a new sibling or a family illness.

When you arrive to take him home, you should be told

Napping in Child Care Settings

Sudden infant death syndrome (SIDS) has gotten plenty of attention in recent years, and many parents now know the importance of placing a baby to sleep on his back to minimize the risk of SIDS. Obviously, this same precaution should be followed in child care settings, where 20 percent of all SIDS cases occur—a disproportionately high amount. In 2006, three years after the American Academy of Pediatrics launched a campaign that stressed the importance of using the back sleeping position to lower the incidence of SIDS during child care, only half of the states in the United States had licensing regulations mandating that child care facilities place infants on their backs to sleep. Fortunately, that statistic has improved, but there is still a long way to go.

If your baby is going to be napping at his child care site, you must discuss this issue with the caregivers before making a final selection about a facility. Make sure that the child care setting you choose routinely follows this simple procedure. (For more information about SIDS, see page 223.)

One other important napping recommendation: For older children, make sure that bedding is clean and hypoallergenic.

about any important events that occurred in your absence, from a change in bowel movements or eating patterns to a new way of playing or his first steps. Also, if he's showing symptoms of a developing illness, you and the caregiver should discuss the situation and agree on what to do if symptoms get worse.

A rivalry may develop between you and the caregiver for your baby's affection and control of his behavior. For example, you may hear "Funny, he never does that for me" when he misbehaves. Don't take this seriously—children usually save their worst behavior for the people they trust most.

If you treat caregivers as partners, they will feel that you respect them and probably will be more enthusiastic about looking after your baby. Here are some ways to build this sense of partnership on a daily basis.

- **Talk to the caregiver** about things your baby has done that are particularly funny or interesting. Explain that sharing this kind of information is important to you, and encourage two-way communication.
- **Extend basic courtesy** to your baby's caregivers.
- **Provide materials and** suggestions for special projects the caregivers can do with your baby and/or the group, or ask if there are ways you can help with already planned activities.
- **Help out before** you leave your child by spending a few minutes getting him settled. If he's in a child care center, help him put away his things and join an activity. If he is being cared for at home, get him involved in an activity before you depart. Make sure your baby always knows you are leaving. Say good-bye before you disappear, but leave without prolonging your departure. Don't just "slip away."
- **Help plan and** carry out special activities with the caregiver.

Periodically, you and the caregiver also should have longer discussions to review your baby's progress, discuss any problems, and plan for future changes in your infant's care. Schedule these extended conversations at a time when you won't be rushing to get somewhere, your baby's caregiver isn't busy tending to other children, or the two of you aren't at a place where there will be distractions. If possible, arrange for someone else to care for your baby while you are talking. Allow enough time to discuss all the facts and opinions that both of you have on your minds, and agree on specific objectives and plans.

Most parents find that this discussion goes more smoothly if they've made a list of important topics beforehand. You also should start the conversation on a positive note by talking about some of the things the caregiver is doing that please you. Then move on to any concerns. After presenting your own thoughts, ask for her opinions and listen carefully. Remember, there is little that's strictly right or wrong when it comes to child rearing, and most situations have several "right" approaches. Be open-minded and flexible in your discussions. Close the conversation with a specific plan of action and follow-up communication. Both of you will be more comfortable if something concrete comes out of the meeting, even if it's only a decision to stay on the same course for another month or two.

Resolving Conflicts

Let's assume that you've chosen a child care setting carefully. So what can you now expect?

Most parents are pleased with the child care they've chosen. Nevertheless, whenever two or more people share responsibility for a child, conflicts sometimes arise. In many cases, you can resolve a disagreement about child care simply by talking through the problem. You may find that the conflict is nothing more than a misunderstanding or a misreading of the situation. Other times, especially when several people are involved in the care of your baby, you may need a more organized approach to resolving problems. The following step-by-step strategy can help.

1. Define the problem clearly. Make sure you understand who is involved, but avoid blaming anyone. For example, what if your baby has been biting other children in his child care program? Find out which caregivers were on hand at the time. Ask what they observed and focus your attention on what realistic measures can be taken to prevent or decrease the likelihood of further incidents. Maybe you can suggest an alternate way in which the caregivers can respond if the incident recurs.
2. Listen to everyone's ideas in order to find other possible solutions.
3. Agree on a specific plan of action with clearly defined time limits and assignments to each of the caregivers—including you.

Tips for Transitioning

Getting the day started can be a challenge. So here are some suggestions to make your separation at the child care setting a little easier for both of you.

Your Child's Developmental Stage	Your Response
0 to 7 months In early infancy your baby primarily needs love, comforting, and good basic care to satisfy his physical needs.	Although this period may be a difficult time of separation for you, young infants generally will transition to a consistent child care worker in almost any setting. Be patient during this initial settling-in period.
7 to 12 months Stranger anxiety normally occurs at this time. Suddenly your baby may be reluctant to stay with anyone outside his family. The unfamiliar setting of a child care center also may upset him.	If possible, do not start child care during this period, or just ease into it. If your child is already in a program, take a little extra time each day before you say good-bye. Create a short good-bye ritual, perhaps letting him hold a favorite stuffed animal. Say good-bye and then quietly leave. Above all, be consistent from day to day.

4. Consider everything that could go wrong with the plan you've devised, and decide how these problems might be avoided or handled if they occur.

5. Put the plan into action.

6. Meet again at a specified time to decide whether the plan is working. If it's not, go through the process again to decide what changes need to be made.

What to Do When Your Baby Is Sick

If your baby is like most others, he'll get his share of illnesses, whether he's in a child care program or not. In most cases these illnesses will be colds or other respiratory infections, which tend to occur more often between early fall and late spring. At times he may get one infection right after another and be sick for weeks. If both parents have full-time jobs, this can be a big problem and cause a great deal of stress since often one of the parents will need to stay home with the ill baby.

Even infants who seem to be only mildly ill may be sent home from child care programs, and, if based on good policies, for good reason. A sick baby may be contagious and risks giving his illness to another child. Also, a sick baby may need more individual care and attention than a child care provider or program can reasonably be expected to provide without interfering with the care of others.

States often have regulations that actually require child care programs to send sick children home. This makes sense, particularly when a baby has a fever and is acting sick, is sneezing or coughing, is vomiting, or has diarrhea, since it is under those circumstances that contagious diseases are spread to others. The ultimate goal is to both provide your baby with the care he needs and to limit the spread of contagious illnesses in the child care setting.

Ideally, you'll be able to stay home when your baby is sick. However, there may be times when this option is particularly difficult or simply not possible. Be sure to talk to your employer ahead of time to see what arrangements you can make in the event that your baby is ill. You might suggest taking your work home with you, or try to identify in advance coworkers who can substitute for you when this situation arises. Spouses, other family members, and trusted friends may be able to help in caring for your infant.

If your job and your spouse's employer require full-time attendance, you'll have to make other arrangements for a sick baby. These are days when you might arrange alternate care for him, preferably where both the caregiver and the setting are familiar. If you rely on a relative or hire a sitter to stay with him, make sure the caregiver understands the nature of the illness and how it should be treated.

If your baby requires any medication, confirm your child care provider's policies regarding giving medication to children, and always obtain written instructions from your pediatrician to give to your caregiver. Don't expect your caregiver to follow your instructions without a pediatrician's authorization. Also, both prescription and over-the-counter medications should have a pharmacy or drugstore label on them with the baby's name, the medication dosage, and the expiration date. Giving medication to children is a significant responsibility, and can be quite a challenge for caregivers. It should be requested only when it is necessary.

Your baby's caregiver will need to know why the medication is being given, how it should be stored and administered (in what doses, at what intervals, and for how long), and what side effects to look for and what to do if they occur. Again, this should all be put in writing. Explain that medicine should not be disguised as food or described as candy; instead, your baby should be told what the medicine is and why he needs to take it. Ask the caregiver to record the time each dose is given.

If your baby is in a child care center, you should be prepared to sign a consent form, authorizing the staff to administer the medication. Also, you should expect your baby's medications to be sent home each evening (since regulations typically do not allow them to be kept in the child care facility overnight).

A few communities have services that specialize in care for mildly ill babies and older children. These include the following:

HOME-BASED PROGRAMS

- Family child care homes that are equipped to care for both sick and well children. If a baby becomes ill in such a program, he can continue attending in a segregated area, if necessary. Not all infections are contagious.
- Family child care homes that care only for sick children. Some of these are associated with well-child care centers.
- Agencies or child care centers that provide caregivers who can work in your home.

CENTER-BASED PROGRAMS

- Regular child care centers that have trained staff members to care for sick babies in the usual child care setting, but apart from the main group of well children.
- Centers that offer a separate "get-well room" for sick babies, staffed by a caregiver.
- Sick-child care centers that are set up specifically to care for ill babies and older children.

In sick-child programs, caregivers adjust the activity level of the children to the child's ability to participate, and the children receive a lot of cuddling and personal attention. These programs should pay extra attention to hygiene for both caregivers and babies. The premises and equipment, especially toys, should be cleaned thoroughly and often. Disposable toys may be necessary in some situations, depending on the nature of the illnesses involved. A pediatrician and public health consultant should be on call for every sick-child care facility.

Controlling Infectious Diseases

Whenever children gather in groups, their risk of getting sick increases. Infants are particularly affected, since they can be expected to place their toys and their hands in their mouths, making it even easier to spread infectious diseases.

While it's impossible for adults to keep toys and other objects in the child care center in perfect sanitary condition, many precautions and practices can help control the spread of infection. Child care programs should be extremely careful about maintaining good hygiene. Children and teachers should have easy access to sinks. They should be reminded, and children should be assisted if necessary, to wash their hands after going to the bathroom. Staff members also should wash at all the times listed earlier in this chapter, and especially after changing diapers. Both the caregiver's and the baby's hands should at least be wiped during diaper changing after removing the soiled diaper, and then both should wash their hands at the end of the diaper change routine. Hand-washing after blowing or wiping noses and before handling food or food surfaces can also significantly reduce the spread of infection.

If a center cares for infants, toddlers, and toilet-trained children, each of these groups should have a separate area, each with its own accessible sink for hand-washing. The facility and all equipment should be cleaned at least daily. Changing tables and toilets should be washed and disinfected.

As a parent, you can help control the spread of disease in your baby's center by keeping him at home when he has an illness that's contagious or requires extra attention. Also notify her caregiver as soon as anyone in your family is diagnosed as having a particular illness, and request that all parents be alerted when any child in the program has a serious or highly contagious infectious illness.

Immunizations can greatly reduce outbreaks of serious infectious diseases. Centers should require children to be immunized (at appropriate ages) against hepatitis B, rotavirus, diphtheria, tetanus, pertussis, polio, influenza (flu), *Haemophilus influenzae* type b, pneumococcus, measles, mumps, rubella, hepatitis A, chickenpox, and meningococcus. The immunity of your baby's caregivers should be checked as well, and if there is any doubt, they should receive appropriate immunizations.

Remember, teach your child proper hygiene and hand-washing habits so that he's less likely to spread illnesses himself. Finally, educate yourself about the illnesses that are most common in child care settings, so you know what to expect and how to respond if they occur in your child's program. These include the following.

Colds and Flu

The most common infections are caused by viruses that produce the symptoms of a cold or the flu. Children in child care typically have an average of seven to nine colds each year, and are more likely to get these infections than infants cared for at home.

Fortunately, the chances of contracting some of the most severe illnesses or complications associated with the common cold can be decreased by immunizing children with the vaccines mentioned earlier. In child care centers, toys, tables, doorknobs, and other surfaces that are touched by hands should be sanitized frequently.

The symptoms of colds can include a runny nose, cough, sore or scratchy throat, sneezing, and watery eyes. Colds are spread by direct or close contact with the mouth or nose secretions of an infected individual, or by touching contaminated objects. Children can be taught to wash their hands frequently, and when that's not possible, to "give their sneezes the cold shoulder" by sneezing into their upper arm rather than their hands. They also should be taught proper disposal of tissues and not to share cups or eating utensils.

Cytomegalovirus (CMV) and Parvovirus Infection

Cytomegalovirus and parvovirus usually do not cause any (or cause only mild) illness in babies, older children, and adults. However, these viruses can be dangerous to a pregnant woman who is not immune to them, because an infection sometimes can cause a serious infection in her unborn child. The infection can be transmitted through direct contact with body fluids (tears, urine, saliva). Fortunately, most adult women are already immune to these diseases, but if you are pregnant, have a baby in child care, or work in a child care home or center yourself, you have an increased risk of exposure to CMV and parvovirus, and you should discuss this concern with your obstetrician.

Diarrheal Diseases

Gastrointestinal diseases are less common than respiratory infections. The average baby has one or two episodes of diarrhea a year. These illnesses can spread easily in child care homes and centers.

If your infant has diarrhea, do not take him to child care unless all of his stool can be controlled by using the toilet. Children with loose stools who wear diapers or who cannot make sure that all of their stool ends up in the toilet should not be in child care unless your pediatrician has determined that the cause is not infectious. If he has a mild form of the illness, then several days away from the center should minimize the chances that he'll transmit it to other children. But if a more serious cause is suspected, further tests to identify the responsible agent (bacteria, virus, or parasite) may need to be done before the child returns. (See *Diarrhea,* page 440.)

Hepatitis A Virus

Hepatitis A vaccines are universally recommended and given to children over one year of age (ages twelve to twenty-three months old) with a second booster dose at least six months after the first. Because of the success of the vaccine, Hepatitis A infection in child care settings is less common than it once was.

If a child in a care program gets hepatitis A, a viral infection of the liver, it can spread easily to other children and caregivers. In infants and preschool children, most infections are asymptomatic or cause mild, nonspecific symptoms. Older infected children may have only mild fever, nausea, vomiting, diarrhea, or jaundice (a yellowish skin color). However, adults who get this illness usually experience these symptoms to a much greater degree.

Hepatitis can be controlled through gamma globulin injections, but several staff members and parents may be infected before anyone realizes there's a problem. For this reason, whenever hepatitis A is diagnosed in anyone even remotely connected with the program, parents and staff should be alerted and the public health department consulted to decide how best to stop the disease from spreading. (See *Hepatitis,* page 449.)

Hepatitis B Virus

Infants receive the hepatitis B vaccine shortly after birth to protect them from catching this virus. Thanks to the success of this vaccine, rates of hepatitis B in children have significantly decreased.

Hepatitis B virus can cause a chronic infection of the liver that sometimes progresses to cirrhosis (disease of the liver which can turn into liver failure) or cancer of the liver. The virus can be acquired during birth from an infected mother or after birth by exposure to infected blood such as during a needle stick. This type of exposure to blood rarely occurs in a child care setting; thus, there is no need to exclude a child with hepatitis B infection from group child care.

Human Immunodeficiency Virus (HIV)/AIDS

HIV (the AIDS virus) can produce a serious chronic infection when it develops into full-blown AIDS, which can be fatal if not properly treated. Children acquire HIV from their infected mothers before or during birth. HIV also can be transmitted from one child to another by passage of blood from an infected child into the body of someone not infected. Because this does not occur in usual child care activities, children with these infections do *not* present a danger to others.

Some parents are hesitant to let people know that their baby is HIV positive. The American Academy of Pediatrics believes that the decision on whether to disclose this information should be made by the parent (with the advice of the child's pediatrician), and certainly with the baby's best interests in mind. There is no need to restrict placing an HIV-infected baby in child care in the belief that this would protect others, since the risk of HIV transmission in this setting is extremely low when standard appropriate blood and body fluid precautions are used.

If an injury involving blood occurs, the caregiver should put on gloves and wash the wound, administer first aid, and apply a bandage. All blood-contaminated surfaces or clothing should be washed and disinfected. Diluted bleach kills HIV. All blood should be dealt with as if it were contaminated.

Also, since human milk can transmit HIV and other

viruses, be sure that the child care facility has procedures to prevent feeding milk of one mother to another mother's baby. If such an incident occurs, the situation should be handled following the national standards described in *Caring for Our Children* (published by the National Resource Center for Health and Safety in Child Care and Early Education; http://nrc.uchsc.edu).

Preventing Injuries and Promoting Car Safety

Many injuries that occur at home or in child care settings are predictable and preventable. These issues are described earlier in this chapter on pages 360–365 in sections on assessing and selecting child care for your baby. Safety for children (and adults) in and around cars is a special concern. The center should have well-marked pickup and drop-off points where babies, older children, and adults are protected from street traffic, with signs such as CHILDREN AT PLAY placed in the pickup/drop-off areas as well as along nearby streets. The center should never allow a child to be in these areas, or in any area where cars come and go, unless he is being picked up or dropped off and is accompanied by an adult. Children also should never be permitted behind vehicles that could move and back over them. Also keep in mind that adults may need assistance when dealing with more than one child in the car. Cars should also not be left running, and should always be driven slowly.

If your baby shares a ride to and from child care, be sure the other drivers have good driving records, and are using appropriate car seats for all children in their vehicles. The driver must check the vehicle to be sure that everyone is properly buckled in a car safety seat, booster seat, or seat belt before pulling away and that everyone has left the vehicle before locking up at the parking spot. School buses and vans also need to follow measures that ensure the safety of children while they are being transported.

If your child care program includes swimming, make sure appropriate safety precautions are followed. Any pool, lake, creek, or pond used by children should first be checked by public health authorities. If the pool is at or near the child

Car-Pool Safety

If you drive children in a car pool, you must be as responsible for every child in the car as you are for your own. This means making sure that everyone is properly restrained in car safety seats appropriate for his size, not overloading the car, and checking that your insurance covers everyone on board. In addition, make sure that you and other drivers observe the following precautions, many of which will apply even when you, your spouse, or other family member (e.g., grandparent) are driving only your own child to his care setting.

- Pick up and drop off children only at the curb or in a driveway where the children are protected from other cars.
- If possible, have each child's own parents or another responsible adult buckle him into the car and take him out when he returns home.
- Turn all children over to the direct supervision of a parent or child care staff member.
- Close and lock all car doors, but only after checking that fingers and feet are inside.
- Open passenger windows only a few inches, and lock all power window and door controls from the driver's seat if possible.
- Remind children about safety rules and proper behavior before starting out.
- Plan your routes to minimize travel time and avoid hazardous conditions.
- Pull over if any child in the group gets out of control or misbehaves. If any child consistently presents a problem, discuss the difficulty with his parents and

exclude him from the car pool until his conduct improves.

- Have available emergency contact information for each child who rides in the car.
- Ideally, equip each vehicle with a fire extinguisher and first-aid kit.
- Be sure that no child is ever left in the car without a supervising adult.

care center itself, it should be entirely surrounded by a four-foot-high, four-sided childproof fence with a locked gate that completely separates the center from the pool. For hygienic reasons, portable wading pools should be avoided.

Care for Babies with Special Needs

If your baby has a developmental disability or a chronic illness, don't let that keep him out of child care. In fact, quality child care may be good for him. He is likely to benefit from the social contact, physical exercise, and variety of experiences of a group program. Although the most common special health needs include asthma and allergies, there are a variety of developmental and behavioral issues that also fall into this category.

The time your baby spends in a child care program will be good for you, too. Tending a baby with special needs often places great demands on time, energy, and emotions. The challenge is to find a program that encourages normal childhood activities and at the same time meets his special needs; however, these are more widely available than in the past.

Federal law (the Individuals with Disabilities Education Act [IDEA], formerly known as the Amendments to the Education for All Handicapped Children Act) requires all states to develop special education programs for preschool (three- to five-year-old) children with developmental disabilities. This act also gives states the option to develop special education programs for infants and toddlers with developmental

> ### *Where We Stand*
>
> To ensure the safety of children while they are being transported to school, the American Academy of Pediatrics strongly recommends that all children travel in age-appropriate and properly secured child restraint systems in all motor vehicles.

disabilities or delays. Parents should check with their pediatrician or their state Education or Health Department regarding the availability of these early intervention programs.

Start your search with your pediatrician by asking about the best type of group programs for your baby to participate in. Also ask her for referrals to suitable centers. Your pediatrician can help you draft an individualized "care plan" to address your baby's special healthcare needs and help your child care providers understand what your baby will need. Although only one appropriate site may be available in some smaller communities, you will have several to choose from in many communities. The one you select should meet the same basic requirements outlined earlier in this chapter for other child care programs, plus the following.

1. The program should include babies and older children with and without chronic illnesses and special needs, to the extent possible. Having relationships with typically developing playmates helps a child with a disability feel more relaxed and confident socially, and helps build his self-esteem. The arrangement also benefits the typically developing child and those with no special health needs by teaching them to look past the surface differences and helping him develop sensitivity and respect for *all* people.
2. The staff should be trained to provide the specific care your baby requires. Some of the training needs can be specified in your baby's care plan.
3. The program should have at least one physician consultant who is active in the development of policies and procedures affecting the type of special needs present

Safety Walk Checklist

Next time you walk through your baby's child care home or center, use the following checklist to make sure the facility is safe, clean, and in good repair. If there is a problem with any item on the list, bring it to the attention of the director or caregiver and follow up later to be sure it was corrected.

Indoors in All Programs

- Floors are smooth, clean, and have a nonskid surface.
- Medicines, cleaning agents, and tools are locked up and out of children's reach.
- First-aid kit is fully supplied and out of children's reach.
- Windowsills, walls, and ceilings are clean and in good repair, with no peeling paint or damaged plaster. (Windowsills are the highest risk areas for lead poisoning.)
- Children are never left unattended.
- Electrical outlets are covered with childproof caps that are not a choking hazard.
- Electric lights are in good repair, with no frayed or dangling cords.
- Heating pipes and radiators are out of reach or covered so children cannot touch them.
- Ask if the hot water is set at or below 120 degrees Fahrenheit (48.9 degrees Celsius) to lessen the risk of a scald burn.
- There are no poisonous plants or disease-bearing animals (e.g., turtles or iguanas).
- Trash containers are covered.

- Exits are clearly marked and easy to reach.
- No smoking is allowed in the child care facility.
- Windows at or above the second story have guards on them to prevent falls; and all window blind or drapery cords are secured out of children's reach.
- Leaks are fixed promptly and any mold is properly treated.

Outdoors in All Programs

- Grounds are free of litter, sharp objects, and animal droppings.
- Play equipment is smooth, well anchored, and free of rust, splinters, and sharp corners. All screws and bolts are capped or concealed.
- Outdoor playground equipment is mounted over impact-absorbent surfaces for a distance of at least 6 feet (1.8 meters) on all sides of the equipment. Playground surfaces should be made of at least 12 inches (30 cm) of wood chips, mulch, sand, pea gravel, or other impact-absorbing material under and around areas where falls are more likely to occur (under monkey bars, slides).
- Swing seats are lightweight and flexible, and there are no open or S-shaped hooks.
- Slides have wide, flat, stable steps with good treads, rounded rims along the sides to prevent falls, and a flat area at the end of the slide to help children slow down.
- Metal slides are shaded from the sun.
- Sandboxes are covered when not in use.
- Childproof barriers keep babies and older children out of hazardous areas.

Infant Programs

- Toys do not contain lead or have any signs of chipping paint, rust, or small pieces that could break off. (The weight or softness of the material may provide clues that the toys are made of lead.)
- High chairs have wide bases and safety straps.
- Babies are not allowed to walk around with bottles or to take bottles to bed.
- Infant walkers are not used.
- Beds and playpens meet safety standards.
- No recalled products or old products with broken or missing parts are used. Recalled products can be determined by checking the website of the Consumer Product Safety Commission: www.cpsc.gov.

among the children in the group. Your own pediatrician should also play an active role. Give permission for your child care providers to discuss questions and issues with your pediatrician.

4. All children should be encouraged to be as independent as their abilities allow, within the bounds of safety. They should be restricted only in activities that might be dangerous for them or that have been prohibited by doctor's orders.

5. The program should be flexible enough to adapt to slight variations in the children's abilities. For example, this may include altering some equipment or facilities for physically challenged or visually or hearing-impaired children.

6. The program should offer special equipment and activities to meet the special needs of babies, such as breathing treatments for children with asthma. The equipment should be in good repair, and the staff should be trained to operate it correctly.

7. The staff should be familiar with each child's medical and developmental status. The staff should be able to recognize symptoms and determine when the child needs medical attention.

8. If the program includes off-site field trips or activities, the staff should be trained in safe transportation of children with special needs.

9. The staff should know how to reach each child's physician in an emergency and should be qualified to administer any necessary emergency medications. Emergency planning should be specified in your baby's care plan.

These are very general recommendations. Because special needs vary so widely, it's impossible to tell you more precisely how to determine the best program for your own baby. If you're having trouble deciding among the programs your pediatrician has suggested, go back and discuss your concerns with her. She will work with you to make the right choice.

Whatever your baby's special needs, how he will be cared for in your absence is an important decision. The information you have just read should help. However, remember that you know your baby better than anyone, so rely most heavily on your needs and impressions when choosing or changing a child care arrangement.

11

KEEPING YOUR CHILD SAFE

Everyday life is full of well-disguised dangers for babies: sharp objects, shaky furniture, reachable hot water faucets, hot tubs, swimming pools, and busy streets. By adulthood we've learned to navigate this minefield so well that we no longer think of things like scissors and stoves as hazards. To protect your baby from the dangers she'll encounter in and out of your home, you have to see the world as she does, and you must recognize that she cannot yet distinguish hot from cold or sharp from dull.

Keeping your baby physically safe is your most basic responsibility—and a never-ending one. Each year, children experience over 6 million emergency department visits because of unintentional injury and over 5,000 under the age of fifteen die.

As might be expected, automobile crashes account for a large number of the injuries and deaths. But many babies are injured and killed by equipment designed specifically for their use. In one recent twelve-month period, high chair–related injuries sent almost 10,000 children to the hospital. In 2001, toys caused more than 200,000 injuries serious enough to require treatment in hospital emergency rooms in children under the age of fifteen. Even cribs account for about 32 deaths annually.

These are grim statistics, but they are not inevitable. In the past, injuries were called "accidents" because they seemed unpredictable and unavoidable. Today we know that injuries are not random. By understanding how a baby grows and develops, and the risk of injury at each developmental stage, parents can take precautions that will prevent most, if not all, of these injuries.

Why Children Get Injured

Every childhood injury involves three elements: factors related to the baby, the object that causes the injury, and the environment in which it occurs. To keep your baby safe, you must be aware of all three.

Let's start with your baby. His age makes a tremendous difference in the kind of protection he needs. The three-month-old who sits cooing in an infant seat requires quite different supervision from that needed by the ten-month-old who's started walking or the toddler who has learned to climb. So at each stage of your baby's life, you must think again about the hazards that are present and what you can do to eliminate them. Repeatedly, as your baby grows, you must ask: How far can he move and how fast? How high can he reach? What objects attract his attention? What can he do today that he couldn't do yesterday? What will he do tomorrow that he can't do today?

During the first six months of life, you can secure your infant's safety by never leaving him alone, even for a moment, in a dangerous situation such as on a bed or changing table where he might wiggle or roll off. As he grows, he'll create dangers of his own—perhaps by first rolling or crawling off the bed, then by creeping into places he shouldn't be, and finally by actively seeking out things to touch and taste that may be dangerous.

As your child begins to move about, you certainly will tell him "no" whenever he approaches something potentially hazardous, but he will not really understand the significance of your message. Many parents find the ages between six months and twelve months extremely frustrating, because the baby doesn't seem to learn from these reprimands. Even if you tell him twenty times a day to stay away from the toilet, he's still in the bathroom every time you turn your back. At this age your baby is not being willfully disobedient; his memory just isn't developed enough for him to recall your warning the next time he's attracted by the forbidden object or activity. What looks like naughtiness is actually the testing and retesting of reality—the normal way of learning for a baby of this age.

Young children are extraordinary mimics, so they may try to take medicine just as they've seen Mom doing, or they may play with a razor just like Dad. Unfortunately, their notions of cause and effect aren't as advanced as their motor skills. Yes, your baby may realize that tugging on the cord pulled the iron down on his head after it falls, but his ability to anticipate many similar consequences is still months away.

Your child's temperament also may determine his vulnerability. Studies suggest that children who are extremely active and unusually curious have more than their share of injuries. At certain stages of development, your baby is likely to be stubborn, easily frustrated, aggressive, or unable to concentrate—all characteristics associated with injuries. So when you notice that your baby is having a bad day or is going through a difficult phase, be especially alert: That's when he's most likely to test safety rules, even those he ordinarily follows.

Since you can't change your child's age, and you have little influence over his basic temperament, most of your efforts to prevent injury should focus on objects and surroundings. By designing an environment in which the obvious hazards have been removed, you can allow your baby the freedom he needs to explore.

Some parents feel they don't need to childproof their homes because they intend to supervise their baby closely. And in fact, with constant vigilance, most injuries *can* be avoided. But even the most conscientious parents can't watch a baby every moment. Most injuries occur not when parents are alert and at their best, but when they are under stress. The following situations are often associated with injuries:

- Hunger and fatigue (i.e., the hour or so before dinner)
- Mother's pregnancy
- Illness or death in the family
- Changes in the baby's regular caregiver
- Tension between parents
- Sudden changes in the environment, such as moving to a new home or going on vacation

All families experience at least some of these stresses some of the time. Childproofing eliminates or reduces the opportunities for injury so that even when you are momentarily distracted—for example, by the ring of the telephone or doorbell—your baby is less likely to encounter situations and objects that can cause him harm.

The pages that follow include advice about how to minimize dangers in and out of the home. The intention is to alert you to hazards—particularly those that, on the surface, might seem harmless—so you can take the sensible precautions that will keep your baby safe and allow him the freedom he needs to grow up happy and healthy.

Safety Inside Your Home

Room to Room

Your lifestyle and the layout of your home will determine which rooms should be childproofed. Examine every room in which your baby spends any time. (For most families, that means the entire house.) It's tempting to exclude a formal dining or living room that remains behind closed doors when not in use; but remember, the rooms that are forbidden to your baby are the ones she'll want most to explore as soon as she's old enough. Any areas not childproofed will require extra vigilance on your part, even if their entrances are normally locked or blocked.

At the very least, your baby's room should be a place where everything is as safe as it can be.

Nursery

Cribs. Your baby usually will be unattended when in his crib, so this should be a totally safe environment. Falls are the most common injury associated with cribs, even though they are the easiest to prevent. Babies are most likely to fall out of the crib when the mattress is raised too high for their height or when the side rail is left down.

If you use a new crib or one manufactured since 1990, it should meet current safety standards; look for one with Juvenile Product Manufacturer's Association (JPMA) certification. No matter what the age of your crib, inspect it carefully for the following features:

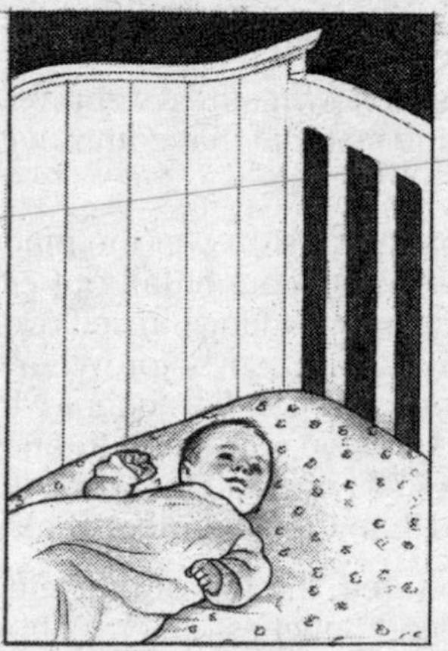

- Slats should be no more than 2⅜ inches (6 cm) apart so a baby's head cannot become trapped between them.
- There should be no cut-outs in the headboard or footboard, as your baby's head could become trapped in them.
- If the crib has corner posts (sometimes called finials), unscrew them or cut them off. Loose clothing can become snagged on these and choke your baby.
- All screws, bolts, and hardware must be tightly in place to prevent the crib from coming apart. A baby's activity can cause the crib to collapse, trapping and suffocating her.
- Before each assembly and weekly thereafter, inspect the crib for damage to hardware, loose joints, missing parts, or sharp edges. Do not use a crib if any parts are missing or broken. Do not substitute parts; instead, obtain replacements from the manufacturer.

You can prevent other crib hazards by observing the following guidelines.

1. The mattress should fit snugly so your baby cannot slip into the crack between it and the crib side. If you can insert

two fingers between the mattress and the sides or ends of the crib, replace the mattress with one that fits snugly.

2. If you purchase a new mattress, remove and destroy all plastic wrapping material that comes with it, because it can suffocate a baby.
3. Before your baby can sit, lower the mattress of the crib to the level where he cannot fall out either by leaning against the side or by pulling himself over it. Set the mattress at its lowest position before your baby learns to stand. The most common falls occur when a baby tries to climb out, so move your baby to another bed when he is 35 inches (89 cm) tall, or when the height of the side rail is less than three-quarters of his height.
4. When fully lowered, the top of the side rail of the crib should be at least 9 inches (23 cm) above the mattress, even when the mattress is set at its highest position. Be sure the locking latch that holds the side up is sturdy and can't be released by your baby. Always leave the side up when your baby is in the crib.
5. Periodically check the crib to be sure there are no rough edges or sharp points on the metal parts, and no splinters or cracks in the wood. If you notice tooth marks on the railing, cover the wood with a plastic strip (available at most children's furniture stores).
6. If you use a crib bumper, be sure it goes all the way around the crib and is secured with at least six straps or ties, to keep the bumper from falling away from the sides. To prevent strangulation, the ties should be no more than 6 inches (15 cm) long. *Do not use soft, pillowlike bumpers.*
7. If you use a crib bumper, remove it as soon as your baby can pull to a standing position.
8. Pillows, quilts, comforters, sheepskins, stuffed animals, and other soft products should not be placed in a crib.
9. If you hang a mobile over your baby's crib, be sure it is securely attached to the side rails. Hang it high enough so your baby cannot reach it to pull it down, and remove it when he is able to get up on his hands and knees, or when he reaches five months, whichever comes first.

10. Crib gyms should be removed as soon as your baby can get up on all fours. Even though these gyms are designed to withstand a baby's grabbing and tugging, he could fall forward onto the gym and become injured.

11. To prevent the most serious of falls and to keep babies from getting caught in cords from hanging window blinds or draperies and strangling, don't place a crib—or any other baby's bed—near a window.

Changing Tables. Although a changing table makes it easier to dress and diaper your baby, falls from such a high surface can be serious. Don't trust your vigilance alone to prevent falls; you should also consider the following recommendations.

1. Choose a sturdy, stable changing table with a 2-inch (5 cm) guardrail around all four sides.

2. The top of the changing table should be concave, so that the middle is slightly lower than the sides.

3. Buckle the safety strap, but don't depend on it alone to keep your baby secure. Never leave an infant unattended on a dressing table, even for a moment, even if he is strapped.

4. Keep diapering supplies within your reach—but out of your infant's reach—so you don't have to leave your baby's side to get them. Never let him play with a powder container. If he opens and shakes it, he's likely to inhale particles of powder, which can injure his lungs.

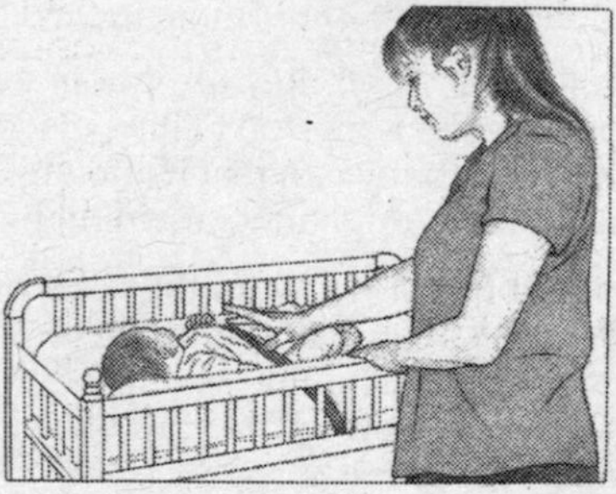

5. If you use disposable diapers, store them out of your infant's reach and cover them with clothing when he wears them. Babies can suffocate if they tear off pieces of the plastic liner and swallow them.

Kitchen

The kitchen is such a dangerous room for young children that some experts recommend they be excluded from it. That's a difficult rule to enforce, because parents spend so much time there and most young children want to be where the action is. While he's with you in the kitchen, sit him in a high chair or playpen so he can watch you and others in the room. He should be securely strapped in and within your vision. Keep a toy box or drawer with safe play items in the kitchen to amuse him. You can eliminate the most serious dangers by taking the following precautions.

1. Store strong cleaners, lye, furniture polish, dishwasher soap, and other dangerous products in a high cabinet, locked and out of sight. If you must store some items under the sink, buy a child safety lock that refastens automatically every time you close the cupboard. (Most hardware and department stores have them.) Never transfer dangerous substances into containers that look as if they might hold food as this may tempt a baby to taste it.
2. Keep knives, forks, scissors, and other sharp instruments separate from "safe" kitchen utensils, and in a latched drawer. Store sharp cutting appliances such as food processors out of reach and/or in a locked cupboard.
3. Unplug appliances when they are not in use so your infant cannot turn them on. Don't allow electrical cords to dangle where your baby can reach and tug on them, possibly pulling a heavy appliance down on himself.
4. Always turn pot handles toward the back of the stove so your child can't reach up and grab them. Whenever you have to walk with hot liquid—a cup of coffee, a pot of soup—be sure you know where your baby is so you don't trip over him.

5. When shopping for an oven, choose one that is well insulated to protect your baby from the heat if he touches the oven door. Also, never leave the oven door open.
6. If you have a gas stove, turn the dials firmly to the off position, and if they're easy to remove, do so when you aren't cooking so that your baby can't turn the stove on. If they cannot be removed easily, use child-resistant knob covers and block the access to the stove as much as possible.
7. Keep matches out of reach and out of sight.
8. Don't warm baby bottles in a microwave oven. The liquid heats unevenly, so there may be pockets of milk hot enough to scald your baby's mouth when he drinks. Also, some overheated baby bottles have exploded when they were removed from the microwave.
9. Keep a fire extinguisher in your kitchen. (If your home has more than one story, mount an extinguisher in a place you will remember on each floor.)
10. Do not use small refrigerator magnets that your baby could choke on or swallow.

Bathroom

The simplest way to avoid bathroom injuries is to make this room inaccessible unless your baby is accompanied by an adult. This may mean installing a latch on the door at adult height so the infant can't get into the bathroom when you aren't around. Also, be sure any lock on the door can be unlocked from the outside, just in case your baby locks himself in.

The following suggestions will prevent injuries when your baby is using the bathroom.

1. Babies can drown in only a few inches of water, so *never leave a young child alone in the bath, even for a moment.* If you can't ignore the doorbell or the phone, wrap your infant in a towel and take him along when you go to answer them. Bath seats and rings are meant to be bathing *aids* and will not prevent drowning if the infant is left unattended. Never leave water in the bathtub when it is not in use.

2. Install no-slip strips on the bottom of the bathtub. Put a cushioned cover over the water faucet so your baby won't be hurt if he bumps his head against it.

3. Get in the habit of closing the lid of the toilet, and get a toilet lid lock. A curious baby who tries to play in the water can lose his balance and fall in.

4. To prevent scalding, the hottest temperature at the faucet should be no more than 120 degrees Fahrenheit (48.9 degrees Celsius). In many cases you can adjust your hot water heater. When your baby is old enough to turn the faucets, teach him to start the cold water before the hot.

5. Keep all medicines in containers with safety caps. Remember, however, that these caps are child-*resistant*, not childproof, so store all medicines and cosmetics high and out of reach in a locked cabinet. Don't keep toothpaste, soaps, shampoos, and other frequently used items in the same cabinet. Instead, store them in a hard-to-reach cabinet equipped with a safety latch or locks.

6. If you use electrical appliances in the bathroom, particularly hair dryers and razors, be sure to unplug them and store them in a cabinet with a safety lock when they aren't in use. It is better to use them in another room where there is no water. An electrician can install special bathroom wall sockets (ground-fault circuit interrupters) that can lessen the likelihood of electrical injury when an appliance falls into the sink or bathwater.

All Rooms

Certain safety rules and preventive actions apply to every room. The following safeguards against commonplace household dangers will protect not only your baby, but your entire family.

1. Install smoke detectors throughout your home, at least one on every level and outside bedrooms. Check them monthly to be sure they are working. It is best to use smoke detectors with long-life batteries, but if these are not available, change the batteries annually on a date

you will remember. Develop a fire escape plan and practice it so you'll be prepared if an emergency does occur.

2. Put safety plugs that are not a choking hazard in all unused electrical outlets so your baby can't stick her finger or a toy into the holes. If your baby won't stay away from outlets, block access to them with furniture. Keep electrical cords out of reach and sight.

3. To prevent slipping, carpet your stairs where possible. Be sure the carpet is firmly tacked down at the edges. When your baby is just learning to crawl and walk, install safety gates at both top and bottom of stairs. Avoid accordion-style gates, which can trap an arm or a neck.

4. Certain houseplants may be harmful. Your regional Poison Help Line will have a list or description of plants to avoid. You may want to forego house plants for a while or, at the very least, keep all house plants out of reach.

5. Check your floors constantly for small objects that a baby might swallow, such as coins, buttons, beads, pins, and screws. This is particularly important if someone in the household has a hobby that involves small items, or if there are older children who have small items.

6. If you have hardwood floors, don't let your baby run around in stocking feet. Socks make slippery floors even more dangerous.

7. Attach cords for window blinds and drapes to floor mounts that hold them taut, or wrap these cords around wall brackets to keep them out of reach. Use safety stop devices on the cords. Cords with loops should be cut and equipped with safety tassels. Babies can strangle on them if they are left loose.

8. Pay attention to the doors between rooms. Glass doors are particularly dangerous, because a baby may bang into them, so fasten them open if you can. Swinging doors can knock an infant down, and folding doors can pinch little fingers, so if you have either, consider removing them until your baby is old enough to understand how they work.

9. Check your home for furniture pieces with hard edges and sharp corners that could injure your baby if she fell

against them. (Coffee tables are a particular hazard.) If possible, move this furniture out of traffic areas, particularly when your baby is learning to walk. You also can buy cushioned corner- and edge-protectors that stick onto the furniture.

10. Test the stability of large pieces of furniture, such as floor lamps, bookshelves, and television stands. Put floor lamps behind other furniture and anchor bookcases and TV stands to the wall. Deaths and injuries can occur when children climb onto, fall against, or pull themselves up on large pieces of furniture.

11. Keep computers out of reach so that your baby cannot pull them over on herself. Cords should be out of sight and reach.

12. Open windows from the top if possible. If you must open them from the bottom, install operable window guards that only an adult or older child can push out from the inside. Never put chairs, sofas, low tables, or anything else a child might climb on in front of a window. Doing so gives him access to the window and creates an opportunity for a serious fall.

13. Never leave plastic bags lying around the house, and don't store children's clothes or toys in them. Dry-cleaning bags are particularly dangerous. Knot them before you throw them away so that it's impossible for your child to crawl into them or pull them over his head.

14. Think about the potential hazard of anything you put into the trash. Any trash container into which dangerous items will go—for example, spoiled food, discarded razor blades, or batteries—should have a child-resistant cover or be kept away and out of the baby's reach.

15. To prevent burns, check your heat sources. Fireplaces, woodstoves, and kerosene heaters should be screened so that your baby can't get near them. Check electric baseboard heaters, radiators, and even vents from hot-air furnaces to see how hot they get when the heat is on. They, too, may need to be screened.

16. A firearm should not be kept in the home or environment of a child. If you must keep a firearm in the house,

keep it unloaded and locked up. Lock ammunition in a separate location. If your baby plays or is cared for in other homes, ask if guns are present there, and if so, how they are stored. (Also see *Where We Stand*, below.)

17. Alcohol can be very toxic to a baby. Keep all alcoholic beverages in a locked cabinet and remember to empty any unfinished drinks immediately.

Baby Equipment

During the past thirty years, the Consumer Product Safety Commission has taken an active role in setting standards to assure the safety of equipment manufactured for children and infants. Because many of these rules went into effect in the early 1970s, you must pay special attention to the safety of furniture made before then. The following guidelines will help you select the safest possible baby equipment, whether used or new, and utilize it properly.

Where We Stand

The most effective way to prevent firearm-related injury to children is to keep guns out of homes and communities. The American Academy of Pediatrics strongly supports gun-control legislation. We believe that handguns, deadly air guns, and assault weapons should be banned.

Until handguns are banned, we recommend that handguns and handgun ammunition be regulated, that restrictions be placed on handgun ownership, and that the number of privately owned handguns be reduced. Firearms should be removed from the environments where children live and play, but if they are not, they *must* be stored locked and unloaded. Loaded firearms and unloaded firearms and ammunition represent a serious danger to children.

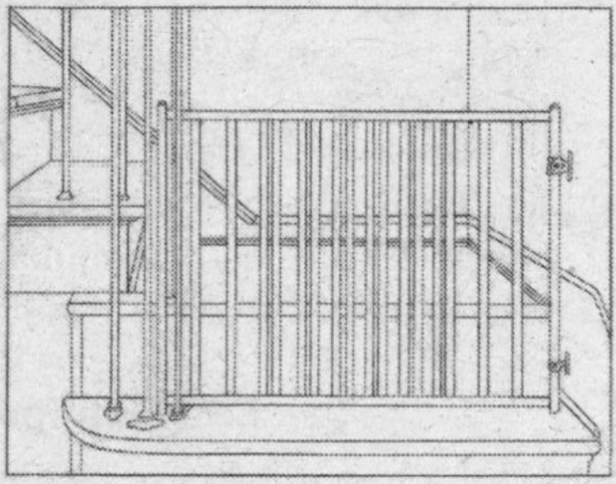

Safe, horizontal-type gate with slats 2⅜ inches (6 cm) apart

High Chairs

Falls are the most serious danger associated with high chairs. To minimize the risk of your baby falling:

1. Select a chair with a wide base, so it can't be tipped over if someone accidentally bumps against it.
2. If the chair folds, be sure the locking device is secure each time you set it up.
3. Strap your baby in with the shoulder, waist, and crotch safety straps whenever he sits in the chair. Never allow him to stand in the high chair.
4. Don't place the high chair near a counter or table or within reach of a hot or dangerous object. Your baby may be able to push hard enough against these surfaces to tip the chair over.
5. Never leave your baby unattended in a high chair, and don't allow older children to climb or play on it, as this could cause it to tip over.
6. A high chair that hooks onto a table is *not* a substitute for a more solid one. But if you plan to use such a model when you eat out or when you travel, look for one that locks onto the table. Be sure the table is heavy enough to support your baby's weight without tipping. Also, check to see whether his feet can touch a table support. If he can push against it, he may be able to dislodge the seat from the table.

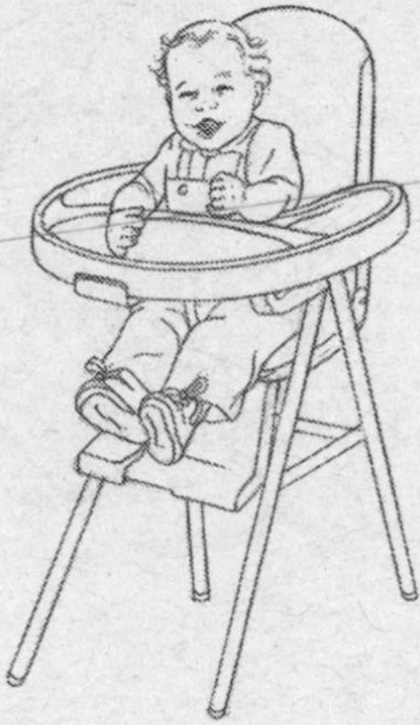

7. Check that all caps or plugs on chair tubing are firmly attached and cannot be pulled off; these could be choking hazards.

Infant Seats

Infant seats are not car safety seats, so not all the same regulations apply. Use care in selecting an infant seat. Check the weight guidelines provided by the manufacturer, and don't use the seat after your baby has outgrown it. Here are some other safety guidelines to follow.

1. Never leave a baby unattended in an infant seat.

2. Never use an infant seat as a substitute for a car safety seat. Infant seats are designed only for propping a baby up, so that she can see or be fed more easily.

3. Always use the safety strap and harness when your baby is in the seat.

4. Choose a seat with an outside frame that allows the infant to sit deeply inside. Be sure the base is wide, so it is difficult to tip over.

5. Look at the bottom of the infant seat to see whether it's covered with a nonskid material. If it isn't, cut thin pieces

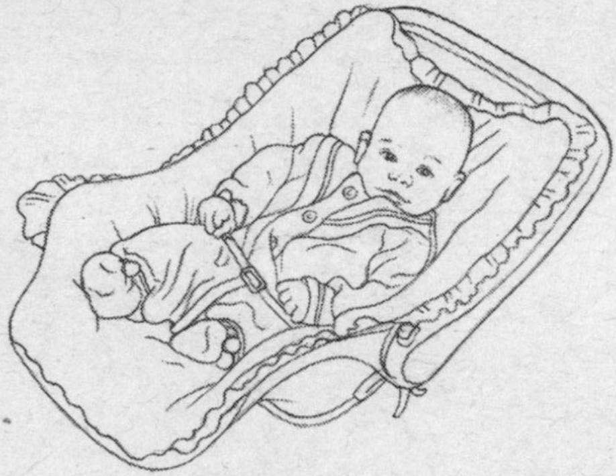

of rubber, and glue them to the base so that the seat is less likely to slip when it's on a smooth surface.

6. Always carry your baby securely strapped into the seat, and use both your arms under the frame to hold it. Although some infant seats have carrying handles, using them alone will allow the seat to tip if the baby's weight is distributed unevenly. Even with the safety strap on, the weight of his head could pull him down and out.
7. The most serious injuries associated with infant seats occur when a baby falls from a high surface. Even small infants can jiggle a seat or carrier off a surface and fall. Therefore, do not put the seat above floor level. To keep an active, squirming baby from tipping the seat over, place it on a carpeted area near you and away from sharp-edged furniture. Infant seats also may tip over when placed on soft surfaces, such as beds or upholstered furniture; these are not safe places for infant seats.
8. Never place a baby in an infant seat or a car safety seat on the roof or back of a car, even for a moment.

Playpens

Most parents depend on playpens (sometimes called play yards) as a safe place to put a baby when Mom or Dad isn't available to watch him every moment. Yet playpens, too, can be dangerous under certain circumstances. To prevent mishaps:

1. Never leave the side of a mesh playpen lowered. An infant who rolls into the pocket created by the slack mesh can become trapped and suffocate.

2. Once your baby is able to sit or get up on all fours or when he reaches five months, whichever comes first, remove any toys that have been tied across the top of the playpen, so he cannot become entangled in them.

3. If your playpen has a raised changing table, always remove the changing table when your infant is in the playpen so he cannot become entrapped in the space between the changing table and the side rail of the playpen.

4. When your baby can pull himself to a standing position, remove all boxes and large toys that he could use to help him climb out.

5. Babies who are teething often bite off chunks of the vinyl or plastic that cover the top rails, so you should check them periodically for tears and holes. If the tears are small, repair them with heavy-duty cloth tape; if they are more extensive, you may need to replace the rails.

6. Be sure that a playpen's mesh is free of tears, holes, or loose threads and that the openings are less than ¼ inch (0.6 cm) across, so that your infant cannot get caught in it. The mesh should be securely attached to the top rail and floor plate. If staples are used, they should not be missing, loose, or exposed. Slats on wooden playpens should be no more than 2⅜ inches (6 cm) apart, so your baby's head cannot become trapped between them.

7. Circular enclosures made from accordion-style fences are extremely dangerous, because babies can get their heads caught in the diamond-shaped openings and the V-shaped border at the top of the gate. Never use such an enclosure, either indoors or out.

Walkers

The American Academy of Pediatrics does not recommend infant walkers. Children can fall down stairs, and head injuries are common. Walkers do not help a baby learn to walk, and they can delay normal motor development. A stationary walker or activity center is a better choice. These do not have wheels, but seats that rotate and bounce. You may also want to consider a sturdy wagon or a "kiddie push car." Be sure the toy has a bar he can push and that it's weighted so it won't tip over when he pulls himself up on it.

Pacifiers

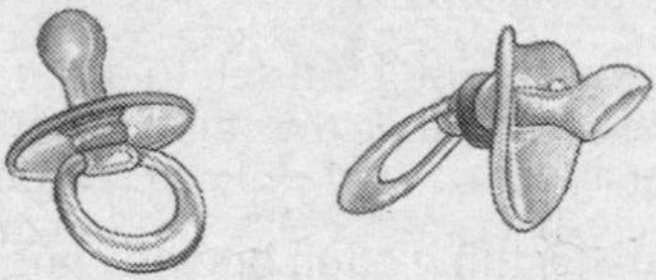

Pacifiers will not harm your baby. In fact, there is some evidence that pacifiers may help reduce the risk of sudden infant death syndrome (SIDS). However, for maximum safety use the following tips when giving your baby a pacifier:

1. Do not use the top and nipple from a baby bottle as a pacifier, even if you tape them together. If the baby sucks hard, the nipple may pop out of the ring and choke her.
2. Purchase pacifiers that cannot possibly come apart. Those molded of one solid piece of plastic are particularly safe. If you are in doubt, ask your pediatrician for a recommendation.
3. The shield between the nipple and the ring should be at least 1½ inches (3.8 cm) across, so the infant cannot take the entire pacifier into her mouth. Also, the shield should be made of firm plastic with ventilation holes.

4. Never tie a pacifier to your child's crib or around your child's neck or hand. This is very dangerous and could cause serious injury or even death.
5. Pacifiers deteriorate over time. Inspect them periodically to see whether the rubber is discolored or torn. If so, replace them. In addition, follow the recommended age range on the pacifier, as older children can sometimes fit an entire newborn pacifier in their mouth and choke.

Toy Boxes and Toy Chests

A toy box can be dangerous for two reasons: A baby could become trapped inside, or a hinged lid could fall on your baby's head or body while he's searching for a toy. If possible, store toys on open shelves so that your baby can get them easily. If you must use a toy box:

1. Look for one with no top, or choose one that has a lightweight removable lid or sliding doors or panels. Little fingers can easily become caught and injured under lids and between sliding doors and panels.
2. If you use a toy box with a hinged lid, be sure it has lid support that holds the lid open at any angle to which the lid is opened. If your toy box didn't come with such a support, install one yourself—or remove the lid.
3. Look for a toy box with rounded or padded edges and corners, or add the padding yourself, so your baby won't be injured if he falls against it.
4. Children occasionally get trapped inside toy boxes, so be sure your box has ventilation holes or a gap between the lid and the box. Don't block the holes by pushing the box tight against a wall. Be sure the lid doesn't latch.

Toys

Most toy manufacturers are conscientious in trying to produce safe toys, but they cannot always anticipate the way a baby might use—or abuse—their products. In 2006, there were an estimated 220,500 toy-related injuries treated in U.S. hospital emergency rooms. Of these, 36 percent (78,400) involved children under the age of five years. If your baby is injured by an unsafe product or if you would like to report a product-related injury, refer to the information in the box on page 405. The Consumer Product Safety Commission keeps a record of complaints and initiates recalls of dangerous toys, so your phone call may protect not only your baby but others.

When selecting or using toys, always observe the following safety guidelines.

1. Match all toys to your baby's age and abilities. Manufacturers' guidelines on packaging may be helpful.
2. Rattles—probably your baby's first toys—should be at least 1⅝ inches (4 cm) across. An infant's mouth and throat are very flexible, so one that's smaller than that could cause choking. Also, rattles should have no detachable parts.
3. All toys should be constructed of sturdy materials that won't break or shatter even when a baby throws or bangs them.
4. Check squeeze toys to be sure the squeaker can't become detached from the toy.
5. Before giving your baby a stuffed animal or a doll, be certain its eyes and nose are firmly attached, and check them periodically. Remove all ribbons. Don't allow your infant to suck on a pacifier or any other accessory that comes packaged with a doll and is small enough to be swallowed.
6. Swallowing and/or inhaling small parts of toys are serious dangers to babies. Inspect toys carefully for small parts that could fit in your infant's mouth and throat. Look for toys labeled for children three and under, because they must meet federal guidelines requiring that they have no small parts likely to be swallowed or inhaled.
7. Toys with small magnets are especially dangerous for babies. If more than one magnet is swallowed, the magnets can attract each other in the infant's body and cause intestinal blockages, perforations, and even death. Keep toys with small magnets away from children under age six.

How to Report Unsafe Products

If you become aware of an unsafe product used by children—or if your own baby suffers an injury related to a particular product—report it to the Consumer Product Safety Commission (CPSC). For more information, go to the CPSC website (www.cpsc.gov), and look for the link for reporting unsafe products. Or call the CPSC's toll-free hotline (1–800–638–2772); when prompted, press ext. 300 to speak with a hotline representative.

8. Toys with small parts that are purchased for older children should be stored out of the reach of babies. Impress on your older child the importance of picking up all the pieces from such toys when she's finished playing with them. You should check that there are no items dangerous for your baby left out.

9. Don't let a baby play with balloons; she may inhale a balloon if she tries to blow it up. If a balloon pops, be sure to pick up and discard all the broken pieces.

10. To prevent both burns and electrical shocks, don't give young children (under age ten) a toy that must be plugged into an electrical outlet. Instead, buy toys that are battery-operated. Be sure that the battery cover is securely fastened, though, to prevent a loose battery from becoming a choking hazard.

11. Carefully inspect toys with mechanical parts for springs, gears, or hinges that could trap a child's fingers, hair, or clothing.

12. To prevent cuts, check toys before you purchase them to be sure they don't have sharp edges or pointed pieces. Avoid toys with parts made of glass or rigid plastic that could shatter.

13. Don't allow your baby to play with very noisy toys, including squeeze toys with unexpectedly loud squeakers.

Noise levels at or about 100 decibels—the sound of the typical cap gun at close range—can damage hearing.

14. Projectile toys are not suitable for babies and older children, because they can so easily cause eye injuries. Never give your child a toy that actually fires anything except water.

SAFETY OUTSIDE THE HOME

Even if you create the perfect environment for your baby inside your home, she'll be spending a lot of time outside, where surroundings are somewhat less controllable. Obviously, your personal supervision will remain the most valuable protection. However, even a well-supervised child will be exposed to many hazards. The information that follows will show you how to eliminate many of these hazards and reduce the risk that your baby will be injured.

Car Safety Seats

Each year, car crashes claim the lives of many babies and older children. Many of these deaths could be prevented if the children were properly restrained. Contrary to what many people believe, a parent's lap is actually the most dangerous place for a baby to ride. In case of a car crash, sudden stop, or swerve, you wouldn't be able to hold on to your baby, and your body would crush hers as you were thrown against the dashboard and windshield. The single most important thing you can do to keep your baby safe in the car is to buy,

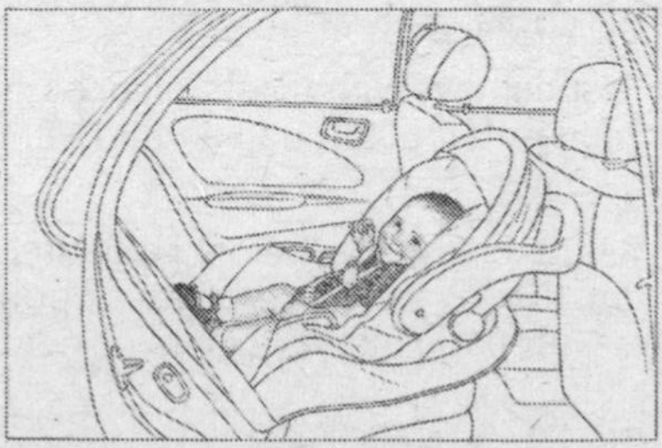

Infant-only car safety seat

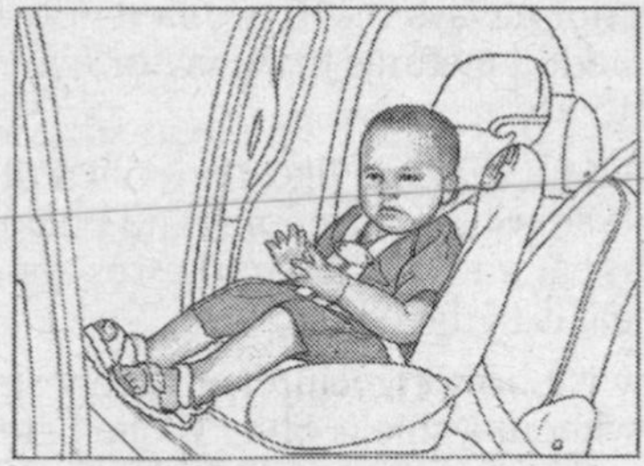

Forward-facing car safety seat

install, and use an approved car safety seat, appropriate for the age and size of your child, every time she rides in the car.

Car safety seats are required by law in all fifty states, the District of Columbia, and U.S. territories. Unfortunately, studies consistently show that many parents do not use them properly. The most common mistakes are placing rear-facing seats in front of an air bag, facing car safety seats in the wrong direction, failing to harness the baby into the seat, and failing to securely fasten the infant's car safety seat to the vehicle seat. Also, some parents don't use the car seat on short trips. They are not aware that most fatal crashes occur within five miles (8 km) of home and at speeds of less than twenty-five miles (40 km) per hour. For all these reasons, babies continue to be at risk. It's not enough to have a car safety seat—you must use it correctly, every time.

Choosing a Car Safety Seat

Here are some guidelines you can use to help you select a car safety seat.

1. The American Academy of Pediatrics annually publishes a list of car safety seats that are available; "Car Safety Seats: A Guide for Families" can be found online at www.aap.org.
2. No one seat is "safest" or "best." The "best" car safety seat is one that fits your baby's size and weight, and can be installed correctly in your car and used correctly on every trip.

3. Price does not always make a difference. Higher prices can mean added features that may or may not make the seat easier to use.

4. When you find a seat you like, try it out. Put your child in the seat and adjust the harnesses and buckles. Make sure it fits in your car and that the harnesses are easy to adjust when the seat is in the car.

5. If your baby is born premature, or is very small, use a car safety seat without a shield. Shields often are too high and too far from the body to fit correctly. A small baby's face could hit a shield in a crash. Before you bring your baby home from the hospital, she should be observed in her car safety seat by hospital staff to make sure the semireclined position does not cause low heart rate, low oxygen, or other breathing problems. If your baby needs to lie flat during travel, use a crash-tested car bed. If possible, an adult should ride in the backseat next to your baby to watch her closely.

6. Babies with special health problems may need other restraint systems. Discuss this with your pediatrician. More information about safe transportation of children with special health needs is available from the Automotive Safety for Children Program at 1–317–274–2977.

7. Do not use a car safety seat that is more than ten years old. Look on the label for the date it was made. Many manufacturers recommend that seats be used for only six years. Check with the manufacturer to find out when the company recommends getting a new seat.

8. If a car safety seat was in a moderate or severe crash, it may have been weakened and should not be used, even if it looks fine. Seats that were in a minor crash may still be safe to use. A crash is considered minor if the vehicle can be driven away from the crash, the door closest to the car safety seat was not damaged, no one in the vehicle was injured, the airbags did not go off, and you can't see any damage to the car safety seat. Do not use a seat if you do not know its full history. Call the car safety seat manufacturer if you have questions about the safety of your seat.

9. Do not use a car safety seat that does not have a label with the date of manufacture and seat name or model number. Without these, you cannot check on recalls.

10. Do not use a car safety seat if it does not come with instructions. You need them to know how to use the car safety seat. Do not rely on the former owner's directions. Get a copy of the instruction manual from the manufacturer before you use the seat.

11. Do not use a car safety seat that has any cracks in the frame of the seat or is missing parts.

12. You can find out if your car safety seat has been recalled by calling the manufacturer or the Auto Safety Hot Line at 1–888–DASH–2–DOT (1–888–327–4236), from 8 a.m. to 10 p.m. ET, Monday through Friday. This information is also available on the National Highway Traffic Safety Administration website: www.nhtsa.gov. If the seat has been recalled, be sure to follow instructions to fix it or get the necessary parts. You also may get a registration card for future recall notices from the hotline.

Types of Car Safety Seats

Infant-Only Seats

- Can be used only rear-facing.
- Are used for babies from birth or 4–5 pounds (1.8–2.25 kg), and who weigh up to 22–32 pounds (10–15 kg), depending on the model.
- Are small and portable.
- Come with a five-point or three-point harness.

Infant-Only Seat Features

Detachable base
Most infant-only seat models come with detachable bases. The base attaches to the car, and the car safety seat easily snaps into the base. This way you can carry your baby in and out of the car without needing to reinstall the seat. After buckling your baby into the seat, you simply lock the seat into the installed base. Some bases are adjustable to make it easier to recline newborns correctly. You can buy additional bases for other cars; however, this feature is helpful only if

the base fits tightly into your car. These seats also can be installed in the vehicle without the base, and in some cases, the seat may fit better without the base.

Higher weight and height limits

Several infant-only seats are available for use up to 22 pounds (10 kg), and a few up to 30–32 pounds (10–15 kg). Most convertible seats also now have higher weight and height limits, 30–35 pounds (14–16 kg) in the rear-facing position for heavier or taller babies. Keep in mind that some babies may reach the top height limits of the seat before they reach the top weight limits. If your infant's weight or height exceeds the limits of the seat before a year, use an infant-only seat or a rear-facing convertible seat that has a higher rear-facing limit.

Harness slots

Infant-only seats that come with more than one harness slot provide more room for growing babies. In the rear-facing position, the harness slots usually should be at or below your baby's shoulders. Check the car safety seat manufacturer's instructions to be sure.

Handles

Carrying handles on car safety seats vary greatly in style and ease of use. Check the instructions for how to adjust the handle during travel.

Other features

Angle indicators, built-in angle adjusters, harness adjusters, and head-support systems are other features that may make correct installation and use easier to achieve.

Convertible Seats

- Are bigger and heavier than infant-only seats, but can be used longer and for larger children.
- May not fit newborns as well as some infant-only seats fit. Make sure that your baby can recline comfortably in the

seat. Check the car safety seat manufacturer's instructions to be sure that harnesses can be adjusted properly.

- Can be used rear-facing up to 30–35 pounds, as long as the top of the head is below the top of the seat back. At a minimum they should be used rear-facing to 12 months *and* 20 pounds.
- Have the following two types of harnesses:
  1. Five-point harness—five straps: two at the shoulders, two at the hips, one at the crotch
  2. Overhead shield—a padded, traylike shield that swings down around the child

Note: If you are using a convertible seat for a small infant, the best choice for a more secure fit is the five-point harness. A small baby's face can hit a shield in a crash.

Convertible Seat Features

Adjustable buckles and shields

Many convertible seats have two or more buckle positions to give you extra room for a growing child or bulky clothing. Many overhead shields can be adjusted, as well.

Higher weight limits

Several convertible seats are available with higher rear-facing weight limits for bigger babies. For larger babies, look for a seat that can be used rear-facing up to 30 to 35 pounds (14 kg to 16 kg).

Installing a Car Safety Seat

1. Read your vehicle owner's manual for important information on how to install the car safety seat correctly in your vehicle.
2. The safest place for all children to ride is in the backseat.
3. Never place a baby in a rear-facing car safety seat in the front seat of a vehicle that has a passenger air bag. Most new cars have air bags. When used with seat belts, air bags work very well to protect older children and adults. How-

ever, air bags are very dangerous when used with rear-facing car safety seats. If your car has a passenger air bag, infants in rear-facing seats *must* ride in the backseat. Even in a low-speed crash, the air bag can inflate, strike the car safety seat, and cause serious brain injury and death. Toddlers who ride in forward-facing car safety seats also are at risk from air bag injuries. Remember, *all* babies and older children, even through school age, are safest in the backseat. If you must put an older child in the front seat because all backseat positions are occupied, slide the vehicle seat back as far as it will go. Make sure your child is buckled and stays in the proper position at all times. Doing so will help prevent the air bag from striking your child. For most families, air bag on/off switches are not necessary. Air bags that are turned off cannot protect other passengers riding in the front seat. Air bag on/off switches should be used only if *all* of the following are true:

- Your baby has special healthcare needs.
- Your pediatrician recommends constant supervision of your infant during travel.
- No other adult is available to ride in the backseat with your baby.

On/off switches also must be used if you have a vehicle with no backseat or a backseat that is not made for passengers.

4. Place the seat facing the correct direction for the size and age of your baby. Route the seat belt through the correct path on the car safety seat (check your instructions to make sure), and pull it tight. Before each trip, check to make sure the car safety seat is installed tightly enough by pulling on the car safety seat where the seat belt passes through. It should not move easily side to side or toward the front of the car.

5. If your infant's head flops forward, the seat may not be reclined enough. Tilt the seat back until it is reclined as close as possible to a 45-degree angle (according to manufacturer's instructions). Your seat may have a built-in recline adjuster for this purpose. If not, you may wedge firm padding, such as a rolled towel, under the front base of the seat.

6. Check the seat belt buckle. Make sure it does not lie just at the point where the belt bends around the car safety seat. If it does, you will not be able to make the belt tight enough. If you cannot get the belt tight, look for another set of belts in the car that can be tightened properly.

7. Many lap/shoulder belts allow passengers to move freely even when they are buckled. Read your car owner's manual to see if your seat belts can be locked into position or if you will need to use a locking clip. Locking clips come with all new car safety seats. (Some have them built in.) Read your instructions for information on how to use the locking clip, if needed.

8. Some lap belts need a special, heavy-duty locking clip, available from the vehicle manufacturer. Check your car owner's manual for more information.

9. A car safety seat attachment system has been developed to make car safety seats easier to use and safer. The system is called LATCH, which stands for *L*ower *A*nchors and *T*ethers for *Ch*ildren. This anchor system is intended to make correct installation much easier because you no longer need to use seat belts to secure the car safety seat. Starting in model year 2002, most new vehicles and new safety seats have been equipped with these lower anchors and attachments. However, unless both the vehicle and the car safety seat have this new anchor system, you still will need to use seat belts to secure the car safety seat. Check the car safety seat and vehicle instructions for information on using LATCH, including the weight limits for the lower anchors and attachments and which seating positions can be used for LATCH installation.

10. New car safety seats that can be used facing forward come with top tethers, straps that hook the top of the car safety seat to a special permanent anchor in the vehicle. Most anchors are located on the rear window ledge, the back of the vehicle seat, or the floor or ceiling of the vehicle. Tethers give extra protection by keeping the car safety seat from being thrown forward in a crash. Tether retrofit kits are available for most older car safety seats. Check with the car safety seat manufacturer to find out

how to get a top tether for your seat if it doesn't have one. Be sure to install it according to instructions. The tether strap may help make some seats that are difficult to install fit more tightly. Since September 2000, all new cars, minivans, and light trucks have been required to have upper tether anchors for securing the tops of car safety seats.

11. For specific information about installing your car safety seat, consult a certified Child Passenger Safety (CPS) Technician. A list of certified CPS Technicians is available by state or ZIP code at www.seatcheck.org. A list of inspection stations staffed by certified CPS Technicians is also available on the Internet at www.nhtsa.dot.gov/people/injury/childps/CPSFitting/Index.cfm. The information also can be accessed by telephone on the NHTSA Auto Safety Hot Line at 1–888–DASH–2–DOT (1–888–327–4236), from 8 a.m. to 10 p.m. ET, Monday through Friday.

12. Lap belts work fine with infant-only, convertible, and forward-facing seats. They cannot be used with belt-positioning boosters (which are safest for children who have outgrown forward-facing seats and who are not big enough to fit in adult seat belts). If your car has lap belts only, use a forward-facing seat with a harness approved for use to higher weights or check with your dealer or the car manufacturer to see if shoulder harnesses can be installed. Or consider buying another car with lap/shoulder belts in the backseat.

13. Avoid driving more children than can be buckled safely in the backseat. However, if a child must ride in front in an emergency, place the child most likely to sit in the proper forward-facing position in the front seat, with the vehicle seat moved as far back as possible. A child in a forward-facing car safety seat may be the best choice to ride in the front seat, because a child who is in a booster seat or using a regular seat belt can move out of position more easily and be at greater risk for injuries from the air bag.

Using the Car Safety Seat

1. A car safety seat can protect your baby only if she is buckled securely in it *every* time she rides in the car—no exceptions, beginning with your baby's first ride home from the hospital. Help your baby form a lifelong habit of buckling up by *always* using your own seat belt. If you have two cars, buy two seats or transfer the seat to the car in which your infant will be traveling. Remember to never place a rear-facing car safety seat in the front seat if there is an air bag. The safest place for all children to ride is in the back.

2. Read and follow the car safety seat manufacturer's instructions, and always keep them with the car safety seat. If you lose the instructions, call or write the manufacturer and ask for a new set. In many cases, you can download the instructions from the manufacturer's website.

3. Most babies go through a stage when they protest whenever you put them in the car safety seat. Explain firmly that you cannot drive until everyone is buckled up. Then back up your words with action.

4. Be sure to use the correct harness slots for the baby.

5. Be sure the harness straps are snug against your infant's body. Dress your baby in clothes that allow the straps to go between her legs. Keep the straps snug by adjusting them to allow for the thickness of your baby's clothes, making sure that the harness still holds her securely. Be certain the straps lie flat and are not twisted.

6. To keep your newborn from slouching, pad the sides of the seat and behind the crotch strap with rolled-up diapers or receiving blankets, if needed. Do not use add-on products that go behind the baby or between the baby and the harness straps; these can cause the straps not to restrain the baby properly in a crash. Never use any add-on products unless they came with your car safety seat or are specifically allowed by the manufacturer's instructions.

7. In cold weather, dress your baby in thinner layers rather than thickly padded clothes, and tuck blankets around your baby *after* adjusting the harness straps snugly.

8. In hot weather, drape a towel over the seat when you leave the car in the sun. Before putting your baby in the seat, touch the vinyl and the metal buckle with your hand to be sure they aren't hot.

9. No matter how short your errand is, *never* leave an infant or child alone in a car. She can get overheated or too cold very quickly, even if the temperature outside seems mild, or she may become frightened and panicky when she realizes she's alone. Children who have been left alone in a car in hot weather have died from hyperthermia (overheating). Any child alone in a car is a target for abduction.

Air Bag Safety

An air bag can save your life. However, air bags and babies do not mix. The following information will help keep you and your baby safe. (You've already read some of this information, but it's worth repeating.)

- The safest place for all infants to ride is in the backseat.
- Never put a rear-facing car safety seat in the front seat of a car with an air bag.
- Infants always must ride in rear-facing car safety seats in the backseat until they are at least one year of age *and* weigh at least 20 pounds (9 kg). It is safest to ride rear-facing to the highest weight or height allowed by the manufacturer.
- All babies should be properly secured in car safety seats correct for their age and size.
- When purchasing a car, look for one with an air bag on the front passenger side for your family's safety. Keep in mind, however, that infants—as well as children of any age—should ride in the backseat. Even if your baby's safety seat is rear-facing, he can suffer a serious injury from the impact of the air bag against the back of the safety seat. Although the backseat is the safest place for children of any age to ride, all passengers in the front seat should be positioned as far back as possible from the front air bag on the passenger side.

Keeping Your Baby Happy and Safe on the Road

As hard as you may try to enforce car safety seat and seat belt use, your baby may resist these constraints as he gets older. Here are some tips to keep him occupied and content—and also safe—while the car is in motion.

Birth to Nine Months

- Ensure your newborn's comfort by padding the sides of his car safety seat with receiving blankets to prevent slouching.
- If needed, place a small rolled-up cloth diaper or receiving blanket between the crotch strap and your baby to prevent his lower body from sliding too far forward.
- If your infant's head flops forward, double-check to see if the seat has been reclined enough. Tilt the seat backward until it is reclined as close as possible to a 45-degree angle, following the manufacturer's instructions. Your seat may have a built-in recline adjuster for this purpose. If not, you may wedge firm padding, such as a rolled towel, under the front of the base of the seat.

Nine Months to Twelve Months

- Babies this age may want desperately to get out of the car safety seat. If this describes your infant, remind yourself that this is only a phase. As mentioned earlier, in a calm but stern voice, insist that he stay in his seat whenever the car is on the road. Let him know that the car cannot move unless everyone is buckled up, and then follow through if he tries to escape his seat.

- Entertain your baby by talking or singing with him as you drive. However, never do this to the point that it distracts you from paying attention to your driving.

- Side air bags improve safety for adults in side impact crashes. When children ride next to side air bags, it is essential that they be restrained in the proper position. Read your car safety seat manual for guidance on placing the seat next to a side air bag, and refer to your vehicle owner's manual for recommendations that apply to your vehicle.

Kids Around Cars

Babies and other young children are not safe around streets and should not be playing near them. While they may have the skills to get to roads and streets, they do not have the

Where We Stand

All fifty states require that children ride in car safety seats. The American Academy of Pediatrics urges that all newborns discharged from hospitals be brought home in infant car safety seats. The AAP has established car safety seat guidelines for low–birth-weight infants, which include riding in a rear-facing seat and supporting the infant with ample padding around the sides, outside the harness system. A convertible car safety seat is recommended as a child gets older.

Infants and young children always should ride in car safety seats—preferably in the backseat—because it is safest. Never use a rear-facing car safety seat in the front seat of a vehicle equipped with a passenger-side air bag. An infant or child should never ride in an adult's arms.

ability to recognize that streets and cars are dangerous. Children move quickly and impulsively. They are curious. Yet they have difficulty seeing cars in their peripheral vision, localizing sounds, and understanding traffic and the meaning of signs and signals. They cannot judge speed and vehicle distance. Couple this with drivers who may be multitasking and not looking out for young children who may run into the street, and a disaster could be in the making.

If young children are near streets, "hands-on" supervision is necessary so you can quickly intervene if they dart into the street to get a ball or run after an older child or adult.

To avoid injuries from vehicle backovers, driveways, alleyways, and any adjacent unfenced front yards should not be used as play areas. Parents should be reminded of the large blind spot behind the car (especially in bigger, elevated vehicles) and the need to walk completely around the car before getting in and starting the engine.

Baby Carriers—Backpacks and Front Packs

Back and front carriers for infants are very popular, although most babies outgrow front carriers by the age of three months. For your baby's—and your own—comfort and safety, follow these guidelines when purchasing and using baby carriers.

1. Infants born prematurely or with respiratory problems should not be placed in backpacks or other upright positioning devices as it may make it harder for them to breathe.

2. Take your baby with you when you shop for the carrier so that you can match it to his size. Make sure the carrier supports his back and that the leg holes are small enough so he can't possibly slip through. Look for sturdy material.

3. If you buy a backpack, be sure the aluminum frame is padded, so that your baby won't be hurt if he bumps against it.

4. Check the pack periodically for rips and tears in the seams and fasteners.

5. When using a baby carrier, be sure to bend at the knees, not the waist, if you need to pick something up. Otherwise, the baby may tip out of the carrier and you may hurt your back.

6. Babies over five months old may become restless in the back carrier, so continue to use the restraining straps. Some babies will brace their feet against the frame, changing their weight distribution. You should be certain that your infant is seated properly before you walk.

Strollers

Look for safety features and take the following precautions.

1. If you use bumpers in your stroller, or if you string toys across it, fasten them securely so they can't fall on top of the baby. Remove such toys as soon as the baby can sit or get on all fours.

2. Strollers should have brakes that are easy to operate. Use the brake whenever you are stopped, and be sure your

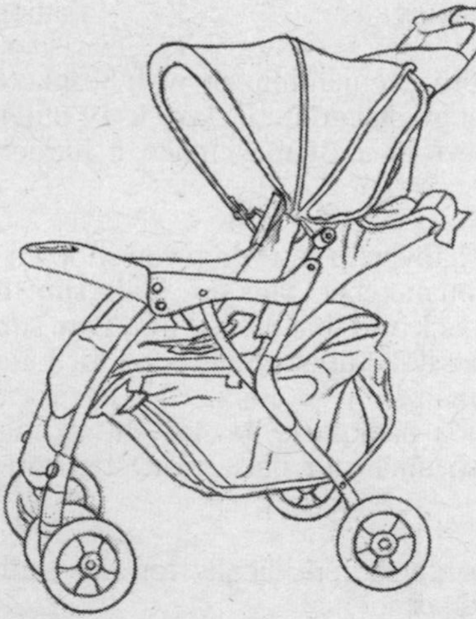

baby can't reach the release lever. A brake that locks two wheels provides an extra measure of safety.

3. Select a stroller with a wide base, so it won't tip over.

4. Babies' fingers can become caught in the hinges that fold the stroller, so keep your baby at a safe distance when you open and close it. Make sure the stroller is securely locked open before putting your infant in it. Check that your baby's fingers cannot reach the stroller wheels.

5. Don't hang bags or other items from the handles of your stroller—they can make it tip backward. If the stroller has a basket for carrying things, be sure it is placed low and near the rear wheels.

6. The stroller should have a seat belt and harness, and it should be used whenever your infant goes for a ride. Use rolled-up baby blankets as bumpers on either side of the seat.

7. Never leave your baby unattended.

8. If you purchase a side-by-side twin stroller, be sure the footrest extends all the way across both sitting areas. An infant's foot can become trapped between separate footrests.

9. There are also strollers that allow an older child to sit or stand in the rear. Be mindful of weight guidelines and especially careful that the child in the back doesn't become overly active and tip the stroller.

Shopping Cart Safety

An estimated 20,700 children under five years old were treated in emergency rooms for shopping cart–related injuries in 2005. The most frequent kinds of injuries were contusions, abrasions, and lacerations, and most injuries are to the head or neck. Shopping cart–related injuries can be serious enough to require hospitalization, often because of head injuries and serious fractures. Some deaths have even occurred.

The design of shopping carts makes it easier for them to tip over when a baby is in the cart or in the seat designed to fit on the cart. Until shopping carts are redesigned to be more stable, you need to know that seats attached to the top of shopping carts or built into them won't prevent a baby from falling out if she isn't properly restrained; these seats also won't prevent the cart from tipping over even if the infant is restrained.

If possible, you should seek an alternative to placing your baby in a shopping cart. If you must do so, make sure she is restrained at all times. Never allow her to stand up in the cart or be transported in the basket. Do not snap an infant car safety seat onto the built-in cart seat, as this can make the cart even more unstable. If one is available, use a shopping cart designed to carry infants in a seat that is lower to the ground. Never leave a baby alone in a shopping cart, even for a moment.

Your Backyard

Your backyard can be a safe play area for your baby if you eliminate potential hazards. Here are some suggestions for keeping your yard safe.

1. If you don't have a fenced yard, teach your child the boundaries within which she should play. Always have a responsible person supervise outdoor play.
2. Check your yard for dangerous plants. Plants are a leading cause of poisoning. If you are unsure about any of the plants in your yard, call your local Poison Help Line (1–800–222–1222) and request a list of poisonous plants common to your area. If you have any poisonous plants, either replace them or securely fence and lock that area of the yard away from your child.
3. Teach your baby never to pick and eat anything from a plant, no matter how good it looks, without your permission. This is particularly important if you let her help out in a vegetable garden where there's produce that could be eaten.
4. If you use pesticides or herbicides on your lawn or gar-

den, read the instructions carefully. Don't allow infants to play on a treated lawn for at least forty-eight hours.

5. Don't use a power mower to cut the lawn when babies are around. The mower may throw sticks or stones with enough force to injure them. Never have your baby on a riding mower even when you are driving. It is safest to keep infants indoors while the lawn is being mowed.
6. When you cook food outdoors, screen the grill so that your baby cannot touch it, and explain that it is hot like the stove in the kitchen. Store propane grills so your infant cannot reach the knobs. Be sure charcoal is cold before you dump it.

Water Safety

Water is one of the most ominous hazards your infant will encounter. Babies can drown in only a few inches of water. Swimming lessons are not a way to prevent drowning in young children. Although swimming classes for young children are widely available, the American Academy of Pediatrics does not recommend them for babies and young children until after their fourth birthday for several reasons:

1. You may be lulled into being less cautious because you think your child can swim, and children themselves may unwittingly be encouraged to enter the water without supervision.
2. Babies and young children who are repeatedly immersed in water may swallow so much of it that they develop water intoxication. This can result in convulsions, shock, and even death.
3. Children are generally not developmentally ready for formal swimming lessons until after their fourth birthday. Children can learn swimming skills more quickly once their motor development has reached the five-year-old level.
4. Safety training does not result in a significant increase in poolside safety skills of babies and young children.

If you do enroll a baby or child under four years old in a swimming program, particularly a Daddy- or Mommy-and-me class, think of it primarily as an opportunity to enjoy playing in the water together. Be sure the class you choose adheres to guidelines established by the national YMCA. Among other things, these guidelines forbid submersion of young children and encourage parents to participate in all activities. Remember that even a child who knows how to swim needs to be watched constantly. Whenever your baby is near water, follow these safety rules.

1. Be aware of small bodies of water your infant might encounter, such as fishponds, ditches, fountains, rain barrels, watering cans—even the bucket you use when you wash the car. Empty containers of water when you're done using them. Babies are drawn to places and things like these and need constant supervision to be sure they don't fall in.
2. Children who are swimming—even in a shallow toddler's pool—always should be watched by an adult, preferably one who knows CPR. (See *Cardiopulmonary Resuscitation and Mouth-to-Mouth Resuscitation,* page 575.) The adult should be within arm's length, providing "touch supervision" whenever infants are in or around water. Empty and put away inflatable pools after each play session.
3. Enforce safety rules: Children should never run near the pool or push others underwater.
4. Don't use inflatable toys or mattresses to keep your baby afloat. These toys may deflate suddenly, or your infant may slip off them into water that is too deep for him.
5. Be sure the deep and shallow ends of any pool your child uses are clearly marked. Never allow her to dive into the shallow end.
6. If you have a swimming pool at home, it should be completely surrounded with at least a four-foot (1.2 meters)-high fence that has a self-latching and self-locking gate that opens away from the pool. Check the gate frequently to be sure it is in good working order. Keep the gate closed and locked at all times. Be sure your children

cannot manipulate the lock or climb the fence. No opening under the fence or between uprights should be more than four inches (10 cm) wide. Keep toys out of the pool area when not in use so that children are not tempted to try to get through the fence.

7. If your pool has a cover, remove it completely before swimming. Also, never allow your baby to crawl or walk on the pool cover; water may have accumulated on it, making it as dangerous as the pool itself. Your infant also could fall through and become trapped underneath. Do not use a pool cover in place of a four-sided fence because it is not likely to be used appropriately and consistently.
8. Keep a safety ring with a rope beside the pool at all times. If possible, have a phone in the pool area with emergency numbers clearly marked.
9. Spas and hot tubs are dangerous for babies, who can easily drown or become overheated in them. Don't allow babies to use these facilities.
10. Your baby should always wear a life preserver when he swims or rides in a boat. A life preserver fits properly if you can't lift it off over your baby's head after he's been fastened into it. It also should have a flotation collar to keep the head upright and the face out of the water.

Where We Stand

The American Academy of Pediatrics feels strongly that parents should never—even for a moment—leave children alone near open bodies of water, such as lakes or swimming pools, nor near water in homes (bathtubs, spas). For backyard pools, rigid, motorized pool covers are not a substitute for four-sided fencing, since pool covers are not likely to be used appropriately and consistently. Parents should learn CPR and keep a telephone and emergency equipment (i.e., life preservers) at poolside.

11. Adults should not drink alcohol when they are swimming. It presents a danger for them as well as for any children they might be supervising.

12. Be sure to eliminate distractions while children are in the water. Talking on the phone, working on the computer, and other tasks need to wait until children of any age are out of the water.

Safety Around Animals

Babies and other children are more likely than adults to be bitten by domesticated animals, including your own family pet. This is particularly true when a new baby is brought into the home. At such times, the pet's response should be observed carefully, and it should not be left alone with the infant. After a two- or three-week get-acquainted period, the animal usually ignores or actually enjoys the baby. However, it is always wise to be cautious when the animal is around, regardless of how much your pet seems to enjoy the relationship.

If you are getting a pet as a companion for your baby, wait until she is mature enough to handle and care for the animal—usually around age five or six. Babies and young children have difficulty distinguishing an animal from a toy, so they may inadvertently provoke a bite through teasing or mistreatment. Remember that you have ultimate responsibility for your baby's safety around any animal, so take the following precautions.

1. Look for a pet with a gentle disposition. An older animal is often a good choice for a child, because a puppy or kitten may bite out of sheer friskiness. Avoid older pets raised in a home without children, however.

2. Treat your pet humanely so it will enjoy human company. Don't, for example, tie a dog on a short rope or chain, since extreme confinement may make it anxious and aggressive.

3. Never leave a baby alone with an animal. Many bites occur during periods of playful roughhousing, because the child doesn't realize when the animal gets overexcited.

4. Teach your baby not to put her face close to an animal.
5. Don't allow your baby to tease your pet by pulling its tail or taking away a toy or a bone. Make sure she doesn't disturb the animal when it's sleeping or eating.
6. Have all pets—both dogs and cats—immunized against rabies.
7. Obey local ordinances about licensing and leashing your pet. Be sure your pet is under your control at all times.
8. Find out which neighbors have dogs, so your baby can meet the pets with which she's likely to have contact. Teach your child how to greet a dog: The child should stand still while the dog sniffs her; then she can slowly extend her hand to pet the animal.
9. Warn your baby to stay away from yards in which dogs seem high-strung or unfriendly.
10. Wild animals can carry very serious diseases that may be transmitted to humans. You (and your family pets) need to avoid contact with rodents and other wild animals (raccoons, skunks, foxes) that can carry diseases ranging from hantavirus to plague, from toxoplasmosis to rabies. To avoid bites by wild creatures, notify the health department or Animal Control whenever you see an animal that seems sick or injured, or one that is acting strangely. Don't try to catch the animal or pick it up. Teach your baby to avoid all undomesticated animals. Fortunately, most wild animals come out only at night and tend to shy away from humans. A wild animal that is found in your yard or neighborhood during the daylight hours might have an infectious disease like rabies, and you should contact the local authorities.

In the Community and Neighborhood

Many parents worry about keeping their baby safe in and around the neighborhood. Fortunately, child abductions are rare, although they understandably get plenty of media attention when they occur. Most abductions occur when children are taken by noncustodial parents, although a smaller number of stranger abductions do take place each year.

Here are some suggestions to help keep your baby safe.

- When you're shopping with your child, keep an eye on him at all times, as he can move quickly and out of your line of vision in an instant.
- When choosing a day care center, ask about safety issues. Make sure a policy is in place where your baby can be picked up only by his parent or someone else you designate.
- Although your child should be supervised by a trusted adult at all times, it is still important to teach him (when he's able to understand) to never get into a car or go along with someone unfamiliar to him.
- When hiring babysitters, always check references and/or ask for recommendations from friends and family members.
- For more information, contact the National Center for Missing & Exploited Children (1–800–843–5678; www.missingkids.com).

When planning ways to keep your baby safe, remember that she is constantly changing. Strategies that protect her from danger when she's one year old may no longer be adequate as she becomes stronger, more curious, and more confident in later months and years. Review your family's home and habits often to make sure your safeguards remain appropriate for your infant's age.

A Message for Grandparents

As a grandparent, your grandchild's well-being and safety are extremely important to you. Particularly when she is under your care—at your home, in her own home, in the car, or elsewhere—make sure that you've taken every step possible to ensure that she's safe and secure.

Take the time to read this chapter from beginning to end. It will provide you with guidelines to protect your grandchild in the situations that she's most likely to encounter. Before you have your grandchild visit or stay at your home, make certain that you've reviewed and adopted the recommendations you'll find here.

In this special section, you'll find the most important safety points for grandparents to keep in mind.

Safety Inside the Home

There are plenty of safety measures you should implement in your home to protect your grandchild. To keep some of these guidelines in the forefront of your mind, use the acronym SPEGOS to help remind you of the following:

Smoke detectors should be placed in the proper locations throughout the house.

Pets and pet food should be stored out of a baby's reach.

Escape plans should be thought about in advance, and fire extinguishers should be readily available.

Gates should be positioned at the top and bottom of stairs.

Outlet covers that are not a choking hazard should be placed over sockets to prevent your grandchild from putting herself at risk of an electrical shock. Use furniture or other objects to block access to electrical outlets, wherever possible.

Soft covers or bumpers should be positioned around sharp or solid furniture.

In addition to these general rules, be sure to keep important phone numbers by the telephone. In an emergency, you'll not only want to call 911 when appropriate, but certain specific family members. Another safety consideration: Your special chairs or walking aids could be unstable and present a risk; if possible, move them into the closet or a room that your grandchild won't be able to enter when he visits.

Read on to review safety measures for specific areas of your home.

Nursery/Sleeping Area

- If you saved your own child's crib, stored in your attic or garage, perhaps awaiting the arrival of a grandchild someday, review the crib guidelines in this chapter (see pages 388–391). Guidelines for baby's furniture and equipment have changed dramatically. There is a good chance the old crib no longer meets today's safety standards and you will need to invest in a new one. (Use the same approach for other saved and aging furniture that could pose risks to infants, such as an old playpen.)
- Buy a changing table (see page 391), use your own bed, or even a towel on the floor to change the baby's diapers. As she gets a little older, and she becomes more likely to squirm, you may need a second person to help in changing her diaper.
- Don't allow your grandchild to sleep in your bed.
- Keep the diaper pail emptied.

Kitchen

- Put "kiddy locks" on the cabinets; to be extra safe, move unsafe cleansers and chemicals so they're completely out of reach.
- Remove any dangling cords, such as those from the coffeepot or toaster.

- Take extra precautions before giving your grandchild food prepared in microwave ovens. Microwaves can heat liquids and solids unevenly, and they may be mildly warm on the outside but *very hot* on the inside.

Bathrooms

- Store pills, inhalers, and other prescription or nonprescription medications, as well as medical equipment, locked and out of the reach of your grandchild.
- Put nonslip material in the bathtub to avoid dangerous falls.
- If there are handles and bars in the bathtub for your own use, cover them with soft material if you're going to be bathing the baby there.
- Never leave a baby unattended in a tub or sink filled with water.

Baby Equipment

- Never leave your grandchild alone in a high chair or in an infant seat located in high places, such as a table or countertop.
- Do not use baby walkers.

Toys

- Buy new toys for your grandchild that have a variety of sounds, sights, and colors. Simple toys can be just as good as more complex ones. Remember, no matter how fancy the toys may be, your own interaction and play with your grandchild are much more important.
- Toys, CDs, and books should be age-appropriate and challenge children at their own developmental level.

- Avoid toys with small parts that the baby could put into her mouth and swallow.
- Because toy boxes can be dangerous, keep them out of your home, or look for one without a top or lid.

Garage/Basement

- Make sure that the automatic reversing mechanism on the garage door is operating.
- Keep all garden chemicals and pesticides as well as tools in a locked cabinet and out of reach.

Safety Outside the Home

Buy a car safety seat that you can keep inside your own car. Make sure you install it properly (or have a trained professional install it for you) and that you can strap your grandchild into it easily. Experiment with the buckles and clasps before you buy the car seat since their ease of use varies. Make sure you know that your grandchild is out of harm's way before backing your car out of the garage or down the driveway.

- Purchase a stroller to use when taking the baby for a walk in your neighborhood.
- On shopping trips, whenever possible choose stores that offer child-friendly shopping carts with seats that are low to the ground. Don't place your own car seat into a shopping cart.
- If you have a tricycle or bicycle at your home for your grandchild, make sure you also have a helmet for her. Let her choose a helmet in a special design or color.
- Although playgrounds can be fun, they also can be dangerous. Select one that has been designed to keep children as safe as possible; those at schools

or at community-sponsored parks are often good choices.

- Inspect your own backyard for anything hazardous or poisonous.
- If you have a backyard swimming pool, or if you take your grandchild to another home or a park where there is a pool, *carefully read the water safety guidelines in this chapter (see pages 423–426). There should be a four-foot-high fence with a locking gate surrounding the pool.* Make sure that neighbors' pools are enclosed by fences, as well.

PART II

The information and policies in this part are constantly changing. Ask your pediatrician or other qualified health professional for the latest information on these procedures.

It is rare for children to become seriously ill with no warning. Based on your child's symptoms, you should usually contact your child's pediatrician for advice. Timely treatment of symptoms can prevent an illness from getting worse or turning into an emergency.

12

Abdominal/ Gastrointestinal Tract

Abdominal Pain

Children of all ages experience abdominal pain occasionally, but the causes of such pain in infants tend to be quite different from what they are in older children. So, too, is the way babies react to the pain. An older child may rub her abdomen and tell you she's having a "bellyache" or "tummyache," while a very young infant will show her distress by crying and pulling up her legs or by passing gas (which is usually swallowed air). Vomiting or excessive burping also may accompany crying in babies.

Fortunately, most stomachaches disappear on their own, and are not serious. However, if your baby's complaints continue or worsen over a period of three to five hours, or if she has a fever, severe sore throat, or extreme change in appetite or energy level, you should notify your pediatrician immediately. These symptoms may indicate a more serious disorder.

In this section, you'll find descriptions of problems that lead to abdominal pain in children, from colic to intestinal infections. You'll be referred to other sections of this and other chapters in the book, as well, for more detailed descriptions of some of these disorders.

Abdominal Pain in Infants

Colic usually occurs in infants between the ages of ten days and three months of age. While no one knows exactly what causes it, colic seems to produce rapid and severe contractions of the intestine that probably are responsible for the baby's pain. The discomfort often is more severe in the late afternoon and early

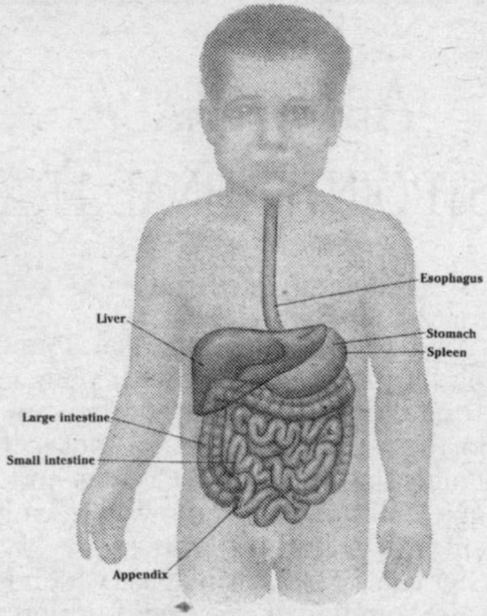

Abdomen/Gastrointestinal Tract

evening, and may be accompanied by inconsolable crying, pulling up of the legs, frequent passage of gas, and general irritability. You can try a variety of approaches to colic, which might include rocking your baby, walking with her in a baby carrier, swaddling her in a blanket, or giving her a pacifier. (For more information about colic, see page 190 in Chapter 6, *The First Month*).

Intussusception is a rare condition that may cause abdominal pain in young infants (usually between eight months and fourteen months of age). This problem occurs when one part of the intestine slides inside another portion of the intestine, creating a blockage that causes severe pain. The baby will intermittently and abruptly cry and pull her legs toward her stomach. This will be followed by periods without stomach pain and often without any distress. These infants also may vomit and have dark, mucousy, bloody stools that often look like blackberry jelly.

It is important to recognize this cause of abdominal pain and to talk to your pediatrician immediately. She will want to see your baby and perhaps order an X-ray called an air or barium enema. Sometimes doing this test not only enables the diagnosis but also unblocks the intestine. If the enema does not unblock the intestine, an emergency operation may be necessary to correct the problem.

Viral or bacterial infections of the intestine (gastroenteritis) are usually associated with diarrhea and/or vomiting. On and off abdominal pain is often also present. Most cases are viral, require no treatment, and will resolve on their own over a week or so; the pain itself generally lasts one or two days and then disappears. One exception is an infection caused by the *Giardia lamblia* parasite. This infestation may produce periodic recurrent pain not localized to any one part of the abdomen. The pain may persist for a week or more and can lead to a marked loss of appetite and weight. Treatment with appropriate medication can cure this infestation and the abdominal pain that accompanies it. (For more information, see *Diarrhea,* page 440, and *Vomiting,* page 458.)

Constipation

Bowel patterns vary in children just as they do in adults. Because of this, it is sometimes difficult to tell if your baby is truly constipated. In general, it is best to watch for the following signals if you suspect constipation.

- In a newborn, firm stools less than once a day, though this can be normal in some exclusively breastfed infants
- Stools that are large, hard and dry, and associated with painful bowel movements
- Episodes of abdominal pain relieved after having a large bowel movement
- Blood in or on the outside of the stools
- Soiling between bowel movements

The tendency toward constipation seems to run in families. It may start in infancy and remain as a lifetime pattern, becoming worse if the child does not establish regular bowel habits or withholds stool.

Treatment

Mild or occasional episodes of constipation may be helped by the following suggestions.

Constipation due to breastmilk is unusual, but if your breastfed infant is constipated, it is probably due to a reason other than diet. Consult your doctor before substituting formula for breastmilk. (Keep in mind that the American Academy of Pediatrics recommends breastfeeding and avoiding cow's milk for the first twelve months of life.)

For infants, ask your pediatrician about giving small amounts of water or prune juice. In addition, fruits (especially prunes and pears) can often help a constipated infant.

Prevention

Parents should become familiar with their baby's normal bowel patterns and the typical size and consistency of their stools. Doing this is helpful in determining when constipation occurs and how severe the problem is. If the infant does not have regular bowel movements each day or two, or is uncomfortable when they are passed, talk with your pediatrician about dietary changes that may help his bowel habits become more regular.

DIARRHEA

Normally your baby's bowel movements will vary in number and consistency, depending on her age and diet. Breastfed newborns may have up to twelve small bowel movements a day, but by the second or third month, they may have some days without any. Most babies under one year of age produce less than 5 ounces (150 ml) of stool per day, while older children can produce up to 7 ounces (210 ml).

An occasional loose stool is not cause for alarm. If, however, your baby's bowel pattern suddenly changes to loose, watery stools that occur more frequently than usual, he has diarrhea.

Diarrhea occurs when the inner lining of the intestine is injured. The stools become loose because the intestine does not properly digest or absorb the nutrients from the foods that your child eats and drinks. Also, the injured lining tends to leak fluid. Minerals and salt are lost along with the fluid. This loss can be made even worse if your infant is fed food or beverages that contain large amounts of sugar such as found in fruit juice and sweetened beverages, since unabsorbed sugar draws even more water into the intestine, increasing the diarrhea.

When the body loses too much water and salt, dehydration results. This can be prevented by replenishing losses due to the diarrhea with adequate amounts of fluid and salt, as described under *Treatment* (page 442).

The medical term for intestinal inflammation is *enteritis*. When the problem is accompanied by or preceded by vomiting, as it often is, there is usually some stomach and small-intestinal inflammation, as well, and the condition is called *gastroenteritis*.

Causes of Diarrhea

In young children, the intestinal damage that produces diarrhea is caused most often by viruses called enteroviruses. Other causes are:

- Rotavirus infections
- Bacteria (salmonella, shigella, *E. coli*, campylobacter)
- Parasitic infections (*Giardia*)
- Food poisoning (from things such as mushrooms, shellfish, or contaminated food)
- Side effects from oral medication (most commonly antibiotics)
- Food or milk allergy
- Infections outside the gastrointestinal tract, including the urinary tract, the respiratory tract, and even the middle ear (If your child is taking an antibiotic for such an infection, the diarrhea may become more severe.)

The causes of diarrhea are described in the box on the previous page (*Causes of Diarrhea*; page 441), and include viral or bacterial infections of the intestine. Babies with viral diarrheal illnesses often have symptoms such as vomiting, fever, and irritability, as well. (See *Vomiting*, page 458; Chapter 23, *Fever*.) Their stools tend to be greenish yellow in color and have a significant amount of water with them. (If they occur as often as once an hour, they usually won't have any solid stool at all.) If the stools appear red or blackish, they might contain blood; this bleeding may arise from the injured lining of the intestine or, more likely, simply may be due to irritation of the rectum by frequent, loose bowel movements. In any event, if you notice this or any other unusual stool color, you should notify your pediatrician.

Treatment

There are no effective medications for treating viral intestinal infections, which cause most cases of diarrhea in infants. Prescription medications should be used only to treat certain types of bacterial or parasitic intestinal infections, which are much less common. When the latter conditions are suspected, your pediatrician will ask for stool specimens to be tested in the laboratory; other tests also may be done.

Over-the-counter antidiarrheal medications are not recommended for babies. They often worsen the intestinal injury and cause the fluid and salt to remain within the intestine. With these medications, your infant can become dehydrated without your being aware of it, because the diarrhea appears to stop. Always consult your pediatrician before giving your baby any medication for diarrhea.

Mild Diarrhea If your baby has a small amount of diarrhea but is not dehydrated (see the box on page 443 for signs of dehydration), does not have a high fever, and is active and hungry, you may not need to change her diet and you can continue breastmilk or formula.

If your baby has mild diarrhea and is vomiting, substitute a commercially available electrolyte solution for her normal diet. Your pediatrician will recommend these solutions to be given in small amounts, frequently to maintain normal body water and salt levels until the vomiting has stopped. In most

Signs and Symptoms of Dehydration (Loss of Significant Amounts of Body Water)

The most important part of treating diarrhea is to prevent your baby from becoming dehydrated. Be alert for the following warning signs of dehydration, and notify the pediatrician immediately if any of them develop.

Mild to Moderate Dehydration:

- Plays less than usual
- Urinates less frequently (for infants, fewer than six wet diapers per day)
- Parched, dry mouth
- Fewer tears when crying
- Sunken soft spot of the head in an infant
- Stools will be loose if dehydration is caused by diarrhea; if dehydration is due to other fluid loss (vomiting, lack of fluid intake), there will be decreased bowel movements

Severe Dehydration (in addition to the symptoms and signals already listed):

- Very fussy
- Excessively sleepy
- Sunken eyes
- Cool, discolored hands and feet
- Wrinkled skin
- Urinates only one to two times per day

cases, they're needed for only one to two days. Once the vomiting has subsided, gradually restart the normal diet.

Never give boiled milk (skimmed or otherwise) to any baby with diarrhea. Boiling the milk allows the water to evaporate, leaving the remaining part dangerously high in salt and mineral content. In fact, you should never give boiled milk even to a well baby.

Significant Diarrhea If your baby has a watery bowel movement every one to two hours, or more frequently, and/or has signs of dehydration (see the box on page 443), consult his pediatrician. She may advise you to withhold all solid foods for at least twenty-four hours and to avoid liquids that are high in sugar (Jell-O, soft drinks, full-strength fruit juices, or artificially sweetened beverages), high in salt (packaged broth), or very low in salt (water and tea). She probably will have you give him only commercially prepared electrolyte solutions, which contain the ideal balance of salt and minerals. (See the table *Estimated Oral Fluid and Electrolyte Requirements by Body Weight* on page 446.) Breastfed babies usually are treated in a similar fashion except in very mild cases, when breastfeeding may be continued.

Remember, if your baby has diarrhea, keeping him hydrated is very important. If he shows any signs of dehydration (such as decreased wet diapers, no tears, sunken eyes or fontanel), call your pediatrician right away and withhold all foods and milk beverages until she gives you further instructions. Also contact your doctor if your infant looks sick, and the symptoms aren't improving with time. *Take your baby to the pediatrician or nearest emergency department immediately if you think he is moderately to severely dehydrated.* In the meantime, give your baby a commercially prepared electrolyte solution.

For severe dehydration, hospitalization is sometimes necessary so that your infant can be rehydrated intravenously. In milder cases, all that may be necessary is to give your baby an electrolyte replacement solution according to your pediatrician's directions. The table on page 446 indicates the approximate amount of this solution to be used.

Exclusively breastfed infants are less likely to develop severe diarrhea. If a breastfed infant does develop diarrhea, generally you can continue breastfeeding, giving additional electrolyte solution only if your doctor feels this is necessary. Many breastfed babies can continue to stay hydrated with frequent breastfeeding alone.

Once your infant has been on an electrolyte solution for twelve to twenty-four hours and the diarrhea is decreasing, you gradually may expand the diet to include foods such as applesauce, pears, bananas, and flavored gelatin, with a goal of returning to his usual diet over the next few days as he tolerates.

It is usually unnecessary to withhold food for longer than twenty-four hours, as your baby will need some normal nutrition to start to regain lost strength. After you have started giving him food again, his stools may remain loose, but that does not necessarily mean that things are not going well. Look for increased activity, better appetite, more frequent urination, and the disappearance of any of the signs of dehydration. When you see these, you will know your infant is getting better.

Diarrhea that lasts longer than two weeks (chronic diarrhea) may signify a more serious type of intestinal problem. When diarrhea persists this long, your pediatrician will want to do further tests to determine the cause and to make sure your baby is not becoming malnourished. If malnutrition is becoming a problem, the pediatrician may recommend a special diet or special type of formula.

If your infant drinks too much fluid, especially too much juice or sweetened beverages as mentioned earlier, a condition commonly referred to as toddler's diarrhea could develop. This causes ongoing loose stools but shouldn't affect appetite or growth or cause dehydration. Although toddler's diarrhea is not a dangerous condition, the pediatrician may suggest that you limit the amounts of juice and sweetened fluids your infant drinks (limiting fruit juice is always a good idea). You can give plain water to babies whose thirst does not seem to be satisfied by their normal dietary and milk intake.

When diarrhea occurs in combination with other symptoms, it could mean that there is a more serious medical problem. Notify your pediatrician immediately if the diarrhea is accompanied by any of the following:

- Fever that lasts longer than twenty-four to forty-eight hours
- Bloody stools
- Vomiting that lasts more than twelve to twenty-four hours
- Vomited material that is green-colored, blood-tinged, or like coffee grounds in appearance

Estimated Oral Fluid and Electrolyte Requirements by Body Weight
1 pound = 0.45 kilograms
1 ounce = 30 ml

Body Weight in Pounds	*Minimum Daily Fluid Requirements (in ounces)**	*Electrolyte Solution Requirements for Mild Diarrhea (in ounces for 24 hours)*
6–7	10	16
11	15	23
22	25	40
26	28	44

*NOTE: This is the *smallest* amount of fluid that a normal baby requires. Most infants drink more than this.

- A distended (swollen-appearing) abdomen
- Refusal to eat or drink
- Severe abdominal pain
- Rash or jaundice (yellow color of skin and eyes)

If your baby has another medical condition or is taking medication routinely, it is best to tell your pediatrician about any diarrheal illness that lasts more than twenty-four hours without improvement, or anything else that really worries you.

Probiotics and Prebiotics

Probiotics are types of "good" bacteria. These living organisms inhabit the intestines, and may have beneficial health effects, although the evidence is not yet conclusive. Some studies have shown that foods or infant formula containing probiotics can prevent or even treat diarrhea in children, whether this condition is chronic or acute, or is associated with the use of antibiotics. To date, the strongest evidence suggests that probiotics may help avoid or improve viral gastroenteritis (see page 441); they also may strengthen a child's disease-fighting immune system and thus help fight off a number of infections that could lead to diarrhea. Ongoing research will provide more guidance on the role of probiotics in infants, but if your baby has diarrhea, you may wish to talk to your doctor about the use of these organisms.

Probiotics are available in many forms. Many infant formulas are now supplemented with probiotics. Some dairy products such as yogurt and kefir contain them, too. So do miso, tempeh, and soy beverages. Probiotic supplements (powders, capsules) are sold in health food stores; pediatricians are still debating the most appropriate use of these commercial probiotics—for example, what are the best dosages, how frequently should they be taken, and should they be used at all for preventing or managing certain health conditions?

Foods containing probiotics appear to be safe for most babies, although they can cause mild bloating or gas in some cases. If products like probiotic supplements have been exposed to heat or moisture, the living "good" bacteria may be killed, and thus the products will become useless. For now, if you're interested in trying probiotics, talk to your pediatrician first. (For more information about probiotics, see page 142.)

Some doctors recommend that rather than giving your infant *pro*biotics, you should consider using *pre*biotics instead. While probiotics are living bacteria, prebiotics are nondigestible food components (such as sugars and fiber). They promote the growth of beneficial bacteria that are already present in the intestines, thus increasing the number of these good bacteria while also suppressing the growth of unhealthy strains. They also may decrease the levels of inflammation in the intestines and stimulate the absorption of calcium.

Breastmilk is a good source of prebiotics. So are foods like bran, legumes, and barley, as well as certain vegetables (asparagus, spinach, onion) and fruits (berries, bananas.)

Prevention

The following guidelines will help lessen the chances that your baby will get diarrhea.

1. Most forms of infectious diarrhea are transmitted from direct hand-to-mouth contact following exposure to contaminated fecal (stool) material. This happens most often in children who are not toilet trained. Promote personal hygiene (i.e., hand-washing after using the toilet or changing diapers and before handling food) and other sanitary measures in your household and in your baby's child care center or preschool.
2. Avoid drinking raw (unpasteurized) milk and eating foods that may be contaminated.
3. Avoid unnecessary medications, especially antibiotics.
4. If possible, breastfeed your baby through early infancy.
5. Limit the amount of juice and sweetened beverages.
6. Make sure your infant has received the rotavirus vaccine

as it protects against the most common cause of diarrhea and vomiting in babies.

(See also *Abdominal Pain,* page 437; *Malabsorption,* page 456; *Milk Allergy,* page 485; *Rotavirus,* page 688; and *Vomiting,* page 458.)

Hepatitis

Hepatitis is an inflammation of the liver that, in children, is almost always caused by one of several viruses. In some babies it may cause no symptoms, while in others it can provoke fever, jaundice (yellow skin), loss of appetite, nausea, and vomiting. There are at least six forms of hepatitis, each categorized according to the type of virus that causes it. The most common forms include:

1. Hepatitis A, also called infectious hepatitis or epidemic jaundice. Routine vaccination is recommended for all children at one year of age with a booster dose six to twelve months later.
2. Hepatitis B, also known as serum hepatitis or transfusion jaundice. Routine vaccination is now recommended for all infants at birth, with two booster doses given.
3. Hepatitis C, which is an important cause of chronic hepatitis. Currently there is no vaccine.

About one half of all cases of hepatitis are caused by hepatitis B; of the remainder, slightly less than one half are caused by hepatitis A, and nearly all of the rest are hepatitis C. Fortunately, with the routine vaccination now of nearly all children against hepatitis A and B (see above), the cases of hepatitis are decreasing.

Children, especially those in low socioeconomic groups, have the highest incidence of hepatitis A infection. However, because they often have no symptoms, their illnesses may go unrecognized.

Hepatitis A can be transmitted directly from person to person or through contaminated food or water. Commonly, human feces contain the virus, so in a child care or household setting, the infection can be spread when hands are not washed after having a bowel movement or after changing the diaper of an infected infant. Anyone who drinks water contaminated with infected human feces or who eats raw shellfish taken from polluted areas also may become infected. A baby infected with hepatitis A virus will become ill two to six weeks after the virus is transmitted. The illness usually disappears within one month after it begins.

Although hepatitis A is rarely transmitted via contaminated blood or semen, hepatitis B is usually spread through these body fluids. The incidence of hepatitis B infection is now greatest among adolescents, young adults, and in the newborns of women who are infected with the virus. When a pregnant woman has acute or chronic hepatitis B, she may transmit the infection to her newborn at the time of delivery. Therefore, all pregnant women should be tested for exposure to hepatitis. Among adults and adolescents, the virus can be transmitted during sexual activity, and young children sometimes contract the infection through nonsexual, person-to-person contact.

In the past, hepatitis C was acquired from contaminated blood transfusions. With screening of all donors using new, sensitive tests, however, blood contaminated with the hepatitis C virus is now detectable and discarded. Hepatitis C also can be acquired by intravenous (IV) drug abusers who use contaminated needles. However, the use of sterile disposable needles and the screening of all blood and blood products has essentially eliminated the risk of transmission of hepatitis B and C in hospitals and doctors' offices.

Infection with the hepatitis C virus commonly produces no symptoms, or only mild symptoms of fatigue and jaundice. In many cases, however, this form of hepatitis becomes chronic and can result in severe liver disease, liver failure, cancer of the liver, and death.

Signs and Symptoms

A baby could have hepatitis without anyone being aware of it, since many affected children have few, if any, symptoms. In some babies the only signs of disease may be malaise and fatigue for several days. In others there will be a fever followed by jaundice (the sclera, or whites of the eyes, and the skin develop noticeable yellowish color). This jaundice is due to an abnormal increase in bilirubin (a yellow pigment) in the blood, caused by liver inflammation.

With hepatitis B, fever is less likely to occur, although the baby may suffer loss of appetite, nausea, vomiting, abdominal pain, and malaise, in addition to jaundice.

If you suspect that your baby has jaundice, notify your pediatrician. She will order blood tests to determine if hepatitis is causing the problem, or if it is due to another condition. You should contact your doctor anytime vomiting and/or abdominal pain persist beyond a few hours, or if appetite loss, nausea, or malaise continue for more than a few days. These may be indicators of hepatitis.

Treatment

In most settings, there is no specific treatment for hepatitis. As with most viral infections, the body's own defense mechanisms usually will overcome the infecting agent. Although you do not need to rigidly restrict the diet or activity of your child, you may need to make adjustments depending on his appetite and energy levels. Avoid aspirin and acetaminophen, because of the risk of toxicity due to inadequate liver function. Also, babies on certain medications for long-term illnesses should have their dosages carefully reviewed by the pediatrician, again to avoid the toxicity that might result because the liver is unable to handle the usual medication load.

A few medications are available for patients with hepatitis B and hepatitis C. If your baby's hepatitis becomes a chronic condition, your pediatrician will refer you to a pediatric gastroenterologist to help decide on appropriate follow-up care and to consider whether medications should be used.

Most babies with hepatitis do not need to be hospitalized. However, if loss of appetite or vomiting is interfering with your baby's fluid intake and posing a risk of dehydration, your pediatrician may recommend that he be hospitalized. You should contact your doctor immediately if your baby appears very lethargic, unresponsive, or delirious, as these may indicate that his illness is worsening and hospitalization is indicated.

Many infants with hepatitis B develop chronic hepatitis.

Cirrhosis (scarring of the liver) may follow recovery in some of these babies. Death, however, occurs rarely. There is no chronic infection following hepatitis A; in comparison, about ten of every hundred children under five years of age infected with hepatitis B become chronic carriers of the virus. A much higher percentage of infants who are born to mothers with acute or chronic hepatitis B become chronic carriers if they are not properly immunized after birth with the vaccine developed for protection against the hepatitis B virus. As chronic hepatitis B carriers, they would be at risk for the development of liver cancer many years later.

Prevention

Hand-washing before eating and after using the toilet is the most important preventive measure against hepatitis. Children should be taught as young as possible to wash their hands at these times. If your baby is in child care, check to be sure that members of the staff wash their hands after handling diapers and before feeding the children.

Hepatitis is not transmitted simply by being in the same school or room with an infected person, or by talking to him, shaking his hand, or playing with him. A hepatitis A infection can occur if there has been a direct exposure to food or water contaminated with feces from a person infected with hepatitis A. It might be transmitted during the mouthing of toys or sharing food or utensils. For hepatitis B, there must be direct contact with the blood or bodily fluids of an infected person.

If you find out that your baby has been exposed to a person with hepatitis, immediately contact your pediatrician, who will determine if the exposure has placed your infant at risk. If there's a chance of infection, the doctor may administer an injection of gamma globulin or a hepatitis vaccine, depending on which hepatitis virus was involved.

Prior to foreign travel with your baby, consult your physician to determine the risk of exposure to hepatitis in the countries you plan to visit. In certain situations, gamma globulin and/or a hepatitis A vaccine may be indicated.

It is now recommended that all newborn infants, children, and adolescents be immunized against hepatitis B. A hepatitis A vaccine, first licensed in 1995, is recommended for all children at twelve to twenty-three months of age, as well as older children and adolescents who have not yet been vaccinated. (See immunization schedule on pages 734–735.)

INGUINAL HERNIA

If you notice a small lump or bulge in your baby's groin area or an enlargement of the scrotum, you may have discovered an inguinal hernia. This condition, which is present in up to five of every hundred children (most commonly in boys), occurs when an opening in the lower abdominal wall allows the infant's intestine to squeeze through. This inguinal hernia is frequently confused with a more benign condition, a communicating hydrocele (see section below).

The testicles of the developing male fetus grow inside his abdominal cavity, moving down through a tube (the inguinal canal) into the scrotum as birth nears. When this movement takes place, the lining of the abdominal wall (peritoneum) is pulled along with the testes to form a sac connecting the testicle with the abdominal cavity. A hernia in a baby is due to a failure of this normal protrusion from the abdominal cavity to close properly before birth, leaving a space for a small portion of the bowel to later push through into the groin or scrotum.

Most hernias do not cause any discomfort, and you or the pediatrician will discover them only by seeing the bulge. Although this kind of hernia must be treated, it is not an emergency condition. You should, however, notify your doctor, who may instruct you to have the baby lie down and elevate his legs. Sometimes this will cause the bulge to disappear. However, your doctor will still want to examine the area as soon as possible.

Rarely, a piece of the intestine gets trapped in the hernia, causing swelling and pain. (If you touch the area, it will be tender.) Your son may have nausea and vomiting as well. This condition is called an incarcerated (trapped) hernia and *does* require immediate medical attention. Call your pediatrician immediately if you suspect an incarcerated hernia.

Treatment

Even if the hernia is not incarcerated, it still should be surgically repaired as soon as possible. The surgeon also may check the other side of the abdomen to see if it, too, needs to be corrected, since it is very common for the same defect to be present there.

If the hernia is causing pain, it may indicate that a piece of intestine has become trapped or incarcerated. In that case, consult with your pediatrician immediately. He may try to move the trapped piece of intestine out of the sac. Even if this can be done, the hernia still needs to be surgically repaired soon thereafter. If the intestine remains trapped despite your doctor's efforts, emergency surgery must be performed to prevent permanent damage to the intestine.

Communicating Hydrocele

If the opening between the abdominal cavity and the scrotum has not closed properly and completely, abdominal fluid will pass into the sac around the testis, causing a mass called a communicating hydrocele. As many as half of all newborn boys have this problem; however, it usually disappears within one year without any treatment. Although most common in newborns, hydroceles also can develop later in childhood, most often with a hernia (see preceding section).

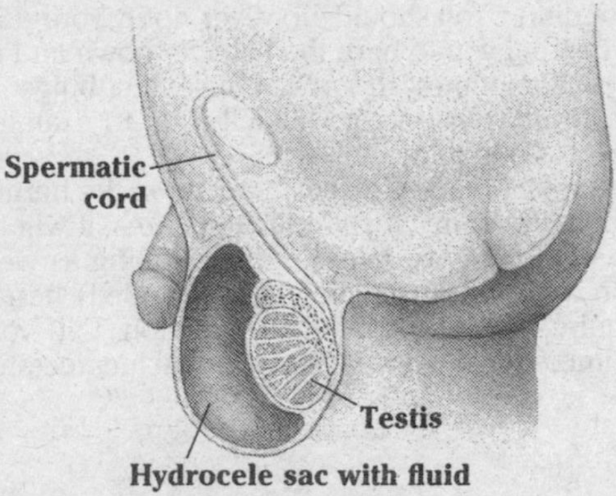

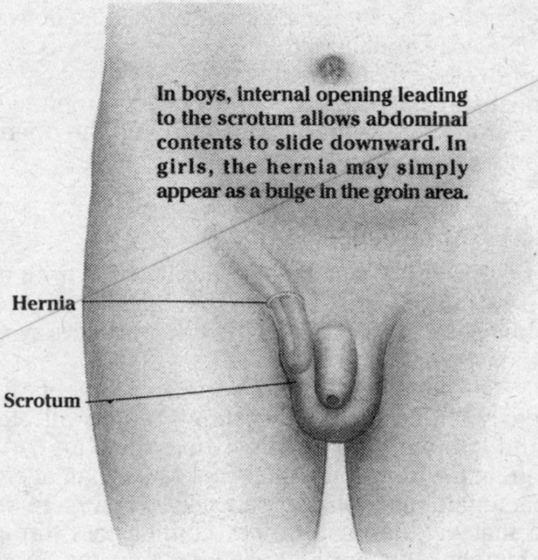

In boys, internal opening leading to the scrotum allows abdominal contents to slide downward. In girls, the hernia may simply appear as a bulge in the groin area.
Hernia
Scrotum

If your son has a hydrocele, he probably will not complain, but you or he will notice that one side of his scrotum is swollen. In an infant this swelling decreases at night or when he is resting or lying down. When he gets more active or is crying, it increases, then subsides when he quiets again. Your pediatrician may make the final diagnosis by shining a bright light through the scrotum, to show the fluid surrounding the testicle. Your doctor also may request an ultrasound examination of the scrotum if it is very swollen or hard.

If your baby is born with a hydrocele, your pediatrician will examine it at each regular checkup until around one year of age. During this time your infant should not feel any discomfort in the scrotum or the surrounding area. But if it seems to be tender in this area or he has unexplained discomfort, nausea, or vomiting, call the doctor at once. These are signs that a piece of intestine may have entered the scrotal area along with abdominal fluid. (See *Inguinal Hernia,* page 453.) If this occurs and the intestine gets trapped in the scrotum, your baby may require immediate surgery to release the trapped intestine and close the opening between the abdominal wall and the scrotum.

If the hydrocele persists beyond one year without causing pain, a similar surgical procedure may be recommended. In this operation, the excess fluid is removed and the opening into the abdominal cavity closed.

Malabsorption

Sometimes babies who eat a balanced diet suffer from malnutrition. The reason for this may be malabsorption, the body's inability to absorb nutrients from the digestive system into the bloodstream.

Normally the digestive process converts nutrients from the diet into small units that pass through the wall of the intestine and into the bloodstream, where they are carried to other cells in the body. If the intestinal wall is damaged by a virus, bacterial infection, or parasites, its surface may change so that digested substances cannot pass through. When this happens, the nutrients will be eliminated through the stool.

Malabsorption commonly occurs in a normal baby for a day or two during severe cases of stomach or intestinal flu. It rarely lasts much longer since the surface of the intestine heals quickly without significant damage. In these cases, malabsorption is no cause for concern. However, chronic malabsorption may develop, and if two or more of the following signs or symptoms persist, notify your pediatrician.

Signs and Symptoms

Possible signs and symptoms of chronic malabsorption include the following:

- Persistent abdominal pain and vomiting
- Frequent, loose, bulky, foul-smelling stools
- Increased susceptibility to infection
- Weight loss with the loss of fat and muscle
- Increase in bruises
- Bone fractures

- Dry, scaly skin rashes
- Personality changes
- Slowing of growth and weight gain (may not be noticeable for several months)

Treatment

When an infant suffers from malnutrition, malabsorption is just one of the possible causes. She might be undernourished because she's not getting enough of the right types of food, or she has digestive problems that prevent her body from digesting them. She also might have a combination of these problems. Before prescribing a treatment, the pediatrician must determine the cause. This can be done in one or more of the following ways.

- **You may be** asked to list the amount and type of food your baby eats.
- **The pediatrician may** test the child's ability to digest and absorb specific nutrients. For example, the doctor might have her drink a solution of milk sugar (lactose) and then measure the level of hydrogen in her breath afterward. This is known as a lactose hydrogen breath test.
- **The pediatrician may** collect and analyze stool samples. In healthy people, only a small amount of the fat consumed each day is lost through the stool. If too much is found in the stool, it is an indication of malabsorption.
- **Collection of sweat** from the skin, called a sweat test, may be performed to see if cystic fibrosis (see page 521) is present. In this disease, the body produces insufficient amounts of certain enzymes necessary for proper digestion and an abnormality in the sweat.
- **In some cases** the pediatrician might request that a pediatric gastroenterologist obtain a biopsy from the wall of the small intestine, and have it examined under the microscope for signs of infection, inflammation, or other injury.

Ordinarily, these tests are performed before any treatment is begun, although a seriously sick baby might be hospitalized in order to receive special feedings while her problem is being evaluated.

Once the physician is sure the problem is malabsorption, she will try to identify a specific reason for its presence. When the reason is infection, the treatment usually will include antibiotics. If malabsorption occurs because the intestine is too active, certain medications may be used to counteract this, so that there's time for the nutrients to be absorbed.

Sometimes there's no clear cause for the problem. In this case, the diet may be changed to include foods or special nutritional formulas that are more easily tolerated and absorbed.

VOMITING

Because many common childhood illnesses can cause vomiting, you should expect your baby to have this problem several times during these early years. Usually it ends quickly without treatment, but this doesn't make it any easier for you to watch. That feeling of helplessness combined with the fear that something serious might be wrong and the desire to do something to make it better may make you feel tense and anxious. To help put your mind at ease, learn as much as you can about the causes of vomiting and what you can do to treat your infant when it occurs.

First of all, there's a difference between real vomiting

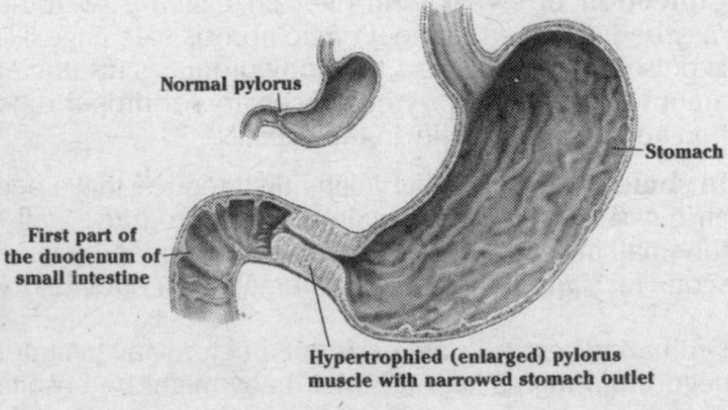

and just spitting up. Vomiting is the forceful throwing up of stomach contents through the mouth. Spitting up (most commonly seen in infants under one year of age) is the easy flow of stomach contents out of the mouth, frequently with a burp.

Vomiting occurs when the abdominal muscles and diaphragm contract vigorously while the stomach is relaxed. This reflex action is triggered by the "vomiting center" in the brain after it has been stimulated by:

- Nerves from the stomach and intestine when the gastrointestinal tract is either irritated or swollen by an infection or blockage
- Chemicals in the blood (e.g., drugs)
- Psychological stimuli from disturbing sights or smells
- Stimuli from the middle ear (as in vomiting caused by motion sickness)

The common causes of spitting up or vomiting vary according to age. During the first few months, for instance, most infants will spit up small amounts of formula or breastmilk, usually within the first hour after being fed. This "cheesing," as it is often called, is simply the occasional movement of food from the stomach, through the tube (esophagus) leading to it, and out of the mouth. It will occur less often if a baby is burped frequently and if active play is limited right after meals. This spitting up tends to decrease as the baby becomes older, but may persist in a mild form until ten to twelve months of age. Spitting up is not serious and doesn't interfere with normal weight gain. (See *Spitting Up,* page 148.)

Occasional vomiting may occur during the first month. If it appears repeatedly or is unusually forceful, call your pediatrician. It may be just a mild feeding difficulty, but it also could be a sign of something more serious.

Around two weeks to four months of age, persistent forceful vomiting may be caused by a thickening of the muscle at the stomach exit. Known as hypertrophic pyloric stenosis, this thickening prevents food from passing into the intestines. It requires *immediate* medical attention. Surgery usually is required to open the narrowed area. The important sign of this condition is forceful vomiting occurring approximately fifteen to thirty minutes or less after every feeding. Anytime you notice this, call your pediatrician as soon as possible.

Occasionally the spitting up in the first few weeks to months of life gets worse instead of better—that is, even though it's not forceful, it occurs all the time. This happens when the muscles at the lower end of the esophagus become overly relaxed and allow the stomach contents to back up. This condition is known as gastroesophageal reflux disease, or GERD. This condition usually can be controlled by doing the following:

1. Thicken the milk with small amounts of baby cereal as directed by your pediatrician.
2. Avoid overfeeding or give smaller feeds more frequently.
3. Burp the baby frequently.
4. Leave the infant in a safe, quiet, upright position for at least thirty minutes following feeding.

If these steps are not successful, your pediatrician may refer you to a pediatric gastrointestinal (GI) specialist.

Infectious Causes. After the first few months of life, the most common cause of vomiting is a stomach or intestinal infection. Viruses are by far the most frequent infecting agents, but occasionally bacteria and even parasites may be the cause. The infection also may produce fever, diarrhea, and sometimes nausea and abdominal pain. The infection is usually contagious; if your child has it, chances are good that some of her playmates also will be affected.

Rotaviruses are a leading cause of vomiting in infants and young children, with symptoms often progressing to diarrhea and fever. These viruses are very contagious, but are becoming less common than in the past, due to the availability of a vaccine that can prevent the disease. The rotavirus is one of the viral causes of gastroenteritis, but other types of viruses—such as noroviruses, enteroviruses, and adenoviruses—can cause it as well. (For more information about gastroenteritis, see page 441.)

Occasionally infections outside the gastrointestinal tract will cause vomiting. These include infections of the respiratory system (also see discussions of otitis media, page 557; pneumonia, page 505), infections of the urinary tract (see page 660), and meningitis (see page 663). Some of these conditions require immediate medical treatment, so be alert for the following trouble signs, whatever your baby's age, and call your pediatrician if they occur.

- Blood or bile (a green-colored material) in the vomit
- Severe abdominal pain
- Strenuous, repeated vomiting
- Swollen or enlarged abdomen
- Lethargy or severe irritability
- Convulsions
- Signs or symptoms of dehydration (see below under *Treatment,* as well as *Signs and Symptoms of Dehydration,* on page 443.)
- Inability to drink adequate amounts of fluid
- Vomiting continuing beyond twenty-four hours

Treatment

In most cases, vomiting will stop without specific medical treatment. The majority of cases are caused by a virus and will get better on their own. You should never use over-the-counter or prescription remedies unless they've been specifically prescribed by your pediatrician for your baby and for this particular illness.

When your infant is vomiting, keep her lying on her stomach or side as much as possible. Doing this will minimize the chances of her inhaling vomit into her upper airway and lungs.

When there is continued vomiting, you need to make certain that dehydration doesn't occur. *Dehydration* is a term used when the body loses so much water that it can no longer function efficiently (see *Signs and Symptoms of Dehydration,* page 443). If allowed to reach a severe degree, it can be serious and life-threatening. To prevent this from happening, make sure your baby consumes enough extra fluids to restore what has been lost through throwing up. If she vomits these fluids, notify your pediatrician.

For the first twenty-four hours or so of any illness that causes vomiting, keep your baby off solid foods, and encourage her to suck or drink small amounts of electrolyte solution (ask your pediatrician which one), clear fluids such as water, sugar water (½ teaspoon [2.5 ml] sugar in 4 ounces [120 ml] of water), Popsicles, gelatin water (1 teaspoon [5 ml] of flavored gelatin in 4 ounces of water), instead of eating. Liquids not only help to prevent dehydration, but also are less likely than solid foods to stimulate further vomiting.

Be sure to follow your pediatrician's guidelines for giving your baby fluids. Your doctor will adhere to requirements like those described in the box on page 446 (*Estimated Oral Fluid and Electrolyte Requirements by Body Weight*).

In most cases, your baby will just need to stay at home and receive a liquid diet for twelve to twenty-four hours. Your pediatrician usually won't prescribe a drug to treat the vomiting, but some doctors will prescribe antinausea medications to infants.

If your baby also has diarrhea (see page 440), ask your pediatrician for instructions on giving liquids and restoring solids to her diet.

If she can't retain any clear liquids or if the symptoms become more severe, notify your pediatrician. She will examine your baby and may order blood and urine tests or imaging tests such as X-rays to make a diagnosis. Occasionally hospital care may be necessary.

Until your infant feels better, remember to keep her hydrated, and call your pediatrician right away if she shows signs of dehydration. If your child looks sick, the symptoms aren't improving with time, or your pediatrician suspects a bacterial infection, he may perform a culture of the stool, and treat appropriately.

13

ALLERGIES

ASTHMA

Asthma is a chronic disease of the breathing tubes that carry air to the lungs. In the last twenty years, there has been a major increase in the number of people with asthma, especially young children and those living in urban areas. In fact, asthma is now one of the most common chronic diseases of childhood, affecting about 5 million children. We don't know what caused this increase, but the main reasons seem to be air pollution, exposure to allergens, obesity, and respiratory illnesses.

Asthma symptoms can be different for each infant, but wheezing is a hallmark sign. Wheezing is the high-pitched sound that occurs when the airways in the lungs are narrowed, typically due to inflammation. In asthma, wheezing occurs when breathing out, most often at night or in the early morning. Still, not everyone who wheezes has asthma. Although no specific test can determine asthma, the diagnosis is often made after a baby has had three or more wheezing attacks; between these episodes, the wheezing often goes away.

Asthma is commonly diagnosed after developing bronchiolitis (see page 494). Following the initial wheezing attack, wheezing reoccurs during a cold. In between these attacks babies do well, but since they often get colds, the attacks can be as frequent as every month. If an infant has no other allergies—meaning that she does not have eczema and neither parent has asthma—wheezing will likely decrease between three and six years of age. If these children begin wheezing in the first years of life and have repeated wheezing attacks, they are diagnosed with asthma.

For many parents this provokes anxiety. But each

case is different and it is important to discuss your infant's health with your primary physician or specialist. At this time it will be difficult to predict how the condition will impact your baby. Asthma is such a variable disease that some infants and children may wheeze without much distress while others have such severe wheezing and breathing difficulty that it may create an emergency situation.

If there is a history of asthma or allergy, an infant who frequently wheezes is likely to continue wheezing for a number of years. It is not possible to cure asthma, so a child will receive treatment to reduce wheezing and prevent future attacks. Asthma also occurs in infants who are not allergic. Babies who are not allergic may begin wheezing from exercise, stress, and exposure to irritants—or triggers—such as pollution, household cleaners (especially bleach), perfumes, and cold air. Cigarette smoke also is a major risk factor.

Many things can trigger an asthma attack, but in babies and other children under five, it's most common after a viral respiratory infection, including the common cold.

Other common asthma triggers include:

- Dust, dust mites, cockroaches, animal dander, pollens, and molds
- Inhaling cold air

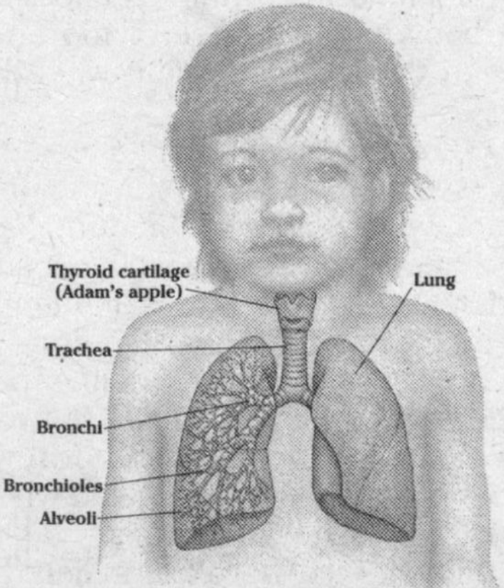

Chest and Lungs

- Certain medications
- Certain foods like milk, eggs, and wheat
- Gastroesophageal reflux

Some less common triggers are:

- Sinus infections
- Previous injury to the airways (e.g., in babies who have had an endotracheal tube inserted or who have inhaled cigarette smoke)

Signs and Symptoms

When your baby has an asthma attack, the major symptom will be a cough that gets worse at night, with physical activity, or after contact with an irritant (i.e., cigarette smoke) or an allergen (i.e., animal dander, mold, dust mites, or cockroaches). As the attack progresses, the wheezing actually may decrease, as less air is able to move in and out. She also may experience shortness of breath during an asthma episode, breathe fast, and have “retractions” when the chest and neck pull in while she works to take in air.

Many infants with asthma have chronic symptoms, such as daily (or nightly) cough, or cough with certain daily exposures to pets, dust, and pollens. Asthma is considered “persistent” if there is a need for “rescue” medication (see *Treatment* section below) more than twice a week, or if there are more than two awakenings at night for asthma symptoms per month.

In some babies, the physician may hear wheezing (especially when the child blows out hard) even without symptoms.

When to Call the Pediatrician

Most babies with asthma can do the same activities as other infants, including play outdoors and be active. At the same time, watch your baby closely when she's outside or active and if symptoms develop or worsen, talk to your pediatrician.

For an infant with asthma, you should know the situations that require *immediate* medical attention. As a rule, call your pediatrician immediately or consider going to the emergency room if:

- Your baby has *severe* trouble breathing and seems to be getting worse, especially if she is breathing rapidly and there is pulling in of the chest wall when she inhales and forceful grunting when she exhales.
- Your baby's mouth or fingertips appear blue.

You also should call your pediatrician without delay if:

- Your baby has a fever and persistent coughing or wheezing that is not responding to treatment.
- Your infant is vomiting, and cannot take oral medication.
- Your child has difficulty sleeping because of wheezing, coughing, or troubled breathing.

Treatment

Asthma always should be treated under your pediatrician's supervision. The goals of treatment are to:

1. Decrease the frequency and severity of attacks, and reduce or prevent the chronic symptoms of coughing and difficulty breathing.
2. Develop a sensible "plan of response" for any serious asthma attack to minimize emergency medical treatment.
3. Allow your baby to grow and develop normally, and take part in normal childhood activities as fully as possible.
4. Control your infant's symptoms with the smallest amount of medication possible to decrease the risk of drug side effects.
5. Decrease trips to the emergency room and the need for "rescue" treatments.

With these goals in mind, your pediatrician will prescribe medication and may refer you to a specialist who can evaluate your infant's lungs. Your doctor also will help you plan your baby's specific home treatment program. **This will**

include learning how to use the medicines and treatments that are prescribed and developing a plan to avoid the irritants and allergens that may be causing your baby to wheeze. It may be helpful to write down this asthma management plan that you can read over now and then, which should describe your baby's medications, when and how she should take them, and any other instructions that your pediatrician has given for caring for your infant's condition.

If your baby's asthma seems to be triggered by severe allergies, your pediatrician may refer you to a pediatric allergist or pulmonologist (lung specialist).

The medication prescribed for your baby will depend on the nature of the asthma. There are two main types of asthma drugs. One type opens up the breathing tubes and relaxes the muscles causing the obstruction. These quick-relief or "rescue" medicines are called bronchodilators. The second type are controller or maintenance medications, which are used to treat the airway inflammation.

- **Quick-relief or rescue medications are intended for short-term use.** If your baby has an asthma attack, with coughing and/or wheezing, a rescue medication should be given. Medicines such as albuterol are a common choice. By opening up her narrowed airways, these rescue medicines can relieve the tightness in her chest, and ease her wheezing and feelings of breathlessness. They are prescribed on an as-needed basis, and you need to follow your doctor's instructions on when and how to use them. Should an attack become severe, your doctor may prescribe an additional medication—such as an oral or inhaled corticosteroid drug—for moderate to severe asthma attacks. It is important to note that if there is no improvement or change after giving the rescue medicine, the baby may need further evaluation. Usually breathing will improve for a few hours before the wheezing comes back. Some infants continue to wheeze despite the treatment, and as long as your baby is feeding and not in distress this may be okay.

  The rescue medication can be given by nebulizer (see next section). Your doctor should clearly explain the number of doses that can be given. Discuss with your doctor and nurse when it is necessary to give the rescue medication and how you will know that it is working.

- **Controller medications are intended to be used every day.** They are designed to control your baby's asthma and lower the number of days and nights that he has asthma symptoms. In general, controller medicines are appropriate for infants who have symptoms two or more times a week, or who awaken with symptoms more than twice a month. These drugs can reduce underlying inflammation but are not used to directly relieve symptoms.

  The controller medication most often prescribed by doctors is an inhaled corticosteroid. There are several different steroids but they all work by preventing inflammation in the airway, which has the potential to reduce the number and severity of asthma episodes.

When delivering medication by nebulizer, a compressor (also known as a breathing machine) connects by tubing to a device that is like a small cup into which the medication is placed. The compressor converts the liquid into a mist that is then breathed in. In small children a mask is used and needs to be on the face. If the mask is not on the face the medication escapes into the air and never reaches the lungs. Unfortunately babies and small children do not like having the mask on and so sometimes the medication is given during sleep.

Also, when a baby cries, instead of getting more medicine with the nebulizer, she gets less. That is why it is so important to try and give the medication when your infant is not crying.

Because asthma can be a complicated disease and differ from one person to another, your doctor will individualize your baby's treatment. If your infant's symptoms occur on an intermittent basis, your pediatrician might prescribe a bronchodilator only when there is coughing or wheezing. If the asthma is chronic or recurrent, he usually will prescribe certain medications for regular daily use. These medicines may take some time (even up to a few weeks) to provide their full effect.

Anti-inflammatory medications—most commonly inhaled corticosteroids—are recommended for all asthmatic children who have persistent symptoms. They are very effective and safe, but must be used regularly to be effective. Often they fail because they are not taken consistently. Because they do not have an immediate effect, it is often tempting to stop using them. Doing so, however, will leave your baby's airway unprotected, and she may experience an asthma attack.

Also, after taking an inhaled steroid, it is important for your child to rinse her mouth by drinking something or brushing her teeth.

Be sure to give medications according to your pediatrician's (pulmonologist's or allergist's) directions. *Do not stop medicines too soon,* give them less often than recommended, or switch to other drugs or treatments without first discussing the change with the doctor. In some babies, pediatricians may begin treatment by prescribing several medicines at the same time to get the asthma controlled, and then the number of medications will be reduced. Or he may change the dose or switch to a different medicine altogether, depending on whether your baby's symptoms improve or worsen. If you do not understand why a particular treatment has been recommended, or how it should be given, ask for an explanation.

In some cases, babies do not experience any improvement in their symptoms when they're using asthma medications. When that happens, more asthma medication may be needed, they might not have asthma after all, or other medical conditions may be interfering with their treatment. Your pediatrician will examine your infant and check for problems that could be making her asthma worse, such as allergic rhinitis, sinus infections, and heartburn (gastroesophageal reflux disease).

Prevention

After a careful and detailed exam, it may become clear that your baby has allergies. In this situation the first thing to consider is how to avoid the allergic triggers, the most common being dust and the dust mite. While you cannot eliminate dust, there are some things that can be done to reduce exposure and lower your baby's chances of having asthma attacks. For example, in your home you can:

- Cover your infant's bed mattress with special asthma-allergy-proof covers.

- Wash sheets, blankets, pillows, throw rugs, and stuffed animals every one to two weeks in hot water to kill dust mites.
- Limit stuffed animals in your baby's room (or reduce the time your infant spends playing with stuffed animals).
- Consider removing pets (especially cats and dogs) from your home.
- Keep your infant out of rooms while you're vacuuming carpets and dusting furniture.
- Consider investing in a special air filter (called a high-efficiency particulate air filter, or HEPA) to keep your baby's room clean.
- Maintain the humidity in your house below 50 percent when possible; dust mites and mold grow best in damp areas.
- Avoid perfumes, scented cleaning products, and other items with scents that could become irritants.
- Reduce mold in your house by repairing leaky plumbing.
- Keep your baby away from cigarette, cigar, or pipe smoke, as well as smoke from a fireplace.
- Don't allow anyone to smoke in your home or car.

Eczema

Eczema is a general term used to describe a number of different skin conditions. It may appear as reddened skin that is dry and peeling or may start oozing, occasionally resulting in small, fluid-filled bumps. When eczema becomes chronic (persists for a long time), the skin tends to thicken, dry out, and become scaly with coarse lines.

Eczema (also known as atopic dermatitis) and contact dermatitis are the two main types of skin conditions.

Eczema or Atopic Dermatitis Atopic dermatitis often occurs in infants who have allergies or a family history of allergy or eczema, although the problem is not necessarily or always caused by an allergy. Eczema usually develops in different phases, with the first occuring between two and six months of age, with itching, redness, and the appearance of small bumps on the cheeks, forehead, or scalp. This rash then may spread to the arms or trunk. Although eczema often is confused with other types of dermatitis, especially seborrheic dermatitis, severe itching and additional allergy problems are clues that atopic dermatitis is the problem. In many cases the rash disappears or improves by two or three years of age.

Contact Dermatitis. Contact dermatitis can occur when the skin comes in contact with an irritating substance or allergen. One form of this problem results from repeated contact with irritating substances such as citrus juices, bubble baths, strong soaps, certain foods and medicines, and woolen or rough-weave fabrics. In addition, one of the most common irritants is the infant's own saliva. Contact dermatitis doesn't itch as much as atopic dermatitis and usually will clear when the irritant is no longer present and improves when babies no longer drool on their skin.

Another form of contact dermatitis develops after skin contact with substances to which the baby is allergic. The most common of these are:

- Nickel jewelry or snaps on jeans or pants
- Certain flavorings or additives to toothpastes and mouthwashes (These cause a rash around or in the mouth.)
- Glues, dyes, or leather used in the manufacture of shoes (They produce a reaction on the tops of the toes and feet.)
- Dyes used in clothing (These cause rashes in areas where the clothing rubs or where there is increased perspiration.)
- Plants, especially poison ivy, poison oak, and poison sumac. This rash usually appears within several hours after contact (one to three days with poison ivy); as well as being itchy, it may cause small blisters.
- Medications such as neomycin ointment

Treatment

If your baby has a rash that looks like eczema, your pediatrician will need to examine it to make the correct diagnosis and prescribe the proper treatment. In some cases he may arrange for a pediatric dermatologist to examine it.

Although there is no cure for eczema, it generally can be well controlled and often will go away after several months or years. The most effective treatment is to prevent the skin from becoming dry and itchy and to avoid substances that cause the condition to flare. To do this:

- **Use skin moisturizers** (e.g., creams or ointments) regularly and frequently to decrease the dryness and itchiness.
- **Give your baby** frequent soaking baths in lukewarm water. After a bath, rinse twice to remove any residual soap (which might be an irritant). Then apply the cream or ointment within three minutes of getting out of the bath to lock in the moisture.
- **Avoid harsh or** irritating clothing (wool or coarse-weave material).
- **If there is** oozing or exceptional itching, use tepid (lukewarm) compresses on the area, followed by the application of prescribed medications.

There are many types of medicated prescription creams and ointments available, so ask your pediatrician to suggest one that he prefers to control inflammation and itching. These preparations often contain a form of cortisone, but there are also several types of nonsteroidal medications. These creams or ointments should be used on an as-needed or daily basis, but only under the direction of your baby's doctor. In addition, other lotions or bath oils might be prescribed. It's important to continue to apply the medications for as long as your pediatrician recommends their use. Stopping too soon will cause the condition to recur.

In addition to the skin preparations, your baby also may need to take an antihistamine by mouth to control the itching, and antibiotics (sometimes by mouth and sometimes as a cream) if the skin becomes infected.

Treating allergic contact dermatitis is similar, although your pediatric dermatologist or allergist also will want to find the cause of the rash by taking a careful history or by conducting a series of patch tests. These tests are done by placing small patches of common irritants (or allergens) against your infant's skin. If the skin reacts with redness and itching, that substance should be avoided.

Alert your pediatrician if any of the following occurs:

- Your baby's rash is severe and is not responding to home treatment.
- There is any evidence of fever or infection (i.e., blisters, redness, yellow crusts, pain, or oozing of fluid).
- The rash spreads or another rash develops.

Food Allergy

While many foods can cause allergic reactions, true food allergies are less common than you might think. Currently, they affect 2 percent of the general population and 6 to 8 percent of children.

Food allergies are most likely to happen in infants and children younger than six years old, as well as in children with other allergies or whose family members (parents, siblings) have allergies. When food allergies do occur, they may be in response to any food, although particular items are more likely to cause reactions (see the list below). While food allergies cause only mild symptoms in many cases, they can trigger more serious reactions in some children, and in very rare instances, even be life-threatening.

While any food can trigger a food allergy, several cause the vast majority of cases in children. Cow's milk is among them (see *Milk Allergy,* page 485). Other common foods associated with allergies include:

- Eggs
- Soy
- Wheat

- Fish (such as tuna, salmon, and cod) and shellfish (such as shrimp, crab, and lobster)
- Chocolate

If your baby has a food allergy, her immune system responds in an exaggerated way to otherwise harmless proteins in foods. When this food is consumed, her immune system manufactures antibodies that attempt to fight off the "offending" food. In the process, substances called "histamines" and other chemicals (called "mediators") are released that cause allergic symptoms. However, you may be able to reduce your baby's likelihood of ever developing food allergies by exclusively breastfeeding her for a minimum of four months, but preferably for six months or more (see also *How Allergies Develop,* below).

Another condition, called *food intolerance* or *food sensitivity,* occurs more often than true food allergies. Although the terms are often confused and sometimes used interchangeably, food intolerance is a digestive problem that is triggered by food but does not involve the immune system. For example, a baby with lactose intolerance (a condition of food sensitivity) is deficient in an enzyme required to digest milk sugar, leading to stomachaches, bloating, and diarrhea.

How Allergies Develop

If your child has a tendency to develop allergies, he probably has inherited it from you and your spouse. When an allergic-prone child is exposed to an allergen, his immune system produces an antibody (called IgE) in a process called allergic sensitization. Then the IgE sticks to so-called mast cells in the skin and the linings of the airways, stomach, and intestines. The next time she comes in contact with allergens, these cells release chemicals (e.g., histamine and leukotrienes) that cause allergic symptoms.

Symptoms

While food intolerance may produce gas, bloating, and abdominal pain, a true food allergy is more likely to develop suddenly, with symptoms such as a rash, hives, vomiting, or stomach pain soon after eating, as well as chronic skin or stomach problems. Symptoms like these should make you and your pediatrician suspect that a food allergy is present.

Specific indications of a possible food allergy in some babies include:

- Skin problems (itchy skin rashes, hives, swelling)
- Breathing problems (sneezing, wheezing, throat tightness)
- Stomach problems (nausea, vomiting, diarrhea)
- Circulation problems (pale skin, light-headedness, loss of consciousness)

While most babies do have an immediate reaction to certain foods within minutes, others may have symptoms that are delayed for up to two hours or, in rare cases, even days. The intensity of the allergic reaction can range from mild to severe, with its strength intensified if several areas of the body are affected. At the same time, if your baby is highly allergic, even small amounts of the food can trigger a violent and potentially dangerous allergic response.

Fortunately, the most severe reactions to food—called anaphylactic reactions—are very rare. But when they occur, they can develop without warning, progress rapidly, and must be treated immediately. They may trigger symptoms such as:

- Swelling of the throat and tongue
- Difficulty breathing
- Wheezing
- A sudden drop in blood pressure
- Swelling in the head and neck
- Turning blue
- Loss of consciousness

(See the box, *Anaphylactic Reactions: What You Should Do,* on page 479.)

Sometimes the acids in foods, such as in orange juice or tomato products, can cause reactions like a rash around the mouth that is mistaken for food allergies. Certain other conditions can be confused with food allergies as well, such as food poisoning that is usually caused by bacteria in spoiled or undercooked food, and that can trigger diarrhea or vomiting. Also, when small children consume too much sugar in fruit juices, they may develop diarrhea, which might be mistaken for an allergic reaction.

Diagnosis and Management

Because some food allergies can be serious, talk to your pediatrician if you suspect that your baby has one. To help make the diagnosis, your pediatrician will review your concerns and may perform some tests or refer you to an allergist, who may recommend additional testing. Sometimes the presence of a food allergy is obvious, like when a baby gets hives and lip swelling after eating an orange. But some tests, including a skin prick test and blood tests, can confirm your doctor's suspicions:

- With the *skin prick test* (or *scratch test*), the doctor will place a drop of a liquid extract of the suspicious food on your child's back or forearm. Then he'll make a tiny, painless scratch on the skin, allowing a bit of the substance to enter the skin. If your baby is allergic to this food, she may experience a reaction such as swelling or itching at the site within fifteen minutes.

- **A blood test** can measure allergic antibodies to foods as well; these antibodies are called immunoglobulin E, or IgE. A sample of your baby's blood will be drawn and sent to the laboratory, where it will be mixed with a number of food extracts to see if antibodies to that food develop. Results are usually available in one to two weeks.

Although your pediatrician or allergist may recommend these tests, they are not perfect tests. Your doctor should discuss with you the specifics of your baby's diet, including any of your concerns about reactions to particular foods, to know what tests to consider and how to interpret the results. He may ask you to keep a diary of everything your child eats and whether she appears to respond to foods with any symptoms. Make a note of this in the diary and let your allergist and pediatrician know.

In some children, the allergist may recommend placing them on an "elimination diet." You'll be asked to remove for a period of time those foods that are suspected of causing your child's allergic symptoms, and then you'll monitor whether symptoms subside when those foods are no longer being eaten. Several weeks later, the foods can be returned to your child's meals, one at a time, and you can determine whether symptoms have come back when a particular food is consumed again. This elimination diet should be done only under the guidance of an allergist or your pediatrician to ensure that your child is still receiving proper nutrition. In addition, sometimes returning a specific food to the diet requires a doctor-supervised feeding test; some allergists might even want to watch your child eat certain foods to see how her body reacts.

The main way to treat food allergies is to simply avoid foods that cause them. For example, if an allergy to eggs has been detected, your pediatrician or allergist may urge you to avoid feeding them to your child until she is older, when your doctor may recommend retesting your child to see if she is still allergic. Even though egg allergies are caused by a protein present only in egg whites, the yolks can become contaminated with egg whites, and thus it is safer to avoid this food entirely early in life, including products that contain eggs.

Even once you're successful in keeping allergy-prone foods out of your refrigerator and off your dining room table, it may be more difficult to keep your baby away from those items when she is out of your care. As your child gets older you'll have to educate her, as well as her friends and their parents, teachers, and child care workers, about the importance of avoiding specific foods that could trigger allergy symptoms. Every time you shop, read food labels and look for major allergens that your baby is allergic to such as eggs, milk, peanuts, and wheat. Also, when your family is eating in restaurants, ask questions about the ingredients of menu items. While the waiter may be helpful, confirm the information by speaking with the chef.

As you make adjustments in your baby's diet, talk to your pediatrician regularly about compensating for the missing foods and keeping her diet balanced. For example, if your child is allergic to milk, you will need to include other calcium-rich foods (like green leafy vegetables and calcium-fortified drinks) in her diet.

Keep in mind that there is no "cure" for food allergies, and no medication to treat them, although avoidance of certain foods can effectively keep them under control. Fortunately, children often outgrow allergies with the maturing of their immune systems. With the passage of time, problem foods like eggs and milk can be reintroduced into the diet. However, do so only with your doctor's consent and guidance. Certain food allergies—like those to peanuts and fish—are less likely to be "outgrown." At some point, your pediatrician may decide to repeat allergy testing to confirm whether particular food allergies have run their course.

HIVES

If your baby has an itchy rash that consists of raised red bumpy areas, perhaps with pale centers and no flaking skin over the lesions, he probably has hives. This rash may look like mosquito bites, and can occur all over the body or just in one region, such as the face. The location may change, with the hives disappearing in one area of the body and appearing in another, often in a matter of hours.

Among the most common causes of hives are:

- Response to an infection, most commonly a virus
- Foods (most commonly egg whites, milk, shellfish, and sesame)
- Medications, either over-the-counter or prescription
- Bites or stings from bees or other insects

In at least half of the cases, it is not possible to identify the cause.

Anaphylactic Reactions: What You Should Do

An anaphylactic reaction is always an emergency. It is potentially fatal, and requires immediate medical attention. If symptoms such as swelling of the face or throat and wheezing occur, call 911 or go to the emergency department immediately. To avoid such problems from ever occurring, make sure your child does not eat any food that has previously caused such a reaction. In the case of an insect sting causing a serious reaction, make sure she stays away from such insects that may cause serious stings.

If your baby has had an anaphylactic reaction or is susceptible to one, your pediatrician will strongly recommend that you keep a prescribed emergency injectable medication (called epinephrine, that is packaged in penlike form), to be administered using a preloaded auto-injector. For infants prone to severe reactions, these devices (which go by names such as EpiPen or Twinject) should be kept on hand at all times. When used properly and promptly, they can control the most serious reactions and allow you enough time to get to an emergency room for further treatment. In most cases, they reduce symptoms rapidly, but if they don't, another injection should be given in five to thirty minutes.

To use an auto-injector, you'll press the device against your baby's thigh, and hold it there for a few seconds. Make sure to ask your doctor or nurse to give you precise instructions on its use. At the same time, your child care center should have written instructions on how to recognize and react to a severe allergic reaction that may be life-threatening; and epinephrine should be available to them, along with a step-by-step guide on how to administer it. Keep in mind that unused medication in these auto-injectors should be replaced at regular intervals, so check the expiration date and replace them as recommended by your doctor.

If your baby has an anaphylactic reaction, see your pediatrician afterward, and find out exactly why the reaction happened and how to avoid another one. Your child should also wear a medical identification bracelet if she has had an anaphylactic episode in the past. This bracelet should give information about the allergies that your baby has.

Treatment

An oral antihistamine should relieve or at least help reduce the itching of hives. It can be obtained without a prescription. You may need to use this type of medication for several days. Some of this medicine may need to be given to your baby as often as every four to six hours while others can be given once or twice a day. Applying cool compresses to the area of itching and swelling also may help.

Other treatments may be necessary if internal parts of the body are involved in the allergic reaction. If your child is wheezing or having trouble swallowing, seek emergency treatment. The doctor usually will prescribe a more effective antihistamine and may even give an injection of epinephrine to stop the allergic response. If the allergy causing the hives also results in severe breathing difficulties, your pediatrician will help you obtain a special emergency injection kit containing epinephrine for possible use at home, or in child care, in case of such reactions in the future. (For more information about these emergency kits, see the box *Anaphylactic Reactions: What You Should Do,* above.)

Prevention

In order to prevent subsequent outbreaks of hives, your doctor will try to determine what is causing the allergic reaction. If the rash is confined to a small area of skin, it probably was caused by something your baby touched. (Plants and soaps are frequent culprits.) But if it spreads all over her body, something she ingested (a food or medication) or possibly an infection is most likely to blame.

Often the pattern to the appearance of the hives provides a clue to the allergy. For example, does it usually happen after meals? Does it seem to occur more during certain seasons, or when traveling to particular places? If you discover a specific pattern, alter your routine to see if your baby improves. Sometimes hives will occur if your child eats an unusually large amount of a food to which she is only mildly allergic. If you discover the cause of the problem, try keeping her away from it as much as possible.

INSECT BITES AND STINGS

Your baby's reaction to a bite or sting will depend on her sensitivity to the particular insect's venom. While most babies have only mild reactions, those who are allergic to certain insect venoms can have severe symptoms that require emergency treatment.

In general, bites are usually not a serious problem, but in some cases, stings may be. While it is true that most stings (from yellow jackets, wasps, and fire ants, for example) may cause pain and localized swelling, severe anaphylactic reactions are possible, although uncommon.

Treatment

Although insect bites can be irritating, they usually begin to disappear by the next day and do not require a doctor's treatment. To relieve the itchiness that accompanies bites by mosquitoes, flies, fleas, and bedbugs, apply a cool compress and/or calamine lotion freely on any part of your baby's body *except* the areas around her eyes and genitals. If your baby is stung by a wasp or bee, soak a cloth in cold water and press it over the area of the sting to reduce pain and swelling. Call your pediatrician before using any other treatment, including creams or lotions containing antihistamines or home remedies. If the itching is severe, the doctor may prescribe oral antihistamines.

If your baby disturbs a beehive, get him away from it as quickly as possible. The base of a honeybee's stinger emits an alarm pheromone (hormone) that makes other bees more likely to sting as well.

It is very important to remove a bee stinger quickly and completely from the skin. The quick removal of a bee stinger will prevent a large amount of venom from being pumped into the skin. If the stinger is visible, remove it by gently scraping it off horizontally with a credit card or your fingernail. Avoid squeezing the stinger with a pair of tweezers; doing this may release more venom into the skin. The skin may be more swollen on the second or third day after a bee sting or mosquito bite.

Keep your baby's fingernails short and clean to minimize the risk of infection from scratching. If infection does occur, the bite will become redder, larger, and more swollen. In some cases you may notice red streaks or yellowish fluid near the bite or your child may get a fever. Have your pediatrician examine any infected bite right away, because it may need to be treated with antibiotics.

Call for medical help immediately if your baby has any of these other symptoms after being bitten or stung:

- Sudden difficulty in breathing
- Weakness, collapse, or unconsciousness
- Hives or itching all over the body
- Extreme swelling near the eyes, lips, or penis that makes it difficult for the baby to see, eat, or urinate

Prevention

Some babies with no other known allergies may have severe reactions to insect stings. But if you suspect that your baby is allergy-prone, discuss the situation with your doctor. He may recommend a series of shots (hyposensitization injections) to decrease your baby's reaction to future insect stings (but not bites). In addition, he will prescribe a special auto-injection kit containing epinephrine for you to keep on hand for use if your baby is stung (see the box *Anaphylactic Reactions: What You Should Do* on page 479).

It is impossible to prevent all insect bites, but you can minimize the number your baby receives by following these guidelines.

- Avoid areas where insects nest or congregate, such as garbage cans, stagnant pools of water, uncovered foods and sweets, and orchards and gardens where flowers are in bloom.
- When you know your baby will be exposed to insects, dress her in long pants and a lightweight long-sleeved shirt.
- Avoid dressing your baby in clothing with bright colors or flowery prints, because they seem to attract insects.
- Don't use scented soaps, perfumes, or hair sprays on your baby, because they also are inviting to insects.

Insect repellents are generally available without a prescription, but they should be used sparingly on infants and young babies. In fact, the most common insecticides include DEET (N,N-diethyl-m-toluamide), which is a chemical *not* recommended for use in children under two months of age. Do not apply DEET-containing repellents more than once a day on older children.

The concentrations of DEET vary significantly from product to product—ranging from less than 10 percent to over 30 percent—so read the label of any product you purchase. Some products have concentrations much higher than 30 percent, and the higher the concentration of DEET, the longer the duration of action. Its effectiveness peaks at a concentration of 30 percent, however, which is also *the maximum concentration currently recommended for children*. The safety of DEET does not appear to be related to its level of concentration; therefore, a prudent approach is to select the lowest effective concentration for the amount of time your baby spends outdoors. You should avoid products that include DEET plus a sunscreen, because sunscreen needs to be applied frequently while DEET should be applied only once a day. If you apply DEET more frequently, it may be associated with toxicity. Also be sure to wash off the DEET with soap and water at the end of the day.

An alternative to DEET is a product called picaridin (KBR 3023). While it has had wider use in Europe, picaridin has more recently become available in the U.S. It is a generally pleasant-smelling product without the oil residue associated

Insect Bites and Stings

Insect/ Environment	Characteristics of Bite or Sting	Special Notes
Mosquitoes Water (pools, lakes, birdbaths)	Stinging sensation followed by small, red, itchy mound with tiny puncture mark at center.	Mosquitoes are attracted by bright colors and sweat.
Flies Food, garbage, animal waste	Painful, itchy bumps; may turn into small blisters.	Bites often disappear in a day but may last longer.
Fleas Cracks in floor, rugs, pet fur	Multiple small bumps clustered together; often where clothes fit tightly (waist, buttocks).	Fleas are most likely to be a problem in homes with pets.
Bedbugs Cracks of walls, floors, crevices of furniture, bedding	Itchy red bumps occasionally topped by a blister; usually 2–3 in a row.	Bedbugs are most likely to bite at night and are less active in cold weather.
Fire ants Mounds in pastures, meadows, lawns, and parks in southern states	Immediate pain and burning; swelling up to ½ inch (1.2 cm); cloudy fluid in area of bite.	Fire ants usually attack intruders.

Bees and wasps Flowers, shrubs, picnic areas, beaches	Immediate pain and rapid swelling.	A few children have severe reactions, such as difficulty breathing and hives/swelling all over the body.
Ticks Wooded areas	May not be noticeable; hidden on hair or on skin.	Don't remove ticks with matches, lighted cigarettes, or nail polish remover; grasp the tick firmly with tweezers near the head; gently pull the tick straight out.

with DEET, and is available in concentrations of 5 to 10 percent.

The American Academy of Pediatrics recommends that repellents used in babies over six months of age have 30 percent DEET or 5 to 10 percent picaridin repellent, applied once before going outdoors. These repellents are effective in preventing bites by mosquitoes, ticks, fleas, chiggers, and biting flies, but have virtually no effect on stinging insects such as bees, hornets, and wasps. Contrary to popular belief, giving antihistamines continuously throughout the insect season does not appear to prevent reactions to bites.

The adjacent table summarizes information about common stinging or biting insects.

MILK ALLERGY

A true milk protein allergy usually appears in the first year of life, when an infant's digestive system is still quite immature.

Symptoms

Milk allergy symptoms may appear anywhere from a few minutes to a few hours after the baby consumes a milk product, but the most severe symptoms usually occur within half an hour. The most common symptoms are:

- Rashes
- Gastrointestinal/stomach upset
- Vomiting and/or diarrhea (see pages 458 and 440)

Less common symptoms include blood in the stool.

In babies, if the milk allergy affects their respiratory system, they also may have chronic nasal stuffiness, a runny nose, cough, wheezing, or difficulty in breathing. The allergy also can cause eczema, hives, swelling, itching, or a rash around the mouth and on the chin due to contact with milk. (See *Cough,* page 497; *Eczema,* page 470; *Hives,* page 478.)

If you suspect your baby has an allergy to milk, tell your pediatrician, and be sure to mention whether there's a family history of allergy. Take your infant to the doctor's office or emergency room *immediately* if he

- Has difficulty breathing
- Turns blue
- Is extremely pale or weak
- Has generalized hives
- Develops swelling in the head and neck region
- Has bloody diarrhea

Treatment

Breastfed babies. If your breastfed infant develops a milk allergy, your pediatrician may recommend that you follow a milk-free diet yourself. (You should take an extra calcium supplement in addition to the prenatal vitamin that you are already taking.) As you wean your baby, delay feeding him cow's milk as long as possible, and give it very cautiously at first, at the direction of your doctor.

Formula-fed babies. Infants with milk allergy should be given alternatives like soy formula or elemental formula, according to your pediatrician's guidelines. Ask your doctor to recommend a brand of hypoallergenic formula made with extensive hydrolysate protein, which is processed in a way to avoid allergic reactions. He can not only offer guidance on which formulas to select, but also where to buy them (they're not available in all stores). (Also see *Choosing a Formula,* pages 131–133).

As your baby gets older, and if your pediatrician suspects that a milk allergy is present, first he will try eliminating milk and milk products completely for a period of time to see if there is any improvement. If there is, your child may then be given a milk trial—that is, a controlled introduction of milk to the diet. This will reveal whether the symptoms decrease or disappear when milk is avoided and if they reappear when it's introduced again. *This trial of milk should be carried out cautiously and under the supervision of a doctor; don't experiment by trying to introduce milk on your own—talk with your pediatrician.* Infants who are allergic to milk can become sick quickly, even if exposed to only a small amount.

Your pediatrician can use several appropriate medications to treat a reaction to milk; these include antihistamines and antiasthma medication (if wheezing is among your child's allergy symptoms). However, the main "treatment" is to eliminate milk and milk products from the diet. Most children eventually will outgrow the allergy by ages two to five years; this allergy seldom lasts until adolescence.

By the way, be sure to tell all of your baby's caregivers (including babysitters and those in child care settings) of your child's milk allergy so he is not given milk by mistake.

Prevention

As mentioned earlier, breastfeeding a baby is the best way to prevent a milk allergy from developing in a newborn. Particularly if anyone in your immediate family is allergy-prone, you should plan to breastfeed your baby; research has shown that breastfeeding for at least four months (some recommend exclusive breastfeeding to six months or longer) can prevent or delay the development of allergies to cow's milk. When you eventually introduce other foods to your baby, you'll want to do it gradually (a new one at one- or two-week intervals), watching for the signs of allergy.

If you cannot breastfeed, ask your pediatrician to guide you in selecting an appropriate formula (as discussed above).

14

BEHAVIOR

There are many times when your baby's behavior warms and embraces your heart. But there are other times when it probably drives you a little crazy. From temper tantrums to dancing around your living room, she's expressing her feelings and needs, although not always in ways that you'd prefer.

Your child's behavior is partly innate; in a real sense, she was born to act this way. In fact, every baby has her own temperament. For example, some infants are very active and engaged with the world around them, seemingly from the moment of birth. But others are quite different, and are much quieter. As you read earlier, neither type of temperament is "better" than the other—both are normal and occur in perfectly healthy infants—but their unique temperament can set them apart from other children, including their own siblings. They may be easygoing, not seeking much attention, and may sleep for long stretches at a time. But if their temperament is different, they may be much more strong-willed, demanding, and fussy than you'd like, and their erratic sleep habits may leave you more bleary-eyed than you'd prefer; along the way, you may feel that your own patience and parenting skills are being challenged at every turn.

If your baby was born prematurely, it may take longer for these character traits to become apparent. But once you become familiar with your baby's temperament, you may feel the need to make some adjustments in the way you relate to her. Remember, your baby is an individual, and you should respect her personality and uniqueness. But talk to your pediatrician if there are concerns about her temperament.

For more information about temperament, see chapters 6 (page 199) and 8 (page 277).

Stranger Anxiety

Not surprisingly, your baby has become very connected to you. So don't be surprised if she breaks into tears when you leave the room at times, or when she encounters an unfamiliar face. When strangers get too close—even relatives or babysitters who she once seemed comfortable with—she may become anxious and cry out for you.

Don't be upset as your baby moves through this stage (typically starting at about eight to nine months of age); it's a normal part of her development. Be patient, even though it may be unsettling for you to watch—and perhaps upsetting for Grandma when your baby shies away from her. But it will run its course, often during the second year of life.

For more information about stranger anxiety (as well as separation anxiety), see pages 264 and 320.

MEDIA USE: TELEVISION AND COMPUTERS

Your child may view his first television program during infancy. When she's older, a TV set and/or DVD could become an important part of her life and will teach her many life lessons—some positive and some negative.

The same can be said about computers and young children. As she grows computers and the Internet will give her unprecedented access to knowledge and information. But at the same time, you should be involved in your child's use of both the Internet and TV. She needs your experience, judgment, and supervision.

Television When your baby's verbal skills start to expand, she can benefit a great deal from watching educational television programming such as *Sesame Street,* nature programs, and concerts or dances. But during infancy and later in childhood, educational TV is not a substitute for reading, playing, or problem-solving.

However, if your baby is exposed to typical television programming, she will absorb some negative messages. She'll

Where We Stand

The first two years of your child's life are especially important in the growth and development of her brain. During this time, babies and toddlers need positive interaction with other children and adults. This is especially true at these younger ages, when learning to talk and play with others is so important.

Until more research is done about the effects of screen time on very young children, the American Academy of Pediatrics strongly discourages television viewing for children ages two years old or younger, and encourages interactive play. For older children, the Academy advises no more than one to two hours per day of educational, nonviolent programs, which should be supervised by parents or other responsible adults in the home.

frequently see characters hitting, shooting, or otherwise harming each other. Television also exposes children to sexuality, drugs, and alcohol at a time when they are too young to understand the consequences of these issues.

Children who watch a great deal of television are more likely to become obese than are children who watch less and tend to be more physically active. All children need active play, not only for the physical exercise but also for proper mental and social development. Watching TV is passive. It does not help your child acquire the most important skills and experiences she needs such as communication, creativity, fantasy, judgment, and experimentation. The more time your child spends in front of a TV set, the less she'll have left for other, more worthwhile activities.

What You Can Do

Media-wise children and families are equipped to enjoy the positive benefits of television and to minimize the negative effects. Media education includes smart, limited TV time in your home, plus an understanding of how TV programming and advertising work.

As a general policy, the American Academy of Pediatrics advises against *any* TV viewing up to the age of two years. These guidelines apply not only to television, but to videos, movies, and computer games. Never allow the TV to become a babysitter.

Where We Stand

Although the American Academy of Pediatrics does not hold television solely responsible for violence in our society, we believe that televised violence has a clear effect on the behavior of children and contributes to the frequency with which violence is used to resolve conflict. Television also distorts reality on matters such as drugs, alcohol, tobacco, sexuality, and family relations.

The primary goal of commercial children's television is to sell products—from toys to food—to children. Young children in particular cannot distinguish between programs and their commercials, nor do they fully understand that commercials are designed to sell them (and their parents) something.

Together, parents, broadcasters, and advertisers must be held responsible for the television that children see. The American Academy of Pediatrics strongly supports legislative efforts to improve the quality of children's programming. We urge parents to limit the amount of TV that their children view, to monitor what their children are watching, and to watch TV with them to help them learn from what they see.

THUMB AND FINGER SUCKING

Do not be upset if your baby begins sucking his thumb or fingers. This habit is very common and has a soothing and calming effect. Some experts feel that one half or more of all children engage in this activity at some time in their early life. It is largely the result of the normal rooting and sucking reflexes present in all infants at birth. There is evidence that some infants suck their thumbs and fingers even before delivery, and some, particularly finger suckers, will show that behavior immediately after being born.

By definition, a habit is a pattern of behavior that's repeated, and the baby is not even aware that he's doing it. Of course, parents are very aware of it, and many of them worry. But habits like thumb sucking (as well as body rocking or head banging) often calm the baby when he's feeling stress or fatigue. Because sucking is a normal reflex, thumb and finger sucking can be considered a normal habit.

All babies have habits, and the only time thumb or finger sucking should cause you concern is if it continues too long or affects the shape of your baby's mouth or the alignment of his teeth. Over half of thumb or finger suckers stop by age six or seven months.

15

Chest and Lungs

Bronchiolitis

Bronchiolitis is an infection of the small breathing tubes (bronchioles) of the lungs. It occurs most often in infants. (Note: The term *bronchiolitis* sometimes is confused with bronchitis, which is an infection of the larger, more central airways.)

Bronchiolitis is caused by a virus, most commonly the respiratory syncytial virus (RSV). However, several other viruses can cause this condition, including parainfluenza, influenza, and adenovirus. The infection causes inflammation and swelling of the bronchioles, which in turn causes obstruction of air flowing in and out of the lungs.

Most adults and older children who are infected by RSV get only a cold. In infants, however, the infection is more likely to lead to bronchiolitis. It also may cause apnea, which occurs when the baby stops breathing temporarily for more than ten seconds. This most commonly occurs in babies who were born prematurely. Many infants who develop RSV bronchiolitis go on to develop asthma during the first decade of life.

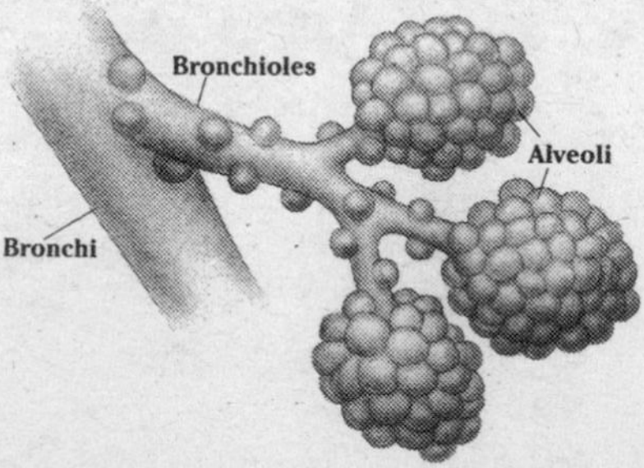

In most parts of the U.S., RSV occurs from October or November through March. During the other months, bronchiolitis usually is caused by other viruses.

RSV is highly contagious and can last on surfaces for several hours. It is spread by contact with an infected person, and can spread easily through families, child care centers, and hospital wards. Careful hand-washing and alcohol hand sanitizers are the best ways to prevent spreading the infection.

Signs and Symptoms

Almost all children get an RSV infection by the time they are three years old. The majority of them develop only an upper respiratory infection (a cold) with a runny nose, mild cough, and sometimes fever, but a small number of infants go on to develop bronchiolitis. After a day or two, the cough becomes more pronounced, and the infant begins to breathe more rapidly and with more difficulty.

If your baby shows any of the following signs of breathing difficulty, or if his fever lasts more than three days (or if it is present at all in an infant under three months), call your pediatrician immediately.

- He makes a high-pitched whistling sound, called a wheeze, each time he breathes out or exhales.
- He may be unable to drink fluids well because he is working so hard to breathe that he has difficulty sucking and swallowing.
- He may develop a bluish tint around his lips and fingertips. This indicates that his airways are so blocked that not enough oxygen is getting into his lungs and subsequently into the blood.

Also call the pediatrician if your baby develops any of the following signs or symptoms of dehydration, which also can appear with bronchiolitis.

- Dry mouth
- Taking less than his normal amount of fluids

- Shedding no tears when he cries
- Urinating less often than normal

If your baby has any of the following conditions, notify your pediatrician as soon as you suspect that he has bronchiolitis.

- Cystic fibrosis
- Congenital heart disease
- Bronchopulmonary dysplasia, seen in some infants who were born prematurely or were on a respirator (breathing machine) as newborns
- Low immunity
- Organ transplant
- Cancer for which he is receiving chemotherapy

Home Treatment

There are no medications to treat RSV infections at home. All you can do during the early phase of the illness is ease your baby's cold symptoms. You can relieve some of the nasal stuffiness with a humidifier and nasal saline drops with or without nasal aspiration.

Also, to avoid dehydration, make sure your baby drinks lots of fluid during this time. (See *Diarrhea,* page 440.) He may prefer clear liquids rather than milk or formula. Because of his breathing difficulty, he also may feed more slowly or eat smaller amounts more frequently, and may not tolerate solid foods very well.

Professional Treatment

If your baby is having mild to moderate breathing difficulty, your pediatrician may try using a bronchodilating medication (one that opens up the breathing tubes), often given by a breathing machine (nebulizer), before considering hospitalization. These drugs seem to help a small number of patients.

Bronchiolitis is the most common reason that infants are hospitalized, either because their breathing is very difficult, they cannot eat normally, or they need to be treated with oxygen and bronchodilating medications. Very rarely, an infant will not respond to these treatments and might have to be placed on a breathing machine (respirator) to help his lungs and body get enough oxygen. This treatment usually is only a temporary measure to help him until his body is able to overcome the infection.

Prevention

The best way to protect your baby from bronchiolitis is to keep him away from the viruses that cause it. When possible, especially while he's an infant, avoid close contact with children or adults who are in the early (contagious) stages of respiratory infections. If he is in a child care center where other children might have the virus, make sure that those who care for him wash their hands thoroughly and frequently.

There are medications that your pediatrician may prescribe that could reduce the risk of developing serious RSV infection. These medications are used only for the small number of babies who are in the highest risk groups for hospitalization. The AAP has developed specific criteria for use of these medications. Ask your pediatrician regarding specific details on who is at highest risk and which high-risk infants are most likely to benefit from receipt of these medications.

Cough

Coughing is almost always an indication of an irritation in your baby's air passages. When the nerve endings in the throat, windpipe, or lungs sense the irritation, a reflex causes air to be ejected forcefully through the passageways.

Coughs usually are associated with respiratory illnesses, such as colds/upper respiratory infection (see page 554), asthma (see page 463), bronchiolitis (see page 494), croup (see page 500), flu (see page 502), or pneumonia (see page 505). If your baby's cough is accompanied by fever, irritability, or difficulty breathing, he probably has such an infection.

When a baby has a cold, the cough may sound wet (productive or congested), or dry and irritating. The cough may last longer than the accompanying runny nose. If he has a cough, a fever, and difficulty breathing (too fast, too slow, noisy, pulling in of the chest muscles), he may have pneumonia. If he has these symptoms, see your doctor immediately.

To a large extent, the location of the problem determines the sound of the cough: An irritation in the larynx (voice box), such as croup, causes a cough that sounds like the bark of a dog or seal. Irritation of the larger airways, such as the trachea (windpipe) or bronchi, is a deeper, raspy cough that gets worse in the morning.

Allergies and sinus infections can cause a chronic cough because mucus drips down the back of the throat, producing a dry, hard-to-stop cough, particularly at night. An infant who coughs only at night may have asthma (see page 463) or gastroesophageal reflux (a condition where the contents of the stomach rise up into the esophagus causing irritation and cough).

Here are some other cough-related issues in the lives of babies:

- **Anything more than** an occasional cough in an infant has to be taken seriously. The most common causes are colds and bronchiolitis, which usually get better in a few days. It is important to watch for signs of breathing difficulties and seek medical help if needed. These signs include not only rapid breathing, especially while asleep, but also drawing in of the skin between and around the ribs and breastbone (sternum).

- **Sometimes babies cough** so hard that they throw up. Usually they vomit liquid and food from the stomach, but there may be a lot of mucus as well, especially during a cold or an asthma attack.

- **Wheezing is a** high-pitched sound during breathing that occurs when there is an obstruction of the airway inside the chest. It is one of the symptoms of asthma, but also can occur if your baby has bronchiolitis, pneumonia, or certain other disorders.

- **Infants with asthma** often cough and wheeze together. This may happen when they are active or playing, or at night. Sometimes their cough can be heard, but the wheezing may be evident only to your doctor when she listens with a stethoscope. The cough and the wheeze usually get better after using asthma medications.

- **A cough is** commonly worse at night. When your baby coughs at night, it may be caused by irritation in the throat or a sinus infection. Asthma is another major reason for a nighttime cough.

- **A sudden cough** can develop in babies who are choking. It could mean that some food or liquid has "gone down the wrong way" and ended up in the lungs. The coughing helps clear the airways. However, if coughing continues for more than a few minutes, or if your infant is having difficulty breathing, seek medical help right away. Don't put your fingers in your baby's mouth to clear the throat because you may push the food or other cause of the obstruction down farther. (See *Choking*, page 576.)

When to Call the Pediatrician

An infant under two months of age who develops a cough should be seen by the doctor. For older infants and children, consult your physician immediately if the coughing:

- Makes it difficult for your baby to breathe.
- Is painful, persistent, and accompanied by whooping, vomiting, or turning blue.
- Interferes with eating and sleeping.
- Appears suddenly and is associated with a fever.
- Begins after your infant chokes on food or any other object. (See *Choking*, page 576.) In about 50 percent of cases, when a foreign body (food or toy) is inhaled into the bronchi and lungs the cough may develop a few hours or days later.

Your pediatrician will try to determine the cause of your baby's cough. When the cough is from a medical problem other than a cold or the flu, such as a bacterial infection or asthma, it will be necessary to treat that condition before the cough will clear. Occasionally when the cause of a chronic cough is not apparent, further tests such as chest X-rays or tuberculosis skin tests may be necessary.

Treatment

Treating a cough depends on its cause. But whatever the cause, it is always a good idea to give extra fluids. Adding moisture to the air with a humidifier or vaporizer also may make your child more comfortable, especially at night.

However, be sure to clean the device thoroughly with detergent and water each morning, so it doesn't become a breeding ground for harmful bacteria or fungi.

Nighttime coughs, particularly those associated with allergies or asthma, can be especially annoying, because they occur when everyone is trying to sleep. In some cases it may help to elevate the head of the baby's bed. If the night cough is due to asthma, use a bronchodilator or other asthma medication as directed by your pediatrician.

Although cough medicines can be purchased without a prescription, the Food and Drug Administration (FDA) recommends that over-the-counter cough medicines should not be given to children under two years of age because of serious and life-threatening side effects. Also several studies show that these products don't work in children younger than six years of age and can have potentially serious side effects.

CROUP

Croup is an inflammation of the voice box (larynx) and windpipe (trachea). It causes a barking cough and a high-pitched sound when breathing in. Although croup is sometimes associated with allergies, it usually is caused by a virus, most commonly the parainfluenza virus. The illness most often is "caught" from someone who is infected, sometimes from air droplets or from your baby's own hand, which he uses to transfer the virus into his nose or eyes.

Croup tends to occur in the fall and winter when your child is between three months and three years old. Initially he may develop nasal stuffiness resembling a cold, and he may have a fever. After a day or two, the sound of the cough

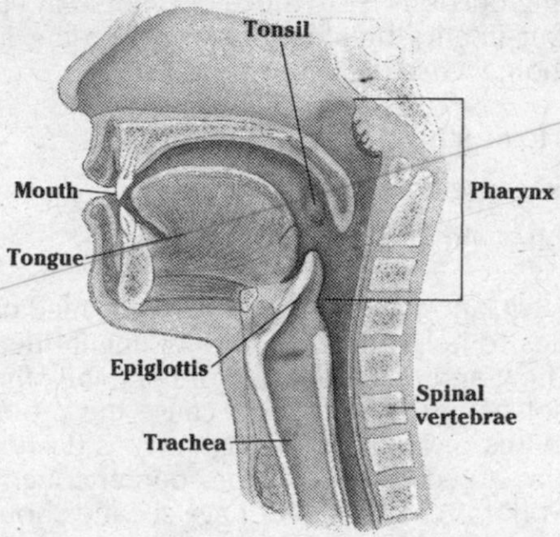

will turn into something resembling barking. The cough tends to become worse at night.

The greatest danger with croup is that your child's airway will continue to swell, further narrowing his windpipe and making it difficult, at times almost impossible, to breathe. As your baby tires from the effort of breathing, he may stop eating and drinking. He also may become too fatigued to cough. Some children are particularly prone to getting a crouplike cough and seem to develop such a cough whenever they have a respiratory illness.

Treatment

If your infant has mild croup symptoms, steam up the bathroom by turning on hot water in the shower, take her into the steamy bathroom, close the door, and sit in the bathroom with your baby. Inhaling the warm, humidified air should ease her breathing within fifteen to twenty minutes. Or, weather permitting, you can take her outside to breathe in the cool, wet night air. While she is sleeping use a cold-water vaporizer or humidifier in your infant's room.

Do *not* try to open your baby's airway with your finger. Her breathing is being obstructed by swollen tissue beyond your reach, so you can't clear it away. She may throw up because of the coughing, but don't try to make her vomit. Pay close attention to your infant's breathing. Take her to the nearest emergency room *immediately* if:

- She seems to be struggling to get a breath.
- She gets excessively sleepy.
- She turns blue when she coughs.

Your pediatrician may prescribe various medications, usually steroids, to help decrease the swelling in the upper airway and throat and make it easier for her to breathe. Antibiotics are not helpful for croup because the problem is caused by a virus or an allergy. Cough syrups do not help, either. In fact, as stated earlier, over-the-counter cough medicines don't work for children under age six and should not be given to children under two years of age as they may pose a health risk.

In the most serious cases, which are quite rare, your baby will have a lot of difficulty breathing, and your pediatrician may admit her to the hospital for a few days until the swelling in the airway gets better.

Flu/Influenza

Flu is the short term for influenza. It is an illness caused by a respiratory virus. Influenza epidemics often occur in the winter months, although the flu season extends from the beginning of October through March. The infection can spread rapidly through communities as the virus is passed from person to person. When someone with the flu coughs or sneezes, the influenza virus gets into the air, and people nearby, including babies, can inhale it. The virus also can be spread when your infant touches a hard surface, such as a door handle, and then places his hand or fingers in his nose or rubs his eye.

When there is an outbreak or epidemic, it usually occurs during the winter months. Adult caregivers are easily exposed and can contract the disease. The virus usually is transmitted in the first several days of the illness.

You can suspect that your infant has the flu if you observe the following signs or symptoms:

- Sudden onset of fever (usually above 101 degrees Fahrenheit, or 38.3 degrees Celsius)
- Chills and shakes accompanying the fever
- Extreme tiredness or fatigue
- Muscle aches and pains
- Dry, hacking cough

After the first few days of these symptoms, a sore throat, stuffy nose, and continuing cough become most evident. The flu can last a week or even longer. A baby with a common cold (see *Colds/Upper Respiratory Infection,* page 554) usually has a lower fever, a runny nose, and only a small amount of coughing. Infants with the flu—or adults, for that matter—usually feel much sicker, more achy, and more miserable.

Healthy people, especially children, get over the flu in about a week or two, without any lingering problems. However, you might suspect a complication if your baby's ear hurts or if he appears congested in his face and head or if his cough and fever persist.

Babies who appear to have the greatest risk of complications from the flu are those with an underlying chronic medical condition, such as heart or lung disease, an immune problem, some blood diseases, or malignancy. As these babies may have more severe disease or complications, they should, when possible, be kept away from children with the flu. Their pediatrician may suggest additional precautions that should be taken. If your infant has flulike symptoms along with any difficulty breathing, seek medical attention right away.

Treatment

For all babies with the flu who don't feel well, lots of tender loving care is in order. Infants can benefit from extra bed rest, extra fluids, and light, easy-to-digest meals. A cool mist humidifier or vaporizer in the room may add additional moisture to the air and make breathing through inflamed mucous membranes of the nose a little easier.

If your baby is uncomfortable because of a fever, acetaminophen or ibuprofen in doses recommended by your pediatrician for his age and weight will help him feel better. (See Chapter 23, *Fever*.) Ibuprofen is approved for use in infants six months of age and older; however, it should never be given to babies who are dehydrated or who are vomiting continuously. *It is extremely important not to give aspirin to an infant who has the flu or is suspected of having the flu. Aspirin during bouts of influenza is associated with an increased risk of developing Reye syndrome.*

Prevention

Since the flu virus is transmitted from person to person, a first step you can take to decrease the chances of family members getting the flu is to practice and teach good hygiene such as frequent hand-washing. If, for example, you have a baby with the flu, do the following to prevent its spread:

- Avoid kissing your infected baby on or around the mouth, although he will need plenty of hugs during the illness.
- Make sure you and other caregivers wash hands both before and after caring for your baby.
- Wash your baby's utensils in hot, soapy water or in the dishwasher.
- Don't allow others to share drinking glasses or utensils, and never share toothbrushes.
- Use disposable paper cups in the bathroom and kitchen.
- Talk with your physician about giving antiviral medication to other household members over one year of age to prevent them from contracting the flu.

There is a vaccine to protect against the flu. The American Academy of Pediatrics recommends that the influenza vaccination be given annually to *all* healthy babies starting at six months of age. Flu vaccines are especially important for infants at high risk for complications from the flu such as those with a chronic disease such as asthma. Adults who live in the same household as someone who has a high risk for flu complications or who care for babies should receive the flu vaccine yearly. The flu vaccine also can be given to any child whose parent requests it, although it is *not* approved for use in infants younger than six months old.

The flu vaccine has few side effects. However, all flu vaccines are produced using eggs, so anyone who has an egg allergy should speak to their pediatrician or allergist about whether or not they should receive the flu vaccine. If a baby has had a serious allergic reaction to eggs or egg products, you should discuss this with your pediatrician.

Antiviral medications to treat an influenza infection are now available by prescription. Such treatments must be initiated within forty-eight hours of the beginning of illness. Also, for chronically ill children, preventing influenza is important. If your infant has not been immunized, using antiviral medication before the exposed baby gets the disease can reduce the risk of infection.

Pneumonia

The word *pneumonia* means "infection of the lung." While such infections were extremely dangerous in past generations, today most children can recover from them easily if they receive proper medical attention.

Most cases of pneumonia follow a viral upper respiratory tract infection. Typically, the viruses that cause these infections (respiratory syncytial virus [RSV], influenza, parainfluenza, adenovirus) spread to the chest and produce pneumonia there. Pneumonia also can be caused by bacterial infections. Some of these are spread from person to person by coughing or by direct contact with the infected person's saliva or mucus. Also, if a viral infection has weakened a baby's immune system, bacteria may begin to grow in the lung, adding a second infection to the original one.

Infants whose immune defenses or lungs are weakened by other illnesses, such as cystic fibrosis, asthma, or cancer (as well as by the chemotherapy used to treat cancer), are more likely to develop pneumonia. Babies whose airways or lungs are abnormal in any other way also have a higher risk.

Because most forms of pneumonia are linked to viral or bacterial infections that spread from person to person, they're most common during the fall, winter, and early spring, when children spend more time indoors in close contact with others. The chance that a baby will develop pneumonia is *not* affected by how she is dressed or by air temperature.

Signs and Symptoms

Like many infections, pneumonia usually produces a fever, which in turn may cause sweating, chills, flushed skin, and general discomfort. The baby also may lose her appetite and seem less energetic than normal. Babies and toddlers may seem pale and limp, and cry more than usual.

Because pneumonia can cause breathing difficulties, you may notice these other, more specific symptoms, too:

- Cough (see page 497)
- Fast, labored breathing
- Increased activity of the breathing muscles below and between the ribs and above the collarbone
- Flaring (widening) of the nostrils
- Pain in the chest, particularly with coughing or deep breathing
- Wheezing
- Bluish tint to the lips or nails, caused by decreased oxygen in the bloodstream

Although the diagnosis of pneumonia usually can be made on the basis of the signs and symptoms, a chest X-ray sometimes is necessary to make certain and to determine the extent of lung involvement.

Treatment

When pneumonia is caused by a virus, usually there is no specific treatment other than rest and the usual measures for fever control (see Chapter 23). Cough suppressants containing codeine or dextromethorphan should not be used, because coughing is necessary to clear the excessive secretions caused by the infection. Viral pneumonia usually improves after a few days, although the cough may linger for several weeks. Ordinarily, no medication is necessary.

Because it is often difficult to tell whether the pneumonia is caused by a virus or by bacteria, your pediatrician may prescribe an antibiotic. All antibiotics should be taken for the full prescribed course and at the specific dosage recommended. You may be tempted to discontinue them early, but you should not do so. Your baby will feel better after just a few days, but some bacteria may remain and the infection might return unless the entire course is completed.

Your baby should be checked by the pediatrician as soon as you suspect pneumonia. Check back with the doctor if your infant shows any of the following warning signs that the infection is worsening or spreading.

- Fever lasting more than a few days despite using antibiotics
- Breathing difficulties
- Evidence of an infection elsewhere in the body: red, swollen joints, bone pain, neck stiffness, vomiting, or other new symptoms or signs

Prevention

Your baby can be vaccinated against pneumococcal infections, a bacterial cause of pneumonia. The American Academy of Pediatrics recommends that all children younger than two years old receive this immunization (called pneumococcal conjugate or PCV7). A series of doses needs to be given at two, four, six, and twelve to fifteen months of age, at the same time that children receive other childhood vaccines.

(See also: *Asthma,* page 463, *Colds/ Upper Respiratory Infection,* page 554; Chapter 23, *Fever.*)

TUBERCULOSIS

Tuberculosis (TB) is an airborne infection that primarily affects the lungs. While TB is less common than it once was, some groups of babies have a higher risk of developing tuberculosis, including:

- Infants living in a household with an adult who has active tuberculosis or has a high risk of contracting TB
- Babies infected with HIV or another condition that weakens the immune system
- Infants born in a country that has a high prevalence of TB
- Babies visiting a country where TB is endemic and who have extended contact with people who live there
- Infants from communities that generally receive inadequate medical care
- Babies living in a shelter or living with someone who has been in jail

Tuberculosis usually is spread when an infected adult coughs the bacteria into the air. These germs are inhaled by the infant, who then becomes infected. Babies with TB of the lungs rarely infect other people, because they tend to have very few bacteria in their mucus secretions and also have a relatively ineffective cough.

Fortunately, most infants exposed to tuberculosis do not become ill. When the bacteria reach their lungs, the body's immune system attacks them and prevents further spread. These children have developed a symptom-free infection indicated only by a positive skin test. (See a description of this test below.) However, the symptom-free baby still must be treated, as noted below, to prevent an active disease from ever occurring. Occasionally, in a small number of children without proper treatment, the infection does progress, causing fever, fatigue, irritability, a persistent cough, weakness, heavy and fast breathing, night sweats, swollen glands, weight loss, and poor growth.

In a very small number of babies (mostly those less than four years old), the tuberculosis infection can spread through the bloodstream, affecting virtually any organ in the body. This illness requires much more complicated treatment, and the earlier it is started, the better the outcome. These infants have a much greater risk of developing tuberculosis meningitis, a dangerous form of the disease that affects the brain and central nervous system.

Babies who are at risk for contracting TB should receive a tuberculin skin test (sometimes called a PPD (purified protein derivative of tuberculin). Your infant may need a skin test if you answer yes to at least one of the following questions:

- Has a family member or contact had tuberculosis disease?
- Has a family member had a positive tuberculin skin test?
- Was your baby born in a high-risk country (countries other than the United States, Canada, Australia, New Zealand, or Western European countries)?
- Has your infant traveled (had contact with resident populations) to a high-risk country for more than one week?

The test is performed in the pediatrician's office by injecting a purified, inactive piece of TB germ into the skin of the forearm. If there has been an infection, your baby's skin will swell and redden at the injection site. Your pediatrician will check the skin forty-eight to seventy-two hours after the injection, and measure the diameter of the reaction. This skin test will reveal a past infection by the bacteria, even if the infant has had no symptoms and even if his body has fought the disease successfully.

If your baby's skin test for TB turns positive, a chest X-ray will be ordered to determine if there is evidence of an active or past infection in the lungs. If the X-ray does indicate the possibility of an active infection, the pediatrician also will search for the TB bacteria in your infant's cough secretions or in his stomach. This is done in order to determine the type of treatment needed.

Treatment

If your baby's skin test turns positive, but he does not have symptoms or signs of active tuberculosis infection, he still is infected. In order to prevent the infection from becoming active, your pediatrician will prescribe a medication called isoniazid (INH). This medication must be taken by mouth once a day every day for a minimum of nine months.

For an *active* tuberculosis infection, your pediatrician will prescribe three or four medications. You will have to give these to your infant every day for six to twelve months. Your baby may have to be hospitalized initially for the treatment to be started, although most of it can be carried out at home.

Prevention

If your baby has been infected with TB, regardless of whether he develops symptoms, it is *very* important to attempt to identify the person from whom he caught the disease. Usually this is done by looking for symptoms of TB in everyone who came in close contact with him, and having TB skin tests performed on all family members, child care providers, and housekeepers; the most common symptom in adults is a persistent cough, especially one that is associated with coughing up blood. Anyone who has a positive skin test should receive a physical examination, a chest X-ray, and treatment.

When an active infection is found in an adult, he will be isolated as much as possible—especially from young children—until treatment is under way. All family members who have been in contact with that person usually are also treated with INH, regardless of the results of their own skin tests. Anyone who becomes ill or develops an abnormality on a chest X-ray should be treated as an active case of tuberculosis.

Tuberculosis is much more common in underprivileged populations, which are more susceptible to disease due to crowded living conditions, poor nutrition, and the probability of inadequate medical care. AIDS patients, too, are at a greater risk of getting TB, because of their lowered resistance.

If untreated, tuberculosis can lie dormant for many years, only to surface during adolescence, pregnancy, or later adulthood. At that time, not only can the individual become quite ill, but he also can spread the infection to those around him. Thus, it's very important to have your baby tested for TB if he comes in close contact with any adult who has the disease and to get prompt and adequate treatment for him if he tests positive.

Whooping Cough (Pertussis)

Pertussis, or whooping cough, is less common in young children than it used to be, as the pertussis vaccine has made most children immune. Before this vaccine was developed, there were several hundred thousand cases of whooping cough each year in the United States. Now there are approximately 1 million cases a year in the U.S., but these are mostly in adults and adolescents.

This illness is caused by pertussis bacteria, which produces a toxin that attacks the lining of the breathing passages (bronchi and bronchioles), producing severe inflammation and narrowing of the airways. Severe coughing is a prominent symptom. If not recognized properly, the bacteria may spread to those in close contact with the infected person, through her respiratory secretions.

Infants under one year of age are at greatest risk of developing severe breathing problems and life-threatening illness from whooping cough. Because the baby is short of breath, she inhales deeply and quickly between coughs. These breaths (particularly in older infants) frequently make a "whooping" sound—which is how this illness got its common name. The intense coughing scatters the pertussis bacteria into the air, spreading the disease to other susceptible persons.

Pertussis often acts like a common cold for a week or two. Then the cough gets worse, and the older baby may start to have the characteristic "whoop"s. During this phase (which can last two weeks or more), the infant often is short of breath and can look bluish around the mouth. She also may tear, drool, and vomit. Infants with pertussis become exhausted and develop complications such as susceptibility to other infections, pneumonia, and seizures. Pertussis can be fatal in some infants, but the usual course is for recovery to begin after two to four more weeks. The cough may not disappear for months, and may return with subsequent respiratory infections.

When to Call the Pediatrician

Pertussis infection starts out acting like a cold. You should consider whooping cough if the following conditions are present.

- The very young infant has not been fully immunized and/or has been exposed to someone with a chronic cough or the disease.
- The baby's cough becomes more severe and frequent, or her lips and fingertips become dark or blue.
- She becomes exhausted after coughing episodes, eats poorly, vomits after coughing, and/or looks "sick."

Treatment

The majority of infants with whooping cough who are less than six months old, and slightly less than one half of older babies with the disease initially are treated in the hospital. This more intensive care can decrease the chances of complications. These complications can include pneumonia, which occurs in slightly less than one fourth of babies under one year old who have whooping cough.

While in the hospital, your baby may need to have the thick respiratory secretions suctioned. His breathing will be monitored, and he may need to have oxygen administered. For several days, your baby will be isolated from other patients to keep the infection from spreading to them.

Whooping cough is treated with antibiotics, usually for two weeks. These medications are most effective when they are given in the first stage of the illness before coughing spells begin. Although antibiotics can stop the spread of the whooping cough infection, they cannot prevent or treat the cough itself. Because cough medicines do not relieve the coughing spells, your pediatrician probably will recommend other forms of home treatment to help manage the cough. Use a cool-mist vaporizer to help soothe your baby's irritated lungs and breathing passages. A vaporizer also will help loosen secretions in the respiratory tract. Ask your pediatrician for instructions on the best position for your baby to help drain those secretions and improve breathing. Also ask your doctor whether antibiotics or vaccine boosters need to be given to others in your household to prevent them from developing the disease.

Prevention

The best way to protect your baby against pertussis is with the DTaP vaccine (immunizations at two months, four months, and six months of age, and booster shots at twelve to eighteen months and at four or five years of age).

16

Chronic Conditions and Diseases

Coping with Chronic (Long-Term) Health Problems

We tend to think of childhood as a carefree and healthy time of life, but some children face chronic health problems during these early years. (By *chronic*, we mean conditions that last for at least three months.) While most long-term health problems in babies are relatively mild, any type of lengthy illness or disability is stressful for both them and their families.

The specific medical treatment of many chronic conditions is discussed elsewhere, under the names of those conditions. (See Index.) The information that follows is aimed at helping parents deal with the emotional and practical challenges of living with any baby who has a long-term illness or disability.

Getting Help

If your infant is born with a serious medical problem or develops a chronic medical condition during her first years, you may face some of the following stressors and decisions.

- **The realization that** your baby is not perfectly healthy often leads to feelings of disappointment and guilt, and fear for her future. In trying to deal with these feelings, you may find yourself struggling with unexplained emotional swings ranging from hopefulness to guilt and depression.
- **You will need** to select and work with a team of medical professionals who can help your baby.

- **You may face** decisions about treatment or surgery.
- **You may have** to be responsible for giving your baby certain medications, guide her in usage of special equipment, or help her perform special therapies.
- **You will be** called on to provide the time, energy, money, and emotional commitment necessary for your baby to receive the best possible treatment.
- **You will need** to learn how to access appropriate services and information to help your infant.
- **In adapting your** life to meet your baby's needs without neglecting other family members, you will face many difficult choices, some of which may require compromise solutions.

To avoid becoming overwhelmed, it is helpful to select one medical person as the overall coordinator of your infant's medical care, taking a lead role in the so-called "medical home" that's a partnership between your family and your baby's healthcare providers. This person may be your pediatrician or another health professional who is most closely involved with your infant's treatment. It should be someone who knows your family well, makes you feel comfortable, and is willing to spend time answering your questions and working with other doctors and therapists involved in your baby's care.

Not all of your infant's special needs will be medical, of course. She may require special therapy. Your family may need outside financial or governmental assistance. The person who coordinates your baby's medical care also should provide some guidance in obtaining this extra help, but the best way to make sure you and your infant get the services and support you need is to learn about the resources and regulations that apply to special services for children with chronic illnesses or disabilities. You also should find out what you can do if the services your family receives do not meet your baby's needs.

Balancing the Needs of Family and Baby

For a while, the infant with special needs may take all your attention, leaving little for other family members and outside relationships. Although this is normal, everyone will suffer unless you find some way to restore a sense of balance and routine to your activities. Neither your sick baby nor the rest of the family—nor your marital relationship—will benefit if the health problem becomes the central and overwhelming issue in your family's life. Eventually your infant's medical care must become a part of your daily routine rather than its focus.

If your infant must be hospitalized, returning her to normal family and community life is vital, not only for the family but also for her health and well-being. The longer she is treated like a "patient" instead of a growing child, the more problems she may have socially and emotionally later on. As she grows, although it's natural to want to protect a sick baby, overprotection may make it more difficult for her to develop the self-discipline she needs. Also, if you have other children, you can't expect them to observe rules that you allow the baby who is sick or disabled to ignore.

Your baby needs your encouragement far more than your protection. Rather than concentrating on what she cannot do, try to focus instead on what she *can* do. If given a chance to participate in normal activities with infants her age, she probably will do things that surprise everyone. Establishing this sense of normalcy is difficult if your infant's condition is uncertain. You may find yourself withdrawing from your friends because you're so worried about your baby, and you may hesitate to plan social activities if you're not sure she'll be well enough to attend. If you give in to these feelings all the time, resentment is bound to build up, so try not to let this happen. Even if there is a chance that your infant's condition may worsen unexpectedly, take the risk and plan special outings, invite friends to your home, and get a babysitter from time to time so you can go out for an evening. Both you and your infant will be better off in the long run if you take this approach.

Special Tips

The following suggestions may help you cope more effectively with your baby's condition.

- **Whenever possible, both** parents should be included in discussions and decisions about your baby's treatment.

Too often, one parent may go alone to the medical appointment and then must explain what was said to the other parent. This may prevent one parent from getting some of his or her questions answered or learning enough about the choices.

- **Keep an open** line of communication with your pediatrician. Express your concerns and ask questions.
- **Do not be** offended if your baby's doctors ask personal questions about your family life. The more they know about your family, the better they can help you manage your infant's care. For example, if your baby will need a wheelchair, the doctor may ask about your home in order to suggest the best places for wheelchair ramps. If you have concerns about the doctor's suggestions, discuss them with him so you can reach an acceptable plan of action together.
- **Remember that although** you and your doctor want to be optimistic about your baby's condition, you must be honest about it. If things are not going well, you should say so. Work with the doctor to adjust the treatment or find a solution that will make the situation as good as possible.
- **As your baby matures, discuss her** condition frankly with her, as well as the other members of your family. If you do not tell your child the truth, she may sense that you are lying; this can lead to feelings of isolation and rejection.
- **Call on friends** and family members for support. You cannot expect to handle the strain created by your baby's chronic condition all by yourself. Asking close friends to help you meet your own emotional needs will in turn help you to meet your infant's.
- **Remember that your** baby needs to be loved and valued as an individual. If you let the medical problems overshadow your feelings for her as a person, they may interfere with the bond of trust and affection between you. Don't let yourself become so worried that you cannot relax and enjoy your baby.

ANEMIA

Blood contains several different types of cells. The most numerous are the red blood cells, which absorb oxygen in the lungs and distribute it throughout the body. These cells contain hemoglobin, a red pigment that carries oxygen to the tissues and carries away carbon dioxide (the waste material). *Anemia* is a condition in which a decreased amount of hemoglobin is available in the red blood cells, making the blood less able to carry the amount of oxygen necessary for all the cells in the body to function and grow.

Anemia may occur for any of the following reasons.

1. The production of red blood cells slows down.
2. Too many red blood cells are destroyed.
3. There is not enough hemoglobin within the red blood cells.
4. Blood cells are lost from the body.

Babies most commonly become anemic when they fail to get enough iron in their diet. Iron is necessary for the production of hemoglobin. This iron deficiency causes a decrease in the amount of hemoglobin in the red blood cells. A young infant may get iron-deficiency anemia if he starts drinking cow's milk too early, particularly if he is not given an iron supplement or food with iron. The deficiency occurs because cow's milk contains very little iron and the small amount is poorly absorbed through the intestines into the body. In addition, cow's milk given to an infant under twelve months of age can irritate the bowel and cause small amounts of blood loss. This results in a decrease in the number of red blood cells, which can cause anemia.

Other nutritional deficiencies, such as a lack of folic acid, also can cause anemia, but this is very rare. It is probably seen most often in children fed goat's milk, which contains very little folic acid.

Anemia at any age can result from excessive blood loss. In rare cases, the blood loss may occur because the blood does not clot properly. A newborn infant with difficulty clotting may bleed heavily from his circumcision or a minor injury and become anemic. Because vitamin K promotes blood clotting and is often lacking in newborns, an injection of this vitamin generally is given right after birth.

Sometimes the red cells are prone to being easily destroyed. This condition, called hemolytic anemia, can result from disturbances on the surface of the red cells or other abnormalities in or outside the cells.

A severe condition called sickle cell anemia involves an abnormal structure of hemoglobin, and is seen most often in children of African heritage. This disorder can be very severe and is associated with frequent "crises," often requiring repeated hospitalizations. (See page 542.)

Disorders called thalassemias are inherited blood conditions, and tend to occur most frequently in children of Asian, African, Middle Eastern, Greek, and Italian heritage. Babies with these disorders have an abnormally low number of red blood cells, or not enough hemoglobin. They can develop anemia, sometimes severe cases.

Finally, certain enzyme deficiencies also can alter the function of the red blood cells, increasing their susceptibility to destruction.

Signs and Symptoms

Anemia frequently causes the skin to be mildly pale, usually most apparent as a decreased pinkness of the lips, the lining of the eyelids (conjunctiva), and the nail beds (pink part of the nails). Anemic babies also may be irritable, mildly weak, or tire easily. Those with severe anemia may have shortness of breath, rapid heart rate, and swelling of the hands and feet. If the anemia continues, it may interfere with normal growth. A newborn with hemolytic anemia may become jaundiced (turn yellow), although many newborns are mildly jaundiced and don't become anemic.

If your infant shows any of these symptoms or signs, or if you suspect he is not getting enough iron in his diet, consult your pediatrician. A simple blood count can diagnose anemia in most cases.

Some babies are not anemic but still are deficient in iron. They may have a decreased appetite and be irritable, fussy, and inattentive, which may result in developmental delays. These problems will reverse when the babies are given iron.

Babies with sickle cell anemia may have unexplained fever or swelling of the hands and feet as infants, and they are extremely susceptible to infection. If there is a history of sickle cell anemia or sickle cell trait in your family, make sure your newborn is tested for it at birth.

Although some cases of thalassemia have no symptoms, more moderate to severe cases can cause lethargy, jaundice, a poor appetite, slow growth, and an enlarged spleen.

Treatment

Since there are so many different types of anemia, it is very important to identify the cause before any treatment is begun. Do not attempt to treat your infant with vitamins, iron, or other nutrients or over-the-counter medications unless it is at your physician's direction. This is important, because such treatment may mask the real reason for the problem and thus delay the diagnosis.

If the anemia is due to a lack of iron, your infant will be given an iron-containing medication. This comes in a drop form for infants. Because "iron overload" occurs when iron is given when it's not needed, your pediatrician will check your baby's blood iron levels at regular intervals. Do not stop giving the medication until the physician tells you it is no longer needed.

Following are a few tips concerning iron medication.

- **It is best** not to give iron with milk because milk blocks iron absorption.
- **Vitamin C increases** iron absorption, so you might want to follow the dose of iron with a glass of orange juice.
- **Iron medications cause** the stools to become a dark black color. Don't be worried by this change.

Safety precautions: Iron medications are extremely poisonous if taken in excessive amounts. (Iron is one of the most common causes of poisoning in children under five.) For that reason, *keep this and all medication out of reach of small children.*

Severe forms of thalassemias are typically treated with

transfusions of red blood cells and supplements of folic acid.

Prevention

Iron-deficiency anemia and other nutritional anemias can be prevented easily by making sure your baby is eating a well-balanced diet and by following these precautions.

- **Do not give** your infant cow's milk until he is over one year old.
- **If your baby** is breastfed, give him iron-fortified foods such as cereal when solid foods are introduced. Before then, he will absorb enough iron from the breastmilk. If you choose to breastfeed solely beyond four months, an iron supplement is recommended. However, introducing iron-poor solid foods will decrease the amount of iron he absorbs from the breastmilk.
- **If your baby** is formula-fed or partially breastfed, the current recommendation is to give him formula with added iron (4.0 to 12 milligrams of iron per liter), beginning at birth and continuing through age twelve months.

Cystic Fibrosis

Cystic fibrosis (CF) is most common in the Caucasian population, where 1 out of every 20 people is a carrier, and 1 out of every 2,000 to 3,000 Caucasian babies has CF. The disease is much less common in African Americans (1 in 17,000 live births) and Hispanics (1 in 11,500 live births), and even rarer among Asians. About 60,000 children and adults worldwide have been diagnosed with CF; approximately half of them (30,000) are in North America.

Considerable progress has been made in treating cystic fibrosis and its symptoms, although there is still no cure. CF is a disease that changes the secretions of certain glands in the body. It is inherited from parents who carry the gene that causes this disease. For a child to get cystic fibrosis, both parents must be carriers of the gene that causes it. Although the sweat glands and the glandular cells of the lungs and pancreas are affected most often, the sinuses, liver, intestines, and reproductive organs also can be involved.

In 1989 researchers discovered the gene that causes CF. Couples planning to have children can undergo genetic testing and counseling to find out if they carry the CF gene. They can also receive prenatal testing to detect the gene in the fetus.

Signs and Symptoms

The majority of CF cases are diagnosed within the first two years of life; in many states, newborn screenings now include mandatory testing for CF. (As mentioned above, CF can be diagnosed even before the baby is born with genetic testing as well as through detection of an abnormality found on an ultrasound in the later stages of pregnancy.) Your pediatrician may suspect CF if your baby is failing to gain weight, which often accompanies this disease. Other signs and symptoms vary with the degree of involvement of organs such as the lungs.

More than half of CF cases are diagnosed because of repeated lung infections. These infections tend to recur because mucus in the airways is thicker than normal and more difficult to cough out. A baby with CF is likely to have a persistent cough that gets worse with colds. Since the secretions of the lungs remain in the airways longer than normal, the airways are more likely to become infected, increasing the chances of pneumonia or bronchitis. Over time, these infections cause damage to the lungs, and are the major cause of death in CF. Diabetes and chronic liver disease are other complications that may occur in children with CF.

Most children with CF are deficient in digestive enzymes, making it difficult for them to digest fats and proteins as well as they should. As a result, these children have large, bulky, foul-smelling stools. Loose stools may result from an inability to digest formula or food, and are one of the reasons CF children fail to gain weight.

To confirm the diagnosis, your pediatrician will order a sweat test to measure the amount of salt your infant loses as he perspires. Children with cystic fibrosis have much more salt in their sweat than do children who do not have CF. Two or more of these tests may be required to ensure an accurate diagnosis, since the results are not always clearly positive or negative. If your baby is diagnosed as having the disease, your pediatrician will help you get the additional specialized medical help that is necessary. At a medical center that specializes in treating children with CF you can find multidisciplinary experts to help your child and family.

Treatment

Treating CF's lung infections is the most important aspect of your baby's care. The goal is to help clear the thick secretions from your infant's lungs, which may involve various techniques that help him cough out the sputum more easily. The lung infections themselves are treated with antibiotics. Periods in which the lung infections worsen are called exacerbations, which are associated with more coughing and sputum production, and may require treatment with the use of intravenous antibiotics.

To treat the lack of digestive enzymes in CF, your child will be prescribed capsules containing enzymes to be taken with every meal and every snack. The amount of enzymes is based on the level of fat in the diet and the weight of your baby. Once the correct amount of enzymes is taken, your infant's stool pattern will become more normal and he'll begin gaining more weight. He also will need to take supplemental vitamins.

Emotional Burden of Cystic Fibrosis

Because CF is a hereditary disease, many parents feel guilty about their baby's illness. Instead, channel your emotional energies into your infant's treatment.

It is important to raise your baby as you would if he did not have this disease. There is no reason to limit his educational or career goals. The majority of children with CF can expect to grow up and lead productive adult lives. Your child needs both love and discipline, and should be encouraged to develop and test his limits.

Balancing the physical and emotional demands created by this disease is hard on both the CF patient and his family, so it is very important that you get as much support as possible. Ask your pediatrician to put you in touch not only with the nearest CF center, but also with CF support groups. The Cystic Fibrosis Foundation also can be of help (www.cff.org; 1-800-344-4823).

Failure to Thrive

At each of your baby's checkups, your pediatrician's office should plot your infant's weight and measurements. In general, you should see a continuous upward trend, although there will be times when she gains very slowly and perhaps some weeks when she actually loses a little weight due to illness. It is not normal for her to stop growing or to lose weight except for the small amount she loses during the first few days of life. If she does lose weight, it is a clear sign either that she is not getting enough to eat or that she is ill. The medical term for this condition is *failure to thrive.* Although it can happen in older children who are seriously ill or undernourished, it is most common and most dangerous during the active growth period of the first three years.

If allowed to continue for a prolonged period, this condition can become serious. Steady weight gain is especially important for infants and toddlers because it means that they are receiving adequate nutrition and care for normal physical, mental, and emotional development.

Usually when a baby stops growing, it is due to a feeding problem that prevents her from getting as many calories as she needs. As a newborn, she may be too fussy to eat as much as she needs, or, if breastfed, she may not be getting enough milk while nursing. Some babies may require more food than their parents are able to provide. These problems must be detected and treated early in order to avoid long-term or permanent damage.

Sometimes failure to thrive signals a medical problem. The newborn may have an infection passed on from her mother during pregnancy, or she may have a hormonal difficulty, an allergy, or a digestive problem that prevents nutrients from being absorbed into the body properly. Diseases such as cystic fibrosis (page 521), or heart disease also can interfere with normal growth. If one of these is present, the baby may need a special diet as well as medical treatment.

When to Get Help

Regularly charting your baby's growth, and comparing her general development with others her age, are the best ways to make sure she is thriving. If she does not gain weight, grow in length, or otherwise develop normally, consult your pediatrician. He will measure and examine your baby, ask about her diet and eating patterns, and review her medical history for signs of illness that may be contributing to her failure to thrive. The physician will try to establish exactly when the growth or weight gain stopped, and ask about anything that may have contributed to this. The pediatrician also may watch your infant's eating or nursing to see how much she consumes and how she responds to food. Sometimes a short period of in-hospital observation may be necessary.

If the doctor discovers a physical cause for the decrease in growth rate, he will recommend the appropriate treatment.

HIV Infection and AIDS

HIV (human immunodeficiency virus) is a virus that can lead to AIDS (acquired immunodeficiency syndrome).

Babies acquire the infection primarily from their HIV-infected mothers, either in utero (as the virus passes across the placenta), during delivery (when the newborn is exposed to the mother's blood and body fluids), or by ingesting infected breastmilk. An HIV infection will develop in 13 to 39 of 100 infants born to HIV-infected mothers who are untreated. Treating the mother and newborn with zidovudine (or AZT) reduces the risk of HIV infection from mothers to babies to about 8 of 100, and more powerful combinations of drugs can reduce this figure to 2 of 100 or less.

Once a baby is infected with HIV, the virus will be in his body for life. Infants with the HIV infection initially may appear well, but problems gradually develop. For example, their weight and height fail to increase appropriately within the first six months to one year. They have frequent episodes of diarrhea or minor skin infections. The lymph nodes (glands) anywhere in the body may enlarge, and there is a persistent fungus infection of the mouth (thrush). The liver and spleen may enlarge. Because neurological development may be affected, children may have a delay in walking and other motor skills, a delay in their ability to think and talk, and diminished head growth during infancy.

Eventually, if the HIV infection progresses as the body's immune system further deteriorates, AIDS-related infections and cancers may occur. The most common of these, *Pneumocystis jirovecii* pneumonia, is accompanied by fever and breathing difficulties. This common infection occurs predominantly in infants between three months and one year of age. It is possible to prevent this infection with antibiotics, and doctors recommend that all babies born to HIV-infected women be placed on preventive antibiotics as early as six weeks of age until tests show that the infant does not have an HIV infection.

Care of an HIV-Infected Baby

Infants who are HIV positive need love and attention like all other children. HIV infections cannot be transmitted by just holding a baby who is HIV positive. These infants need all we can give them, whether it is in a child care center, on a one-to-one basis, or in any group, large or small. Often, in fact, their circumstances have placed them in a situation or an environment that hinders optimum growth and development. We must all do everything we can to counteract those negative factors and contribute to their positive outlook on life.

Common infections can cause serious complications in infants with HIV infection. These babies with HIV should attend child care when they are able. At the same time, they may be accidentally exposed to communicable illnesses like chickenpox, and the child care facility should inform parents of these exposures and report them to their child's doctor. Call the doctor immediately if your HIV-infected child develops a fever, breathing difficulties, diarrhea, swallowing problems, or skin irritation, or if he's been exposed to a communicable disease. In fact, any change in your infant's health status should prompt you to seek medical attention, since the baby with HIV may have few reserves to combat even minor illnesses.

Whenever seeking any medical attention for your infant, be sure to inform the physician of the HIV infection so that she can assess and care for the illness appropriately, as well as give correct immunizations.

As mentioned earlier, approved anti-HIV or "antiretroviral" drugs are available for use in children. Others are in the process of being tested. These medications suppress virus reproduction and improve growth and neurologic development. They also delay the progression of the disease. It is es-

Where We Stand

The American Academy of Pediatrics supports legislation and public policy directed toward eliminating any form of discrimination based on whether a child is infected with HIV (the virus that causes AIDS).

- AIDS in child care: All HIV-infected babies should have the same right as those without the infection to attend child care. The confidentiality of an infant's HIV-infection status should be respected, with disclosure given only with the consent of the parent(s) or legal guardian(s).
- AIDS legislation: As the number of HIV-infected children, adolescents, and young women continues to grow, the Academy supports federal funding for AIDS research and healthcare services for HIV-infected individuals and their families.
- AIDS testing: The Academy recommends that information about HIV infection, prevention of mother-to-child HIV transmission, and HIV antibody testing be routinely provided as part of a comprehensive healthcare program for pregnant women. Documented, routine HIV antibody testing should be performed for all pregnant women in the United States after notifying them that testing will be performed, unless the patient declines HIV testing (called "opt-out" consent or "right of refusal"). The Academy also recommends HIV testing with parental or guardian consent for *newborns* whose mothers' HIV status (whether the virus is present in her blood) is not known.

sential that your doctor knows about the baby's HIV infection as early in life as possible and that you administer antiretroviral therapy as the doctor advises. With more treatments now available, it's possible to completely hold back the virus in many cases. There are specific guidelines for the treatment of HIV-infected babies; and with this treatment well over 90 percent of children with HIV infection can live to adulthood.

Immunizing a Baby Born to an HIV-Infected Mother

Your pediatrician has up-to-date guidelines on which vaccines should and shouldn't be given to a baby with HIV infection. HIV-infected infants may experience especially severe illness due to chickenpox or measles. Following exposure to these infections, notify your physician, as an HIV-infected baby should receive treatment to prevent an infection. This will consist of either an injection of a medicine called immune globulin (which contains antibodies against diseases) or antiviral drugs.

If You're Pregnant

All pregnant women should be tested for HIV infection during every pregnancy. When a pregnant woman is infected with HIV, it is important that she be treated appropriately (with three combinations of anti-HIV drugs) to reduce the likelihood of transmission of the virus from mother to infant. Once the baby is born, women who are HIV-infected should not breastfeed their infant because of the risk of transmitting the virus via breastfeeding; safe alternative sources of infant nutrition are available, such as infant formulas.

In Child Care

There is no risk of HIV transmission in routine child care activities. The virus is not spread through casual contact. It cannot be transmitted through the air, by touching, or via toilet seats. Infants with HIV infection can attend regular child care. You should not be required to disclose the HIV status of

Where We Stand

When infants have a chronic, serious illness or disability, their parents often turn to "natural" therapies. Words that describe these therapies include alternative, complementary, and folk remedy. These treatments can be used in addition to the care their baby is receiving from their pediatrician or other mainstream practitioner, even when they're happy with this traditional care. In some cases, they may have become frustrated with what mainstream medicine offered their infant, and they've turned to natural therapies, which continue to increase in popularity.

If you've made the decision to seek natural therapies for your baby's care, involve your pediatrician in the process. Your doctor may be able to help you better understand these therapies, whether they have scientific merit, whether claims about them are accurate or exaggerated, and whether they pose any risks to your infant's well-being. Keep in mind that a "natural" treatment does not always mean a "safe" one. Your pediatrician can help you determine whether there is a risk of interactions with your baby's other medications.

The American Academy of Pediatrics has encouraged pediatricians to evaluate the scientific merits of natural therapies, determine whether they might cause any direct or indirect harm, and advise parents on the full range of treatment options. If you decide to use a natural therapy, your pediatrician also may be able to assist in evaluating your baby's response to that treatment.

your baby in order for him to attend child care and participate in all school-related activities.

Although HIV transmission has not occurred in child care centers, these settings are required to adopt routine precautionary procedures for handling blood, stool, and bodily secretions. The standard precaution is to wash exposed skin immediately with soap and water after any contact with blood or body fluids. Soiled surfaces should be cleaned with disinfectants such as bleach (a 1-to-10 dilution of bleach to water). Disposable towels or tissues should be used whenever possible. Gloves are recommended when contact with blood or blood-containing body fluids may occur, and therefore gloves should be available in child care centers. It is important for staff members to wash their hands thoroughly after changing diapers, whether gloves are used or not.

17

Developmental Disabilities

It's natural to compare your infant with others his age. When the neighbor's baby walks at ten months, for example, you may worry if yours isn't walking by twelve months, although many children do not walk until they are sixteen or seventeen months of age. Usually, however, such differences are not significant in the long run. Each baby has his own unique rate of development, so some learn certain skills faster than others.

Only when a baby or pre-schooler lags far behind, or fails altogether to reach the developmental milestones outlined in Chapters 6 through 9 of this book, or loses a previously acquired skill, is there reason to suspect a mental or physical problem serious enough to be considered a developmental disability. Developmental disabilities that can be identified during childhood include mental retardation (or intellectual disability), language and learning disorders, cerebral palsy, autism, and sensory impairments such as vision and hearing loss. (Some pediatricians include seizure disorders in this category, but a large percentage of children who have seizures develop normally.)

Each of these developmental disabilities can vary greatly in severity. For example, one baby with mild cerebral palsy may have no obvious handicap other than a slight lack of coordination, while another with a severe form may be unable to walk or feed himself. Also, some babies have more than one disability, each requiring different care.

If your baby does not seem to be developing normally, he should have a complete medical and developmental evaluation, perhaps including a consultation with a developmental pediatrician who is a specialist in this field. Doing this will give your pediatrician the information she needs to determine whether a true disability exists and, if so, how it should be managed. Depending on the results of the evaluation, the doctor may recommend physical, speech and language, or occupational therapy at various stages of your baby's life. Educational intervention or psychological counseling also might be necessary. Your pediatrician should be able to help you arrange these consultations. In some states and cities these evaluations are offered free of charge or are partially paid for by local government.

Today, most states offer special early intervention programs for infants and toddlers less than three years old who have developmental delays or disabilities or who are at risk for these difficulties. The families of children with disabilities also need special support and education. It's not easy to accept the fact that a baby has a developmental problem. To understand what your baby is facing and how he can realize his full potential, each member of your family should be educated about the specific problem and counseled about how to deal with it.

Autism Spectrum Disorders

Autism spectrum disorders (ASDs) are a group of conditions that can cause significant problems with social, communication, and behavioral skills. The number of children diagnosed with ASDs has been increasing for reasons that are unclear. Usually, ASDs cannot reliably be diagnosed until a child is 18 months or older. However, some early warning signs may indicate an increased risk for autism. Because all children are unique, any child who shows these signs should be evaluated by their pediatrician first. These are some of the early signs:

By 12 Months of Age the Child

- Does not respond to his or her name
- Avoids eye contact
- Says no single words (like "mama" or "dada")
- Does not learn to use gestures, such as waving good-bye or shaking head

- Does not point to objects or pictures
- Lacks warm, joyful expressions
- Does not share interest or enjoyment
- Has repetitive movements with objects, like spinning the wheels of a toy car
- Has repetitive movements or unusual positioning of body, arms, hands, or fingers
- Does not search for objects that are hidden while he or she watches

A child who shows one or more of these signs does not necessarily have an ASD, but should be evaluated for possible developmental problems. The American Academy of Pediatrics encourages doctors to be aware of the signs of ASD, and to be on the lookout for these signs during every well-child visit. At the same time, the Academy urges parents to always let their pediatricians know of any concerns they may have about their child's behavior and development. If a specific diagnosis cannot be made, the child should be followed over time (developmental surveillance) to monitor his or her development.

Cerebral Palsy

Babies with cerebral palsy have an impairment in the area of the brain that controls movement and muscle tone. Many of these infants have normal intelligence, even though they have difficulty with motor control and movement. The condition causes different types of motor disability, which can vary from quite mild and barely noticeable to very profound. Depending on the severity of the problem, a child with cerebral palsy may simply be a little clumsy or awkward, or he may be unable to walk. Some children have weakness and poor motor control of one arm and one leg on the same side of the body (called hemiparesis). Many have problems with paralysis of both upper or lower extremities; this is called diplegia. In some children the muscle tone generally is increased (called spasticity or hypertonia), while others are abnormally limp (called hypotonia). While many of these children understand language, their ability to produce speech may be affected.

Cerebral palsy is caused by malformation or damage to the brain, usually during pregnancy, but occasionally during delivery, or immediately after birth. A report by the American Academy of Pediatrics and the American College of Obstetricians and Gynecologists concluded that the majority of cerebral palsy cases are not the result of events during labor and delivery, such as an insufficient supply of oxygen (hypoxia).

Premature birth is associated with an increased risk of cerebral palsy. A baby also can get cerebral palsy from very severe jaundice after birth, or later on in infancy from an injury or illness affecting the brain.

Although it may be challenging, it is important to focus your energy on optimizing your baby's development and remember that in many cases a cause cannot be identified.

Signs and Symptoms

The signs and symptoms of cerebral palsy vary tremendously because there are many different types and degrees of disability. The main clue that your baby might have cerebral palsy is a delay in achieving the motor milestones listed in Chapters 5 through 9 of this book. Here are some specific warning signs.

In a Baby over Two Months

- **His head lags** when you pick him up while he's lying on his back.
- **He feels stiff.**
- **He feels floppy.**
- **When held cradled** in your arms, he seems to overextend his back and neck—constantly acts as if he is pushing away from you.
- **When you pick** him up, his legs get stiff and they cross or "scissor."

In a Baby over Six Months

- **He continues to** have the asymmetrical tonic neck reflex (Chapter 6, see page 184).
- **He reaches out** with only one hand while keeping the other fisted.

In a Baby over Ten Months

- **He crawls in** a lopsided manner, pushing off with one hand and leg while dragging the opposite hand and leg.
- **He scoots around** on his buttocks or hops on his knees, but does not crawl on all fours.

If you have any concerns about your baby's development, talk to your pediatrician at your routine visit. Because children's rates of development vary widely, it is sometimes difficult to make a definite diagnosis of mild cerebral palsy in the first year or two of life. Often a consultation with a developmental pediatrician or pediatric neurologist will assist in the diagnosis. A CT (computed tomography) or MRI (magnetic resonance imagery) of the head may be recommended to determine whether a brain abnormality exists. Even when a firm diagnosis is made during these early years, it often is difficult to predict how severe the disability will be in the future.

Treatment

If your pediatrician suspects that your baby has cerebral palsy, you will be referred to an early intervention program. These programs are staffed by early childhood educators; physical, occupational, and speech and language therapists; nurses; social workers; and medical consultants. In such a program you'll learn how to become your child's own teacher and therapist. You will be taught what exercises to do with your infant, what positions are most comfortable and beneficial to him, and how to help with specific problems such as feeding difficulties. You'll be introduced to some of the newer treatment options, such as the medication baclofen, that may be able to manage the spasticity associated with cerebral palsy, and botulinum toxin type A (called Botox), which is a muscle-relaxing drug that can help relieve the toe-walking that is related to muscle tightening. You'll receive information about so-called adaptive equipment that can help your child participate in everyday activities despite the physical problems he may have; this equipment includes special utensils to make eating easier, pencils that can be held more easily, wheelchairs, and walkers. Through these programs you also can meet parents of other children with similar disabilities and share experiences, concerns, and solutions.

The most important thing you can do for your child is to help him develop skills, become resilient, and gain positive self-esteem. When he is old enough to ask or understand, explain to him that he has a disability and reassure him that he'll be able to make adjustments in order to succeed in life. Encourage him to perform the tasks he is ready for, but do not push him to do things at which he might fail. The professionals at early intervention centers can help you evaluate your child's abilities and teach you how to reach appropriate goals.

Although it may be tempting, be careful about wasting time, energy, and money searching for magical cures or undertaking controversial treatments. Instead, ask your pediatrician, or contact the United Cerebral Palsy Association at www.ucp.org, for information about resources and programs available in your area.

Associated Problems

Seizures One out of every three people with cerebral palsy has or will develop seizures. (Some start having them years after the brain is damaged.) Fortunately, these seizures usually can be controlled with anticonvulsant medications. (See also page 666.)

Vision Difficulties Because the injury to the brain often affects eye muscle coordination, more than three out of four children with cerebral palsy have strabismus, a problem with one eye turning in or out. If this problem is not corrected early, the vision in the affected eye will get worse and eventually will be lost permanently. Thus it is extremely important to have your baby's eyes checked regularly by your pediatrician. (See also *Strabismus*, page 620.)

Limb Shortening and Scoliosis Of those babies with cerebral palsy affecting only one side of the body, over half will develop a shortening of the involved leg and arm. The difference between the legs is rarely more than two inches (5 cm), but an orthopedic surgeon should be consulted if shortening is noticed. Depending on the degree of difference between the legs, a heel or sole lift may be prescribed to fit into the shoe on the shorter side. This is done to prevent a tilt of the pelvis, which can lead to curvature of the spine (scoliosis) when standing or walking. Sometimes surgery is required to correct a serious degree of scoliosis. Scoliosis also can develop in the other forms of cerebral palsy involving both sides of the body.

Hearing Loss Some infants with cerebral palsy have a complete or partial hearing loss. This happens most often when the cerebral palsy is a result of severe jaundice or anoxia (a deficiency of oxygen) at birth. If you find that your baby does not blink at loud noises by one month, is not turning his head toward a sound by three to four months, or is not saying words by twelve months, discuss it with your pediatrician. (See also *Hearing Loss*, page 549.)

Joint Problems In children with spastic forms of cerebral palsy, it is often difficult to prevent "contracture," an extreme stiffening of the joints caused by the unequal pull of one muscle over the other. A physical therapist, developmental pediatrician, or physiatrist (doctor of physical medicine) can teach you how to stretch the muscles to try to prevent the onset of contracture. Sometimes braces, casting, or medication may be used to improve joint mobility and stability.

Problems with Spatial Awareness Over half the children with cerebral palsy affecting one side of the body cannot sense the position of their arm, leg, or hand on the affected side. (For example, when a child's hands are relaxed, he cannot tell whether his fingers are pointing up or down without looking at them.) If this problem exists, the child rarely will attempt to use the involved hand, even if the motor disability is minimal. He acts as if it is not there. Physical or occupational therapy can help him learn to use the affected parts of his body, despite this disability.

Congenital Abnormalities

Congenital abnormalities are caused by problems during the fetus's development before birth. Thanks to improved medical care during pregnancy and to progress in early detection of chromosomal and other genetic abnormalities through amniocentesis, chorionic villus sampling, and other newer diagnostic tests, there are fewer and fewer newborns with congenital problems. About three of every hundred babies born in the United States have congenital abnormalities that will affect the way they look, develop, or function—in some cases for the rest of their lives.

There are five categories of these abnormalities, grouped according to the cause.

Chromosome Abnormalities Chromosomes are the structures that carry the genetic material inherited from one generation to the next. Normally, twenty-three chromosomes come from the father and twenty-three from the mother, and all are found in the center of every cell in the body except the red blood cells. The genes carried on the chromosomes determine how the baby will grow, what she will look like, and to a certain extent how she will function.

When a baby does not have the normal forty-six chromosomes, or when pieces of the chromosomes are missing or duplicated, she may look and behave differently from others her age, and she may develop serious health problems, as well. Down syndrome is an example of a condition that can occur when a baby is born with an extra chromosome.

Single-Gene Abnormalities Sometimes the chromosomes are normal in number, but one or more of the genes on them are abnormal. Some of these genetic abnormalities can be passed on to the baby if one of the parents is affected with the same abnormality. This is known as autosomal dominant inheritance.

Other genetic problems can be passed to the infant only if

both parents carry the same defective gene. (Cystic fibrosis, Tay-Sachs disease, and sickle cell anemia are all examples of this type of abnormality.) In these cases both parents are normal, but one in four of their children would be expected to be affected. This is known as autosomal recessive inheritance.

A third type of genetic abnormality is called sex-linked, and generally is passed on to boys only. Girls may carry the abnormal gene that causes these disorders but not show the actual disease. (Examples of this problem include hemophilia, color blindness, and the common forms of muscular dystrophy.)

Conditions During Pregnancy That Affect the Baby Certain illnesses during pregnancy, particularly during the first nine weeks, can cause serious congenital abnormalities—German measles and diabetes, for example. Alcohol consumption and certain drugs during pregnancy significantly increase the risk that a baby will be born with abnormalities. Certain medications, if taken during pregnancy, also can cause permanent damage to the fetus, as can certain chemicals that can pollute air, water, and food. Always check with your doctor before using any medication or supplement while you are pregnant.

Combination of Genetic and Environmental Problems Spina bifida and cleft lip and palate are types of congenital abnormalities that may occur when there is a genetic tendency for the condition combined with exposure to certain environmental influences within the womb during critical stages of the pregnancy.

Unknown Causes The vast majority of congenital abnormalities have no known cause. This situation is particularly troubling for parents who plan to have more children, because there is no way to predict if the problem will recur. If you and your family have experienced such a genetic-related birth abnormality, ask your pediatrician for a referral to a genetic counseling service. These services have expertise with a variety of genetic abnormalities and may be able to advise you as to the proper course of action.

Learning to Live with the Condition

If your newborn has a congenital abnormality, the first hours and days of her life may be very difficult for you. At the same time that you are learning about your infant's condition, you may be mourning the perfect baby you'd imagined she would be. Meanwhile, all your relatives and friends are calling to hear the "good news." One way to relieve the social pressure you're bound to feel is to appoint one family member and one friend to inform other friends and relatives about your newborn's condition.

If you have other children, you'll need to explain the situation to them as soon as possible. It is difficult to predict how siblings will react to such news; but, whether they show it or not, many feel guilty. They may have felt jealous and resentful about the baby during the pregnancy—perhaps even wished secretly that the baby would never come. If so, when they learn that their new brother or sister has a problem, they may feel that their wishes were responsible. Encourage them to ask questions, answer them in terms that they can understand, and be sure to explain that the situation is no one's fault.

Parents may also be tempted to find fault or to blame themselves. In most cases, however, it is likely nothing could have been done to prevent the abnormality. Although you may be tempted, try not to let yourself feel guilty or responsible, because these feelings may prevent you from feeling the very natural love and affection that parents feel for their newborn.

As overwhelmed as you may be by the situation, your infant needs to receive all the nurturing and affection you would give any baby. This is precisely the time when touching, holding, and comforting are especially critical to the child and to you.

Congenital Conditions

Congenital abnormalities are so diverse, and require such different types of treatment, that it would be impossible to discuss them all in this section. Instead, we will look only at the medical management of three conditions: Down syndrome, sickle cell disease, and spina bifida.

Down Syndrome Approximately 1 out of every 800 babies is born with Down syndrome. Fortunately, through amniocentesis, Down syndrome can be detected prenatally. This problem—which is caused by the presence of an extra chromosome—results in a number of physical abnormalities, including up-slanted eyes with extra folds of skin at the inner corners, flattening of the bridge of the nose, a relatively large tongue, and a decrease in the muscle and ligament tone of the body.

A major serious effect of Down syndrome is mental retardation or intellectual disability. All but a very small number of these babies develop more slowly than average, although the extent of the delay can vary widely from one child to the next. Some seem to border on normal development, while others are severely challenged. However, even though children with Down syndrome may be intellectually disabled in development as children and young adults, most eventually are able to feed and dress themselves and to be toilet-trained. Many, with special education, can learn basic job skills.

Detecting Down syndrome early is very important, since many babies with the disorder require early treatment for related abnormalities of the heart, intestinal tract, and/or blood. Early detection also allows parents to adjust to the situation and gather support and information. Once suspected, the condition is confirmed by a blood test, but it usually takes a few days to produce results. Since most of the time newborns with Down syndrome have no medical problems that require immediate treatment, most can leave the hospital after the normal newborn stay.

If you have a newborn with Down syndrome, your pediatrician may recommend a special early-intervention program for you and your baby. If so, you should begin it as soon as possible. These programs employ specially designed services to help your baby make the most of her developmental and physical capabilities.

You may hear about other types of "therapy" that are *not* proven or recommended. These programs may delay effective methods of treatment and be very expensive. If you hear of any treatments that you think may help your baby, always discuss them first with your pediatrician to see if they are valid before spending your money or trying them.

In addition to developmental delay, Down syndrome can

result in physical problems as your baby gets older. Her growth should be closely watched, since extremely slow growth in height and/or excessive weight gain may indicate a lack of thyroid hormone, a problem that affects many children with Down syndrome. Even without thyroid problems, chances are that she'll be shorter and weigh less than average for her age as an infant. When they're older, children with Down syndrome tend to be overweight. One-half of children with Down syndrome also have heart problems that may require medication or surgery. Over one-half have vision and hearing defects.

Another problem, which affects 15 of every 100 children with Down syndrome, is an abnormality in the ligaments of the neck that can cause serious spinal injury if the neck is extended (bent backward) during exercise. For this reason, consult your pediatrician for advice regarding neck X-rays as she gets older and before she's allowed to participate in vigorous athletic activities (especially tumbling and gymnastics). If X-rays show this abnormality, her physical activities should be limited to movements that cannot cause injury.

For all its difficulties, raising a baby with Down syndrome can be deeply rewarding. Children with this condition are usually loving and openly affectionate, and will thrive if nurtured and loved in return. As with all children, each achievement they make can be a triumph shared by everyone in the family.

Sickle Cell Disease Sickle cell disease (SCD) is a group of chronic genetic disorders affecting the red blood cells. In babies with SCD, the red cells in the blood become sickle-shaped (appearing like an icicle under the microscope).

There are several types of sickle cell disease, including the best known, sickle cell anemia. Others include sickle-hemoglobin C disease and 2 types of sickle β-thalassemia. All of these disorders in the SCD complex have similar symptoms such as anemia (shortage of red blood cells), episodes of severe pain, and infections. (See *Signs and Symptoms*.)

In the U.S., about 2,000 newborns each year have SCD (there are about 75,000 people who have SCD in the U.S.). Although it is commonly thought of as affecting only people of African ancestry, it can occur in children of any race or ethnicity, including those whose ancestors come from South and Central America, India, Saudi Arabia, Italy, Greece, or Turkey.

In healthy children, red blood cells are normally round and flexible, and travel easily through blood vessels, transporting oxygen from the lungs to every part of the body. But children with SCD have abnormalities in hemoglobin (a component of every red blood cell), which can distort the shape of these red cells and contribute to the disease process. The irregularly shaped red cells become sticky, clumping together and interfering with the flow of nourishing blood to organs and limbs. These cells also can die prematurely, causing an ongoing deficiency of red blood cells.

Some babies have "sickle cell trait," which is different from SCD. These infants do not have the disease itself, but they carry the sickle cell gene responsible for causing it, and they can pass it along when they have children of their own. If a baby inherits the sickle cell gene from one parent but not the other, pediatricians categorize the child as having sickle cell trait, but with no SCD symptoms.

Signs and Symptoms

In most cases, infants with SCD appear healthy at birth. However, after a baby is a few months old, symptoms may emerge which can range from mild to severe.

Common signs and symptoms of SCD include:

- Inflammation and swelling of the hands and/or feet (called dactylitis or hand-foot syndrome); this is commonly the first symptom of SCD
- Anemia
- Pain
- Fatigue
- Shortness of breath
- Rapid heart rate
- Paleness

- Fever
- Jaundice (yellowing of the skin and eyes)
- Susceptibility to infections
- Delayed growth

A so-called "sickle cell crisis" may occur suddenly when an episode of pain develops, typically affecting the bones, joints, or abdomen. The intensity of pain can vary, and it can last from hours to many weeks. The trigger for these crises is unclear in many cases, although blocked blood flow plays a role, and in some cases, so can infections. Serious SCD complications can develop, including pneumonia, stroke, and organ damage (of the spleen, kidney, liver, or lung). When children with sickle cell trait are flying at high altitudes, "splenic infarction" (death of spleen tissue) can occur. These children also have a greater risk of blood in the stool or urine and urinary tract infections.

Treatment

If your baby has SCD, she should be diagnosed as early as possible so that appropriate treatment can be planned and started. Fortunately, most cases of SCD can be detected through a simple screening blood test that is universally given to infants in most states. SCD is the most common disorder identified by routine blood screening of newborns. Even if your state does not mandate such testing, you can request it from your pediatrician.

Infants with SCD need long-term care, not only to relieve symptoms but also to promptly manage any future "sickle cell crisis." Commonly prescribed treatments include the following:

- **Mild pain can** be relieved with over-the-counter medications such as acetaminophen or nonsteroidal anti-inflammatory drugs (NSAIDs) like ibuprofen. Heating pads also can be used for pain relief. In addition, good hydration is important.
- **Antibiotics should be** prescribed for all babies with SCD, beginning by two months of age and given continu-

ously until at least the age of five years. These medications are a preventive measure to reduce the risk of infections.

- **Babies with SCD** should receive all childhood immunizations as recommended by the American Academy of Pediatrics (see pages 734–735), including an annual influenza immunization.

Your child with SCD can benefit from various lifestyle measures. She should get plenty of rest and sleep. She should drink lots of water (particularly in warm weather) and avoid becoming overly hot or cold. Some doctors recommend folic acid supplements, which can help the body make more red blood cells.

If your baby's pain becomes severe, or she develops other serious symptoms or complications, your pediatrician may recommend hospitalization. While hospitalized, your infant could receive:

- Morphine or other drugs given intravenously (through a vein) for pain relief.
- Intravenous antibiotics that can manage an infection if one develops.
- Blood transfusions that can raise the number of red blood cells.
- Supplemental oxygen given through a mask that can add oxygen to the blood.

Because relatively mild symptoms (fever, pale skin, abdominal pain) can quickly progress to serious illness, parents should talk with their pediatrician in advance to make sure that the family has around-the-clock access to a medical facility experienced in treating SCD. If your baby develops a fever, contact your pediatrician at once because of the risk of a major infection.

Eye involvement. Babies with SCD can develop problems with their eyes and need to be examined by an ophthalmologist or pediatric ophthalmologist on a regular basis to make sure these complications do not occur. If they are found early, treatment is usually possible. Any type of eye injury in a child with SCD needs to be reported to your pediatrician immediately. What appears to be a "minor injury" to the eye might actually be serious, and possibly vision-threatening.

Spina bifida Spina bifida occurs when the spinal bones fail to close properly during early formation. Spina bifida occurs less often than Down syndrome, or in about 1 in 1000 births. It is, however, the most common of the physically disabling congenital abnormalities. A parent who has one child with spina bifida has a greater chance (1 out of 100) of having another. This increased frequency appears to be due to some combined effect of heredity and environment. There are now tests available to screen for spina bifida early in pregnancy.

A newborn with spina bifida appears at first glance to be normal, except for a small sac protruding from the spine. However, the sac contains spinal fluid and damaged nerves that lead to the lower body. Within the first few days, surgery must be performed to remove the sac and close the opening in the spine. Unfortunately, little can be done to repair the damaged nerves.

Most babies with spina bifida develop further problems later on, including the following.

Hydrocephalus. Up to 9 out of 10 babies with spina bifida eventually develop hydrocephalus, caused by an excessive increase in the fluid that normally cushions the brain from injury. The increase occurs because the spina bifida abnormality blocks the path through which the fluid ordinarily flows. This condition is serious and, if not treated, may lead to death.

The pediatrician should suspect hydrocephalus if the baby's head is growing more rapidly than expected. The condition is confirmed by a computerized X-ray of the head, called a CT (computed tomography) scan or magnetic resonance imagery (MRI). If the condition exists, surgery will be required to relieve fluid buildup.

Latex allergies. Infants with spina bifida are more likely to be allergic to latex. You can reduce the chances that he will acquire the sensitivity by avoiding exposure to latex. But be aware that many infant products contain latex (bottle nipples, pacifiers, teething toys, changing pads, mattress covers, and some diapers), so they should be avoided.

Muscle weakness or paralysis. Because the nerves leading to the lower part of the body are damaged, the muscles in the legs may be very weak or even paralyzed in infants with spina bifida. Their joints also tend to be very stiff, and many babies with this disorder are born with abnormalities of the hips, knees, and feet. Surgery can be performed to correct some of these problems, and the muscle weakness can be treated with physical therapy and special equipment, such as braces and walkers. Many children with spina bifida eventually can stand and some do walk, though the learning process is often long and extremely frustrating.

Bowel and bladder problems. Often the nerves that control bowel and bladder function are damaged in infants with spina bifida. As a result, these babies are more likely to develop urinary tract infections and damage to the kidneys due to abnormal urine flow. Special techniques are available to develop urinary control and minimize infections. Your pediatrician will advise you.

Bowel control also is a problem, but usually children with this disorder can achieve it. It may, however, take a great deal of time, patience, careful dietary management (to keep the stools soft), and the occasional use of suppositories, bowel stimulants, or special enemas.

Infection. Parents of babies who have spina bifida and hydrocephalus or urinary tract problems must be ever alert for signs of infection. Fortunately, the types of infections that occur in these cases usually can be treated effectively with antibiotics.

Educational and social problems. Seven out of 10 children with spina bifida have developmental and learning disabilities requiring some sort of special education. Many also need psychological counseling and tremendous emotional support in order to deal with their medical, educational, and social problems.

Parents of a baby with spina bifida need more than one

Where We Stand

In an effort to reduce the prevalence of spina bifida, the American Academy of Pediatrics endorses the recommendation of the U.S. Public Health Service that all women capable of becoming pregnant consume 400 micrograms per day of folic acid (a B vitamin). Folic acid helps to prevent neural tube defects (NTD), which include spina bifida. Although some foods are fortified with folic acid, it is not possible for women to meet the 400 microgram goal through a typical diet. Thus, an Academy policy statement recommends a daily multivitamin tablet that contains folic acid in the recommended dose. Studies show that if all women of childbearing age met these dietary requirements, 50 percent or more of NTDs could be prevented.

Women who are at high risk for an NTD-affected pregnancy (for example because of a previous NTD-affected pregnancy, having diabetes mellitus, or taking antiseizure medications) are advised to discuss their risk with their doctor. This includes possible treatments with very high doses of folic acid (4,000 micrograms per day), beginning one month before becoming pregnant and continuing throughout the first trimester. As the doctor will explain, however, women should not attempt to achieve this very high dose of folic acid by taking multivitamin supplements, but rather only under the care of a physician.

physician to manage their infant's medical care. In addition to the basic care your pediatrician delivers, this disorder requires a team approach that involves neurosurgeons, orthopedic surgeons, urologists, rehabilitation experts, physical therapists, psychologists, and social workers. Many medical centers run special spina bifida clinics, which offer the services of all these health professionals in one location. Having all members of the team together makes it easier for everyone to communicate and usually provides better access to information and assistance when parents need it.

Resources

Information and support for parents are available from various organizations.

March of Dimes
1–914–997–4488
www.marchofdimes.com

The National Down Syndrome Congress
1–800–232–NDSC (6372)
www.ndsccenter.org

The Spina Bifida Association of America
1–800–621–3141
www.spinabifidaassociation.org

United Cerebral Palsy Association
1–800–872–5827
www.ucp.org

HEARING LOSS

Although loss can occur at any age, hearing difficulties at birth or that develop during infancy can have serious consequences. This is because normal hearing is initially needed to understand spoken language and then, later, to produce clear speech. Consequently, if your child experiences hearing loss during infancy and early childhood, it demands immediate attention. Even a temporary but severe hearing loss during this time can make it very difficult for the child to learn proper oral language.

Most babies experience mild hearing loss when fluid accumulates in the middle ear from allergies or colds. This hearing loss is usually only temporary; normal hearing commonly resumes once the cold and allergies subside and the eustachian tube (which connects the middle ear to the throat) drains the remaining fluid into the back of the throat. In many children, perhaps 1 in 10, fluid stays in the middle ear following an ear infection (see page 557) because of problems with the eustachian tube. These infants don't hear as well as they should, and sometimes have delays in talking. Much less common is the permanent kind of hearing loss that always endangers normal speech and language development. Permanent hearing loss varies from mild or partial to complete or total.

There are two main kinds of hearing loss:

Conductive hearing loss. When a baby has a conductive hearing loss, there may be an abnormality in the structure of the outer ear canal or middle ear, or there may be fluid in the middle ear that interferes with the transfer of sound.

Sensorineural hearing loss (also called nerve deafness). This type of hearing impairment is caused by an abnormality of the inner ear or the nerves that carry sound messages from the inner ear to the brain. The loss can be present at birth or occur shortly thereafter. If there is a family history of deafness, the cause is likely to be inherited (genetic). If the mother had rubella (German measles), cytomegalovirus (CMV), or another infectious illness that affects hearing during pregnancy, the fetus could have been infected and may lose hearing as a result. The problem also may be due to a malformation of the inner ear. Most often the cause of severe sensorineural hearing loss is inherited. Still, in most cases, no other family member on either side will have hearing loss because each parent is only a carrier for a hearing loss gene. This is called an "autosomal recessive pattern," rather than "dominant" where it would be expected that other family members on one side would have hearing loss. Future brothers and sisters of the baby have an increased risk of being hearing impaired, and the family should seek genetic counseling if the hearing loss is determined to be inherited.

Hearing loss must be diagnosed as soon as possible, so that your baby isn't delayed in learning language—a process that begins the day she is born. The American Academy of Pediatrics recommends that before a newborn infant goes home from the hospital, she needs to undergo a hearing screening. Thirty-eight states, in fact, now have Early Hearing Detection Intervention (EHDI) programs, which mandate that all newborns be screened for hearing loss before they are discharged from the hospital. At any time during your child's life, if you and/or your pediatrician suspect that she has a hearing loss, insist that a formal hearing evaluation be performed promptly. (See *Hearing Loss: What to Look For* on page 552.) Although some family doctors, pediatricians, and well-baby clinics can test for fluid in the middle ear—a common cause of hearing loss—they cannot measure hearing precisely. Your baby should go to an audiologist, who can perform this service. She may also be seen by an ear, nose, and throat doctor (ENT; an otolaryngologist).

Your baby may be given one of two available screening tests, which are the same tests used for newborn screening. They are painless, take just five to ten minutes, and can be performed while your infant is sleeping or lying still. They are:

- **The auditory brainstem** response test, which measures how the brain responds to sound. Clicks or tones are played into the baby's ears through soft earphones, and electrodes placed on the baby's head measure the brain's response. This allows the doctor to test your baby's hearing without having to rely on her cooperation.

- **The otoacoustic emissions** test, which measures sound waves produced in the inner ear. A tiny probe is placed just inside the baby's ear canal, which then measures the response when clicks or tones are played into the baby's ear.

These tests may not be available in your immediate area, but the consequences of undiagnosed hearing loss are so serious that your doctor may advise you to travel to where one of them can be done. Certainly, if these tests indicate that your baby may have a hearing problem, your doctor should recommend a more thorough hearing evaluation as soon as possible to confirm whether your infant's hearing is impaired.

Treatment

Treating a hearing loss will depend on its cause: If it is a mild conductive hearing loss due to fluid in the middle ear, the doctor may simply recommend that your infant be retested in a few weeks to see whether the fluid has cleared by itself.

When to Call the Pediatrician
Hearing Loss: What to Look For

Here are the signs and symptoms that should make you suspect that your child has a hearing loss and alert you to call your pediatrician.

- Your child doesn't startle at loud noises by one month or turn to the source of a sound by three to four months of age.
- He doesn't notice you until he sees you.
- He concentrates on gargling sounds and other vibrating noises that he can feel, rather than experimenting with a wide variety of vowel sounds and consonants. (See *Language Development* in Chapters 8 and 9.)
- His speech is delayed or hard to understand, or he doesn't say single words such as "dada" or "mama" by twelve to fifteen months of age.
- He doesn't always respond when called. (This is usually mistaken for inattention or resistance, but could be the result of a partial hearing loss.)
- He seems to hear some sounds but not others. (Some hearing loss affects only high-pitched sounds; some babies have hearing loss in only one ear.)
- He seems not only to hear poorly but also has trouble holding his head steady, or is slow to sit or walk unsupported. (In some babies with sensorineural hearing loss, the part of the inner ear that provides information about balance and movement of the head is also damaged.)

Medication such as antihistamines, decongestants, or antibiotics are ineffective in clearing up middle ear fluid.

If there is no improvement in hearing over a three-month period, and there is still fluid behind the eardrum, the doctor may recommend referral to an ENT specialist. If the fluid persists and there is sufficient (even though temporary) conductive hearing impairment from the fluid, the specialist may recommend draining the fluid through ventilating tubes. These are surgically inserted through the eardrum. This is a minor operation and takes only a few minutes, but your baby must receive a general anesthetic for it to be done properly, so he usually will spend part of the day in a hospital or an outpatient surgery center.

Even with the tubes in place, future infections can occur, but the tubes help reduce the amount of fluid and decrease your infant's risk of repeated infection. They will also improve his hearing.

If a conductive hearing loss is due to a malformation of the outer or middle ear, a hearing aid may restore hearing to normal or near-normal levels. However, a hearing aid will work only when it's being worn. You must make sure it is on and functioning at all times, particularly in a very young child. Reconstructive surgery may be considered when the child is older.

Hearing aids will not restore hearing completely to those with significant sensorineural hearing loss, but they will help your child develop spoken or oral language if the hearing impairment is mild or moderate.

Parents of children with sensorineural hearing loss usually are most concerned about whether their child will learn to talk. The answer is that all children with a hearing impairment can be taught to speak, but not all will learn to speak clearly. Some children learn to lip-read well, while others never fully master the skill. But speech is only one form of language. Most children learn a combination of spoken and sign language. Written language also is very important because it is the key to educational and vocational success. Learning excellent oral language is highly desirable, but not all people who are born deaf can master this. Sign language is the primary way deaf people communicate with one another and the way many express themselves best.

18

EARS, NOSE, AND THROAT

COLDS/UPPER RESPIRATORY INFECTION

Your baby probably will have more colds, or upper respiratory infections, than any other illness. If your baby is in child care, or if there are older school-age children in your house, she may have even more, since colds spread easily among children who are in close contact with one another. That's the bad news, but there is some good news, too: Most colds go away by themselves and do not lead to anything worse.

Colds are caused by viruses, which are extremely small infectious organisms (much smaller than bacteria). A sneeze or a cough may directly transfer a virus from one person to another. The virus also may be spread indirectly, in the following manner.

1. A child or adult infected with the virus will, in coughing, sneezing, or touching her nose, transfer some of the virus particles onto her hand.
2. She then touches the hand of a healthy person.
3. This healthy person touches her newly contaminated hand to her own nose, introducing the infectious agent to a place where it can multiply and grow—the nose or throat. Symptoms of a cold soon develop.
4. The cycle then repeats itself, with the virus being transferred from this newly infected child or adult to the next susceptible one, and so on.

Once the virus is present and multiplying, your baby will develop the familiar symptoms and signs:

- Runny nose (first, a clear discharge; later, a thicker, often colored one).

- Sneezing
- Mild fever (101–102 degrees Fahrenheit [38.3–38.9 degrees Celsius]), particularly in the evening
- Decreased appetite
- Sore throat and, perhaps, difficulty swallowing
- Cough
- On-and-off irritability
- Slightly swollen glands in the neck

If your baby has a typical cold without complications, the symptoms should disappear gradually after seven to ten days.

Treatment

A baby older than three months with a cold usually doesn't need to see a doctor unless the condition becomes more serious. If she is three months or younger, however, call the pediatrician at the first sign of illness. With a young baby, symptoms can be misleading, and colds can quickly develop into more serious ailments, such as bronchiolitis (see page 494), croup (see page 500), or pneumonia (see page 505). For a baby older than three months, call the pediatrician if:

- The nostrils are widening with each breath, the skin above or below the ribs sucks in with each breath (retractions), or your baby is breathing rapidly or having any difficulty breathing.
- The lips or nails turn blue.
- Nasal mucus persists for longer than ten to fourteen days.
- The cough just won't go away (it lasts more than one week).
- She has pain in her ear (see *Middle Ear Infections,* page 557).
- Her temperature is over 102 degrees Fahrenheit (38.9 degrees Celsius).
- She is excessively sleepy or cranky.

Your pediatrician may want to see your infant, or he may ask you to watch her closely and report back if she doesn't improve each day and is not completely recovered within one week from the start of her illness.

Unfortunately, there's no cure for the common cold. Antibiotics may be used to combat *bacterial* infections, but they have no effect on viruses, so the best you can do is to make your baby comfortable. Make sure she gets extra rest and drinks a lot of fluids. If she has a fever or is uncomfortable, give her single-ingredient acetaminophen or ibuprofen. Ibuprofen is approved for children six months of age and older; however, it should *never* be given to babies who are dehydrated or who are vomiting repeatedly. (Be sure to follow the recommended dosage for your infant's age and the time interval for repeated doses.)

It's important to note, though, that over-the-counter (OTC) cough and cold medicines should not be given to infants and children under two years old because of the risk of life-threatening side effects. Also, several studies show that cold and cough products don't work in children younger than six years and can have potentially serious side effects. In addition, keep in mind that coughing clears mucus from the lower part of the respiratory tract, and ordinarily there's no reason to suppress it.

If your infant is having trouble breathing or drinking because of nasal congestion, clear her nose with saline (salt water) nose drops or spray, which are available without a prescription. This can then be followed by suction with a rubber suction bulb every few hours or before each feeding or before bed. For the nose drops, use a dropper that has been cleaned with soap and water and rinsed well with plain water. Place two drops in each nostril fifteen to twenty minutes before feeding, and then immediately suction with the bulb. *Never use nose drops that contain any medication, since excessive amounts can be absorbed. Only use normal saline nose drops.*

When using the suction bulb, remember to *squeeze the bulb part of the syringe first, gently stick the rubber tip into one nostril, and then slowly release the bulb.* This slight amount of suction will draw the clogged mucus out of the nose and should allow her to breathe and suck at the same time once again. You'll find that this technique works best when your baby is under six months of age. As she gets older, she'll fight the bulb, making it difficult to suction the mucus, but the saline drops will still be effective.

Placing a cool-mist humidifier (vaporizer) in your baby's room also will help keep nasal secretions more liquid and make her more comfortable. Set it close to her (but safely beyond her reach) so that she gets the full benefit of the additional moisture. Be sure to clean and dry the humidifier thoroughly each day to prevent bacterial or mold contamination. *Hot-water vaporizers are not recommended since they can cause serious scalds or burns.*

Prevention

If your baby is under three months old, the best prevention against colds is to keep her away from people who have them. This is especially true during the winter, when many of the viruses that cause colds are circulating in larger numbers. A virus that causes a mild illness in an older child or an adult can cause a more serious one in an infant.

Middle Ear Infections

Early in your baby's life, there's a good chance that he'll get a middle ear infection. At least 70 percent of the time, middle ear infections occur after colds that have weakened the body's ability to prevent bacteria from entering the middle ear. Doctors refer to this middle ear infection as acute otitis media.

Middle ear infections are one of the most prevalent treatable childhood illnesses, occurring most often in children between six months and three years of age. Two-thirds of all children have at least one ear infection by their second birthday. It's a particularly common problem among babies because they are more susceptible to colds and because of the length and shape of their tiny eustachian tubes, which normally ventilate the middle ear.

Babies under one year of age who spend time in child care programs tend to get more middle ear infections than those cared for at home, primarily because they are exposed to more viruses. Also, infants who self-feed when lying on their backs are susceptible to ear infections since this may allow small amounts of formula to enter the eustachian tube.

Other characteristics may place babies at a higher risk of middle ear infections:

Sex. Although researchers are not sure why, boys have more middle ear infections than girls.

Heredity. Ear infections can run in families. Babies are more likely to have repeated middle ear infections if a parent or a sibling also had numerous ear infections.

Secondhand smoke. Babies who breathe in secondhand tobacco smoke have a markedly increased risk of ear infections as well as respiratory infections, bronchitis, pneumonia, and asthma.

Signs and Symptoms

Middle ear infections are usually, but not always, painful. Babies with ear infections may cry even more during feedings, because sucking and swallowing cause painful pressure changes in the middle ear. A baby with an ear infection may have trouble sleeping. Fever is another warning signal; ear infections sometimes (one out of three) are accompanied by elevated temperatures ranging from 100.4 to 104 degrees Fahrenheit (38–40 degrees Celsius).

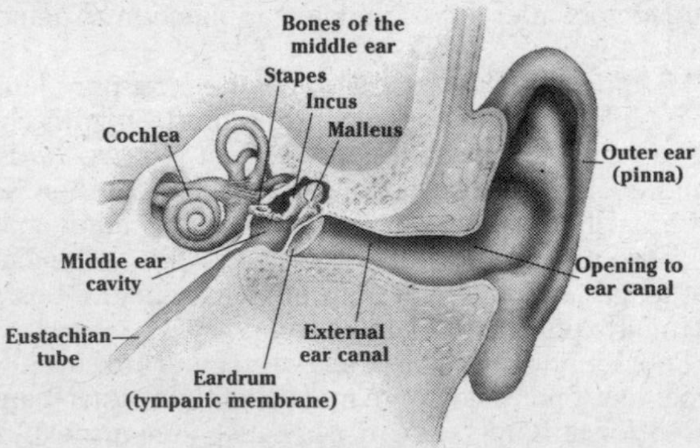

Cross Section of Ear

You might see blood-tinged yellow fluid or pus draining from the infected ear. This kind of discharge means that the eardrum has developed a small hole (called a perforation). This hole usually heals by itself without complications, but you will want to describe the discharge to your pediatrician.

You also may notice that your baby may not hear well. This occurs because the fluid behind the eardrum interferes with sound transmission. But the hearing loss is usually temporary; normal hearing will be restored once the middle ear is free of fluid. Occasionally, when ear infections recur, fluid may remain behind the eardrum for many weeks and continue to interfere with hearing. If you feel your baby's hearing is not as good as it was, including before his ear became infected, consult your pediatrician. If you remain concerned, request a consultation with an ear, nose, and throat doctor (ENT; otolaryngologist). After several months of watchful waiting, your pediatrician may recommend a hearing test if your baby has had middle ear fluid in both ears for more than three months, or in one ear for more than six months.

Ear infections are most common during the cold and flu season of winter and early spring.

Treatment

Whenever you suspect an ear infection, call your pediatrician. In the meantime, follow these steps to make your child more comfortable.

- **If he has** a high fever, cool him using the procedures described in Chapter 23.
- **Give acetaminophen or** ibuprofen in the dose appropriate for his age. (Don't give aspirin to your baby; it has been associated with Reye syndrome, a disease that affects the liver and brain.)

Putting a pain-relieving drop into the ear canal may help reduce pain, but ask your pediatrician whether this should be used. The pediatrician will look into your baby's ears with a lighted magnifying instrument called an otoscope to determine whether there is fluid in the middle ear space behind the eardrum. The doctor may attach a piece of rubber tubing to the otoscope and press on a rubber bulb to gently blow air into the ear to check for sensitivity and eardrum movement. Your doctor may also use a special instrument such as a tympanometer to determine whether there is fluid in the middle ear. He may also perform a test called acoustic reflectometry to detect fluid in the middle ear.

If there's a fever, the doctor will examine your baby to determine whether there are any other problems. Eardrops sometimes are used to relieve pain. Unless your baby's ear infections are associated with allergies, antihistamines and decongestants probably won't help.

An antibiotic is one of the treatment options for ear infections. If recommended, your doctor will specify the schedule for giving it to your baby; it may be two or three times a day. Follow the schedule precisely. There should be clear signs of improvement and disappearance of ear pain and fever within three days.

When your baby starts feeling better, you may be tempted to discontinue the medication—but don't. Some of the bacteria that caused the infection still may be present. Stopping the treatment too soon may allow them to multiply again and permit the infection to return with full force. Your pediatrician may want to see your baby after the medication is finished, to check if any fluid is still present behind the eardrum, which can occur even if the infection has been controlled. This condition (fluid in middle ear), known as otitis media with effusion, is extremely common: 5 out of every 10 children still have some fluid three weeks after an ear infection is treated. In 9 out of 10 cases, the fluid will disappear within three months without additional treatment. Also, this fluid accumulation may be caused by something other than an ear infection, such as swollen adenoid tissue in the upper throat that interferes with drainage; for that reason, seeing a doctor is especially important to determine the cause of and best care for the problem.

Occasionally an ear infection won't respond to the first antibiotic prescribed. If your baby continues to have significant ear pain and still has a high fever for more than two days after starting an antibiotic, call the pediatrician. To determine if the antibiotic is working, your doctor or a consulting ENT specialist may take a sample of the fluid from the ear by inserting a needle through the eardrum. If the analysis of this

Antibiotic Overuse

Antibiotics may be important treatment in managing ear infections. But in recent years pediatricians have been prescribing antibiotics with much more care to minimize the growing problem of "antibiotic resistance." If antibiotics are used when they are not needed—or if patients do not take a complete course of the drug—new strains of bacteria may develop. When that happens, antibiotics eventually may stop working and the infections they're designed to treat will no longer be curable by the use of these medications, because the bacteria have become "resistant" to them.

Here are some important points to keep in mind to reduce the risk of antibiotic resistance.

- Antibiotics work only against bacterial illnesses, not those caused by viruses. So while they may be appropriate for treating ear infections, you should not ask your pediatrician for a prescription for antibiotics to treat your baby's colds and flu (as well as many sore throats and coughs), which are viral infections.
- When your pediatrician recommends antibiotics for an ear infection or other bacterial infection, make sure that your baby takes them exactly as your doctor instructs. That means taking all of the medicine that was prescribed, even if your infant seems well before he has finished the entire course.
- Don't give your baby antibiotics that have been prescribed for another family member or for another illness.

sample reveals that the infection is caused by bacteria resistant to the antibiotic your baby has been taking, your pediatrician will prescribe a different one. In very rare instances, an ear infection may linger even though other drugs are used. In these cases, a baby may be hospitalized so that antibiotics can be given intravenously and the ear can be drained surgically.

Should a baby with an ear infection be kept home? It won't be necessary if he's feeling well, as long as someone at child care can administer his medication properly. Talk with your baby's caregiver, and review the dosage and the times when it should be given. You also should check to be sure that storage facilities are available if the medication must be refrigerated. Medicine that doesn't require refrigeration should be kept in a locked cabinet separate from other items, and its container should be clearly identified with your baby's name and the proper dosage.

If your baby's eardrum has ruptured, he'll be able to engage in most activities. Ordinarily, there's no reason to prevent him from flying in an airplane, although he may have some discomfort from the pressure change.

Prevention

Occasional ear infections cannot be prevented. In some children, ear infections may be related to seasonal allergies, which also can cause congestion and block the natural drainage of fluid from the ear to the throat. If your baby seems to get ear infections more frequently when his allergies flare up, mention this to your pediatrician, who may suggest additional testing or prescribe antihistamines.

If your baby is being bottle-fed, hold his head above the stomach level during feedings. Doing this keeps the eustachian tubes from becoming blocked. You and others also should not smoke around your baby. Again, infants exposed to secondhand tobacco smoke have more respiratory infections, bronchitis, pneumonia, poor lung function, and asthma than children who aren't exposed.

And what about babies who recover from one ear infection only to get another shortly thereafter? If your baby continues to have ear infections, he probably will be referred to an ear specialist, who may recommend that tiny ventilation tubes be inserted in the eardrum under anesthesia. While the tubes are in place, they usually restore hearing to normal, and also prevent fluid and harmful bacteria from

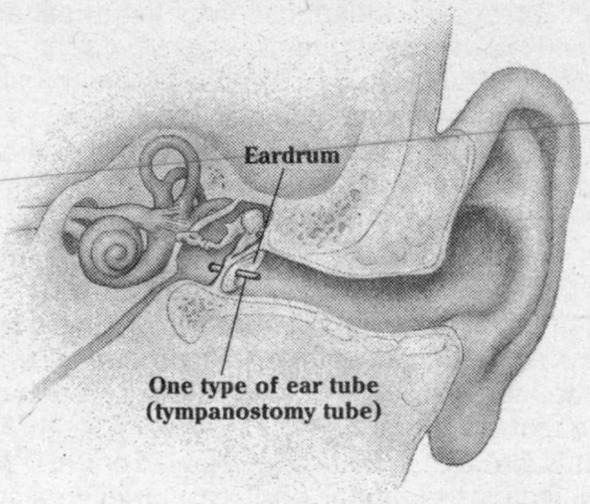

becoming trapped in the middle ear, where they can cause another infection.

Use of tubes has become standard care for the following specific indications: 1) persistent fluid in both middle ears for more than three months with hearing loss; 2) persistent fluid in one middle ear longer than six months; or 3) recurrent ear infections with significant symptoms occurring more than three times in six months or more than four to five times in twelve months. If the placement of ventilation tubes is proposed for your infant, discuss his specific problem with your pediatrician so you fully understand the advantages and disadvantages.

Keep in mind that although ear infections are bothersome and uncomfortable, they are usually minor and clear up without causing any lasting problems.

Sore Throat (Strep Throat, Tonsillitis)

The terms *sore throat, strep throat,* and *tonsillitis* often are used interchangeably, but they don't mean the same thing. Tonsillitis refers to tonsils that are inflamed. Strep throat is an infection caused by a specific type of bacteria, *Streptococcus.* When your child has a strep throat, the tonsils are usually very inflamed, and the inflammation may affect the surrounding part of the throat as well. Other causes of sore throats are viruses and may only cause inflammation of the throat around the tonsils and not the tonsils themselves.

In infants, the most frequent cause of sore throats is a viral infection. No specific medicine is required when a virus is responsible, and the baby should get better over a seven- to ten-day period. Often infants who have sore throats due to viruses also have a cold at the same time. They may develop a mild fever, too, but they generally aren't very sick.

One particular virus (called Coxsackie), seen most often during the summer and fall, may cause the baby to have a somewhat higher fever, more difficulty swallowing, and a sicker overall feeling. If your infant has a Coxsackie infection, she also may have one or more blisters in her throat and on her hands and feet (often called Hand, Foot, and Mouth disease). Infectious mononucleosis can produce a sore throat, often with marked tonsillitis; however, most young children who are infected with the mononucleosis virus have few or no symptoms.

Strep throat is caused by a bacterium called *Streptococcus pyogenes*. To some extent, the symptoms of strep throat depend on the child's age. Infants with strep infections may have only a low fever and a thickened or bloody nasal discharge.

Diagnosis and Treatment

If your baby has a sore throat that persists, whether or not it is accompanied by fever, headache, stomachache, or extreme fatigue, you should call your pediatrician. That call should be made even more urgently if your baby seems extremely ill, or if she has difficulty breathing or extreme trouble swallowing (causing her to drool). This may indicate a more serious infection.

Prevention

Most types of throat infections are contagious, being passed primarily through the air on droplets of moisture or on the hands of infected children or adults. For that reason, it makes sense to keep your baby away from people who have symptoms of this condition. However, most people are contagious before their first symptoms appear, so often there's really no practical way to prevent your baby from contracting the disease.

In the past when a baby had several sore throats, her tonsils might have been removed in an attempt to prevent further infections. But this operation, called a tonsillectomy, is recommended today only for the most severely affected children. Even in difficult cases, where there is repeated strep throat, antibiotic treatment is usually the best solution.

19

EMERGENCIES

The information and policies in this chapter are constantly changing. Ask your pediatrician or other qualified health professional for the latest information on these procedures.

It is rare for babies to become seriously ill with no warning. Based on your infant's symptoms, you should usually contact your pediatrician for advice. Timely treatment of symptoms can prevent an illness from getting worse or turning into an emergency.

At the same time, take steps *before* an emergency occurs to prepare for such an event if it should happen (see guidelines for emergency phone numbers on page 568). Also read the description of how to assemble a first-aid kit (page 581).

A true emergency is when you believe a severe injury or illness is threatening your baby's life or may cause permanent harm. In these cases, an infant needs emergency medical treatment immediately. Discuss with your pediatrician in advance what you should do in case of a true emergency.

Many true emergencies involve sudden injuries. These injuries are often caused by the following:

- Motor vehicle-related injuries (car crashes, pedestrian injuries), or other sudden impacts such as falls from heights
- Poisoning
- Burns or smoke inhalation
- Choking
- "Nonfatal drowning" (once referred to as "near drowning")

- Firearms or other weapons
- Electric shocks

Other true emergencies can result from either medical illnesses or injuries. Often you can tell that these emergencies are happening if you observe that your baby has any of the following symptoms:

- Becoming less alert
- Increasing difficulty with breathing
- Skin or lips that look blue or purple (or gray for darker-skinned children)
- A cut or burn that is large or deep
- Bleeding that does not stop
- Rhythmical jerking and loss of consciousness (a seizure)
- Unconsciousness
- Any change in level of consciousness, confusion, a bad headache, or vomiting several times *after a head injury*
- Major mouth or facial injuries
- Increasing or severe persistent pain
- Decreasing responsiveness when you talk to your baby

Call your baby's pediatrician or the Poison Help Line (1–800–222–1222) at once if your infant has swallowed a suspected poison or another person's medication, even if your baby has no signs or symptoms. You should not make a baby vomit by any means, including giving him syrup of ipecac, making him gag, or giving him saltwater. If you have syrup of ipecac in your home, flush it down the toilet and throw away the container.

Always call for help if you are concerned that your infant's life may be in danger or your baby is seriously hurt.

Emergency Phone Numbers

Keep the following phone numbers and addresses handy by taping them on or near your phone. You might post them on your refrigerator and insert a copy in your wallet:

- Your home phone and address
- Your cell phone or pager number
- A nearby relative's or trusted neighbor's or friend's phone
- Your baby's pediatrician
- Emergency medical services (ambulance) (911 in most areas)
- Police (911 in most areas)
- Fire department (911 in most areas)
- Poison Help Line (1–800–222–1222)
- Hospital
- Dentist

It is important that everyone who cares for your baby, including care providers or sitters, knows where to find emergency phone numbers. If you have 911 service in your area, make sure your older children and your sitter know to dial 911 in case of an emergency. (All the emergency numbers can be programmed into your own cell phone and those of others.) Be certain that they know your home address and phone number, since an emergency operator will ask for or confirm this information. Always leave the phone number and address where you can be located, including your cell phone number. You should also make sure your sitter knows any medications your baby takes and any allergies he may have. Those caring for your infant (including you and your spouse) also should take a CPR class.

Remember, for a medical emergency, always call 911 and/or your baby's pediatrician. If your infant is seriously ill or injured, it may be safer for your baby to be transported by emergency medical services (an ambulance).

In Case of a True Emergency

- Stay calm.
- If it is needed and you know how, start CPR (cardiopulmonary resuscitation). For information on CPR, see page 575.
- If you need immediate help, call 911. If you do not have 911 service in your area, call your local emergency ambulance service or county emergency medical service. Otherwise, call your baby's pediatrician's office and state clearly that you have an emergency.
- If there is bleeding, apply continuous pressure to the site with a clean cloth.
- If your infant is having a seizure, place her on a carpeted floor with her head turned to the side, and stay with her until help arrives.

After you arrive at the emergency room, make sure you tell the emergency staff the name of your baby's pediatrician; he will work closely with the emergency department and can provide them with additional information about your infant. Bring any medication your baby is taking and her immunization record with you to the hospital. Also bring any suspected poisons or other medications your infant might have taken.

Bites

Animal Bites

You need to keep your child safe around animals, including family pets. Review the section *Safety Around Animals* on page 426.

Many parents assume that children are most likely to be bitten by strange or wild animals, but in fact most bites are inflicted by animals the child knows, including the family pet. Although the injury often is minor, biting does at times cause serious wounds, facial damage, and emotional problems.

As many as 1 percent of all visits to pediatric emergency centers during the summer months are for human or animal bite wounds. An estimated 4.7 million dog bites, 400,000 cat bites, 45,000 snake bites, and 250,000 human bites occur annually in the United States. About 6 of 10 of those bitten by dogs are children. About 50 out of every 100 people bitten by a cat get an infection, compared to 15 to 20 of every 100 following dog or human bites.

Treatment

If your baby is bleeding from an animal bite, apply firm continuous pressure to the area for five minutes or until the bleeding stops. Then wash the wound gently with soap and water, and consult your pediatrician.

If the wound is very large, or if you cannot stop the bleeding, continue to apply pressure and call your pediatrician to find out where to take your baby for treatment. If the wound is so large that the edges won't come together, it probably will need to be sutured (stitched). Although this will help reduce scarring, in an animal bite, it increases the chance of infection, so your doctor may prescribe antibiotics.

Contact your pediatrician whenever your baby receives an animal bite that breaks the skin, no matter how minor the injury appears. The doctor will need to check whether your infant has been adequately immunized against tetanus (see Immunization Schedule on pages 734–735) or might require protection against rabies. Both of these diseases can be spread by animal bites.

Rabies is a viral infection that can be transmitted by an infected animal through bites or scratches. It causes a high fever, difficulty in swallowing, convulsions, and ultimately death. Fortunately, rabies in humans is so rare today that no more than five cases have been reported in the United States each year since 1960; the number of human deaths caused by rabies in this country has declined from one hundred or more each year early in the twentieth century to an average of one or two each year today. Nevertheless, because the disease is so serious and the incidence has been increasing in animals, your pediatrician will carefully evaluate any bite for the risk of contracting this disease. The risk probably depends a great deal on the animal and the circumstances surrounding the bite. Bites from wild animals, especially bats but also skunks, raccoons, coyotes, and foxes, are much more dangerous than those from tame, immunized (against rabies) dogs and cats. The health of the animal also is important, so if possible, the animal should be captured and confined for later examination by a veterinarian. For help capturing the animal you may want to contact the animal control in your area or contact your local public health department. Talk to your pediatrician about reporting the incident to your local health department. *Do not destroy the animal.* If it has been killed, however, the brain can be examined for rabies, so call your pediatrician immediately for advice on how to handle the situation.

If the risk of rabies is high as determined by your pediatrician, he immediately will give, or arrange to have given, injections of the rabies vaccine to prevent the disease. If the biting animal is a healthy dog or cat, he will recommend that it be observed for ten days, starting treatment for your baby only if the animal shows signs of rabies. If the animal is a wild one, commonly identified as a rabies risk if captured, it usually is euthanized immediately so that its brain can be examined for signs of rabies infection.

As noted earlier, an animal bite (even when it doesn't cause rabies) can become infected. Notify your pediatrician immediately if you see any of the following signs of infection.

- Pus or drainage coming from the bite
- The area immediately around the bite becoming swollen

and tender (It normally will be red for two or three days, but this in itself is not cause for alarm.)

- Red streaks that appear to spread out from the bite
- Swollen glands above the bite

(See also *Safety Around Animals,* page 426.)

Your pediatrician may recommend antibiotic therapy for a baby who has:

- Moderate or severe bite wounds
- Puncture wounds, especially if the bone, tendon, or joint has been penetrated
- Facial bites
- Hand and foot bites
- Genital area bites

Babies who have a weakened immune system or have no spleen often receive antibiotic treatment.

Your pediatrician may recommend a follow-up visit to inspect any wound for signs of infection within forty-eight hours.

Human Bites

Children often experience a human bite by a sibling or a playmate. If your baby is bitten by another person, call your pediatrician immediately to describe the severity of the injury. Doing this can be especially important if the biter's teeth pierced your infant's skin or if the injury is large enough to require stitches.

Be sure to wash a serious bite carefully with cool water and soap before going to the pediatrician. Your pediatrician will check your baby's tetanus and hepatitis B vaccine status and assess the risk for other infections. For a bite that barely breaks the skin, such as a cut or scrape, a good washing with soap and water, followed by bandaging and close follow-up, is all that is needed. (For more information on human biting, aggressive behavior, or biting in situations with AIDS, see Chapter 10, page 376; Chapter 16, page 525.)

BURNS

Burns are divided into three categories, according to their severity. First-degree burns are the mildest and cause redness and perhaps slight swelling of the skin (like most sunburns). Second-degree burns cause blistering and considerable swelling. Third-degree burns may appear white or charred and cause serious injury, not just to the surface but also to the deeper skin layers.

There are many different causes of serious burns in babies, including sunburn, hot-water scalds, and those due to fire, electrical contact, or chemicals. All of these can cause permanent injury and scarring to the skin.

Treatment

Your *immediate* treatment of a burn should include the following.

1. As quickly as possible, soak the burn in cool water. Don't hesitate to run cool water over the burn long enough to cool the area and relieve the pain immediately after the injury. *Do not use ice on a burn. It may delay healing.* Also, do not rub a burn; it can increase blistering.
2. Cool any smoldering clothing immediately by soaking with water, then remove any clothing from the burned area unless it is stuck firmly to the skin. In that case, cut away as much clothing as possible.
3. If the injured area is not oozing, cover the burn with a sterile gauze pad or a clean, dry cloth.
4. If the burn is oozing, cover it lightly with sterile gauze if available and immediately seek medical attention. If sterile gauze is not available, cover burns with a clean sheet or towel.
5. Do not put butter, grease, or powder on a burn. All of these so-called home remedies actually can make the injury worse.

For anything more serious than a superficial burn, or if redness and pain continue for more than a few hours, consult a physician. *All* electrical burns and burns of the hands, mouth, or genitals should receive immediate medical attention. Chemicals that cause burns also may be absorbed through the skin and cause other symptoms. Call the Poison Help Line (1–800–222–1222) or your pediatrician after washing off all the chemicals. (For treatment of a chemical contact to a baby's eye, see *Poison in the Eye,* page 593.)

If your physician thinks the burn is not too serious, he may show you how to clean and care for it at home using medicated ointments and dressings. Under the following circumstances, however, hospitalization may be necessary.

- If the burns are third degree
- If 10 percent or more of the body is burned
- If the burn involves the face, hands, feet, or genitals, or involves a moving joint

When treating a burn at home, watch for any increase in redness or swelling or the development of a bad odor or discharge. These can be signs of infection, which will require medical attention.

Prevention

Chapter 11, *Keeping Your Child Safe,* provides ways to safeguard your infant against fire and scalding at home. For added protection, here are a few more suggestions.

- **Install smoke detectors** in hallways outside bedrooms, the kitchen, living room, and near the furnace, with at least one on every floor of the house. Test them every month to be sure they work. It is best to use alarms that have long-life batteries, but if these are not available, change batteries at least annually on a specific date that you'll remember (such as January 1 of each year).
- **Practice home fire** drills. Make sure every family member and others who care for your children in your home

know how to leave any area of the home safely in case of a fire.

- **Have several working** fire extinguishers readily available. Place fire extinguishers around the home where the risk of fire is greatest, such as in the kitchen, furnace room, and near the fireplace.
- **Avoid smoking indoors.**
- **Do not leave** food cooking on the stove unattended.
- **Lock up flammable** liquids in the home. It is best to store them outside the home, out of children's reach, and away from heat or ignition sources.
- **Lower the temperature** of your water heater to below 120 degrees Fahrenheit (48.9 degrees Celsius) to prevent hot water scalds and burns.
- **Don't plug appliances** or other electrical equipment into extension cords if they place too much "amperage" or load on the cord, thus creating a potentially unsafe situation.
- **Keep matches and** lighters away from babies and older children, locked and out of reach.
- **Avoid all fireworks,** even those meant for consumer use.

Cardiopulmonary Resuscitation (CPR) and Mouth-to-Mouth Resuscitation

CPR can save your baby's life if his heart stops beating or he has stopped breathing for any reason such as drowning, poisoning, suffocation, smoke inhalation, or choking. Become familiar with the CPR instructions in the Appendix of this book. However, reading about CPR is not enough to teach you how to perform it. *The American Academy of Pediatrics strongly recommends that all parents and anyone who is responsible for the care of children should complete a course in basic CPR and treatment for choking.*

This training is especially vital if you own a swimming pool or live near water, such as a lake or community swimming pool or spa. Contact your local chapter of the American Heart Association or the American Red Cross to find out where and when certified courses are given in your community. Most of the classes teach basic first aid, CPR, and emergency prevention, along with what to do for a choking infant or child.

CHOKING

Choking occurs when a person inhales something other than air into the windpipe or when food or other objects block the windpipe. Among babies, choking often is caused by liquid that "goes down the wrong way." The infant will cough, wheeze, gasp, and gag until the windpipe is cleared, but this type of choking is usually not harmful.

Choking becomes life-threatening when an infant swallows or inhales an object—often food—that blocks air flow to the lungs. This is an emergency that calls for immediate first aid. For specific and complete choking/CPR instructions, familiarize yourself with the chart in the Appendix on page 742, and take a CPR course for children.

A baby who begins to breathe by herself two or three minutes after a choking incident probably will not suffer any long-term damage. The longer she is deprived of oxygen, however, the greater the risk of permanent injury.

Occasionally a choking episode is followed by persistent coughing, gagging, wheezing, excessive salivation, or difficulty in swallowing or breathing. If this occurs, it may mean that an object is still partially blocking the airway—possibly in the lower breathing tubes. In this case, the object can cause continued breathing difficulty, irritation, and possibly pneumonia. Notify your pediatrician if any symptoms persist, so that further tests, such as chest X-rays, can be done. If they show that your baby has inhaled something, she probably will need to be admitted to the hospital for a procedure to remove the object.

Prevention

Choking is a very common cause of unintentional injury or death in children under age one, and the danger remains significant until the age of five. Objects such as safety pins, small parts from toys, and coins cause choking, but food is responsible for most incidents. You must be particularly watchful when babies around the age of one are sampling new foods. Here are some additional suggestions for preventing choking.

- **Don't give babies** hard, smooth foods (i.e., peanuts, raw vegetables) that must be chewed with a grinding motion. Children don't master that kind of chewing until age four, so they may attempt to swallow the food whole. Do not give peanuts to children until age seven or older.
- **Don't give your** infant round, firm foods (like hot dogs and carrot sticks) unless they are chopped completely. Cut or break food into bite-size pieces (no larger than ½ inch [1.27 cm]) and encourage your baby to chew thoroughly.
- **Supervise mealtime for** your infant. Don't let her eat while playing or running. Teach her to chew and swallow her food before talking or laughing.
- **Chewing gum is** inappropriate for babies.

Because infants put everything into their mouths, small nonfood objects are also responsible for many choking incidents. Look for age guidelines in selecting toys, but use your own judgment concerning your baby. Also be aware that certain objects have been associated with choking, including uninflated or broken balloons; baby powder; items from the trash (e.g., eggshells, pop-tops from beverage cans); safety pins; coins; marbles; small balls; pen or marker caps; small, button-type batteries; hard, gooey, or sticky candy or vitamins; grapes; and popcorn. If you're unsure whether an object or food item could be harmful, you can purchase a standard small-parts cylinder at juvenile products stores or test toys using a toilet paper roll, which has a diameter of approximately 1¾ inches.

Cuts and Scrapes

Your baby's natural curiosity and eagerness are likely to produce some scrapes and cuts along the way. His reaction may be far more severe than the actual damage. In most cases, good treatment will require little more than cleansing the injury, protecting it, and providing plenty of reassurance (and perhaps a kiss on the minor bump or bruise).

Scrapes

Most minor injuries in young children are scrapes, or abrasions, which means that the outer layers of skin literally have been scraped off. If the abrasion covers a large area, it may appear to be very bloody, although the actual amount of blood lost is small. The area should be rinsed first with cool water to flush away debris and then washed gently with warm water and soap. Avoid using iodine and other antiseptic solutions. They have little protective value, and can add to the pain and discomfort.

If left alone, most abrasions "scab" over quickly, and this was thought to be the best natural remedy. But scabs actually slow the healing process and can lead to more scarring. Treat large or oozing scrapes with an antibiotic ointment and then cover them with a sterile (germ-free) dressing. These can be obtained at your local pharmacy, either in the form of an adhesive bandage or a separate gauze pad that is held in place by roller gauze or adhesive tape. Antibiotic ointment also helps prevent the dressing from sticking to the healing wound surface. The purpose is to prevent the injury from becoming infected while healing occurs. It is best to keep the bandage in place, except for dressing changes, until the wound heals. Take care that dressings around such areas as fingers or toes are not so tight as to interfere with circulation.

Some dressings are made of materials such as Telfa, which are less likely to adhere to the raw surface of a wound. Examine the wound daily during the dressing change, or whenever it becomes dirty or wet. If a bandage sticks when you try to remove it, soak it off with warm water. Most wounds require a dressing for only two or three days.

Call your pediatrician if you can't get a wound clean or notice drainage of pus, increasing tenderness or redness around the site, or fever. These are signs that the wound may be infected. If necessary, the doctor can use a local anesthetic to prevent severe pain while cleaning out dirt and debris that you are not able to remove. If the wound is infected, she may prescribe antibiotics by mouth or in the form of an ointment or cream.

Cuts, Lacerations, and Bleeding

A cut or laceration is a wound that breaks through the skin and into the tissues beneath. Because the injury is deeper than a scrape, there are more likely to be problems, such as bleeding, and there is the possibility of damage to nerves and tendons. The following simple guidelines will help you prevent serious bleeding and other problems such as scarring when your baby gets a cut.

1. Apply pressure. Almost all active bleeding can be stopped by applying direct pressure with clean gauze or cloth over the site for five or ten minutes. The most common mistake is interrupting the pressure too early in order to peek at the wound. Doing this may result in more bleeding or in the buildup of a clot that can make it harder to control the problem with further pressure. If bleeding starts again after five minutes of continuous pressure, reapply pressure and call your doctor for help. Do *not* use a tourniquet or tie-off on an arm or leg unless you are trained in its use, since this can cause severe damage if left on too long.

2. Stay calm. The sight of blood frightens most people, but this is an important time to stay in control. You'll make better decisions if you are calm, and your baby will be less likely to get upset by the situation. Remember, by using direct pressure you will be able to control bleeding from even the most severe lacerations until help can arrive. Relatively minor cuts to the head and face will bleed more than cuts to other parts of the body because of the greater number of small, superficial blood vessels.

3. Seek medical advice for serious cuts. No matter how much (or how little) bleeding occurs, call your doctor if the laceration is deep (through the skin) or more than ½ inch (1.27 cm) long. Deep cuts can severely damage underlying muscles, nerves, and tendons, even if on the surface the wound does not appear serious. Long lacerations and those on the face, chest, and back are more likely to leave disfiguring scars. In these situations, if the wound is properly closed, the scar probably will be much less apparent. In some circumstances a skin adhesive (a gluelike substance) may be used to close the wound. If in doubt about whether stitches, adhesives, or staples are needed, call your doctor right away for advice as it's important for repair to occur within eight to twelve hours of the injury.

You should be able to treat short, minor cuts yourself, as long as the edges come together by themselves, or with the aid of a "butterfly" bandage, and if there is no numbness beyond the wound and no reduction in sensation or movement. (A butterfly bandage is a strip of adhesive with ends that flare. It's used to keep the edges of a cut together during the healing process.) However, have your doctor examine your baby if there is any possibility that foreign matter, such as dirt or glass, is trapped in the cut. Any injury that you cannot manage should be seen by your pediatrician or emergency medical services as soon as possible to maximize healing. Your baby may not like to let you examine a laceration thoroughly because of the pain involved. The pediatrician, however, can use a local anesthetic, if necessary, to ensure a thorough exam.

4. Clean and dress the wound. If you feel comfortable handling the problem, wash the wound with plain water and examine it carefully to be sure it is clean. Apply an antibiotic ointment, then cover it with a sterile dressing. It's easy to underestimate the extent or severity of a cut, so even if you choose to treat it yourself, don't hesitate to call your pediatrician for advice. If any redness, swelling, or pus appears around the wound, or if bleeding recurs, consult your physician as soon as possible. Antiseptics such as iodine and alcohol are not necessary and increase your baby's discomfort, so do not use them on cuts. If your infant's immunizations are current, tetanus shots are not necessary after most abrasions and lacerations.

See the box *First-Aid Supplies for Your Home and Car* on page 581 for information on assembling items needed to treat your family's wounds and injuries.

First-Aid Supplies for Your Home and Car

You should prepare a first-aid kit for your home as well as one for each of your cars. The kit should contain:

- Acetaminophen or a nonsteroidal anti-inflammatory medication (such as ibuprofen)
- Antibiotic ointment
- Prescription medications (a month's supply)
- Sterile adhesive bandages (in various sizes)
- Gauze pads
- Adhesive tape (hypoallergenic)
- Scissors
- Tweezers
- Soap or another cleansing agent
- Petroleum jelly or another lubricant
- Moistened towelettes
- Thermometer

Prevention

It is almost impossible for a curious and active baby to avoid some scrapes and minor cuts, but there are things you can do to decrease the number your infant will have and to minimize their severity. Keep potentially dangerous objects like sharp knives, easily breakable glass objects, and scissors out of his reach. At regular intervals make a safety check of your house, garage, and yard. If you find objects that are potentially dangerous because your baby is older and can get into them, store them securely out of his reach.

Also see Chapter 11, *Keeping Your Child Safe.*

Drowning

Drowning is a leading cause of death among children, including infants and toddlers. Most infant drownings occur in bathtubs and buckets. It is important to know that children can drown in even one inch of water.

Drowning refers to death that occurs in this way. When a child is rescued before death, the episode is called a nonfatal drowning.

What You Should Do

Get your baby out of the water immediately, then check to see if she is breathing on her own. If she is not, begin CPR immediately (see Appendix). If someone else is present, send him or her to call for emergency medical help, but don't spend precious moments looking for someone, and don't waste time trying to drain water from your baby's lungs. Concentrate instead on giving her rescue breathing and CPR until she is breathing on her own. Vomiting of swallowed water is very likely during CPR. Only when the infant's breathing has resumed should you stop and seek emergency help. Call 911. Once the paramedics arrive, they will administer oxygen and continue CPR if necessary.

Any baby who has come close to drowning should be given a complete medical examination, even if she seems all right. If she stopped breathing, inhaled water, or lost consciousness, she should remain under medical observation for at least twenty-four hours to be sure there is no damage to her respiratory or nervous system.

A baby's recovery from a nonfatal drowning depends on how long she was deprived of oxygen. If she was underwater only briefly, she is likely to recover completely. Longer periods without oxygen can cause damage to the lungs, heart, or brain. An infant who doesn't respond quickly to CPR may have more serious problems, but it's important to keep trying, because sustained CPR has revived babies who have appeared lifeless or who have been immersed in very cold water for lengthy periods.

Prevention

For infants and children through four years of age, parents and caregivers should never—even for a moment—leave them alone or in the care of another child, while in or near bathtubs, pools, spas, or wading pools, or near irrigation ditches or other open bodies of water. With babies of this age, practice "touch supervision"; that means that a supervising adult should be within an arm's length of the infant with full attention focused on the baby at all times when she is in or near water. The supervising adult should not be engaged in distracting activities, such as talking on a telephone, socializing, or tending to household chores.

Home swimming pools should be surrounded by a fence that prevents a baby from getting to the pool from the house. There is no substitute for at least a four-foot-high, nonclimbable, four-sided fence with a self-closing, self-latching gate. Parents, caregivers, and pool owners should learn CPR and keep a telephone and equipment approved by the U.S. Coast Guard (life preservers, life jackets, shepherd's crook) at poolside.

Electric Shock

When the human body comes in direct contact with a source of electricity, the current passes through it, producing what's called an electric shock. Depending on the voltage of the current and the length of contact, this shock can cause anything from minor discomfort to serious injury to death.

Babies experience electric shock most often when they bite into electrical cords or poke metal objects such as forks or knives into unprotected outlets or appliances. These injuries also can take place when electric toys, appliances, or tools are used incorrectly, or when electric current makes contact with water in which an infant is sitting or standing. Lightning accounts for about 20 percent of the cases that occur. Christmas trees and their lights are a seasonal hazard.

What You Should Do

If your baby comes in contact with electricity, *always* try to turn the power off first. In many cases you'll be able to pull the plug or turn off the switch. If this isn't possible, consider an attempt to remove the live wire—but *not with your bare hands,* which would bring you in contact with the current yourself. Instead, try to cut the wire with a wood-handled ax or well-insulated wire cutters, or move the wire off the child using a dry stick, a rolled-up magazine or newspaper, a rope, a coat, or another thick, dry object that won't conduct electricity.

If you can't remove the source of the current, try to pull the baby away. Again, *do not touch the infant with your bare hands* when he's attached to the source of the current, since his body will transmit the electricity to you. Instead, use a nonconducting material such as rubber (or those described above) to shield you while freeing him. (*Caution:* None of these methods can be guaranteed safe unless the power can be shut off.)

As soon as the current is turned off (or the baby is removed from it), check the infant's breathing, skin color, and ability to respond to you. If his breathing or heartbeat has stopped, or seems very rapid or irregular, immediately use cardiopulmonary resuscitation (CPR; see page 575) to restore it, and have someone call for emergency medical help. At the same time, avoid moving the baby needlessly, since such a severe electrical shock may have caused a spinal fracture.

If the baby is conscious and it seems the shock was minor, check him for burned skin, especially if his mouth was the point of contact with the current. Call 911. Electric shock can cause internal organ damage that may be difficult to detect without a medical examination. For that reason, *all* infants who receive a significant electric shock should see a doctor.

In the pediatrician's office, any minor burns from the electricity will be cleansed and dressed. The doctor may order laboratory tests to check for signs of damage to internal organs. If the baby has severe burns or any sign of brain or heart damage, he will need to be hospitalized.

Prevention

The best way to prevent electrical injuries is to use outlet covers that are not a choking hazard, make sure all wires are properly insulated, tuck wires away from your baby's reach, and provide adult supervision whenever babies are in an area with potential electrical hazards. Small appliances are a special hazard around bathtubs, sinks, or pools. (See also Chapter 11, *Keeping Your Child Safe.*)

FINGERTIP INJURIES

Children's fingertips get smashed frequently, usually getting caught in closing doors. The baby is unable to recognize the potential danger, or doors are shut by parents unaware that little fingers are in danger. Fingers also sometimes get crushed when youngsters play with a hammer or other heavy object, or when they're around a car door.

Because fingertips are exquisitely sensitive, your baby will let you know immediately that she's been injured. Usually the damaged area will be blue and swollen, and there may be a cut or bleeding around the cuticle. The skin, tissues below the skin, and the nail bed—as well as the underlying bone and growth plate—all may be affected. If bleeding occurs underneath the nail, it will turn black or dark blue, and the pressure from the bleeding may be painful.

Home Treatment

When the fingertip is bleeding, wash it with soap and water, and cover it with a soft, sterile dressing. An ice pack or a soaking in cold water may relieve the pain and minimize swelling.

If the swelling is mild and your baby is comfortable, you can allow the finger to heal on its own. But be alert for any increase in pain, swelling, redness, or drainage from the injured area, or a fever beginning twenty-four to seventy-two hours after the injury. These may be signs of infection, and you should notify your pediatrician.

When there's excessive swelling, a deep cut, blood under the fingernail, or if the finger looks as if it may be broken, call your doctor immediately. Do not attempt to straighten a fractured finger on your own.

Professional Treatment

If your doctor suspects a fracture, he may order an X-ray. If the X-ray confirms a fracture—or if there's damage to the nail bed, where nail growth occurs—an orthopedic consultation may be necessary. A fractured finger can be straightened and set under local anesthesia. An injured nail bed also must be repaired surgically to minimize the possibility of a nail deformity developing as the finger grows. If there's considerable blood under the nail, the pediatrician may drain it by making a small hole in the nail, which should relieve the pain.

Although deep cuts may require stitches, often all that's necessary is sterile adhesive strips (thin adhesive strips similar to butterfly bandages). A fracture underneath a cut is considered an "open" fracture and is susceptible to infection in the bone. In this case, antibiotics will be prescribed. Depending on your baby's age and immunization status, the doctor also may order a tetanus booster.

HEAD INJURY/CONCUSSION

It's almost inevitable that your child will hit her head every now and then. Especially when she's a baby, these blows may upset you, but your anxiety is usually worse than the bump. Most head injuries are minor, causing no serious problems. Even so, it's important to know the difference between a head injury that warrants medical attention and one that needs only a comforting hug.

If your baby suffers a brief, temporary loss of consciousness after a hard blow to the head, she is said to have had a concussion. By definition, a concussion is a hard strike to the head resulting in temporary confusion or a change in behavior, and sometimes with a loss of consciousness. Particularly if a baby has significant disorientation, altered speech, or vomiting after a head injury, call 911 and contact your pediatrician. In fact, with *any* loss of consciousness, your baby should be examined by her doctor.

Treatment

If a baby's head injury has been mild, she'll remain alert and awake after the incident, and her color will be normal. She may cry out due to momentary pain and fright, but the crying should last no more than ten minutes and then she'll go back to playing as usual.

Occasionally a minor head injury also will cause slight dizziness and headache, and the baby might vomit once or twice. Even so, if the injury seems minor and there's not a significant cut (one that's deep and/or actively bleeding) that might require immediate medical attention or possibly stitches (see *Cuts and Scrapes,* page 577), you may be able to treat your baby at home. Just wash the cut with soap and water. If there's a bruise, apply a cold compress. This will help minimize the swelling if you do it in the first few hours after the injury. Even in these cases, however, it's wise to call your pediatrician and explain the circumstances and your child's condition.

Even after a minor head injury, you should observe your baby for twenty-four to forty-eight hours to see if she develops any signs that the injury was more severe than it first appeared. Although it's very rare, babies can develop a serious brain injury after a seemingly minor bump on the head that causes no immediate obvious problems. Brain injuries after such an apparently insignificant head bump are usually due to internal bleeding and almost always show up within one to two days of the original incident. If your baby develops any of the following symptoms, be sure to consult your pediatrician immediately or seek prompt attention from the nearest emergency room.

- **She seems excessively** sleepy or lethargic during her usual wakeful hours, or you cannot awaken her while she's asleep at night. (You should try to awaken her once or twice during the first night if she's had a hard blow to the head.)
- **She has a** headache that won't go away (even with acetaminophen) or vomits more than once or twice. Headache and vomiting occur commonly after head trauma, but they are usually mild and last only a few hours. (Babies won't be able to let you know that they have a headache so they may cry or be inconsolable.)

- **She's persistently and/or** extremely irritable. With an infant who cannot tell you what she's feeling, this may indicate a severe headache.

- **Any significant change** in your child's mental abilities, coordination, sensation, or strength warrants immediate medical attention. Such worrisome changes would include weakness of arms or legs, clumsy walking, slurred speech, crossed eyes, or difficulty with vision.

- **She becomes unconscious** again after being awake for a while, or she has a seizure (convulsion) or starts to breathe irregularly. These are signs of disturbed brain activity and may indicate a serious head injury.

If your baby loses consciousness *at any time* after hitting her head, notify the pediatrician. If she doesn't awaken within a few minutes, she needs *immediate medical attention.* Call 911 for help while you follow these steps.

1. Move your infant as little as possible. *If you suspect that she might have injured her neck, do not attempt to move her. Changing the position of her neck might make her injuries worse.* One exception: Move her only if she's in danger of being injured further where she is (e.g., on a ledge or in a fire), but try to avoid bending or twisting her neck.
2. Check to see if she's breathing. If she isn't, perform CPR (see page 742).
3. If she's bleeding severely from a scalp wound, apply direct pressure with a clean cloth over the wound.
4. After calling 911, wait for the ambulance's arrival rather than taking your baby to the hospital yourself.

Loss of consciousness following a head injury may last only a few seconds or as long as several hours. If you find the baby after the injury happened, and you are not sure if she lost consciousness, notify the pediatrician.

Most babies who lose consciousness for more than a few minutes will be hospitalized overnight for observation. Hospitalization is essential for infants with severe brain injury and irregular breathing or convulsions. Fortunately, with modern pediatric intensive care, many babies who have suffered serious head injury—and even those who have been unconscious for several weeks—eventually may recover completely.

Poisoning

About 2.2 million people swallow or have contact with a poisonous substance each year. More than half of these poison exposures occur in children under six years of age.

Most babies who swallow poison are not permanently harmed, particularly if they receive immediate treatment. If you think your baby has been poisoned, stay calm and act quickly.

You should suspect poisoning if you ever find your baby with an open or empty container of a toxic substance, especially if she is acting strangely. Be alert for these other signs of possible poisoning.

- Unexplained stains on her clothing
- Burns on her lips or mouth
- Unusual drooling, or odd odors on her breath
- Unexplained nausea or vomiting
- Abdominal cramps without fever
- Difficulty in breathing
- Sudden behavior changes, such as unusual sleepiness, irritability, or jumpiness
- Convulsions or unconsciousness (only in very serious cases)

Treatment

Anytime your baby has ingested a poison of any kind, you should notify your pediatrician. However, your regional Poison Center will provide the immediate information and guidance you need when you first discover that your infant has been poisoned. These centers are staffed twenty-four

Poison-Proofing Your Home

- Store drugs and medications in a medicine cabinet that is locked or out of reach. Do not keep toothpaste, soap, or shampoo in the same cabinet. If you carry a purse, keep potential poisons out of your purse, and keep your baby away from other people's purses.
- Buy and keep medications in their own containers with child safety caps. (Remember, however, that these caps are child-resistant, not childproof, so keep them in a locked cabinet.) Safely dispose of leftover prescription medicines when the illness for which they were prescribed has passed, even taking them back to your pharmacy where they can be discarded.
- Do not take medicine in front of small children; they may try to imitate you later. Never tell a child that a medicine is candy in order to get him to take it.
- Check the label every time you give medication, to be sure you are giving the right medicine in the correct dosage. Mistakes are most likely to occur in the middle of the night, so always turn on the light when handling any medication.
- Read labels on all household products before you buy them. Try to find the safest ones for the job, and buy only what you need to use immediately.
- Store hazardous products in locked cabinets that are out of your baby's reach. Do not keep detergents and other cleaning products under the kitchen or bathroom sink unless they are in a cabinet with a safety latch that locks every time you close the cabinet. (Most hardware stores and department stores sell these safety latches.)

- Never put poisonous or toxic products in containers that were once used for food, especially empty drink bottles, cans, or cups.
- Always open the garage door before starting your car, and never run the car in a closed garage. Be sure that coal, wood, or kerosene stoves are properly maintained. If you smell gas, turn off the stove or gas burner, leave the house, and then call the gas company.
- Post the Poison Help Line number, 1–800–222–1222, near every telephone in your home and in your cell phone, along with other emergency numbers. Be sure that your child care provider and anyone else caring for your child knows when and how to use these numbers.

hours a day with experts who can tell you what to do without delay. Call the national toll-free number for Poison Help Line at 1–800–222–1222, which will provide immediate and free access around the clock to your regional Poison Center. *If there's an emergency and you cannot find the number, dial 911 or Directory Assistance and ask for the Poison Help Line.*

The immediate action you need to take will vary with the type of poisoning. The Poison Help Line can give you specific instructions if you know the particular substance your baby has swallowed. However, carry out the following instructions before calling them.

Swallowed Poison First, get the poisonous substance away from your baby. If she still has some in her mouth, make her spit it out, or remove it with your fingers. Keep this material along with any other evidence that might help determine what she swallowed.

Next, check for these signs:

- Severe throat pain
- Excessive drooling

- Breathing difficulty
- Convulsions
- Excessive drowsiness

If any of these are present, or if your baby is unconscious or has stopped breathing, start emergency procedures and get medical help immediately by calling 911. Take the poison container and remnants of material with you to help the doctor determine what was swallowed. *Do not make your baby vomit by any means*—even if the label on the container suggests it—as this may cause further damage.

If your baby is not showing these serious symptoms, call the Poison Help Line number, 1–800–222–1222, which will direct your call to your regional Poison Center. The person answering the phone will need the following information in order to help you:

- **Your name and** phone number.
- **Your baby's name,** age, and weight. Also be sure to mention any serious medical conditions she has or medications she is taking.
- **The name of** the substance your baby swallowed. Read it off the container, and spell it if necessary. If ingredients are listed on the label, read them, too. If your infant has swallowed a prescription medicine, and the drug is not named on the label, give the center the name of the pharmacy and its phone number, the date of the prescription, and its number. Try to describe the tablet or capsule, and mention any imprinted numbers on it. If your child swallowed another substance, such as a part of a plant, provide as full a description as possible to help identify it.
- **The time your** baby swallowed this poison (or when you found her), and the amount you think she swallowed.

If the poison is extremely dangerous, or because of the age of your child, you may be told to take her directly to the nearest emergency department for medical evaluation. Otherwise, you will be given instructions to follow at home.

Vomiting may be dangerous, so never make a baby vomit. Strong acids (i.e., toilet bowl cleaner) or strong alkalis (i.e., lye, drain or oven cleaner, or dishwasher detergent) can burn the throat—and vomiting will only increase the damage. Syrup of ipecac is a drug that was used in the past to make children vomit after they had swallowed a poison; although this may seem to make sense, it is no longer considered a good poison treatment. If you have syrup of ipecac in your home, flush it down the toilet and throw away the container. Do not make a baby vomit by any means, whether by giving him syrup of ipecac, making him gag, or giving him salt water. Instead, you may be advised to have the baby drink milk or water.

Poison on the Skin If your infant spills a dangerous chemical substance on her body, remove her clothes and rinse the skin with lukewarm—not hot—water. If the area shows signs of being burned, continue rinsing for at least fifteen minutes, no matter how much your baby may protest. Then call the Poison Help Line for further advice. Do not apply ointments or grease.

Poison in the Eye Flush your baby's eye by holding her eyelid open and pouring a steady stream of lukewarm water into the inner corner. A baby is sure to object to this treatment, so get another adult to hold her while you rinse the eye. If that's not possible, wrap her tightly in a towel and clamp her under one arm so you have one hand free to hold the eyelid open and the other to pour in the water.

Continue flushing the eye for fifteen minutes. Then call the Poison Help Line, 1–800–222–1222, for further instructions. Do not use an eyecup, eyedrops, or ointment unless the Poison Center tells you to do so. If there is any question of continued pain or severe injury, seek emergency assistance immediately.

Poison Fumes In the home, poisonous fumes are most likely to be produced by an idling automobile in a closed garage; leaky gas vents; wood, coal, or kerosene stoves that are improperly vented or maintained; or space heaters, ovens, stoves, or water heaters that use gas. If your baby is exposed to fumes or gases from these or other sources, get her into fresh air immediately. If she is breathing, call the Poison Help Line,

1–800–222–1222, for further instructions. If she has stopped breathing, start CPR (see page 575), and don't stop until she breathes on her own or someone else can take over. If you can, have someone call 911 for emergency medical help immediately; otherwise, try one minute of CPR and then call for emergency assistance.

Prevention

Young children, especially those between ages one and three, are commonly poisoned by things in the home such as drugs, even those sold over the counter, and medications, cleaning products, plants, cosmetics, pesticides, paints, solvents, antifreeze, windshield wiper fluid, gasoline, kerosene, and lamp oil. This happens because tasting and mouthing things is a natural way for children to explore their surroundings, and because they imitate adults without understanding what they are doing.

Most poisonings occur when parents are distracted. If you are ill or under a great deal of stress, you may not watch your baby as closely as usual. The hectic routines at the end of the day cause so many lapses in parental attention. So keep all poisons, medications, and toxins high out of children's reach. The best way to prevent poisonings is to store all toxic substances in a locked cabinet where your child cannot possibly get to them, even when you are not directly watching her. Also, supervise her even more closely whenever you're visiting a store or a friend or relative's home that has not been childproofed. (See also Chapter 11, *Keeping Your Child Safe.*)

20

Environmental Health

All babies are potentially exposed to environmental toxins in the world in which we live. But even though you can't protect your infant from every environmental hazard that exists, you can lower his exposure by taking the steps described in this chapter.

Air Pollution and Secondhand Smoke

The outdoor air contains several substances that could be harmful to babies. One of the most worrisome is ozone, which is a colorless gas that can cause harm when it is present near the ground. Ozone is formed when certain chemicals (nitrogen oxides, reactive hydrocarbons) are released by automobiles and industry and are acted on by sunlight. Ozone concentrations are likely to be greatest in the summer on warm, sunny days, peaking in the mid- to late afternoon.

Because babies spend time playing outdoors, they are particularly susceptible to ozone's effects, with breathing difficulties most likely to occur in babies with asthma. Infants also breathe more rapidly than adults and inhale more pollutants per pound of body weight.

Another common air pollutant is secondhand (or environmental) cigarette smoke. According to the Centers for Disease Control and Prevention, about 25 percent of children ages three to eleven years old live in a household with at least one smoker. If you or others in your home use cigarettes, pipes, or cigars, your baby is being exposed to their smoke. This smoke contains thousands of chemicals, some of which have been shown to cause cancer and other illnesses, including respiratory infections, bronchitis, and pneumonia. Infants exposed to cigarette smoke also have a greater likelihood of developing ear infections and asthma, and they may have a more difficult time getting over colds. They are more susceptible to headaches, sore throats, hoarseness, irritated eyes, dizziness, nausea, lack of energy, and fussiness. In fact, children who are exposed to as few as ten cigarettes per day have an increased chance of getting asthma, even if they've never had any symptoms.

If a parent smokes around her newborn, the baby has a greater risk of dying from sudden infant death syndrome (SIDS). In addition, nicotine and other dangerous chemicals from cigarettes are in the breastmilk of nursing mothers, who thus expose their babies.

When babies are exposed to tobacco smoke, they might develop life-threatening illnesses later in life, including lung cancer and heart disease. They also may be more likely to have cataracts as adults.

When you smoke in your home, you create a risk of fires and burns to your infant and others. Babies can suffer burns if they find and play with a lit cigarette or with matches or a lighter.

As your infant grows, keep in mind that you are a role model. If your baby sees you smoking, she may want to try it as well, and you could be laying the foundation for a lifetime of smoking.

Prevention

To protect your infant from air pollution, limit his playtime outdoors when local agencies have issued health advisories or smog alerts. Newspapers and TV news programs often provide information about the air quality in the community.

To reduce the air pollution from automobiles on smoggy days, keep your car in the garage and use public transportation or carpools instead. Do not use gasoline-powered lawn mowers on high pollution days and limit their use at other times. Work with your local, state, and national governments to enforce and tighten air pollution laws and regulations.

To reduce your baby's exposure to environmental tobacco smoke, here are some steps you can take:

- **If you or** other family members smoke, stop! If you've been unable to quit, talk to your doctor, who can refer you to low-cost stop-smoking programs available in your community. Or contact the American Lung Association (www .lungusa.org); the American Cancer Society (www .cancer.org); or the American Heart Association (www .americanheart.org), and inquire about smoking cessation classes.

- **Don't allow anyone** to smoke in your home or your car, particularly when children are present. Don't place ashtrays around your house that may encourage people to light up. Your home and car should always remain smoke-free.
- **Store matches and** lighters out of reach of children.
- **When selecting a** babysitter or child care provider, make it clear that no one is permitted to smoke around your baby.
- **When you're in** public places with your infant, ask others not to smoke around you and your baby. Choose restaurants that don't allow smoking.

Asbestos

Asbestos is a natural fiber that was widely used as a spray-on material for fireproofing, insulation, and soundproofing in schools, homes, and public buildings from the 1940s through the 1970s. It does ***not*** pose health risks unless it deteriorates and becomes crumbly, when it can release microscopic asbestos fibers into the air. When asbestos fibers are inhaled, they can cause chronic health problems to the lungs, throat, and gastrointestinal tract, including a rare type of chest cancer (called mesothelioma) that can occur as long as five decades after asbestos exposure.

Today, schools are mandated by law to either remove asbestos or otherwise ensure that children are not exposed to it. However, it is still in some older homes, especially as insulation around pipes, stoves, and furnaces, as well as in walls and ceilings.

Prevention

Follow these guidelines to keep your baby safe from asbestos.

- **If you think** there may be asbestos in your home, have a professional inspector check for it. Local health departments and regional offices of the Environmental Protection Agency (EPA) can provide the names of individuals and labs certified to inspect homes for asbestos. To locate the regional EPA office nearest you, go to www.epa.gov/asbestos.

- **Do not let** your baby play near any exposed or deteriorating materials that could contain asbestos.
- **If asbestos is** found in your home, it may be acceptable to leave it there if it is in good condition. But if it is deteriorating, or if it might be disturbed by any renovations you're planning, have a properly accredited and certified contractor remove the asbestos, which must be taken off in a safe manner. Again, ask the local health department or the EPA for information on finding a certified contractor in your community.

Carbon Monoxide

Carbon monoxide is a toxic gas that is a by-product of appliances, heaters, and automobiles that burn gasoline, natural gas, wood, oil, kerosene, or propane. It has no color, no taste, and no odor. It can become trapped inside your home if appliances are not working, if a furnace, stove, or fireplace has a clogged vent or chimney, or if a charcoal grill is used in an enclosed area. Carbon monoxide also might enter your home when an automobile is left running in an attached garage.

When your baby breathes carbon monoxide, it harms the ability of his blood to transport oxygen. Although everyone is at risk for carbon monoxide poisoning, it is particularly dangerous for infants because they breathe faster and inhale more carbon monoxide per pound of body weight. Symptoms may include headaches, nausea, shortness of breath, fatigue, confusion, and fainting. Persistent exposure to carbon monoxide can lead to personality changes, memory loss, severe lung injury, brain damage, and death.

Prevention

You can reduce your baby's risk of carbon monoxide poisoning by:

- **Buying and installing** carbon monoxide detectors in your home, particularly near the bedrooms, or near a furnace or woodstove
- **Never leaving your** car running in an attached garage (even if the garage door is open)
- **Never using a** charcoal or propane grill, hibachi, or portable camping stove indoors or in an enclosed area
- **Scheduling an annual** inspection and servicing of oil and gas furnaces, woodstoves, gas ovens and ranges, gas water heaters, gas clothes dryers, and fireplaces
- **Never using your** nonelectric oven to heat your kitchen or your house

CONTAMINATED FISH

Fish is a protein-rich food that is healthy for both children and adults. It contains a good type of fat (omega-3 fatty acids), as well as nutrients such as vitamin D. It also is low in saturated fat. At the same time, a lot of attention has focused on the contaminants that may be in fish and that could pose health risks.

One of the most widely discussed contaminants is mercury, which at high levels can be toxic. It gets into oceans, rivers, lakes, and ponds, and can end up in the fish we eat. Mercury in bodies of water like lakes and streams—some of it discharged from industrial plants—can be converted by bacteria into mercury compounds such as methylmercury. As a result, certain predatory fish (including shark and swordfish) can contain high quantities of mercury, which when consumed can have a serious negative effect on a young child's developing nervous system.

Other environmental pollutants have been found in fish and other foods, including polychlorinated biphenyls (PCBs) and dioxins. Although PCBs are chemicals that were manufactured primarily for use as fire retardants and in electrical transformers, they were banned in the U.S. in the late 1970s. However, they have remained in the environment in water, soil, and air, and have been found in fish. PCBs have been associated with thyroid problems, lowered IQ, and memory impairment in young children.

Dioxin is another pollutant that has been detected in fish. It is the by-product of certain chemicals by incineration and can interfere with the developing nervous system and other organs, particularly when the exposure is long term. Fortunately, PCBs and dioxins have decreased significantly in recent years.

Prevention

You need to make an effort to reduce your baby's exposure to toxic substances in food. Government agencies are recommending that young children reduce their intake of certain fish that may contain high levels of mercury. Specifically, young children should not consume king mackerel, swordfish, shark, and tilefish. At the same time, other types of fish and shellfish are low in mercury, including canned light tuna, salmon, shrimp, cod, catfish, clams, flatfish, crab, scallops, and pollock, so these are much better choices for your child. Nevertheless, you should limit your child's intake of even these safer selections to less than twelve ounces per week.

For information about the safety of fish and shellfish caught in your area, contact state and local health departments. Also check fish advisories on the Environmental Protection Agency's website: http://www.epa.gov/waterscience/fish/. The health department in your state also can provide any advisories issued about the presence of other toxins in fish in your area.

DRINKING WATER

Children drink much more water for their size than adults. Most of this water comes from the tap, and the quality of this water is regulated by standards instituted by Congress, included in the Safe Drinking Water Act of 1974. Subsequent laws have set drinking water standards for chemicals that were known to be in some water supplies.

Today the drinking water in the United States is among the safest in the world, although problems can occur from time to time. Violations in water safety standards are most likely to occur in small systems that serve less than a thousand people. Also, keep in mind that private wells are not

Bisphenol A (BPA)

Many food and liquid containers, including baby bottles, are made of polycarbonate, or have a lining that contains the chemical bisphenol A (BPA). BPA is used to harden plastics, keep bacteria from contaminating foods, and prevent cans from rusting.

There are concerns, though, over the possible harmful effects BPA may have on humans, particularly on infants and children. Animal studies have shown effects on the endocrine functions in animals related to BPA exposure. Additional studies will determine what level of BPA exposure might cause similar effects in humans.

As research continues, concerned parents can take the following precautionary measures to reduce babies' exposure to BPA:

- Avoid clear plastic baby bottles or containers with the recycling number 7 and the letters "PC" imprinted on them. Many contain BPA.
- Consider using certified or identified BPA-free plastic bottles.
- Use bottles made of opaque plastic. These bottles (made of polyethylene or polypropylene) do not contain BPA. You can also look for the recycle symbols with the number 2 or 5 in them.
- Glass bottles can be an alternative, but be aware of the risk of injury to you or your baby if the bottle is dropped or broken.
- Because heat may cause the release of BPA from plastic, consider the following:
    - Do not boil polycarbonate bottles
    - Do not heat polycarbonate bottles in the microwave
    - Do not wash polycarbonate bottles in the dishwasher

Breastfeeding is another way to reduce potential BPA exposure. The AAP recommends exclusive breastfeeding for a minimum of four months but preferably for six months. Breastfeeding should be continued, with the addition of complementary foods, at least through the first twelve months of age and thereafter as long as mutually desired by mother and infant.

If you are considering switching from canned liquid to powdered formula, note that the mixing procedures may differ, so pay special attention when preparing formula from powder.

If your baby is on specialized formula to address a medical condition, you should not switch to another formula, as the known risks would outweigh any potential risks posed by BPA.

Risks associated with giving infants inappropriate (home-made condensed milk) formulas or alternative (soy or goat) milk are far greater than the potential effects of BPA.

federally regulated, and should be tested for nitrates and other environmental toxins if appropriate (see *Where We Stand*).

Contaminants that can cause illness in the drinking water include: germs, nitrates, man-made chemicals, heavy metals, radioactive particles, and by-products of the disinfecting process.

Although bottled water can be purchased in markets, many brands are just tap water that has been bottled for sale. Bottled water is generally much more expensive than tap water, and unless there are known contamination problems in your community's water supply, it is not necessary. Bottled water also may contain undesirable chemicals that come out of the plastic and into the water; and using bottled water generates a lot of plastic waste.

Where We Stand

In the U.S., about 15 million families get their drinking water from private, unregulated wells. Studies show that a significant number of these wells have concentrations of nitrates that exceed federal drinking-water standards. These nitrates are a natural component of plants and nitrate-containing fertilizers that can seep into well water, and don't pose any toxic risk to humans on their own. But in the body, they can be converted to nitrites, which are potentially hazardous. In infants, they can lead to a condition called methemoglobinemia, a dangerous and often fatal blood disorder that interferes with the circulation of oxygen in the blood.

Babies whose formula is prepared using well water may have a high risk of nitrate poisoning. The AAP recommends that if your family drinks well water, the well should be tested for nitrates. If the well water contains nitrates (above a level of 10 mg/L), it should not be used for infant formula or food preparation. Instead, you should prepare food or formula by using purchased water, public water supplies, or water from deeper wells with minimal nitrate levels.

How often should well water be tested? Tests should be done every three months for at least one year to determine the levels of nitrates. If these tests show safe levels, then a follow-up test once a year is recommended.

Breastfeeding is another important and safe way to nourish your infant, since high levels of nitrates are not passed through breastmilk.

Prevention

To ensure that your baby is consuming safe drinking water, you can check the water quality by contacting the county health department, the state environment agency, or the Environmental Protection Agency's Safe Drinking Water Hotline (1–800–426–4791). Local water companies are mandated to report what is in the water on an annual basis. Well water should be tested yearly.

Other guidelines include:

- **Use cold water** for cooking and drinking. Contaminants can accumulate in hot water heaters.
- **If you are** concerned about the quality of your plumbing, run the faucet for two minutes each morning prior to using the water for cooking or drinking. This will flush the pipes and lower the likelihood that contaminants will end up in the water you consume.
- **Have well water** tested for nitrates before giving it to infants under one year of age.
- **Drinking water that** may be contaminated with germs should be boiled and then allowed to cool before drinking. Boil for no more than one minute. However, it is important to remember that boiling water only kills bacteria and other germs; it does ***not*** remove toxic chemicals. If you don't like the taste or smell of your tap water, filters made with activated carbon will remove the off-taste or smell. Such filters will also remove undesirable chemicals without removing fluoride that prevents tooth decay.

Lead Poisoning

During infancy your baby goes through a phase of putting things other than food into his mouth. He'll chew on his toys, taste the sand in the playground, and sample the cat's food if given the opportunity. As annoying as this behavior can be, few of these things will cause him any serious harm, as long as you keep poisons and sharp objects out of his reach. Lead is one dangerous substance, however, that your baby can consume without your knowledge.

Contrary to popular belief, lead poisoning is not caused by chewing on a pencil or being stabbed with its point. The so-called lead in a pencil actually is harmless graphite, and there is no lead in the paint coating the outside. Lead poisoning is caused most often by eating lead contained in dust, bits of old paint or dirt, by breathing lead in the air, or by drinking water from pipes lined or soldered with lead. There also may be lead in hobby materials such as stained glass, paints, solders, and fishing weights. It might be in mini-blinds manufactured outside the United States prior to July 1997. If you buy new mini-blinds, look for those that have a label that says "new formulation" or "nonleaded formula." Lead also might be in food cooked or stored in some imported ceramic dishes. Do not serve acidic substances (e.g., orange juice) in these dishes, since the acids can leach lead from the dishes into the food. Although food cans with soldered seams could add lead to the food inside them, these cans generally have been replaced by seamless aluminum containers in the United States.

Lead was an allowable ingredient in house paint before 1978 and so may be on the walls, doorjambs, and window frames on many older homes. As the paint ages, it chips, peels, and comes off in the form of dust. Babies and toddlers may be tempted by such bite-size pieces and will taste or eat them out of curiosity. Even if they don't intentionally eat the material, the dust can get on their hands and into their food. Sometimes the lead-containing finish has been covered with other layers of newer, safer paints. This can give you a false sense of reassurance, however, since the underlying paint still may chip or peel off with the newer layers and fall into the hands of infants.

Although there has been a decline in high lead levels in children's blood, somewhere between half a million and one million children in the United States still have unacceptably high levels. Living in a city, being poor, and being African American or Hispanic are all risk factors that increase the chances of having an elevated blood-lead level.

Where We Stand

Lead causes serious damage to children's brains even at relatively low levels of exposure—the effects of which are largely irreversible. The American Academy of Pediatrics supports widespread lead screening of children, as well as funding programs to remove lead hazards from the environment.

But even infants living in rural areas or who are in well-to-do families still can be at risk.

As a baby continues consuming lead, it accumulates in the body. Although it may not be noticeable for some time, ultimately it can affect many areas of the body, including the brain. Lead poisoning can cause learning disabilities and behavioral problems. Very high levels will likely cause the most severe problems, but the extent of damage for any individual baby cannot be predicted. Lead also can cause stomach and intestinal problems, loss of appetite, anemia, headaches, constipation, hearing loss, and even short stature. Iron deficiency increases the risk for lead poisoning in infants, which is why these two disorders are often found together in children. (See *Abdominal Pain,* page 437.)

Prevention

If your home was built after 1977, when federal regulations restricted the amount of lead in paint, the risk for having dangerous amounts of lead in the dust, paint, or soil of your residence is low. However, if your home is older, the likelihood of having dangerous amounts of lead there can be very high, especially for the oldest homes (those built before 1960). If you think your home may contain lead, clean up any paint dust or chips using water. During this cleanup, if you add a detergent to the water, it will help bind the lead into the water. Also, keeping surfaces (floors, window areas, porches, etc.) clean may lower your child's chance of being exposed to lead-containing dust. Older windows are of particular concern since paint on wood frames frequently is damaged and the action of opening and closing windows can produce lead-containing dust. Do not vacuum the chips or dust as the vacuum will spread the dust out through its exhaust hole. It's also a good idea to wash your baby's hands often, particularly before he eats.

Another step is to identify surfaces in your home with lead-contaminated paint, or areas with dangerous amounts of lead in the dust or dirt. A home inspection is necessary to do this, and you can get help from your local or state health department to find a lead inspector in your area. Sometimes, health departments will provide the inspection themselves, but most often you will have to pay for it.

If you live in an older home that needs repairs, you should assume that the repair process could potentially generate dangerous amounts of lead dust. So unless you know positively that any paint that will be disturbed does not contain lead, you need to seek expert advice before starting repairs. Renovation projects that disturb lead paint need to be done by individuals with special training in lead-safe work practices. Sanding and scraping of paint can generate large amounts of dust, and exposure to this dust during or following renovation is a common way that babies get lead poisoning. The safest approach is for the family to move out while the renovation is ongoing and until the final cleaning has been completed. Contact your state or local health department for more detailed information.

Incidentally, in a rented home, the landlord is responsible for all maintenance, and this includes necessary repainting and repairs. If you suspect unhealthy lead levels in the building, and your landlord is unresponsive or is not using lead-safe work practices when doing repairs, ask your community's health department for help. Sometimes legal actions can compel the landlord to make safe repairs.

Also, call your local health department, to see if lead in the water is a problem in your community. Or contact the Environmental Protection Agency's Safe Drinking Water Hotline (1–800–426–4791) to find out whether your local water supply presents a risk of lead exposure.

Treatment

Children who have lead poisoning rarely show any physical symptoms. However, learning and behavior problems from lead may show up in a preschool child or may not show up until a child reaches school age. At that point they need to learn more complicated tasks like reading or arithmetic and may have trouble keeping up with class work. Some may even seem overly active, due to the effects of the lead. For this reason, the only sure way to know if your baby has been exposed to excessive lead is to have him tested. A blood test for lead at age one year is recommended for infants at high risk for lead exposure. In communities where high blood lead risk is low, a series of questions will determine whether a blood test is necessary. Local and state health departments have developed guidelines based on the risks for their areas.

The most common screening test for lead poisoning uses a drop of blood from a finger prick. If the results of this test indicate that a baby has been exposed to excessive lead, a second test will be done using a larger sample of blood obtained from a vein in the arm. This test is more accurate and can measure the precise amount of lead in the blood.

Infants who have lead poisoning should immediately be moved from the home where they are being exposed to this toxic substance. In rare instances, they may require treatment with a drug that binds the lead in the blood and greatly increases the body's ability to eliminate it. When treatment is necessary, usually oral medicines are used on an outpatient basis. Much less frequently, the treatment may involve hospitalization and a series of injections.

Some babies with lead poisoning require more than one course of treatment. Unfortunately, standard treatments for lead-poisoned children produce only a short-term or marginal lowering of the body's lead levels and do not lower the chance of developing lead-related behavioral or learning problems. Children who have had lead poisoning will need to have their physical health, behavior, and academic performance monitored for many years and should receive special schooling and therapy to help them overcome learning and behavior problems.

The best treatment for lead poisoning is prevention.

PESTICIDES/HERBICIDES

Pesticides and herbicides are used in a variety of settings, including homes, schools, parks, lawns, gardens, and farms. While they may kill insects, rodents, and weeds, some are toxic to people when consumed in food and water.

More research is needed to determine the short- and long-term effects of pesticides and herbicides on humans. Although some studies have found connections between some childhood cancers and an exposure to pesticides, other studies have not reached the same conclusions. Many pesticides disrupt the nervous system of insects, and research has shown that they have the potential to damage the neurological system of children.

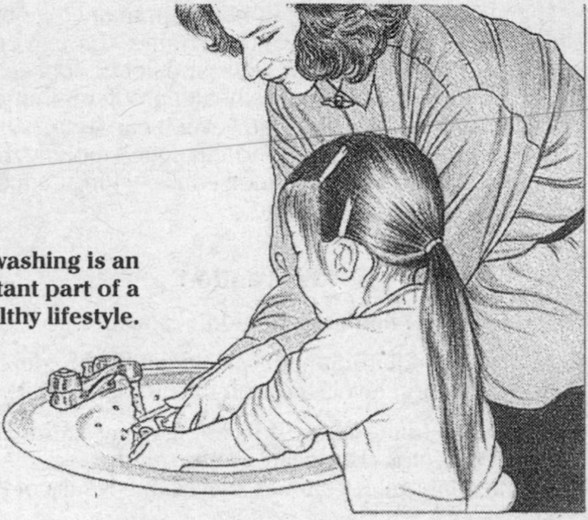

Handwashing is an important part of a healthy lifestyle.

Prevention

Try to limit your baby's unnecessary exposure to pesticides or herbicides. To reduce such exposure:

- Minimize using foods in which chemical pesticides or herbicides were used by farmers.
- Wash all fruits and vegetables with water before your baby consumes them.
- For your own lawn and garden, use nonchemical pest control methods whenever possible. If you keep bottles of pesticides in your home or garage, make sure they're out of the reach of babies to avoid any accidental poisoning.
- Avoid routinely spraying homes or schools to prevent insect infestations.

RADON

Radon is a gas that is a product of the breakdown of uranium in soil and rock. It also may be in water, natural gas, and building materials.

High levels of radon are in homes in many regions of the United States. It makes its way into homes through cracks or openings in the foundation, walls, and floors, or occasionally in well water. It does not cause health problems immediately upon inhalation. Over time, however, it can increase the risk of lung cancer. In fact, next to cigarette smoking, radon is thought to be the most common cause of lung cancer in the United States.

Prevention

To reduce your baby's risk of radon exposure:

- Ask your pediatrician or the local health department whether radon levels are high in your community.
- Have your home tested for radon, using an inexpensive radon detector. (Hardware stores sell these detectors.) A certified laboratory should analyze the results of this test.
- If the levels are too high in your home, call the Radon Hotline (operated by the National Safety Council in conjunction with the Environmental Protection Agency) at 1–800–767–7236; this is also a good resource for information on reducing the radon risk in your home.

21

EYES

Your baby relies on the visual information he gathers to help him develop throughout infancy and childhood. If he has difficulty seeing properly, he may have problems in learning and relating to the world around him. For this reason it is important to detect eye deficiencies as early as possible. Many vision problems can be corrected if treated early but become much more difficult to care for later on.

Your infant should have his first eye examination at your first visit with your pediatrician to check for problems that may be present. Routine vision checks then should be part of every visit to the pediatrician's office. If your family has a history of serious eye diseases or abnormalities, your pediatrician may refer your baby to an ophthalmologist (an eye specialist with a medical degree) for an early examination and follow-up visits if necessary.

If an infant is born prematurely, he will be checked for a vision-threatening condition called retinopathy of prematurity, especially if he required oxygen over a prolonged period of time during his early days of life. The risk is greater in the premature infant with a birth weight of less than 1500 grams (3.3 pounds). This condition may not be prevented even with ideal neonatal care, but in many cases, if detected early, it can be treated successfully. All neonatologists are aware of potential problems resulting from retinopathy and will let parents know about the necessity for evaluation by an ophthalmologist. Parents also should be told that all premature children are at greater risk for developing astigmatism, myopia, and strabismus (these medical eye conditions are described below), and that they therefore should be screened periodically throughout childhood.

How much does a newborn baby see? Until fairly

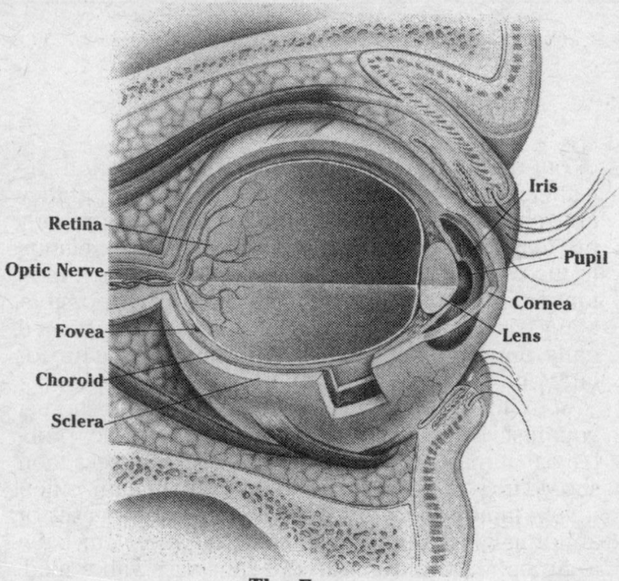

The Eye

recently, doctors thought that a newborn infant could see very little; however, newer information indicates that even during the early weeks of life, an infant can see light and shapes and can detect movement. Far vision remains quite blurry, with the optimal focal length being 8 to 15 inches (20 to 38 cm), which is roughly the distance from his eyes to yours as you are nursing or feeding your baby.

Until your baby learns to use both eyes together, they may "wander," or move randomly. This random movement should be decreasing by two to three months of age. Around three months old, your baby probably will focus on faces and close objects and follow a moving object with his eyes. By four months of age, he should be using his vision to detect various objects close to him, which he probably will reach for and grasp. By six months old he should be able to visually identify and distinguish between objects.

If regular eye checks during pediatric visits indicate that

your baby's eyes are developing normally, he should not need more formal testing until three to four years of age.

Vision Screening Recommendations

Vision screening is a very important factor in identifying vision-threatening conditions. The American Academy of Pediatrics recommends that babies be screened in two stages:

1. In the newborn nursery: Pediatricians should examine all infants prior to their discharge from the nursery to check for infections and structural defects (page 616), cataracts (page 615), or congenital glaucoma. If a problem is suspected, a pediatric ophthalmologist should see the newborn. All children with multiple medical problems or with a history of prematurity and/or oxygen exposure should be examined by an ophthalmologist.

2. By the age of six months: Pediatricians should screen infants at the time of their well-baby visits to check for alignment (eyes working together) and the presence of any eye disease.

When to Call the Pediatrician

Routine eye checks can detect hidden eye problems, but occasionally you may notice obvious signs that your baby is having trouble seeing or that his eyes are not normal. Notify the pediatrician if your infant shows any of the following warning signs.

- A white appearance of the pupil (a condition called leukocoria) in one or both eyes
- Persistent (lasting more than twenty-four hours) redness, swelling, crusting, or discharge in his eyes or eyelids
- Excessive tearing
- Sensitivity to light, especially a change in the baby's light sensitivity
- Eyes that look crooked or crossed, or that don't move together

- Head held in an abnormal or tilted position
- Frequent squinting
- Drooping of one or both eyelids
- Pupils of unequal size
- Continuous eye-rubbing
- Eyes that "bounce" or "dance"
- Inability to see objects unless he holds them close
- Eye injury (see page 617)
- Cloudy cornea

Depending on the symptoms your baby displays, your pediatrician probably will check for vision difficulties and/or some of the other problems discussed in the remainder of this chapter.

AMBLYOPIA

Amblyopia, or lazy eye, is a fairly common eye problem (affecting about 2 out of 100 children) that develops when a child has one eye that doesn't see well or is injured, and he begins to use the other eye almost exclusively. The idle eye then relaxes and becomes even weaker. In general, the problem must be detected by the age of three in order to treat and restore normal vision in the affected eye by age six. If this situation persists for too long (past seven to nine years of age), vision may be lost permanently in the unused eye.

Once an ophthalmologist diagnoses the problems in the unused eye, your baby may need to wear a patch over the "good" eye for periods of time. This forces her to use and strengthen the eye that has become "lazy." Patching therapy will be continued for as long as necessary to bring the weaker eye up to its full potential. This could take weeks, months, or even up to age ten or older. As an alternative to the patch, the ophthalmologist might prescribe eye drops or ointment to blur the vision in the good eye, thereby forcing your child to use the amblyopic eye.

Cataracts

Although we usually think of cataracts as affecting elderly people, they also may be found in infants and young children, and are sometimes present at birth. A cataract is a clouding of the lens (the transparent tissue inside the eye that helps bring light rays to focus on the retina). While rare, congenital cataracts are nonetheless a leading cause of visual loss and blindness in children.

Cataracts in infants need to be detected and treated early so their vision can develop normally. A cataract usually shows up as a white reflection in the center of the baby's pupil. If a baby is born with a cataract that blocks most of the light entering the eye, the affected lens has to be removed surgically to permit the baby's vision to develop. Most pediatric ophthalmologists recommend that this procedure be performed during the first month of life. After the clouded lens is removed, the baby must be fitted with a contact lens or with an eyeglass correction. At the age of about one year, the placement of a lens within the eye is recommended. In addition, visual rehabilitation of the affected eye will almost always involve use of a patch until the child's eyes are fully mature (at age ten or older).

Occasionally a baby will be born with a small cataract that will not initially impede visual development. These cataracts often do not require treatment; however, they need to be monitored carefully to ensure that they do not become large enough to interfere with normal vision. In addition, even if too small to pose a direct threat to visual development, cataracts may cause secondary amblyopia (loss of vision), which will need to be treated by your ophthalmologist.

In most cases, the cause of cataracts in infants cannot be determined. Cataracts may be attributed to a tendency inherited from parents; they may result from trauma to the eye; or they may occur as a result of viral infections such as German measles and chickenpox or an infection from other microorganisms, such as those that cause toxoplasmosis. To protect the unborn child from cataracts and from other serious disorders, pregnant women should take care to avoid unnecessary exposure to infectious diseases. In addition, as a precaution against toxoplasmosis (a disease caused by parasites), pregnant women should avoid handling cat litter or eating raw meat, both of which may contain the organism that causes this disease.

Eye Infections

If the white of your baby's eye and the inside of his lower lid become red, he probably has a condition called conjunctivitis. Also known as pinkeye, this inflammation, which can be painful and itchy, usually signals an infection, but may be due to other causes, such as an irritation, an allergic reaction, or (rarely) a more serious condition. It's often accompanied by tearing and discharge, which is the body's way of trying to heal or remedy the situation.

If your baby has a red eye, he needs to see the pediatrician as soon as possible. Eye infections typically last seven to ten days. The doctor will make the diagnosis and prescribe necessary medication if it is indicated. *Never put previously opened medication or someone else's eye medication into your baby's eye. It could cause serious damage.*

In a newborn baby, serious eye infections may result from exposure to bacteria during passage through the birth canal—which is why all infants are treated with antibiotic eye ointment or drops in the delivery room. Such infections must be treated early to prevent serious complications. Eye infections that occur after the newborn period may be unsightly, because of the redness of the eye and the yellow discharge that usually accompanies them, and they may make your child uncomfortable, but they are rarely serious. Several different viruses, or bacteria, may cause them. If your pediatrician feels the problem is caused by bacteria, antibiotic eyedrops are the usual treatment. Conjunctivitis caused by viruses should not be treated with antibiotics.

Eye infections are very contagious. Except to administer drops or ointment, you should avoid direct contact with your infant's eyes or drainage from them until the medication has been used for several days and there is evidence of clearing of the redness. Carefully wash your hands before and after touching the area around the infected eye. If your baby is in a child care program, you should keep him home until the pinkeye is no longer contagious. Your pediatrician will tell you when you can safely send her back to child care or nursery school.

EYE INJURIES

When dust or other small particles get in your baby's eyes, the cleansing action of tears usually will wash them out. If that fails to occur, or if a serious accident affecting the eye takes place, call your pediatrician or take your infant to the nearest emergency room after heeding the following emergency guidelines.

Chemicals in the Eye (see further discussion, Chapter 19) Flush the eye with water, making sure you get the water into the eye itself. Then take the baby to the emergency room.

Large Particle in the Eye If the particle won't come out with tears or by flushing with water, or if your infant still appears to be in pain after an hour, call your pediatrician. The doctor will remove the object or, if necessary, refer you to an ophthalmologist. Sometimes such particles cause scratches on the cornea (corneal abrasions), which are quite painful but heal rapidly with proper treatment. Corneal injuries also can be caused by blows or other injuries to the eye.

Cut Eyelid Minor cuts usually heal quickly and easily, but a deep cut requires emergency medical attention and probably will need stitches. (See *Cuts and Scrapes,* page 577.) Even if the cut is minor, check to make sure it isn't on the border of the eyelid or near the tear duct. If it is, call your pediatrician right away for advice on how to handle the situation.

Black Eye To reduce swelling, apply a cold pack or towel to the area for ten to twenty minutes. Then consult the doctor to make sure there is no internal damage to the eye or the bones surrounding the eye.

EYELID PROBLEMS

Droopy eyelid (ptosis) may appear as an enlarged or heavy upper lid; or, if it is very slight, it may be noticed only because the affected eye appears somewhat smaller than

Preventing Eye Injuries

Nine out of ten eye injuries are preventable, and almost half occur around the home. To minimize the risk of such accidents in your family, follow these safety guidelines.

- Keep all chemicals out of reach. That includes detergents, ammonia, spray cans, Super Glue, and all other cleaning fluids.
- Choose your infant's toys carefully. Watch out for sharp or pointed parts, especially when your baby is too young to understand their danger.
- Keep your infant away from darts and pellet and BB guns.
- Keep your baby away from power lawn mowers, which can hurl stones or other objects.
- Don't let your infant near you when you're lighting fires or using tools.
- Never allow your baby near fireworks of any kind. The American Academy of Pediatrics encourages children and their families to enjoy fireworks at public fireworks displays rather than purchasing fireworks for home use. In fact, the Academy would support a ban on public sales of all fireworks.

the other eye. Ptosis usually involves only one eyelid, but both may be affected. Your baby may be born with a ptosis, or it may develop later. The ptosis may be partial, causing your baby's eyes to appear slightly asymmetrical; or it may be total, causing the affected lid to cover the eye completely. If the ptotic eyelid covers the entire pupillary opening of your infant's eye, or if the weight of the lid causes the cornea to assume an irregular shape (astigmatism), it will threaten normal vision development and must be corrected as early as possible. If vision is not threatened, surgical intervention, if necessary, is usually delayed until the child is four or five years of age or older, when the eyelid and surrounding tissue are more fully developed and a better cosmetic result can be obtained.

Most **birthmarks** and growths involving the eyelids of the newborn or young child are benign; however, because they may increase in size during the first year of life, they sometimes cause parents to become concerned. Most of these birthmarks and growths are not serious and will not affect your baby's vision. Many decrease in size after the first year of life and eventually disappear entirely without treatment. However, any irregularity should be brought to the attention of your child's pediatrician so that it can be evaluated and monitored.

Some children will develop lumps and bumps on their lids that can impair development of good eyesight. In particular, a blood vessel tumor called a capillary or strawberry hemangioma can start out as a small swelling, and rapidly enlarge. They will enlarge over the first year of life, and then start to spontaneously resolve over the next few years of life. If they become large enough, they can interfere with your baby's development of good vision in the affected eye and will need to be treated. Because of their potential to cause vision problems, any child who starts to show any lumps or bumps around either eye should be examined by an ophthalmologist.

A baby might also be born with a flat, purple-colored lesion on their face called a port wine stain, because of its resemblance to a dark red wine. If this birthmark involves the eye, especially the upper lid, the baby may be at risk for development of glaucoma (a condition where pressure increases inside the eyeball) or amblyopia (a weak eye muscle). Any infant born with this birthmark needs to be examined by an ophthalmologist shortly after birth.

Small dark moles, called **nevi,** on the eyelids or on the white part of the eye itself rarely cause any problems or need to be removed. Once they have been evaluated by your pediatrician, these marks should cause concern only if they change in size, shape, or color.

Small, firm, flesh-colored bulges on your baby's eyelids or underneath the eyebrows are usually **dermoid cysts.** These are noncancerous tumors that usually are present from birth. Dermoids will not become cancerous if not removed; however, because they tend to increase in size during puberty, their removal during preschool years is preferred in most cases.

Two other eyelid problems—**chalazia** and **hordeola** or **sties**—are common, but not serious. A chalazion is a cyst resulting from a blockage of an oil gland. A sty, or hordeolum, is a bacterial infection of the cells surrounding the sweat glands or hair follicles on the *edge* of the lid. Call your pediatrician regarding treatment of these conditions. He probably will tell you to apply warm compresses directly to the eyelid for twenty or thirty minutes three or four times a day until the chalazion or sty clears. The doctor may want to examine your infant before prescribing additional treatment, such as an antibiotic ointment or drops.

Once your baby has had a sty or chalazion, she may be more likely to get them again. When chalazia occur repeatedly, it's sometimes necessary to perform lid scrubs to reduce the bacterial colonization of the eyelids and open the oil gland pores.

Impetigo is a very contagious bacterial infection that may occur on the eyelid. Your pediatrician will advise you on how to remove the crust from the lid and then prescribe an eye ointment and oral antibiotics.

STRABISMUS

Strabismus is a misalignment of the eyes caused by an imbalance in the muscles controlling the eye.

A newborn baby's eyes commonly and normally wander. However, within a few weeks, he learns to move his eyes together, and the wandering should disappear within a few months. If this intermittent wandering continues, or if your baby's eyes don't turn in the same direction (if one turns in, out, up, or down), he needs to be evaluated by a pediatric ophthalmologist. This condition, called strabismus, makes it impossible for the eyes to focus on the same point at the same time.

If your baby is born with strabismus, it's important for his eyes to be realigned early in life so he can focus them together on a single object. Eye exercises alone cannot

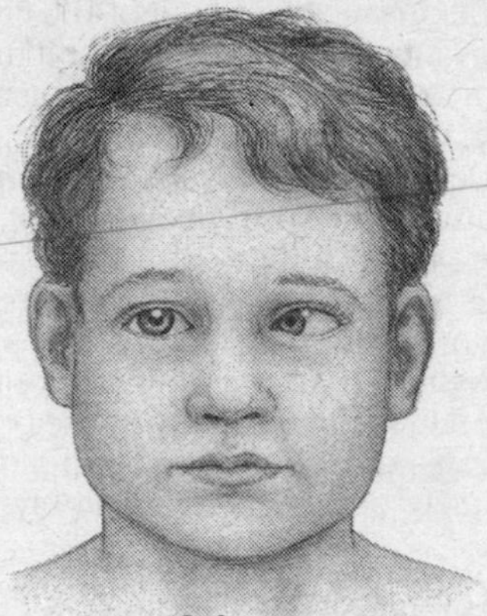

Left eye turning inward

accomplish this, so the treatment usually involves eyeglasses, eyedrops, or surgery.

If your baby needs an operation, this surgery is frequently done between six and eighteen months of age. The operation is usually safe and effective, although it's not uncommon for a child to need more than one procedure. Even after surgery, your child still may need glasses.

Some babies look as if they have strabismus because of the way their faces are structured, but in fact their eyes are perfectly aligned. These infants may have a flat nasal bridge and broad skin folds alongside the nose, termed *epicanthus*, which can distort the appearance of the eyes, making these babies appear cross-eyed when they really aren't. This condition is called pseudostrabismus (meaning false eye turning). The baby's vision is not affected, and, in most cases, as the child grows and the nasal bridge becomes more prominent, he loses the appearance of crossed eyes.

Because of the importance of early diagnosis and treatment of a true misalignment (or true strabismus), if you have any suspicion that your baby's eyes may not be perfectly aligned and working together, you should bring it to the attention of your pediatrician, who can best determine whether your baby has an actual problem.

Strabismus occurs in about 4 out of 100 children. It may be present at birth (infantile strabismus), or it may develop later in childhood (acquired strabismus). Strabismus can develop if your baby has another visual impairment, sustains an eye injury, or develops cataracts. Always report the sudden onset of strabismus to your pediatrician immediately. Although very rare, it may indicate the development of a tumor or other serious nervous system problem. In all cases, it is important to diagnose and treat strabismus as early in your infant's life as possible. If a turned eye is not treated early, the baby may never develop the ability to use both eyes together (binocular vision); and if both eyes are not used together, it is common for one to become "lazy," or amblyopic.

Tear (or Lacrimal) Production Problems

Tears play an important role in maintaining good eyesight by keeping the eyes wet and free of particles, dust, and other substances that might cause injury or interfere with normal vision. The so-called lacrimal system maintains the continuous production and circulation of tears, and depends on regular blinking to propel tears across the surface of the eye, finally draining into the nose.

This lacrimal system develops gradually over the first three or four years of life. Thus, while a newborn will produce enough tears to coat the surface of the eyes, it probably will

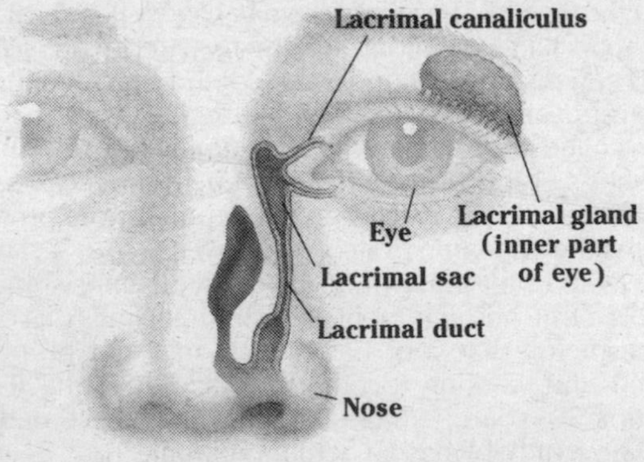

be about seven to eight months after birth before he "cries real tears."

Blocked tear ducts, which are very common among newborns and young babies, can cause the appearance of excessive tearing in one or both eyes, because the tears run down the cheek instead of draining through the duct and into the nose and throat. In newborns, blocked tear ducts usually occur when the membrane covering them at birth fails to disappear. Your pediatrician will demonstrate how to massage the tear duct. She'll also show you how to clean the eye with moist compresses to remove all secretions. Until the tear duct finally opens, the purulent infectious discharge may not go away. Since this is not a true infection or pinkeye, antibiotics should not be used.

Sometimes a membrane or small cyst can cause blocked or inflamed tear ducts. When this occurs and the methods described above are unsuccessful, the ophthalmologist may decide to open the blocked tear duct surgically. Rarely, this procedure must be repeated more than once.

Vision Difficulties Requiring Corrective Lenses

Nearsightedness

The inability to see distant objects clearly is the most common visual problem in young children. This inherited trait occasionally is found in newborns, especially premature infants, but it's more often detected after two years of age.

Nearsightedness is usually the result of an eyeball that's longer, causing the image not to be focused properly. Less frequently, it's due to a change in the shape of the cornea or lens.

The treatment for nearsightedness is corrective lenses—either eyeglasses or contact lenses. Keep in mind that when your child grows rapidly, so do his eyes, so he may need new lenses as often as every six months or less. Nearsightedness usually changes very rapidly for several years and then stabilizes before or during adolescence.

Farsightedness

This is a condition in which the eyeball is shorter than its focusing ability. Most babies are actually born farsighted, but as they grow, their eyeballs get longer and the farsightedness diminishes. Glasses or contact lenses rarely are needed unless the condition is excessive.

Astigmatism

Astigmatism is an uneven curvature of the surface of the cornea and/or lens. (Think of the eye as having the shape of a football.) If your baby has an astigmatism, vision both near and far may be blurred. Astigmatism can be corrected with either glasses or contact lenses.

22

FAMILY ISSUES

ADOPTION

If you are about to adopt or have just adopted a baby, you are likely experiencing conflicting emotions. Along with excitement and delight, you also may feel some anxiety and apprehension. These are emotions common to all parents, regardless of whether an infant joins their family by birth or by adoption. Having an understanding and supportive pediatrician will be helpful as you begin your new job as a parent. Even before a baby joins your family, a pediatrician can discuss your feelings about impending parenthood. If you are adopting an infant internationally or domestically, a pediatrician will also be able to address any medical issues that may arise.

Once your baby is home with you, schedule a visit to a pediatrician as soon as possible. Similar to an initial newborn exam, this initial postadoptive visit can provide an opportunity to ask any questions you have about your infant's health and development. Schedule future exams as required by the baby's age and medical needs. Many families find that they benefit from additional visits with their pediatrician during the first year to help address concerns that may arise as parents and baby start to develop a relationship.

In addition to the typical challenges of parenting, adoptive parents also face several issues and questions that nonadoptive parents do not. They include the following:

How and When Should I Tell My Child She Is Adopted? Your child should learn the truth about her birth family and her adoptive family as early as she is able to understand, which probably will be between ages two and four. It is important to adjust the information to her maturity level, so that she can make sense of it. For example: "Your parents loved you very much, but they knew they could not take care of you. So they looked for someone who also loved little children and was looking to have a bigger family." As she gets older and asks more specific questions, give her honest answers, but do not press information on her if she seems uncomfortable, fearful, or disinterested about it.

Are There Special Problems to Watch For? Adopted children have the same problems that other children of the same age and background have. However, if you adopt an older child, you will need to learn as much as possible about her previous experiences, so you can provide the support and understanding she requires. Children with a history of living in an orphanage or in foster care before joining their family often benefit from counseling at different times in their life.

Should I Tell Others That My Child Is Adopted? If you are asked, answer the question honestly and straightforwardly. Do not belabor the point or go into extensive detail if your child is nearby, as that may make her uncomfortable. Many professionals believe that your child's "adoption story" is hers to share with others as she gets older; so you may wish to share basic information with those who need to know but not all of the details with people beyond your immediate family.

CHILD ABUSE AND NEGLECT

Child abuse is common. The newspapers and TV news are so full of reports about child mistreatment that you cannot help but wonder how safe your baby really is. Although it is a mistake to become overprotective and make your child fearful, it is important to recognize the actual risks and familiarize yourself with the signs of abuse. Approximately 3 million cases of child abuse and neglect involving almost 5.5 million children are reported each year. The majority of cases reported to Child Protective Services involve neglect, followed by physical and sexual abuse. There is consider-

Where We Stand

Increasing numbers of children have been adopted by gay or lesbian individuals or couples in recent years. In some states this has stimulated political debate and public policy change. A growing body of scientific literature reveals that children who grow up with one or two gay and/or lesbian parents will develop emotionally, cognitively, socially, and sexually as well as children whose parents are heterosexual. Parents' sexual orientation is much less important than having loving and nurturing parents.

The American Academy of Pediatrics recognizes the diversity of families. We believe that children who are born to, or adopted by, one member of a gay or lesbian couple deserve the security of two legally recognized parents. Therefore, we support statutory and legal means to enable children to be adopted by the second parent or coparent in families headed by gay and lesbian couples.

able overlap among children who are abused, with many suffering a combination of physical abuse, sexual abuse, and/or neglect.

Most child abuse occurs within the family. Risk factors include parental depression or other mental health issues, a parental history of childhood abuse, and domestic violence. Child neglect and mistreatment is also more common in families living in poverty and among parents who are teenagers or are drug or alcohol abusers. Although it is certainly true that child abuse occurs outside the home, most often children are abused by a caregiver or someone they know, not a stranger.

Sexual abuse is any sexual activity that a child cannot comprehend or consent to. It includes acts such as fondling, oral-genital contact, and genital and anal intercourse, as well as exhibitionism, voyeurism, and exposure to pornography. Studies have suggested that up to one in four girls and one in eight boys will be sexually abused before they are eighteen years old. Physical abuse occurs when a child's body is injured as a result of hitting, kicking, shaking, burning, or other show of force. One study suggests that about 1 in 20 children has been physically abused in their lifetime.

Child neglect can include physical neglect (failing to provide food, clothing, shelter, or other physical necessities), emotional neglect (failing to provide love, comfort, or affection), or medical neglect (failing to provide needed medical care). Psychological or emotional abuse results from all of the above, but also can be associated with verbal abuse, which can harm a child's self-worth or emotional well-being.

Signs and Symptoms

It is not always easy to recognize when a child has been abused. Children who have been mistreated are often afraid to tell anyone, because they think they will be blamed or that no one will believe them. Sometimes they remain quiet because the person who abused them is someone they love very much, or because of fear, or both. Parents also tend to overlook signs and symptoms of abuse, because they don't want to face the truth. This is a serious mistake. A child who has been abused needs special support and treatment as early as possible. The longer he continues to be abused or is left to deal with the situation on his own, the less likely he is to make a full recovery.

Parents should always be alert to any unexplainable changes in the child's body or behavior. While injuries are often specific for an incident of physical abuse, behavioral change tends to reflect the anxiety that results from a stressful situation of any type. There are no behaviors that pinpoint a particular type of child abuse.

Physical Signs

- Any injury (bruise, burn, fracture, abdominal or head injury) that cannot be explained
- Genital pain or bleeding, as well as a sexually transmitted disease

Behavioral Changes That Raise Concern About Possible Abuse

- Fearful behavior (nightmares, unusual fears)
- Failure to gain weight (especially in infants) or sudden dramatic weight gain

Long-Term Consequences

In most cases, children who are abused or neglected suffer greater emotional than physical damage. Emotional and psychological abuse and neglect deny the child the tools needed to cope with stress, and to learn life's lessons. So a child who is severely mistreated may become depressed or develop suicidal, withdrawn, or violent behavior. As he gets older, he may use drugs or alcohol, try to run away, refuse discipline, or abuse others. As an adult, he may develop marital and sexual difficulties, depression, or suicidal behavior. Identifying a child victim is the first step. Recognizing the importance of early trauma to future development is crucial to assisting the victim.

Not all abuse victims have severe reactions. Usually the younger the child, the longer the abuse continues, and the closer the child's relationship with the abuser, the more serious the emotional damage will be. A close relationship with a very supportive adult can increase resiliency, reducing some of the impact.

Getting Help

If you suspect your baby has been abused, get help immediately through your pediatrician or a local child protective agency. Physicians are *legally obligated* to report all suspected cases of abuse or neglect to state authorities. Your pediatrician also will detect and treat any medical injuries or ailments, recommend a therapist, and provide necessary information to investigators. The doctor also may testify in court if necessary to obtain legal protection for the child or criminal prosecution of a sexual abuse suspect. Criminal prosecution is rarely sought in mild physical abuse cases but will occur in cases involving sexual abuse.

If your baby has been abused, you may be the only person who can help him. There is *no* good reason to delay reporting your suspicions of abuse. Denying the problem will only make the situation worse, allowing the abuse to continue unchecked and decreasing your child's chance for a full recovery.

In any case of abuse, the baby's safety is of primary concern. He or she needs to be in a safe environment free of the potential for continuing abuse.

Preventing Abuse

The major reasons for physical and psychological mistreatment of babies within the family often are parental feelings of isolation, stress, and frustration. Parents need support and as much information as possible in order to raise their children responsibly. They need to be taught how to cope with their own feelings of frustration and anger without venting them on babies. They also need the companionship of other adults who will listen and help during times of crisis. Support groups through local community organizations often are helpful first steps to diminish some of the isolation or frustration parents may be feeling. Parents who were themselves victims of abuse as children are in particular need of support. Confronting, addressing, and healing old wounds take uncommon courage and insight, but doing so is often the best assurance that the cycle of abuse is not passed on to the next generation.

Personal supervision of and involvement in your child's activities are the best ways to prevent physical and sexual abuse outside the home. Any child care program you select for your baby should allow unrestricted and unannounced parental visits without prearrangement. Parents should be allowed to volunteer and be informed about the selection or changes of staff members.

DIVORCE

Every year over one million children in the United States are involved in a divorce. Even those children who had lived with parental conflict and unhappiness for a long time may find the changes that follow divorce more difficult than anything they'd experienced before. At the very least, the child must adjust to living apart from one parent (usually the father) or, if in shared custody, to dividing her life between two homes. Because of financial changes, she also may have to move to a smaller home and a different neighborhood. A mother who stayed at home before now may have to go to work. Even if she doesn't, the stress and depression that accompany divorce may make her less attentive and loving with her child.

No one can predict specifically how divorce will affect your child. Her response will depend on her own sensitivity, the quality of her relationships with each parent, and the parents' ability to work together to meet her emotional needs during this time. It also will depend to some extent on her age and resiliency or vulnerability that her previous life experiences have given her.

In a very general way, you can anticipate how your child will react to divorce based on her age at the time it occurs.

Children under two often revert to more infantile behavior. They may become unusually clingy, dependent, or frustrated. They may refuse to go to sleep and may suddenly start waking up during the night. Under the age of three, they may show signs of sadness and fear of others. They also may have angry outbursts and tantrums, lose interest in eating, and have problems with toilet training.

Your child's response to the divorce probably will be most intense during and immediately following the breakup. As she grows older, she may continue to think about the past and struggle to understand why her parents separated. For years she may have some sense of loss, which might become especially painful during holidays and on special occasions like birthdays and family reunions.

Most children of divorce wish desperately for their parents to get back together. However, it is much more difficult for them if the parents repeatedly attempt to reconcile and then part again than if the initial separation is final. When the parents act indecisively, the child is likely to become suspicious, confused, and insecure.

In some cases, a child's behavior and self-esteem actually improve after the parents' divorce. Sometimes this is because the parents are relieved of the tension and sadness of an unhappy marriage and now can give the child more affection and attention. Sometimes it is because the divorce ends an emotionally or physically abusive situation. Often, however, even children who have been abused by a parent still yearn for that parent's love and for the family to be restored.

In summary, some children have serious and lasting psychological aftereffects from a divorce, but many others do well once the initial shock has subsided, and the family members have adapted to their new life circumstances.

How Parents Can Help the Child

A child integrates and mirrors her parents' emotions. If her parents are angry, depressed, or violent during the separation process, a child is likely to absorb these disturbing feelings and may turn them against herself. If the parents argue about her, or if she hears her name during their disputes, she may believe even more strongly that she is to blame. Secrecy and silence probably won't make her feel much better, however, and actually may intensify the unhappiness and tension she feels around her. If you're divorcing, the best approach is to be honest about your feelings but make a special effort to be loving and reassuring with your child. She will have to accept that her parents no longer love each other—and you shouldn't try to pretend otherwise—but make sure she understands and feels that both parents love her just as much as ever.

When parents are sensitive to what their child is going through, the child has a greater likelihood of coping and rebounding from the turmoil and anxiety of the divorce. But each child is different. Children have their own way of reacting to the situations around them—some respond with resilience and a sense of optimism while others tend to think negatively and disastrously about the present and the future. One of your tasks is to help your child deal with the divorce realistically, and avoid any thoughts that these major life changes will shatter her life.

In the weeks, months, and years after a divorce, keep the dialogue with your child open and appropriate for her age level. Repeatedly encourage her to talk about her feelings. Respond to her questions with clear and simple answers, and don't hesitate to bring up issues that she may have never raised on her own but are common among children of divorce. (She may be thinking, "Is it my fault that Mommy and Daddy are going to be apart?" . . . "If I'm a good girl, will Mommy and Daddy get together again?" . . . "Will Mommy and Daddy still always love me?")

If your child is younger than two years, you can't get these messages across very well with words. You will have to convey them through your actions. When you are with your child, try to put your own pain and worries aside and concentrate on her needs. Keep the daily routine as consistent as possible, and do not expect her to make any other major changes (i.e., toilet training, moving from a crib to a bed, or, if avoidable, adjusting to a new care provider or home arrangement) during this transitional period. In the beginning, try to be understanding and patient if your child's behavior regresses, but if this regression continues even after the divorce is completed and your life has settled back into a regular routine, ask your pediatrician for advice.

SINGLE-PARENT FAMILIES

Single-parent families are becoming more common. Most children of divorce spend at least some years in single-parent households. Another increasingly large group of children live with single parents who were never married or involved in a long-term relationship. A smaller number of children have widowed parents.

From a parent's viewpoint, there are some benefits to being single. You can raise the baby according to your own beliefs, principles, and rules, with no need for conflict or resolving differences. Single parents often develop closer bonds with their children. When the father is the single parent, he may become more nurturing and more active in his child's daily life than some fathers in two-parent households. Children in single-parent households may become more independent and mature because they have more responsibility within the family.

Single parenthood is not easy, though, for parents or children. It generally means less income and a lower standard of living. If you can't arrange or afford child care, getting and holding a job may be difficult. (See Chapter 10, *Early Education and Child Care.*) Without another person to share the day-in, day-out job of raising the infant and maintaining the household, you may find yourself socially isolated.

Here are some suggestions that may help you meet your own emotional needs while raising your infant.

- **Take advantage of** all available resources in finding help in caring for your baby. Use the guide to child care in Chapter 10.
- **Maintain your sense** of humor as much as possible. Try to see the positive or funny side of everyday surprises and challenges.
- **For your family's** sake as well as your own, take care of yourself. See your doctor regularly, eat properly, and get enough rest, exercise, and sleep.
- **Set a regular** time when you can take a break without your child. Relax with friends. Go to a movie. Pursue hobbies. Join groups. Do things that interest you. Pursue a social life of your own.
- **Do not feel** guilty because your child has only one parent. There are plenty of families in the same situation. You didn't "do it to her," and you don't need to penalize yourself or spoil her to make amends. Feeling and acting guilty won't help anyone.
- **Do not look** for problems where none exist. Many children grow up very well in single-parent homes, while others have a great many problems in two-parent homes. Being a single parent does not necessarily mean you'll have more problems or have more trouble resolving them.
- **Praise your baby** often, showing genuine affection and unconditional, positive support.
- **Create as large** a support network for yourself as possible. Keep active lists of relatives, friends, and community services that can help with child care. Establish friendships with other families who will let you know of community opportunities (soccer, cultural events, etc.) and are willing to exchange babysitting.
- **Talk to trusted** relatives, friends, and professionals such

Suggestions for Stepfamilies

Making a smooth transition from a single-parent family to a successful stepfamily requires special sensitivity and effort from the biologic parent and stepparent. Here are some suggestions that may help.

- Inform your former spouse of your marriage plans, and try to work together to make the transition as easy as possible for your child. Make sure everyone understands that the marriage will not change your former spouse's role in your child's life.
- Give your child time to get to know the stepparent (and stepsiblings, if any) before you begin living together. Doing this will make the adjustment easier for everyone and will eliminate a lot of your child's anxiety about the new arrangement.
- Watch for signs of conflict, and work together to correct them as early as possible.
- Parent and stepparent should decide together what will be expected of the child, where and how limits will be set, and what forms of discipline are acceptable.
- Parent and stepparent need to share the responsibilities of parenthood. This means that *both* will give affection and attention and that *both* will have authority in the household. Deciding together how the child should be disciplined, and supporting each other's decisions and actions, will make it easier for the stepparent to assume a role of authority without fear of disapproval or resentment.
- If a noncustodial parent visits the child, these visitations should be arranged and accepted so that they do not create disagreement within the stepfamily.

- Try to involve both biologic parents and stepparent(s) in all major decisions affecting a child. If possible, arrange for all the adults to meet together to share insights and concerns; doing this will let the child know that the grown-ups are willing to overcome their differences for his benefit.
- Be sensitive to your child's wishes and concerns about his role within the stepfamily. Respect his level of maturity and understanding when, for example, you help him decide what to call the stepparent or introduce him to the stepparent's relatives.

as your pediatrician about your child's development, and relationships within the family.

Stepfamilies

A single parent's remarriage can be a blessing for the parent and child alike—restoring the structure and security that were lost through divorce, separation, or death.

Benefits may include additional love and companionship for a parent as well as the children. Often a stepparent becomes as appropriate a role model of the same sex as the former spouse. In addition, there may be financial benefits of having another caregiver in the house.

But creating a stepfamily also requires many adjustments and can be very stressful. Yet with time, most blended families do manage to sort through any conflicts, but it requires a great amount of patience and commitment on the part of the adults, as well as the willingness to get professional help if serious problems should develop.

As difficult as the transition may seem at first, try to keep in mind that relationships between stepparents and stepchildren tend to develop gradually, over a period of one to several years, rather than over weeks or months.

In an atmosphere of mutual respect between biologic and stepparents, the child can derive the benefits of stepfamilies. The baby again has the opportunity of living in a household with two parents. The remarried parent often is happier and thus better able to meet the child's needs. As the baby gets older, her relationship to the stepparent may give her additional support, skills, and perspectives. These benefits, together with the economic advantages of the stepfamily situation, may give the child a broader range of opportunities.

MULTIPLES

Having twins (or other "multiples," such as triplets) means much more than simply having two or more babies at once, and the challenges go beyond having twice or three times the work or pleasure. Twins and other multiples quite frequently are born early and therefore tend to be smaller than the average newborn, so you may need to consult your pediatrician even more frequently than you would with a single baby. Feeding twins, whether by breast or bottle, also requires some special strategies, and the doctor can provide advice and support. There may be added financial pressures upon the family as well, spending a lot more on diapers, clothing, food, car seats, and dozens of other items—and perhaps needing a larger family car or even a larger home. (See Chapter 1.)

The twin birth rate in the U.S. is just over 3 percent. But as your obstetrician and pediatrician may have explained to you, the number of multiple births has risen in recent years. It has increased 42 percent since 1990 and 70 percent since 1980. Some researchers have attributed much of this increase to the more frequent use of infertility treatments and procedures such as in vitro fertilization. In vitro fertilization may involve implanting more than one fertilized egg into the uterus, while using infertility drugs can stimulate the ovaries to release two or more eggs.

This section is written primarily with twins in mind, but most of the same information and guidelines apply to triplets and other multiple births.

Raising Multiples

You should care for your healthy multiples just like any other infants. From the very beginning, it is important that you recognize your babies are separate individuals. If they are identical, it is easy to treat them as a "package," providing

Transporting Your Newborn Multiples

In many cases, twins and other multiples are smaller and weigh less than the average newborn. When bringing your babies home from the hospital and for subsequent trips in the car, keep the same guidelines in mind for choosing and using car safety seats. That means choosing infant-only and rear-facing car seats, and relying on them until your babies have reached at least one year of age *and* weigh at least twenty pounds. These infant-only seats have carrying handles, and may be sold with a base that can stay in your car.

But here's a very important point to keep in mind if your babies were born prematurely: rear-facing convertible car seats may *not* be appropriate for preemies. Before your newborns are discharged from the hospital, make sure they are tested to determine if they can ride safely while reclining in a car seat. If they have certain medical issues related to breathing or heart rate, they may not be able to ride in a semi-reclined position. In these instances, preemies should lie flat when they're riding in a car. Shop for a crash-tested car bed in which your newborns can be transported. (In most cases, the car bed will be purchased through the hospital.) Always use the harnesses and buckle that are part of the car beds, and install the beds lengthwise in the back seat; position your babies so their heads are toward the center of the car.

them with the same clothing, toys, and quality of attention. But as similar as they may appear physically, emotionally they are different, and in order to grow up happy and secure as individuals, they need you to support their differences. As one twin explained, "We're not twins. We're just brothers who have the same birthday!"

Identical twins come from the same egg, are always the same sex, and look very much alike. Fraternal twins come from two separate eggs, which are fertilized at the same time.

They may or may not be the same sex. Whether identical or fraternal, all twins have their individual personalities, styles, and temperament. Both identical and fraternal twins may become either competitive or interdependent as they grow. Sometimes one twin acts as the leader and the other as the follower. Whatever the specific quality of their interaction, most twins develop very intense relationships early in life simply because they spend so much time with each other.

If you also have other children, your twin newborns may prompt more than the usual sibling rivalry. They will require a large amount of your time and energy, and will attract a great deal of extra attention from friends, relatives, and strangers on the street. You can help your other children accept, and perhaps even take advantage of, this unusual situation by offering them "double rewards" for helping with the new babies and encouraging even more involvement in the daily baby care chores. It also becomes even more essential that you spend some special time each day alone with the other children doing their favorite activities.

You may find that your twins do not develop in the same pattern as do other children their age. Some twins seem to "split the work," with one concentrating on motor skills while the other perfects social or communication abilities. Because they spend so much time together, many twins communicate better with each other than with other family members or friends. They learn how to "read" each other's gestures and facial expressions, and occasionally they even have their own verbal language that no one else can understand. (This is particularly true of identical twins.) Because they can entertain each other, they may not be very motivated to learn about the world beyond them. This unique developmental pattern does not represent a problem, but it does make it all the more important to separate your twins occasionally and expose them individually to other playmates and learning situations.

Twins are not always happy about being apart, especially if they have established strong play habits and preferences for each other's company. For this reason, it is important to begin separating them occasionally as early as possible. If they resist strongly, try a gradual approach using very familiar children or adults to play with them individually but in the same room or play area.

As much as you appreciate the individual differences between your twins, you no doubt will have certain feelings for them as a unit. There is nothing wrong with this, since they do share many similarities and are themselves bound to develop a dual identity—as individuals and as twins. Helping them understand and accept the balance between these two identities is one of the most challenging tasks facing you as the parent of twins.

Your pediatrician can advise you on how to cope with the special parenting challenges with twins. He also can suggest helpful reading material or refer you to organizations that help parents with multiples.

At the same time, take care of yourself, getting as much rest as possible. Many parents find that raising twins and other multiples can be much more physically demanding and emotionally stressful than having just one baby. So make an effort to catch up on your own sleep whenever you can. Take turns with your spouse on who's going to handle the "middle-of-the-night" feedings, and who will bathe and feed the babies. If your budget can afford it, get some extra help for routine tasks like bathing the newborns and grocery shopping—or ask friends and family members for help. An extra set of hands, especially when there are more than twins, even for just a few hours a week, can make an enormous difference, and can give you more time not only to enjoy your babies, but also more time for yourself.

23

Fever

Your baby's normal temperature will vary with his age, activity, and the time of day. Infants tend to have higher temperatures than older children, and everyone's temperature is highest between late afternoon and early evening and lowest between midnight and early morning. Ordinarily, a rectal reading of 100.4 degrees Fahrenheit (38 degrees Celsius) or less, or an oral reading of 99 degrees Fahrenheit (37.2 degrees Celsius) or less, is considered normal, while higher readings indicate fever.

By itself, fever is *not* an illness. Rather, it is a sign or symptom of sickness. In fact, usually it is a positive sign that the body is fighting infection. Fever stimulates certain defenses, such as the white blood cells, which attack and destroy invading bacteria. The fever may actually be important in helping your baby fight his infection. However, fever can make your infant uncomfortable. It increases his need for fluids and makes his heart rate and breathing rate faster.

Fever most commonly accompanies respiratory illnesses such as croup or pneumonia, ear infections, influenza (flu), severe colds, and sore throats. It also may occur with infections of the bowel, blood, or urinary tract, inflammation of brain and spinal cord (meningitis), and with a wide variety of viral illnesses.

In children between six months and five years, fever can trigger seizures, called febrile convulsions. These convulsions tend to run in families, and usually happen during the first few hours of a febrile illness. Children may look "peculiar" for a few moments, then stiffen, twitch, and roll their eyes. They will be unresponsive for a short time, and their skin may appear to be a little darker than usual during the episode. The entire convulsion usually lasts less than one minute, and may be over in a few seconds, but it can seem like a lifetime to a frightened parent. Although uncommon, convulsions

Best Ways to Take a Temperature

There are several ways to take your baby's temperature. Use a digital thermometer (which shows the temperature in numbers in a small window), and avoid mercury thermometers (see page 643). Whatever approach you use, clean the thermometer with lukewarm soapy water or rubbing alcohol before each use, and then rinse with cool water.

To take the temperature in your baby's bottom (rectally), turn on the digital thermometer and then put a small amount of lubricant, such as petroleum jelly, on the small end of it. Place your infant across your lap or on something firm, either faceup or facedown (if he's facedown, put one hand on his back; if he's faceup, bend your child's leg to his chest, resting your free hand on the back of his thighs). Then gently insert the small end of the thermometer in your baby's bottom (or rectum), putting it in about ½ inch to 1 inch. Hold the thermometer in place for about one minute, or until the device signals that it's done (by beeping or lighting up). Remove it and read the number.

Taking a rectal or oral temperature is more accurate than taking it under your baby's arm. Also, use one digital thermometer labeled "oral," and another one labeled "rectal." Don't use the same thermometer in both places.

can last for up to fifteen minutes or longer. It is reassuring to know that febrile convulsions almost always are harmless—they do not cause brain damage, nervous system problems, paralysis, mental retardation, or death—although they should be reported promptly to your pediatrician. If your child is having trouble breathing or the convulsion (also referred to as a seizure) does not stop within fifteen minutes, call 911.

Children younger than one year at the time of their first simple febrile convulsion have approximately a 50 percent chance of having another such seizure, while children over one year of age when they have their first seizure have about a 30 percent chance of having a second one. Nevertheless, febrile convulsions rarely happen more than once within a twenty-four-hour (one-day) period. Although many parents worry that a febrile convulsion will lead to epilepsy, keep in mind that epileptic seizures are not caused by a fever, and children with a history of fever-related convulsions have only a slightly higher likelihood of developing epilepsy by age seven.

A rare but serious problem that is easily confused with fever is *heat-related illness,* or *heatstroke.* This is not caused by infection or internal conditions, but by surrounding heat. It can occur when a baby is in a very hot place—for example, a hot beach in midsummer or an overheated closed car on a summer day. Leaving babies unattended in closed cars is the cause of several deaths a year; *never* leave an infant unattended in a closed car, even for a few minutes. Heatstroke also can occur if a baby is overdressed in hot, humid weather. Under these circumstances, the body temperature can rise to dangerous levels (above 105 degrees Fahrenheit [40.5 degrees Celsius]), which must be reduced quickly by cool-water sponging, fanning, and removal to a cool place. After the baby has been cooled, he should be taken immediately to a pediatrician or emergency room. Heatstroke is an emergency condition.

Whenever you think your baby has a fever, take his temperature with a thermometer. (See *Best Ways to Take a Temperature* on page 642.) Feeling the skin (or using temperature-sensitive tape) is not accurate, especially when the infant is experiencing a chill.

What type of thermometer should you select? The American Academy of Pediatrics no longer recommends mercury thermometers because these glass thermometers may break and, as their mercury vaporizes, it can be inhaled, resulting in toxic levels. Digital electronic thermometers are better choices.

- **Digital devices can** measure temperatures in your baby's mouth or rectum. As with any device, some digital thermometers are more accurate than others. Follow the manufacturer's instructions carefully, and be sure the thermometer is calibrated.

Acetaminophen Dosage Chart

Dosages may be repeated every four hours, but should not be given more than five times in twenty-four hours. (*Note*: Milliliter is abbreviated as mL; 5 mL equals 1 teaspoon [tsp]. Don't use household teaspoons, which can vary in size.) Be sure to read the label to make sure you are using the right product.

*Age**	*Weight†*	*Infant Drops 80 mg/0.8 mL*	*Children's Elixir 160 mg/5 mL*	*Chewable Tablets 80 mg tabs*
0–5 mos.	6–11 lbs. (2.7–5 kg)	0.4 mL	—	—
6–11 mos.	12–17 lbs. (5.5–7.7 kg)	0.8 mL	½ tsp	1 tab
1–2 yrs.	18–23 lbs. (8.2–10.5 kg)	1.2 mL	¾ tsp	1½ tabs

**Note: Age is provided as a convenience only. Dosing for fever should be based on current weight.*

†Weight given is representative of the age range.

We do not recommend using aspirin ever to treat a simple fever.

When to Call the Pediatrician

If your infant is *two months or younger* and has a rectal temperature of 100.4 degrees Fahrenheit (38 degrees Celsius) or higher, call your pediatrician immediately. *This is an absolute necessity.* The doctor will need to examine the baby to rule out any serious infection or disease.

You also may need to notify the doctor if your infant is between three and six months and has a fever of 101 degrees Fahrenheit (38.3 degrees Celsius) or greater, or is older than six months and has a temperature of 103 degrees Fahrenheit (39.4 degrees Celsius) or higher. Such a high temperature may indicate a significant infection or dehydration, which may require treatment. However, in most cases, your decision to call the pediatrician should depend on associated symptoms, such as a severe sore throat, a severe earache, a cough, an unexplained rash, or repeated vomiting or diarrhea. Also, if your baby is very fussy or sleeping more than usual, call your doctor. In fact, your baby's activity level tends to be a more important indicator than the height of the fever. Again, fever in and of itself is not a sickness. It is a sign of sickness.

Other circumstances should prompt an immediate call to your pediatrician. For example, contact your doctor if your baby is feverish and has been in an extremely hot place, such as an overheated car. Also, talk to your pediatrician if your baby has a fever and has a condition that suppresses immune responses, such as sickle cell disease or cancer, or if he is taking steroids.

If your baby has a febrile convulsion (or seizure), he should be examined by your pediatrician or taken to the pediatric emergency room after consulting with your pediatrician as soon as possible, particularly if this is the first time it has occurred, or if it is more severe or prolonged than others he has had. You need to be sure that the convulsion is due to fever and not to a more serious condition such as meningitis (see page 663).

Home Treatment

Fevers generally do not need to be treated with medication unless your baby is uncomfortable or has a history of febrile convulsions. The fever may be important in helping your infant fight the infection. Even higher temperatures are not in themselves dangerous or significant unless your baby has a history of seizures or a chronic disease. Even if your infant has a history of a fever-related convulsion and you treat the fever with medication, they may still have this kind of seizure.

Ibuprofen Dosage Chart

Dosages may be repeated every six to eight hours, but should not be given more than four times in twenty-four hours. (*Note*: Milliliter is abbreviated as mL; 5 mL equals 1 teaspoon [tsp]. Don't use household teaspoons, which can vary in size.) Be sure to read the label to make sure you are using the right product.

*Age**	*Weight†*	*Infant Drops 50 mg/ 1.25 mL*	*Children's Elixir 100 mg/5 mL*	*Chewable Tablets 50 mg tabs*
6–11 mos.	12–17 lbs. (5.5–7.7 kg)	1.25 mL	2.5 mL	—
1–2 yrs.	18–23 lbs. (8.2–10.5 kg)	1.875 mL	3.75 mL	1 tab

**Note: Age is provided as a convenience only. Dosing for fever should be based on current weight.*

†Weight given is representative of the age range.

We do not recommend using aspirin ever to treat a simple fever.

It is more important to watch how your baby is behaving. If he is eating and sleeping well and has periods of playfulness, he probably doesn't need any treatment. You should also talk with your pediatrician about when to treat your infant's fever. A good time to do this is at well-child visits.

When your baby has a fever and seems to be quite bothered or uncomfortable by it, you may treat it with the following approaches.

Medication

Several medications can reduce body temperature by blocking the mechanisms that cause a fever. These so-called antipyretic agents include acetaminophen, ibuprofen, and aspirin. All three of these over-the-counter drugs appear to be equally effective at reducing fever. *However, because aspirin may cause or be associated with Reye syndrome, the American Academy of Pediatrics does not recommend using aspirin to treat a simple fever in children.* Acetominophen can be given without a doctor's advice once your baby is older than three months, and ibuprofen can be given to children older than six months of age. However, if your baby has kidney disease, asthma, an ulcer, or other chronic illness, ask your doctor first if ibuprofen is safe. If your infant is dehydrated or vomiting, ibuprofen should only be given under the supervision of a doctor due to risk of kidney damage.

Ideally, the doses of acetaminophen and ibuprofen should be based on a baby's weight, not his age. (See the dosage charts on pages 644 and 646.) However, the dosages listed on the labels of acetaminophen bottles (which are usually calculated by age) are generally safe and effective unless your baby is unusually light or heavy for his age. Keep in mind that at too-high doses of acetaminophen, a toxic response in the liver can develop, although it happens only rarely. When a toxic reaction does occur, the symptoms may include nausea, vomiting, and abdominal discomfort.

As a general guideline, read and follow the instructions on the manufacturer's label when using *any* medication. Following the instructions is important to ensure that your baby receives the proper dosages. Also, other over-the-counter medications, such as cold and cough preparations, may contain acetaminophen. The simultaneous use of more than one acetaminophen-containing product may be dangerous, so read all medication labels to ensure that your infant is not receiving multiple doses of the same medicine. Also, as a general rule, do not give a baby under two years old either acetaminophen or any other medication without the advice of your pediatrician.

Some parents have tried alternating between giving acetaminophen and ibuprofen when their baby is running a fever. This approach, however, can cause medication errors—"Which medicine am I supposed to give him next?"—and could lead to potential side effects. So if your infant is uncomfortable with a fever, choose which medicine to give, and then give it consistently. Either ibuprofen or acetominophen are effective in reducing fever and making your baby feel better. Always consult your doctor before changing the dose schedule, or using these medicines in combination.

Also keep in mind that over-the-counter cough and cold medicines should *not* be given to infants and children under two years of age because of potentially serious side effects. Studies also have shown that these cough and cold products are *not* effective in treating the symptoms of children under six years old, and may even pose health risks.

Other Treatment Suggestions for Fever

- **Keep your baby's** room and your home comfortably cool, and dress him lightly.
- **Encourage him to** drink.
- **If the room** is warm or stuffy, place a fan nearby to keep cool air moving.
- **Your baby does** not have to stay in his room or in bed when he has a fever, but he should not overexert himself.
- **If the fever** is a symptom of a highly contagious disease (e.g., chickenpox or the flu), keep your baby away from other children, elderly people, or people who may not be able to fight infection well, such as those with cancer.

Sponging

In most cases, using oral acetaminophen (over age three months) or ibuprofen (over age six months) is the most convenient way to make your feverish baby more comfortable. However, sometimes you may want to combine this with tepid sponging, or just use sponging alone.

Sponging is preferred over acetaminophen or ibuprofen if:

- Your baby is known to be allergic to, or is unable to tolerate, antipyretic (antifever) drugs (a rare case).

It is advisable to *combine* sponging with acetaminophen or ibuprofen if:

- Fever is making your baby extremely uncomfortable.
- He is vomiting and may not be able to keep the medication in his stomach.

To sponge your baby, place him in his regular bath (tub or baby bath), but put only 1 to 2 inches of tepid water (85–90 degrees Fahrenheit, or 29.4–32.2 degrees Celsius) in the basin. If you do not have a bath thermometer, test the water with the back of your hand or wrist. It should feel just slightly warm. Do not use cold water, since that will be uncomfortable and may cause shivering, which can raise his temperature. If your infant starts to shiver, then the water is too cold. Shivering can make a fever worse; take your baby out of the bath if he shivers.

Seat your infant in the water—it is more comfortable than lying down. Then, using a clean washcloth or sponge, spread a film of water over his trunk, arms, and legs. The water will evaporate and cool the body. Keep the room at about 75 degrees Fahrenheit (23.9 degrees Celsius), and continue sponging him until his temperature has reached an acceptable level. *Never put rubbing alcohol in the water; it can be absorbed into the skin or inhaled, which can cause serious problems, such as coma.*

Usually sponging will bring down the fever by one to two degrees in thirty to forty-five minutes. However, if your baby is resisting actively, stop and let him just sit and play in the water. If being in the tub makes him more upset and uncomfortable, it is best to take him out even if his fever is unchanged. Remember, a fever less than 105 degrees Fahrenheit (40.5 degrees Celsius) is in itself not harmful.

Treating a Febrile Convulsion

If your baby has a febrile convulsion, take the following steps immediately to prevent injury:

- Place him on the floor or bed away from any hard or sharp objects.
- Turn his head to the side so that any saliva or vomit can drain from his mouth.
- Do not put anything into his mouth; he will not swallow his tongue.
- Call your pediatrician.
- Call 911 if the convulsion lasts longer than fifteen minutes.

24

Genital and Urinary Systems

Blood in the Urine (Hematuria)

If your baby's urine has a red, orange, or brown color, it may contain blood. When the urine specifically contains red blood cells, doctors use the medical term *hematuria* to describe this condition. Many things, including a physical injury or inflammation or infection in the urinary tract, can cause it. Hematuria also is associated with some general medical problems, such as defects of blood clotting, exposure to toxic materials, hereditary conditions, or immune system abnormalities.

Sometimes there may be such small amounts of blood in the urine that you cannot see any color change, although it may be detected by a urine test performed by the pediatrician. In some cases the reddish color is not associated with hematuria at all, and the reddishness may be due simply to something your baby has eaten or swallowed. Beets, blackberries, red food coloring, phenolphthalein (a chemical sometimes used in laxatives), pyridium or phenazopyridine (medicine used to relieve bladder pain), and the medicine rifampin may cause the urine to turn red or orange if your child ingests them. Anytime you are not sure that one of these alternative explanations is responsible for the color change, call your pediatrician. Blood in the urine, when accompanied by protein (albumin), is usually due to inflammation of the filtering membranes of the kidney; the general term for this condition is nephritis. Your doctor may recommend further tests to distinguish among several different kinds of nephritis.

Treatment

Your pediatrician will ask you about any possible injury, foods, or health symptoms that might have caused the change in urine color. He will perform a physical exam, checking particularly for any increase in blood pressure, tenderness in the kidney area, or swelling (particularly of the hands or feet or around the eyes) that might indicate kidney problems. He also will conduct tests on a sample of urine and may order blood tests, imaging studies (such as an ultrasound scan or X-rays), or perform other examinations to check your baby's kidneys, bladder, and immune system. If none of these reveals the cause of the hematuria, and it continues to occur, your pediatrician may refer you to a children's kidney specialist, who will perform additional tests. (Sometimes these tests include examining a tiny piece of kidney tissue under the microscope, a procedure known as a biopsy. This tissue may be obtained by surgery or by performing what's called a needle biopsy.)

Once your pediatrician knows more about what is causing the hematuria, a decision can be made whether treatment is necessary. Often no treatment is required. Occasionally medication is used to suppress the inflammation that is the hallmark sign of nephritis. Whatever the treatment, your baby will need to return to the doctor regularly for repeat urine and blood tests and blood pressure checks. This is necessary to make sure that she isn't developing chronic kidney disease, which can lead to kidney failure.

Occasionally hematuria is caused by kidney stones, or, rarely, by an abnormality that will require surgery. If this is the case, your pediatrician will refer you to a pediatric urologist who can perform such procedures.

Circumcision

Circumcision is a common procedure in many infant boys. It involves removing the foreskin covering the tip of the penis. There are benefits and risks to circumcision, and you should discuss them with your pediatrician and your spouse before your baby is born. Although it is not routinely recommended for all newborn boys, there may be medical, religious, and other reasons why you may decide that it is appropriate for

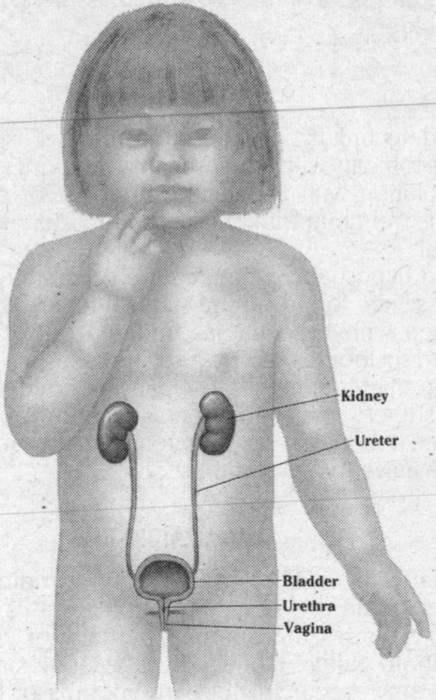

Genitourinary System

your son. Circumcision is discussed in detail on pages 28–29 and 157–159.

Hypospadias

In boys, the opening through which urine passes (the meatus) is located at the tip of the penis. A condition known as hypospadias is a birth defect that leaves the opening on the underside of the penis. There also may be an abnormal bending of the penis called chordee, which may cause sexual problems in adulthood. The meatus (the opening where urine passes) may direct the urinary stream downward and cause the stream to spray. A concern of many parents is the abnormal appearance of the penis in severe hypospadias, which can be a source of embarrassment to boys as they grow older.

Treatment

After detecting hypospadias in your newborn, your pediatrician probably will advise against circumcision until after consultation with a pediatric urologist or surgeon. This is because circumcision makes future surgical repair more difficult.

Mild hypospadias may require no treatment, but moderate or severe forms require surgical repair. At this time, most children with hypospadias undergo outpatient surgery at around six months of age. In severe cases, more than one operation may be needed to repair the condition completely. After surgery your baby's penis will appear nearly normal and he'll be able to urinate normally and—when he's older—have sexual relations.

Labial Adhesions

Ordinarily the lips of skin (labia) surrounding the entrance to the vagina are separated. In rare cases, they grow together to block the opening, partially or completely. This condition, called labial adhesions (sticking together of labia), may occur in the early months of life or, less frequently, later on if there is constant irritation and inflammation in this area. In these latter cases, the problem is usually traceable to diaper irritation, contact with harsh detergents, or underwear made with synthetic fabric. Usually labial adhesions do not cause symptoms, but they can lead to difficulty with urination and increase a girl's susceptibility to urinary tract infections. If the vaginal opening is significantly blocked, urine and/or vaginal secretions will build up behind the obstruction.

Treatment

If the opening of your daughter's vagina appears to have closed or looks partially blocked, notify your pediatrician. He will examine your baby and advise you whether any treatment is necessary. The majority of such adhesions

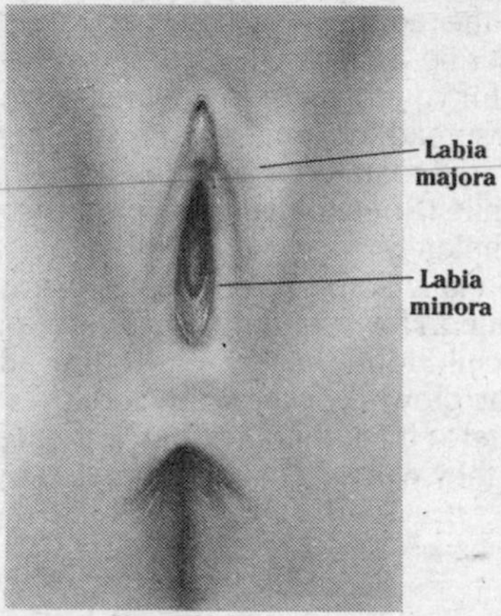

Normal labia

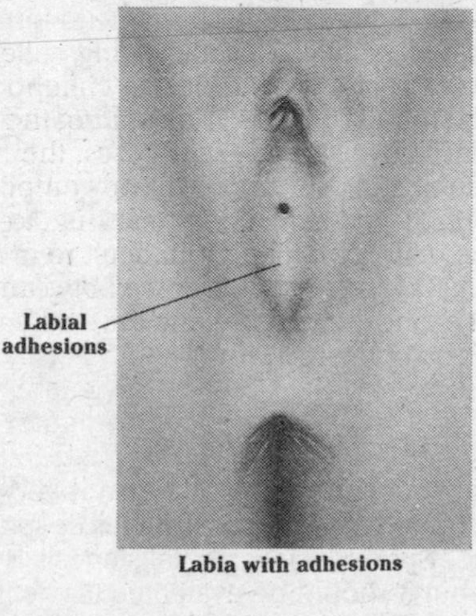

Labia with adhesions

resolve on their own as the child gets older and require no treatment.

At first, your doctor will attempt to spread the labia gently. If the connecting tissue is weak, this mild pressure may expose the opening.

But if the connecting tissue is too strong, the doctor may prescribe a cream that contains the female hormone estrogen for you to apply to the area as you very gently and gradually spread the labia apart over a period of time. Once the labia are separated, you will need to apply the cream for a short while (three to five days) until the skin on both sides heals completely.

Occasionally some adhesions return once the cream is discontinued. However, they usually disappear permanently in early childhood. In rare cases, the adhesions (scarlike tissue that grows between the labia and holds them together) are so thick that they block the flow of urine. In this situation, they will need to be separated by a physician.

Meatal Stenosis

In boys the meatus is the opening through which urine passes. Sometimes, particularly in circumcised boys, irritation of the tip of the penis causes scar tissue to form around the meatus, making it smaller. This narrowing, called meatal stenosis, may develop at any time during childhood, but is most commonly found between ages three and seven. Meatal stenosis is relatively rare.

Boys with meatal stenosis have a narrowed and abnormally directed urinary stream. The stream is directed upward (toward the ceiling), making it difficult to urinate into the toilet without pushing the penis down between the legs. Your son may take longer to urinate, and have difficulty emptying his bladder completely.

Treatment

If you notice that your son's urinary stream is very small or narrow, or if he strains to urinate or dribbles or sprays urine, discuss it with your pediatrician. Meatal stenosis is not a serious condition, but it should be evaluated to see if it needs treatment. In some cases, a steroid cream can be applied to the penis to correct the problem. If an operation is needed, this surgery is very minor and usually requires only local anesthesia. Your baby will have some minor discomfort after the procedure, but this should disappear after a very short period of time.

UNDESCENDED TESTICLES (CRYPTORCHIDISM)

During a woman's pregnancy, the baby boy's testes develop in his abdomen. As he nears birth, they descend through a tube (the inguinal canal) into the scrotum. In a small number of boys, especially those who are premature, one or both testicles fail to descend by the time of birth. In many of these boys, descent will occur during the first few months of life. In some, however, this does not happen.

Most boys will have a normal retraction of the testes under certain situations, such as while sitting in cold water (i.e., the testes "disappear" temporarily up into the inguinal canal). However, in general, when the boy is warm, testes should be low in the scrotum. The cause of most cases of undescended testicles is unknown.

If your baby has undescended testicles, his scrotum may be small and appear underdeveloped. If only one testicle is undescended, the scrotum may look asymmetrical (full on one side, empty on the other). If the testicles sometimes are in the scrotum and at other times (i.e., when he is cold or excited) are absent, and located above the scrotum, they are said to be retractile. This condition usually self-corrects as a boy grows older.

Rarely the undescended testicle may be twisted, and in the process, its blood supply may be stopped, causing pain in the inguinal (groin) or scrotal area. If this situation is not corrected, the testicle can be damaged severely and permanently. If your son has an undescended testicle and complains of pain in the groin or scrotal area, call your pediatrician immediately.

Undescended testicles should be reevaluated at each regular checkup. If they do not descend into the scrotum by one year of age, treatment should be considered.

Treatment

Undescended testicles may be treated with hormone injections and/or surgery. Currently, hormonal treatment is limited to cases of a very low undescended testis or some retractile testes. Many boys with true undescended testes will also have an inguinal hernia (see page 453), and the hernia will

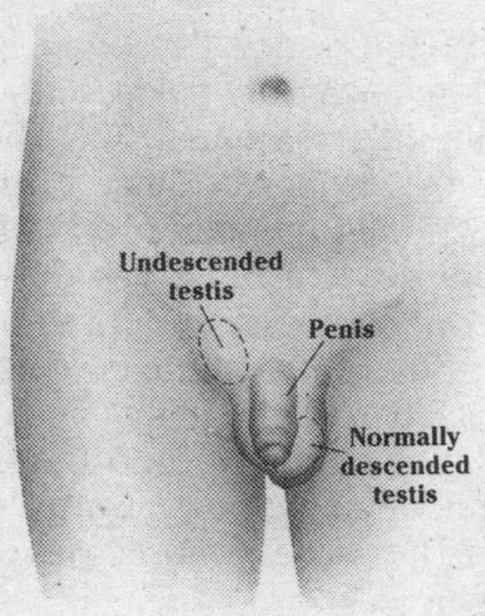

be repaired at the same time that the undescended testis is moved to the scrotum.

If your son's undescended testicle is allowed to remain in that position for over two years, he has a higher than average risk of being unable to father children (infertility). He also has a slightly increased risk of developing testicular tumors in adult life, particularly if the testicle is left in its abnormal position. Fortunately, with early and proper treatment, all of these complications usually can be avoided.

Urethral Valves

Urine leaves the bladder through a tube called the urethra, which in boys passes through the penis. Rarely, small membranes form across the urethra in boys early in pregnancy, and they can block the flow of urine out of the bladder. These membranes are called posterior urethral valves and can have life-threatening consequences by causing blockage of normal urine flow interfering with development of the kidneys. If there is abnormal kidney development, there can be abnormal development of the lungs.

The severity of posterior urethral valves can vary widely. Most cases are diagnosed before birth with a screening

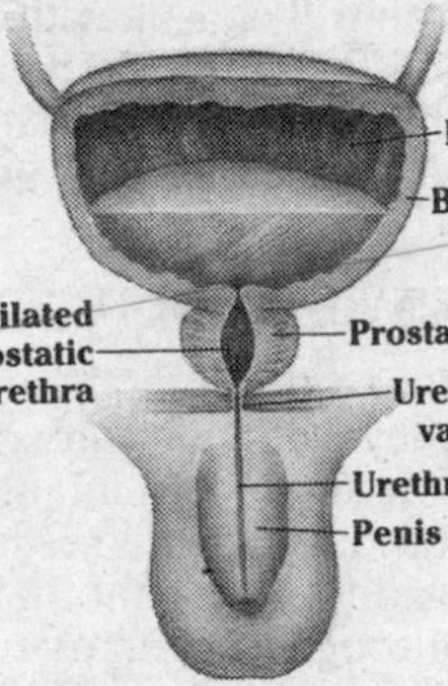

ultrasound. This condition may be suspected in boys if there appears to be a decrease in the amount of amniotic fluid. Consulting a pediatric urology specialist is always advisable before the baby is born.

In boys who are not diagnosed before birth with posterior urethral valve, sometimes the newborn exam may reveal that the baby's bladder is distended and enlarged. Other warning signals include a continual dribbling of urine and a weak stream during urination. More commonly though, posterior urethral valve is diagnosed when the boy develops a urinary tract infection with fever and poor feeding. If you notice these symptoms, notify your pediatrician at once.

Posterior urethral valves require immediate medical attention to prevent serious urinary tract infections or damage to the kidneys. If the blockage is severe, the urine can back up through the ureters (the tubes between the bladder and the kidneys), creating pressure that can damage the kidneys.

Treatment

If your baby has a posterior urethral valve, your pediatrician may pass a small tube (catheter) into the bladder to relieve the obstruction temporarily and allow the urine to flow out of the bladder. Then he'll order X-rays and/or an ultrasound of the bladder and kidneys to confirm the diagnosis and to see if any damage has occurred to the upper urinary tract. Your pediatrician will consult with a pediatric nephrologist (kidney specialist) or urologist, who may recommend surgery to remove the obstructing valves and prevent further infection or damage to the kidneys or urinary system.

URINARY TRACT INFECTIONS

Urinary tract infections are common among young children, particularly girls. They generally are caused by bacteria that enter through the urethra. In infants, though, they may also rarely be caused by bacteria carried through the bloodstream to the kidneys from another part of the body. As the bacteria move through the urinary tract, they may cause an infection in different locations. *Urinary tract infection (UTI)* is a general term used for all the following specific infections.

- *Cystitis:* infection of the bladder
- *Pyelonephritis:* infection of the kidney
- *Urethritis:* infection of the urethra

The bladder is the area most commonly infected. Usually cystitis is caused by bacteria that get into the urinary tract through the urethra. The urethra is very short in girls, so bacteria can get into the bladder easily. Fortunately, these bacteria normally wash out when urinating.

Cystitis can cause lower abdominal pain, tenderness, pain during urination, frequent urination, blood in the urine, recurrence of day- or nighttime wetting in a previously toilet-trained child, and a low fever. Infection of the upper urinary tract (the kidneys) will cause a more general abdominal pain and a higher fever, but is less likely to cause frequent and painful urination. In general, urinary tract infections in infants and young children (up to two years of age) may have few recognizable signs or symptoms other than a fever; they also have a greater potential for causing kidney damage than those occurring in older children.

Urinary tract infections must be treated with antibiotics as quickly as possible, so you should notify your pediatrician promptly if you suspect your baby has developed one. This is especially the case for infants, in whom an unexplained high fever (that is, not explained by a respiratory infection or diarrhea) may be the only indicator of a urinary tract infection. If your child has no symptoms, the American Academy of Pediatrics does not recommend routine urine testing (urinalyses), nor should routine blood pressure checks be performed on well children under the age of three years old.

Diagnosis/Treatment

When a urinary tract infection is suspected, particularly in a child with symptoms, your pediatrician will measure her blood pressure (since an increase in blood pressure can be a sign of a kidney problem) and examine her for lower abdominal tenderness that might indicate a UTI. Your doctor will want to know what your child has been eating and drinking, because certain foods can irritate the urinary tract, causing symptoms similar to those of an infection.

Your pediatrician also will want a urine sample from your child for analysis. Infants who are very sick or have a fever may need to have their urine collected through a small tube called a catheter or, rarely, by draining the urine out of the bladder with a needle inserted through the skin of the lower abdomen. In young infants, the urine will be collected by briefly inserting a catheter into the urethra and when urine is obtained, the catheter is quickly taken out.

The urine will be examined under the microscope for any sign of blood cells or bacteria, and special tests (cultures) will be done to identify the bacteria. An antibiotic will be started if an infection is suspected, although depending on what the final results of the culture show, the particular antibiotic may need to be changed (up to forty-eight hours later).

Your pediatrician may prescribe antibiotics for as long as a ten-day to two-week period. Prompt treatment is important in order to eliminate the infection and prevent its spread, and also to reduce the chances of kidney damage.

Make sure your baby takes the full course of medication prescribed, even if the discomfort goes away after just a few days. Otherwise, the bacteria may grow again, causing further infection and more serious damage to the urinary tract. After the treatment is complete, your doctor may want to obtain and analyze another urine sample to make sure that the infection is completely gone and no bacteria remain, though this is no longer a requirement.

The American Academy of Pediatrics recommends that imaging tests (ultrasound, X-rays, or renal scans) be done in children under age two with their first urinary tract infection. Your pediatrician also may conduct other tests to check the functioning of the kidneys. If any of these examinations indicate a structural abnormality that should be corrected, your doctor will recommend that your child see a pediatric urologist or child kidney specialist (nephrologist).

25

HEAD, NECK, AND NERVOUS SYSTEM

MENINGITIS

Meningitis is an inflammation of the tissues that cover the brain and spinal cord. The inflammation sometimes affects the brain itself. With early diagnosis and proper treatment, a baby with meningitis has a good chance of getting well without any complications.

Thanks to vaccines that protect against serious forms of bacterial meningitis, today most cases of meningitis are caused by viruses. The *viral* form usually is not very serious, except in infants less than three months of age. Once meningitis is diagnosed as being caused by a virus, there is no need for antibiotics and recovery should be complete. *Bacterial* meningitis (several types of bacteria are involved) is a very serious disease. It occurs very rarely (because of the success of vaccines), but when it does occur, babies and toddlers under the age of two are at greatest risk.

The bacteria that cause meningitis often can be found in the mouths and throats of healthy babies. But this does not necessarily mean that these infants will get the disease. That doesn't happen unless the bacteria get into the bloodstream.

We still don't understand exactly why some babies get meningitis and others don't, but we do know that certain groups of children are more likely to get the illness. These include the following:

- Babies, especially those under two months of age (Because their immune systems are not well developed, the bacteria can get into the bloodstream more easily.)

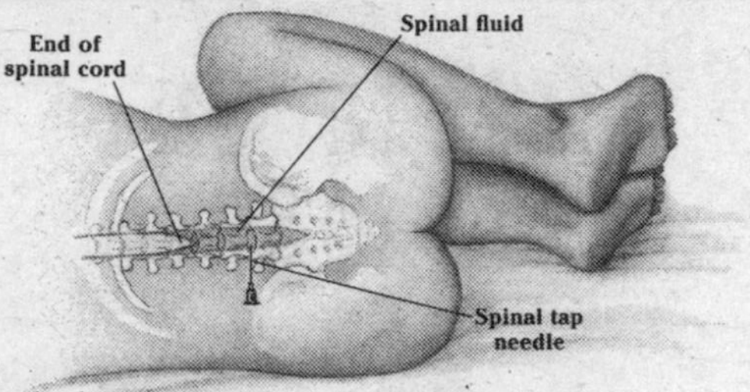

A spinal tap is taken from the space below the spinal cord so that the needle will not touch the spinal cord.

- Children with recent serious head injuries and skull fractures
- Children who have just had brain surgery

With prompt diagnosis and treatment, 7 out of 10 children who get bacterial meningitis recover without any complications. However, bear in mind that meningitis is a potentially fatal disease, and in about 2 out of 10 cases, it can lead to serious nervous-system problems, deafness, seizures, the loss of arms or legs, or difficulties at school. Because meningitis progresses quickly, it must be detected early and treated aggressively. This is why it's so important for you to notify your pediatrician immediately if your baby displays any of the following warning signs:

If your infant is less than two months old: A fever, decreased appetite, listlessness, or increased crying or irritability warrants a call to your doctor. At this age, the signs of meningitis can be very subtle and difficult to detect. It's better to call early and be wrong than to call too late.

If your baby is two months to two years old: This is the most common age for meningitis. Look for symptoms such as fever, vomiting, decreased appetite, excessive crankiness, or excessive sleepiness. (His cranky periods might be extreme and his sleepy periods might make it impossible to arouse him.) Seizures along with a fever may be the first signs of meningitis, although most brief, generalized (so-called tonic-clonic) convulsions turn out to be simple febrile seizures, not meningitis. (See *Seizures, Convulsions, and Epilepsy,* page 666.) A rash also is a symptom of this condition.

Treatment

If, after an examination, your pediatrician is concerned that your baby may have meningitis, she will conduct a blood test to check for a bacterial infection and also will obtain some spinal fluid by performing a spinal tap, or lumbar puncture (LP). This simple procedure involves inserting a special needle into your infant's lower back to draw out spinal fluid. This is a very safe technique in which fluid is sampled from the bottom of the sac surrounding the spinal cord, so there is no risk of injury to the cord itself. Any signs of bacterial infection in this fluid will confirm that your baby has bacterial meningitis. In that case he'll need to be admitted to the hospital for intravenous antibiotics and fluids and for careful observation for complications. During the first days of treatment, your baby may not be able to eat or drink, so intravenous fluids will provide the medicine and nutrition he needs. For certain types of meningitis, this may be necessary for seven to twenty-one days, depending on the age of the baby and the bacteria identified.

Prevention

Some types of bacterial meningitis can be prevented with vaccines. Ask your pediatrician about the following.

Hib (*Haemophilus Influenzae* type b) Vaccine This vaccine will decrease the chance of children becoming infected with *Haemophilus influenzae* type b (Hib) bacteria, which was the leading cause of bacterial meningitis among young children before this immunization became available. The vaccine is given by injection to children at two months, four months, and six months, and then again between twelve and fifteen months of age. (Some combined vaccines may allow your doctor to omit the last injection.)

Pneumococcal Vaccine This vaccine is effective in preventing many serious infections caused by the *pneumococcus* bacteria, including meningitis as well as bacteremia (an infection of the bloodstream) and pneumonia. It is recommended starting at two months of age, with additional doses at four, six, and between twelve and fifteen months of age. Some babies who have an increased susceptibility to serious infections (these high-risk children include those with abnormally functioning immune systems, sickle cell disease, certain kidney problems, and other chronic conditions) may receive an additional pneumococcal vaccine between ages two and five years.

Meningococcal Vaccine There are two kinds of meningococcal vaccines available in the U.S., but the preferred vaccine for children is called the meningococcal conjugate vaccine (MCV4). Although it can prevent four types of meningococcal disease, it is not recommended for very young children, but rather for young adolescents (eleven to twelve years of age), or teenagers at the time they start high school (or at fifteen years old).

Seizures, Convulsions, and Epilepsy

Seizures are sudden temporary changes in physical movement, sensation, or behavior caused by abnormal electrical impulses in the brain. Depending on how many muscles are affected by the electrical impulses, a seizure may cause sudden stiffening of the body or complete relaxation of the muscles, which can make a person appear to be paralyzed temporarily. Sometimes these seizures are referred to as "fits" or "spells." The terms *convulsion* and *seizure* can be used interchangeably.

A convulsion that involves the whole body (sometimes called a "generalized tonic-clonic" or "grand mal" seizure) is the most dramatic type of seizure, causing rapid, violent movements and occasionally loss of consciousness. These sometimes can start with focal movements (those involving one specific part of the body) and progress to generalized (i.e., both sides of the body) movements. Convulsions occur in about 5 out of every 100 people at some time during childhood. By contrast, "absence" seizures (previously called "petit mal" seizures) are momentary episodes with a vacant stare or a brief (one- or two-second) lapse of attention. These occur mainly in young children and may be so subtle that they aren't noticed until they begin affecting schoolwork.

Febrile convulsions (seizures caused by high fever) occur in 3 or 4 out of every 100 children between six months and five years of age, but most often around twelve to eighteen months old. Children younger than one year at the time of their first simple febrile seizure convulsion have approximately a 50 percent chance of having another, while children over one year of age when they have their first seizure have about a 30 percent chance of having a second one. Nevertheless, only a very small number out of 100 children will go on to develop chronic seizures without a fever. A febrile convulsion can cause reactions as mild as a rolling of the eyes or stiffening of the limbs, or as startling as a generalized convulsion with twitching and jerking movements that involve the whole body. Febrile convulsions usually last less than two or three minutes, and ordinarily the baby's behavior shortly returns to normal.

The term *epilepsy* is used to describe seizures that occur repeatedly over time without an acute illness (like fever) or brain injury. Sometimes the cause of the recurring seizures is known (symptomatic epilepsy), and sometimes it is not (idiopathic epilepsy).

Some babies and older children experience sudden episodes that might masquerade as or imitate seizures, but are really not. Examples include breath holding, fainting (syncope), facial or body twitching (myoclonus), and unusual sleep disorders (night terrors, sleepwalking, and cataplexy). They may occur just once or may recur over a limited time period. Again, although these episodes may resemble epilepsy or true seizures, they are not, and they require quite different treatment.

Treatment

Most seizures will stop on their own and do not require immediate medical treatment. If your baby is having a convulsion, protect her from injuring herself by laying her on her side with her hips higher than her head, so she will not choke if she vomits.

If the convulsion does not stop within two or three minutes or is unusually severe (difficulty breathing, choking, blueness of the skin, having several in a row), call 911 for emergency medical help. Do not leave your baby unattended, however. After the seizure stops, call the pediatrician immediately and arrange to meet in the doctor's office or the nearest emergency department. Also call your doctor if your baby is on an anticonvulsant medication, since this may mean that the dosage must be adjusted.

If your infant has a fever, the pediatrician will check to see if there is an infection. If there is no fever and this was your baby's first convulsion, the doctor will try to determine other possible causes by asking if there is a family history of seizures or if your child has had any recent head injury. He will examine your infant and also may order blood tests, pictures of the brain using computed tomography (CAT scan) or magnetic resonance imaging (MRI), or testing with an electroencephalogram (EEG), which measures the electrical activity of the brain. Sometimes a spinal tap will be performed to obtain a specimen of spinal fluid that can be examined for some causes of convulsions such as meningitis, an infection of the lining of the brain (see page 663). If no explanation or cause can be found for the seizures, the doctor may consult a pediatric neurologist, a pediatrician who specializes in disorders of the nervous system.

If your baby has had a febrile convulsion, some parents may try controlling the fever using acetaminophen and sponging. However, these approaches do *not* prevent future febrile seizures, but only make the infant more comfortable. If a bacterial infection is present, your doctor will probably prescribe an antibiotic. If a serious infection such as meningitis is responsible for the seizure, your baby will have to be hospitalized for further treatment. Also, when seizures are caused by abnormal amounts of sugar, sodium, or calcium in the blood, hospitalization may be required so that the cause can be found and the imbalances corrected.

If epilepsy is diagnosed, your infant usually will be placed on an anticonvulsant medication. When the proper dosage is maintained, the seizures can almost always be completely controlled. Your baby may need to have her blood checked periodically after starting some medications to make certain there is an adequate amount present. She also may need periodic EEGs. Medication usually is continued until there have been no seizures for a year or two.

As frightening as seizures can be, it's encouraging to know that the likelihood that your baby will have another one drops greatly as she gets older. (Only 1 in 100 adults ever has a seizure.) Unfortunately, a great deal of misunderstanding and confusion about seizures still exists, so it is important that child care workers become educated about her condition. If you need additional support or information, consult with your pediatrician or contact your local or state branch of the Epilepsy Foundation of America (www.epilepsyfoundation.org; 1–800–332–1000).

Head Tilt (Torticollis)

Head tilt is a condition that causes a child to hold her head or neck in a twisted or otherwise abnormal position. She may lean her head toward one shoulder and, when lying on her stomach, always turn the same side of her face toward the mattress. This can cause her head to flatten on one side and her face to appear uneven or out of line. If not treated, head tilt may lead to permanent facial deformity or unevenness and to restricted head movement.

Most cases of head tilt are associated with a condition called torticollis (described below), although in rare instances a head tilt can be due to other causes such as hearing loss, misalignment of the eyes, reflux (a flowing back of stomach acid), a throat or lymph node infection, or, very uncommonly, a brain tumor.

Congenital Muscular Torticollis By far the most common cause of head tilt among children under age five, this condition is the result of injury to the muscle that connects the breastbone, head, and neck (the sternocleidomastoid muscle). The injury may occur during birth (particularly breech and difficult first-time deliveries), but it also can occur while the baby is still in the womb. Whatever the cause, this condition usually is detected in the first six to eight weeks of life, when the pediatrician notices a small lump on the side of the baby's neck in the area of the damaged muscle. Later the muscle contracts and causes the head to tilt to one side and look toward the opposite side.

Klippel-Feil Syndrome In this condition, which is present at birth, the tilt of the neck is caused by a fusion or bony connection between two or more bones in the neck. Babies with Klippel-Feil syndrome may have a short, broad neck, low hairline, and very restricted neck movement.

Treatment

Each type of head tilt requires a slightly different treatment. It is very important to seek such treatment early, so that the problem is corrected before it causes permanent deformity.

Your pediatrician will examine your baby's neck and may order X-rays of the area in order to identify the cause of the problem. X-rays of the hip also may be ordered, as some children with congenital muscular torticollis also have an abnormality known as developmental dysplasia of the hip. If the doctor decides that the problem is muscular torticollis due to a birth-related injury to the sternocleidomastoid muscle, you will learn an exercise program to stretch the neck muscles. The doctor will show you how to gently move your baby's head in the opposite direction from the tilt. You'll need to do this several times a day, very gradually extending the movement as the muscle stretches.

When your baby sleeps, it is best to place her on her back or side, with her head positioned opposite to the direction of the tilt. She can be placed on her stomach if she allows you to turn her face away from the side of the muscle injury, and if she then keeps her head in this position while sleeping. When she is awake, position her so those things she wants to look at (windows, mobiles, pictures, and activity) are on the side away from the injury. In that way, she'll stretch the shortened muscle while trying to see these objects. These simple

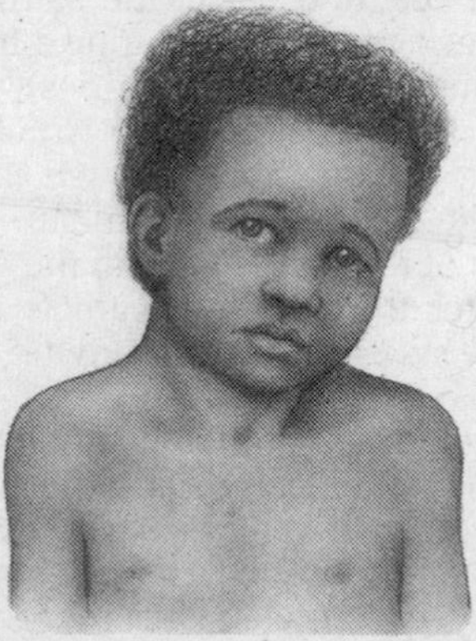

strategies cure this type of head tilt in the vast majority of cases, preventing the need for later surgery.

If the problem is not corrected by exercise or position change, your pediatrician will refer you to a pediatric neurologist or orthopedist. In some cases it may be necessary to lengthen the involved tendon surgically.

If your baby's head tilt is caused by something other than congenital muscular torticollis, and the X-rays show no spinal abnormality, other treatment involving rest, a special collar, traction, application of heat to the area, medication, or, rarely, surgery may be necessary. To treat Klippel-Feil syndrome, a specialist may recommend treatments ranging from physical therapy to an operation. For treating torticollis due to injury or inflammation, your doctor may recommend applying heat, as well as using massage and stretching to ease head and neck pain. Your pediatrician can refer you to a specialist for a definitive diagnosis and treatment program.

26

HEART

CONGENITAL HEART DISEASE

About 8 to 10 of every 1,000 children are born with a congenital heart defect (a heart problem at birth). The defect can range from a structural abnormality of the heart's chambers, to a malfunctioning heart valve, to arteries or veins that are improperly connected or abnormally formed.

Most defects develop early in pregnancy, typically by the eighth to twelfth week of fetal development. About one-third of these babies have a severe heart disorder that requires treatment, with surgery or by catheter, in the first months of life.

The cause of nearly all congenital heart defects is never identified, although researchers are investigating possible roles of genetic and environmental factors. Parents should not blame themselves for their baby's heart condition; it is not caused by anything that the mother or father did or didn't do.

The two most common congenital heart defects are the following:

A *ventricular septal defect* is characterized by a hole in the septum (the wall or partition) between the two ventricles, or pumping chambers, of the heart. This allows blood to pass abnormally from the left side of the heart to the right side. In babies, if the defect is large, the increased workload on the heart may lead to breathing difficulties and poor growth. For these children, surgery is usually necessary. In other children the defect may be small and require no treatment at all.

An *atrial septal defect* occurs when there is a hole in the septum between the atria (upper or receiving chambers) of the heart. Because the pressure in the atrial chambers is lower than in the ventricular

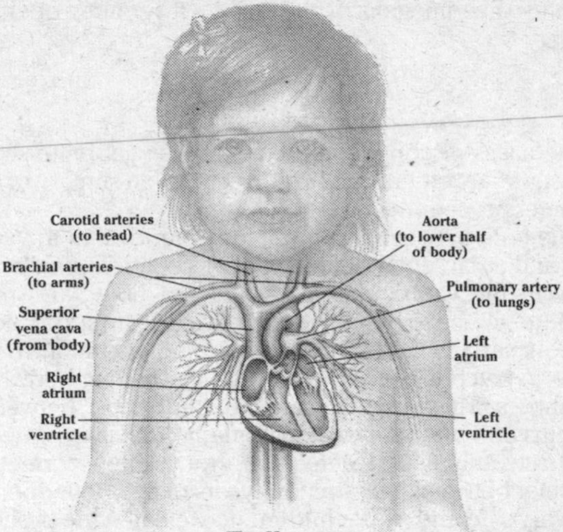

The Heart

chambers, this problem tends to cause less of a workload upon the heart than ventricular septal defects. Many children with this condition have no symptoms and function well, particularly in the early years of life. A pediatrician may detect the problem, however, during a routine physical exam. Eventually, often not until adulthood, those with atrial septal defects may experience symptoms such as irregular heart rhythms, shortness of breath, or stroke. Most patients with an atrial septal defect can have it closed by a catheter procedure, and open heart surgery is not necessary.

There are other, less common types of congenital heart defects. One of them, called *transposition of the great arteries*, occurs when the two arteries coming out of the heart are reversed—that is, the aorta comes from the right ventricle instead of the left one, and the pulmonary artery comes from the left ventricle. Thus, oxygenated blood does not circulate properly through the body. Transposition of the great arteries is the most common cause for a "blue baby," due to the fact that the baby's oxygen level is very low. It can usually be diagnosed immediately after birth because of the baby's blueness, and the diagnosis is confirmed by echocardiography (sound-wave imaging of the heart). It requires open heart surgery.

Treatment

Some cases of congenital heart disease get better without therapy. Many others can be corrected with surgery or with a catheter procedure.

The hole between the pumping chambers in the ventricular and atrial septal defects tends to become smaller on its own; in the ventricular defects, if the hole was small to medium in size to begin with, it may close up spontaneously without surgery. Larger holes require an operation, in which a fabric patch is used to close up the opening between the chambers. This surgery may be performed between six months and one year of age in infants with large defects. By contrast, atrial septal defects are most often corrected by catheter between two and four years of age. Both operations are very safe, and most children do well after the procedure.

Transposition of the great arteries can be corrected with an operation performed about three to four days after birth, before the child ever leaves the hospital. It involves reconnecting the arteries to the appropriate pumping chambers. Refinements in this procedure in recent years have turned this defect into a highly correctable one.

Prevention

Although there is no known way to prevent most congenital heart defects, a pregnant woman can help ensure the health of her baby by avoiding alcohol, cocaine, and other drugs, and by taking steps to avoid contracting rubella (German measles). If you have a family history of congenital heart disease—that is, if you or your spouse or a previously born child has this condition—your doctor may check the fetus for a possible heart problem.

Heart Murmur

Technically, a heart murmur is simply a noise heard between the beats of the heart. When a doctor listens to the heart, she hears a sound something like *lub-dub, lub-dub, lub-dub.* Most often, the period between the *lub* and the *dub* and between the *dub* and the *lub* is silent. If there is any sound during this period, it is called a murmur. Heart murmurs are extremely common, and are usually normal (that is, the sounds are caused by a healthy heart pumping blood normally).

Most children with a murmur require no special care, and the sound eventually disappears. These children have "normal" or so-called functional or innocent heart murmurs.

If your child has such a murmur, it probably will be discovered between the ages of one and five during a routine examination. The doctor then will listen carefully to determine if this is a "normal" heart murmur or one that might indicate a problem. Usually, just by listening to its sound, the pediatrician will be able to tell if a murmur is innocent (normal). If necessary, she will consult a pediatric cardiologist to be certain, but additional tests are usually not needed.

On rare occasions, a pediatrician will hear a murmur that sounds abnormal enough to indicate that something might be wrong with the heart. If the doctor suspects this, your child will be referred to a pediatric cardiologist to enable a precise diagnosis to be made.

When do heart murmurs become a concern? When they occur very early at birth or during the first six months of life. These murmurs are *not* functional or innocent, and most likely they will require the attention of a pediatric cardiologist immediately. They may be due to abnormal connections between the pumping chambers (septal defects) or the major blood vessels coming from the heart (e.g., transposition of vessels). Your infant will be observed for changes in skin color (turning blue), as well as breathing or feeding difficulties. He also may undergo additional tests, such as a chest X-ray, electrocardiogram (ECG), and an echocardiogram. This echocardiogram creates a picture of the inside of the heart by using sound waves. If all of these tests prove normal, then it is safe to conclude that the baby has an innocent murmur, but the cardiologist and pediatrician may want to see him again to be absolutely certain. The cardiologist and pediatrician together will make a decision as to next steps depending on the results of these tests.

When a specific condition called patent ductus arteriosus (PDA) occurs, it is often detected shortly after birth, most commonly in premature babies. It is a potentially serious condition in which blood circulates abnormally between two of the major arteries near the heart, due to the failure of a blood vessel (the ductus arteriosis) between these arteries to properly close. In most cases, the only symptom of PDA is a heart murmur until the ductus closes on its own shortly after birth, which often happens in otherwise healthy, full-term newborns. Sometimes, especially in premature babies, it may not close on its own, or it may be large and permit too much blood to pass through the lungs, which can place extra strain on the heart, forcing it to work harder and causing a rise in blood pressure in the arteries of the lungs. If this is the case, a medication or, rarely, surgery may be needed to help close the PDA.

Treatment

Innocent heart murmurs are normal and therefore require no treatment. Children with these innocent heart murmurs do not need repeated evaluations or long-term follow-up care from cardiologists, nor do they require restrictions on sports or other physical activities.

Innocent heart murmurs generally disappear by midadolescence. Cardiologists don't know why they go away, any more than we know why they appear in the first place. In the meantime, don't be discouraged if the murmur is softer on one visit to the pediatrician and loud again on the next. This may simply mean that your child's heart is beating at a slightly different rate each time. Most likely, this normal murmur will go away eventually.

Patent ductus arteriosus is a self-correcting problem in some cases, or medications can be used to close a PDA. But if the ductus arteriosus remains open, it may need to be corrected surgically or with a catheter.

If other, more serious, heart conditions are diagnosed from birth or shortly thereafter, and the evaluation reveals more serious defects, the pediatric cardiologist and pediatrician will consult a pediatric cardiac surgeon at a regional Pediatric Cardiac Center where complete pediatric cardiac diagnostic and intervention capabilities exist.

Kawasaki Disease

Kawasaki disease is a potentially serious and perplexing disease, the cause of which is unknown. Some researchers believe, however, that it is caused by a virus or bacteria. Signs of this disease include fever, usually quite high, that lasts for at least five days and doesn't respond to antibiotics. Fever should be present to consider a diagnosis of Kawasaki disease in the ill infant.

In addition, four of the six following signs appear in the typical case:

1. Rash over some or all of the body, often more severe in the diaper area, especially in infants under six months of age.
2. Redness and swelling of the palms and soles and/or cracking of the skin around the base of the nails.
3. Red, swollen, and cracked lips and/or a strawberry-colored tongue.
4. Red, inflamed eyes, especially the sclerae (white part).
5. A swollen gland, particularly on one side of the neck.
6. Irritability or listlessness. Infants with Kawasaki disease are usually crankier or more lethargic than usual. They also may complain of abdominal pain, headache, and/or joint pain.

Kawasaki disease causes inflammation of the blood vessels; in some cases this includes the arteries of the heart (the coronary arteries). This inflammation weakens the walls of the blood vessels. In most cases the inflammation in the blood vessels appears to resolve after several months, but in some cases they remain weakened and may even balloon out, causing aneurysms (blood-filled swellings of the blood vessels).

Kawasaki disease occurs most frequently in Japan and Korea and in individuals of Japanese and Korean ancestry, but it can be found among all racial groups and on every continent. The exact number of cases are not known, but there are about 5,000 hospitalizations per year in the U.S., typically among older infants and preschoolers.

Kawasaki disease does not appear to be contagious. It is extremely uncommon for two children in the same household to get the disease. Likewise, it does not spread among children in child care programs, where there is daily close contact. Although Kawasaki disease can occur in community outbreaks, particularly in the winter and early spring, no one knows the cause. The peak age of occurrence in the United States is between six months and five years. Evidence suggests that Kawasaki disease may be linked to a yet-to-be-identified infectious cause, such as a virus or bacteria. However, despite intense research, no bacteria, virus, or toxin has been identified as a cause of the disease. No specific test makes the diagnosis. The diagnosis is made by meeting the signs of illness mentioned above and by excluding other possible diseases.

Treatment

Because the cause of Kawasaki disease is unknown, it can be treated but not prevented. If it is diagnosed early enough, intravenous gamma globulin (a mixture of human antibodies) can minimize the risk of a baby developing coronary aneurysms. In addition to gamma globulin, the child should receive aspirin, initially in high doses. Aspirin can decrease the tendency of blood to clot in damaged blood vessels. Although it's appropriate to use aspirin to treat Kawasaki disease, treating children with minor illnesses (i.e., a cold or influenza) with aspirin has been linked with a serious disease called Reye syndrome. Always consult your pediatrician before giving aspirin to your baby.

27

Immunizations

Immunizations have helped children stay healthy for more than half a century. Routine vaccines have become one of the best weapons available to protect your child against major childhood diseases.

Immunizations, in fact, are one of the greatest public-health success stories of our times. Many diseases that were once a routine part of growing up—some of them life-threatening—are now preventable and relatively rare, thanks to improvements in sanitation, better nutrition, less crowded living conditions, antibiotics—and most importantly, vaccines. At one time, most people did not reach adulthood without someone in their family or circle of friends being touched by a very serious illness or death caused by an infectious disease. But now those same diseases are at record low levels in the United States as well as many other countries in the world—and that's because immunization rates are at record highs. There are now immunizations for fourteen childhood diseases. Vaccines work extremely well—most are 90 to 99 percent effective in preventing diseases—so they are important weapons in keeping children safe and healthy. When parents learn of the risks of these infections—for example, whooping cough causing seizures, brain disease, and even death—the argument in favor of childhood immunizations is persuasive. Although chickenpox, for example, is usually a mild disease, before the vaccine was available, more than 11,000 children were hospitalized each year when chickenpox sores became infected. Before the vaccine, about 100 people died of chickenpox complications each year. But now this disease can be prevented.

IMPORTANT AND SAFE

Because many parents (and even some doctors) have never seen a child with diseases like whooping cough or diphtheria, mothers and fathers sometimes ask their pediatrician whether their baby really needs vaccines at all. But while many of the illnesses that once caused lifelong disabilities or even death are now uncommon, they haven't been wiped out completely. Yes, they are preventable, but the germs that cause many of them are still around, and are constantly being brought into the country by international travelers.

Just consider the case of the *Haemophilus influenzae* type b (Hib) vaccine. It protects children from serious childhood diseases like meningitis (an inflammation and swelling of the tissues that cover the brain and spinal cord) and throat infections that can block the airway (such as epiglottitis). Before this vaccine became available in the 1980s, there were about 20,000 cases of Hib disease in the U.S. every year. *H. influenzae* type b was the most common cause of bacterial meningitis in the United States and it was an important cause of mental retardation. It caused about 12,000 cases of meningitis each year in children younger than five years of age—especially in babies six to twelve months old. Of those children infected, 1 in 20 died from this disease, and 1 in 4 developed permanent brain damage. Today, because Hib disease is not as serious in vaccinated children, there are fewer than 100 cases annually. At the same time, vaccines are very safe—but they're not perfect. Like medications, they can cause occasional reactions, but usually these are mild (see *More About Immunizations* on page 681). Side effects like redness or discomfort at the site of the injection can happen in as many as 1 out of 4 children. They appear soon after the shot is given, and then usually go away within a day or two. Your child also may be fussy afterward. Although more severe reactions can occur, they are much less common. Some children with certain health conditions should not receive vaccines. Talk to your doctor if your child had a serious reaction to a previous vaccine, has any allergies, or is sick on the day of the appointment. This type of information can help your doctor determine if your child should not get a vaccine. In recent years, some critics of immunizations have pointed to a preservative called thimerosal, which for decades had been added to

More About Immunizations

When you have your babies immunized:

- You protect them from dangerous and potentially fatal diseases.
- You lower the severity of the disease if your infants happen to get it.
- You cut down the chances that contagious diseases will spread.
- You safeguard other people in your community who are too young to receive the vaccine or cannot receive vaccinations due to medical issues.

Also of Note

- After receiving a vaccine, some children experience mild symptoms such as a low fever and fussiness, as well as tenderness, swelling, or redness where the shot was given. They also may sleep a little longer than usual in the day or two after receiving the shot.
- On very rare occasions, children may react to a vaccine with a more serious response, such as a high fever, a rash, or seizures. Call your pediatrician if your child develops a fever over 103 degrees Fahrenheit, a generalized rash (including hives), a large amount of swelling in the limb where the shot was given, or any other symptoms that worry you. These guidelines apply to all of the immunizations described in this chapter.

some vaccines to prevent contamination of vaccines by bacteria. Thimerosal has a small amount of organic mercury in it, which also worried some parents. They were concerned about a link between disorders such as autism and vaccines that contain thimerosal. But despite countless studies in the United States and abroad, no scientific data has shown a link

Easing the "Hurt"

Shots can hurt. When your baby receives a vaccine, she can be uncomfortable and may cry for several minutes. But fortunately, any pain is very short-lived. At the moment the immunization is given, you may be able to soften the experience by distracting your infant. Talk soothingly, and make eye contact with her. Afterward, comfort and play with her for a while.

If your baby develops side effects, you may be able to ease any fever or irritability by giving her acetaminophen or ibuprofen. Be sure to discuss the use and proper dosage of these medicines with your pediatrician. If your child has pain at the site where the shot was given, your doctor might recommend applying cool compresses to lessen the discomfort. Certainly, if any reaction makes your baby uncomfortable for more than four hours, notify your pediatrician, who will want to note it in your infant's records and prescribe appropriate treatment.

Before immunizing your baby, it's a good idea to talk with your doctor about what reactions you might expect, if any. If an unusual or severe reaction like a high fever or changes in behavior have occurred, you and your pediatrician should discuss the pros and cons of whether another dose of the same vaccine is appropriate when the next one is scheduled.

As painful as it may be for you to watch your infant experience the discomfort of a shot, don't lose sight of the fact that you're doing enormous good for her by making sure she is protected from the diseases that vaccines can prevent.

between thimerosal and autism. In fact, even though all vaccines manufactured for infants have been thimerosal-free or contain only trace levels since 2001, autism rates continue to rise.

While some parents also worry that their baby is receiving "too many vaccines" at one time, there is plenty of research showing that multiple childhood vaccines can be given at the same time safely. In fact, a vaccine cannot be licensed and recommended until the manufacturers show that it can be given safely with other recommended vaccines. And although children receive more vaccines than in years past, the ones they're receiving have been purified and improved so that children are actually receiving less antigens (substances that help a body build up an immunity) with each shot. These shots are effective and safe when they're given according to the guidelines recommended by the American Academy of Pediatrics.

The important point to remember is that getting these preventable diseases is much more dangerous than getting the vaccines. If you have questions or concerns about immunizations, talk with your pediatrician.

What Shots Does Your Baby Need?

Your infant should be vaccinated according to the schedule of immunizations recommended by the American Academy of Pediatrics. The entire schedule appears in the Appendix, and includes the immunizations described below for young children. Please refer to the chart often for information on the immunizations your child needs and when they should be given. Also, recommendations change as vaccines are improved and new ones are developed; so be sure to speak with your pediatrician or visit www.aap.org for the most current immunization schedule.

Where We Stand

The American Academy of Pediatrics believes that immunizations are the safest and most cost-effective way of preventing disease, disability, and death. We urge parents to make sure that their children are immunized against dangerous childhood diseases since it is always better to prevent a disease than to have to treat it or live with the consequences of having it.

Diphtheria, Tetanus, and Pertussis The DTaP vaccine protects your baby against diphtheria (D), tetanus (T), and pertussis (aP). The diphtheria portion of this vaccine guards against a throat infection that can trigger breathing difficulties, paralysis, or heart failure. The tetanus portion protects against a disease that causes the tightening or "locking" of all of the muscles in the body, especially the jaw, and is potentially fatal. The vaccine for pertussis (also called whooping cough) prevents bacteria from causing severe and violent coughing spells in infants that can make breathing and eating difficult.

What about expected side effects? Redness and tenderness may occur with the diphtheria and tetanus portions of the vaccine. Sometimes the fourth or fifth dose is followed by swelling of the arm or leg in which the shot was given. Severe, but very rare, problems that have been reported after the DTaP vaccine include long-term seizures, coma, and permanent brain damage. Don't keep your child from getting this—or any—vaccine without first speaking with your pediatrician. He can address any concerns you may have. He also may tell you that, rarely, certain children should not receive all of the DTaP series of vaccines, including those who have a severe reaction to the initial shot. But for the vast majority of children, the dangers of the diseases themselves outweigh any risks of the shots; keep in mind, for example, that 2 out of 10 people who get tetanus die from it; and 1 out of 100 babies under two who get pertussis die. More than 1 out of 10 children who get diphtheria die of complications. Immunizations are very important.

Measles, Mumps, and Rubella (MMR) The measles portion of this vaccine protects against an infection that causes an extensive red or brownish blotchy rash, as well as flulike symptoms; the measles can lead to severe diseases such as pneumonia, seizures, and brain damage. The mumps vaccine gives your baby protection against a virus that causes swollen salivary glands, a fever, and headaches, and can lead to deafness, meningitis, and painful swelling of the testicles or ovaries. The rubella (German measles) vaccine guards against an infection of the skin and lymph nodes, in which the child may have a pink rash and swollen, tender glands at the back of the neck.

There has been considerable media attention in recent years about a connection between MMR vaccine and autism. In fact, extensive research shows that there is no connection. There has been confusion because autism is often diagnosed at about the age at which children receive the MMR vaccine. This has led to the erroneous conclusion that the vaccine somehow causes autism. But, in fact, studies are now showing that autism actually begins before a baby is born.

The MMR vaccine should not be given to children who are severely allergic to eggs. Also, if your baby is taking any medication that interferes with the immune system, or if her immune system is weakened for any reason, she generally should not receive this immunization. As for side effects, sometimes, around seven to twelve days after the MMR vaccine, a child may develop mild swelling of the glands in the cheeks or neck, and a fever or mild rash. If this mild vaccine side effect does occur, it is important to note that it is not dangerous or contagious and will resolve on its own. Such findings occur less often after the second dose. Severe problems such as seizures caused by fever occur in 1 out of 3,000 doses. Serious allergic reactions are very rare (about 1 out of 1,000,000 doses).

As with other vaccines, receiving the MMR vaccine is much safer for the overwhelming majority of children than getting the mumps, measles, or rubella disease.

Chickenpox (Varicella) The vaccine to protect against the varicella virus became available in 1995, and protects against not only chickenpox but also shingles in later life. Natural chickenpox infection can cause a fever and a very itchy, blisterlike rash all over the body. There may be as many as 250 to 500 of these blisters. Sometimes, the infection causes serious complications, including skin infections, brain swelling, and pneumonia.

Getting the chickenpox vaccine is much safer than getting chickenpox disease. Soreness or swelling at the site where the shot was given happens in about 1 out of 5 children, and fever occurs in about 1 out of 10. Seizures caused by fever develop in less than 1 individual in 1,000. If your baby has a weakened immune system, or is taking steroids or other drugs that can affect the immune system, check with your doctor before she gets the chickenpox immunization.

Research is being done to see how long the vaccine protects and if a person will need another booster shot in the future. Currently if someone who has been vaccinated does get chickenpox, it is usually very mild. They will have fewer blisters, are less likely to have a fever or serious complications, and will recover faster.

Influenza Influenza (or "the flu") is a respiratory illness caused by a virus. This infection leads to symptoms such as a high fever, muscle aches, sore throat, and cough, and it may take your baby several days of rest to recover. There are two types of influenza vaccine to protect your child:

- The inactivated (killed) vaccine or the "flu shot," given by injection
- The live attenuated (weakened) vaccine, sprayed into the nostrils

Children six months of age and older can receive the inactivated influenza vaccine, while the live attenuated vaccine is approved for healthy children two years of age and older. The influenza immunization is recommended for all children six months of age and older. If your child has asthma, heart disease, diabetes, cystic fibrosis, or any other medical condition that increases their risk of serious complication from influenza, it is especially important for her to receive the influenza vaccine. No matter what your child's age, the influenza vaccine must be given annually since a new formulation is manufactured each year. If your child is under age nine and this is the first year she is receiving the influenza vaccine, she must get two doses one month apart. It is very rare to experience serious problems from the influenza vaccine.

Polio The polio vaccine provides protection from the virus that causes polio. While some infections with the polio virus cause no symptoms, it can cause paralysis and death in other cases. Before the polio vaccine was available, millions of children throughout the world were left paralyzed from polio.

Today, all children need four doses of the polio vaccine before they start school, starting with shots at two months and four months of age. The inactivated polio vaccine is given as shots, and there is no risk of the vaccine causing the disease. An oral form of the vaccine is no longer available in the U.S.

Hib (*Haemophilus influenza* Type b) The Hib vaccine protects your baby from the bacteria that (before the vaccine became available) was the leading cause of meningitis. This serious disease occurs most often in children from ages six months to five years, leading to symptoms such as fever, seizures, vomiting, and a stiff neck. Meningitis also can cause hearing loss, brain damage, and death. These same bacteria can also lead to a rare but serious inflammation of the throat called epiglottitis.

The first Hib vaccine should be given at two months of age, with additional doses to follow. It is important to have your baby immunized with this vaccine in order to lower her risk of getting Hib diseases during the early years of life when she is most vulnerable to these infections. There are no reasons to withhold this vaccine from your infant unless she has had a rare life-threatening allergic reaction to a previous dose of the vaccine.

Hepatitis B The hepatitis B vaccine offers protection against a liver disease that can be spread by infected blood and body fluids. The infection is caused by the hepatitis B virus, and can lead to cirrhosis and liver cancer. The infection can be passed from an infected mother to her baby at the time of birth, or from one household member to another.

The first hepatitis B shot should be given shortly after birth, even before your baby is discharged from the hospital. The hepatitis B vaccine is very safe. Severe problems are rare. Possible mild problems include soreness where the shot was given, and in one out of fifteen people, a temperature of 99.9 degrees Fahrenheit or higher.

Hepatitis A Like the hepatitis B vaccine, the hepatitis A immunization protects against a common liver disease, which your child can catch by eating food or drinking water contaminated with the hepatitis A virus. This common infection can sometimes be spread in child care settings when caregivers do not follow good hand-washing procedures.

The hepatitis A vaccine is very safe. Reactions to this vaccine are very uncommon and usually nothing more than soreness where the shot was given.

Pneumococcal Vaccine The pneumococcal conjugate vaccine protects your baby from meningitis, as well as common forms of pneumonia, blood infections, and certain ear infections. A pneumococcal infection is one of the most common causes of vaccine-preventable deaths in children. Only mild reactions are associated with the vaccine. Some children become fussy or drowsy, lose their appetite, or develop a fever.

Rotavirus The rotavirus vaccine protects against a potentially serious stomach virus, which can cause vomiting, diarrhea, and related symptoms in children. The rotavirus is the most common cause of severe diarrhea in children under the age of two years. In the U.S. about 50,000 children less than five years of age are hospitalized each year because of rotavirus infection.

Some children may experience mild, temporary diarrhea or, rarely, vomiting within seven days of getting a dose of the rotavirus vaccine. There are no severe reactions associated with this vaccine. As with some other vaccines mentioned earlier, talk with your doctor before getting the rotavirus vaccine if your child's immune system might be weakened by conditions like HIV or steroid use.

28

Musculoskeletal Problems

Arthritis

Arthritis is an inflammation of the joints that produces swelling, redness, heat, and pain. Although it is typically thought of as a disease of the elderly, some children also have this condition. Though still very uncommon, bacterial infection of the joint is a familiar form of arthritis among infants.

Bacterial Infection of the Joint When a joint becomes infected with bacteria, it causes pain. This pain makes the child refuse to bear weight on that limb or decrease movement if in an upper extremity. Since this is a bacterial infection, the baby also will typically have a fever. Notify your pediatrician immediately if these signs or symptoms appear. If an infection involves the hip, it can be a serious condition and needs to be properly diagnosed and treated by a specialist (usually an orthopedist). Treatment can include a needle aspiration of the hip joint, surgical drainage, and intravenous (IV) use of antibiotics.

Bowlegs and Knock-Knees

Babies' legs often have a bowed appearance. In fact, many children have bowing of the legs until they are about two years old, then they'll look knock-kneed until they are about six years of age. At times, children may not have straight lower legs until they are nine or ten years old.

Bowlegs and knock-knees usually are variations of normal, and require no treatment. Typically, a child's legs will straighten naturally by the teen years. Bracing, corrective shoes, and exercise are rarely helpful, and may hinder a child's physical development and cause

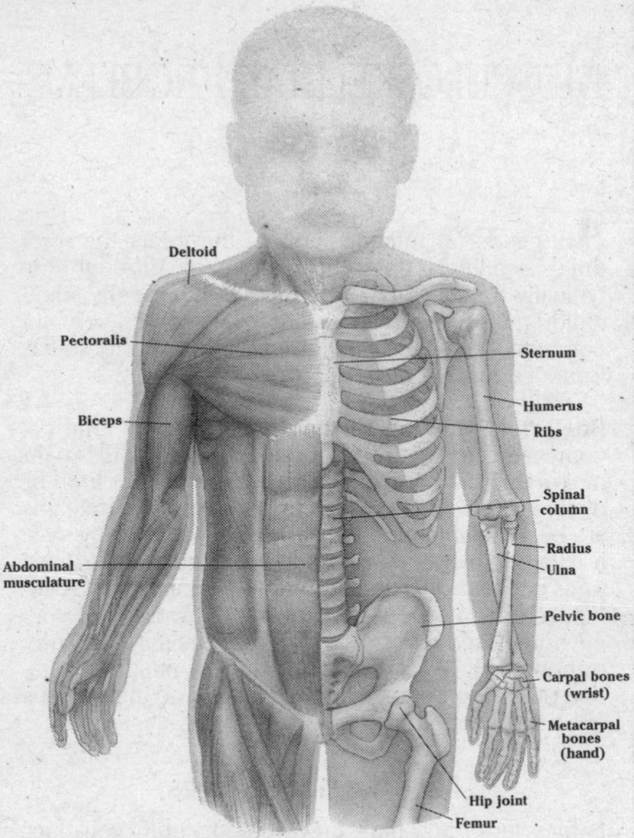

Musculoskeletal System

unnecessary emotional stress. Rarely, bowlegs or knock-knees are the result of a disease. Arthritis, injury to the growth plate around the knee, infection, tumor, Blount's disease (a growth disorder of the shinbone), and rickets all can cause changes in the curvature of the legs.

Here are some signs that suggest a child's bowlegs or knock-knees may be caused by a serious problem:

- The curvature is extreme.
- Only one side is affected.
- Your baby also is unusually short for his age.

If your baby fits any of these descriptions, talk to your pediatrician. In some cases, treatment, including referral to a pediatric orthopedist, may be needed.

Elbow Injuries

A pulled elbow (also known as nursemaid's elbow) is a common, painful injury generally among children under four years old. It occurs when the elbow becomes dislocated or slips out of its joint. This happens because the child's elbow joint is loose enough to separate slightly when her arm is pulled to full length (while being lifted, yanked, or swung by the hand or wrist, or if she falls on her outstretched arm). The nearby tissue slides into the space created by the stretching and becomes trapped after the joint returns to its normal position.

A nursemaid's elbow injury usually doesn't cause swelling, but the child will complain that the elbow hurts, or cry when her arm is moved. A child will typically hold her arm close to the side, with the elbow slightly bent and the palm turned toward the body. If someone tries to straighten the elbow or turn the palm upward, the child will resist because of the pain.

Treating Nursemaid's Elbow

This injury should be treated by a pediatrician or other trained healthcare provider. Since elbow pain can also be due to a fracture, your pediatrician may need to consider this before the elbow is "reduced" or put back into place.

Your doctor will check the injured area for swelling and tenderness and any limitation of motion. If an injury other than nursemaid's elbow is suspected, X-rays may be taken. If no fracture is noted, the doctor will move and twist and flex the arm gently to release the trapped tissue and allow the elbow to return to its normal position. Once he has moved the elbow back in place, the child will generally feel immediate relief and within a few minutes should be using her arm normally without any discomfort. Occasionally, the doctor may recommend a sling for comfort for two or three days, particularly if several hours have passed before the injury is treated successfully. If the injury occurred several days earlier, a hard splint or cast may be used to protect the joint for one to two weeks.

Prevention

Nursemaid's elbow can be prevented by not pulling or lifting your baby by the hands or wrists, or swinging her by the arms. Instead, lift your child by grasping her body under the arms.

FLAT FEET/FALLEN ARCHES

Babies are often born with flat feet, which may persist well into their childhood. This occurs because children's bones and joints are flexible, causing their feet to flatten when they stand. Young babies also have a fat pad on the inner border of their feet that hides the arch. You still can see the arch if you lift your baby up on the tips of the toes, but it disappears when he's standing normally. The foot may also turn out, increasing the weight on the inner side and making it appear even more flat.

Normally, flat feet disappear by age six as the feet become less flexible and the arches develop. Only about 1 or 2 out of every 10 children will continue to have flat feet into adulthood. For children who do not develop an arch, treatment is not recommended unless the foot is stiff or painful. Shoe inserts won't help your child develop an arch, and may cause more problems than the flat feet themselves.

However, certain forms of flat feet may need to be treated differently. For instance, a baby may have tightness of the heel cord (Achilles tendon) that limits the motion of his foot. This tightness can result in a flat foot, but it usually can be treated with special stretching exercises to lengthen the heel cord. Rarely, a baby will have truly rigid flat feet, a condition that can cause problems. These children have difficulty moving the foot up and down or side to side at the ankle. The rigid foot can cause pain and, if left untreated, can lead to

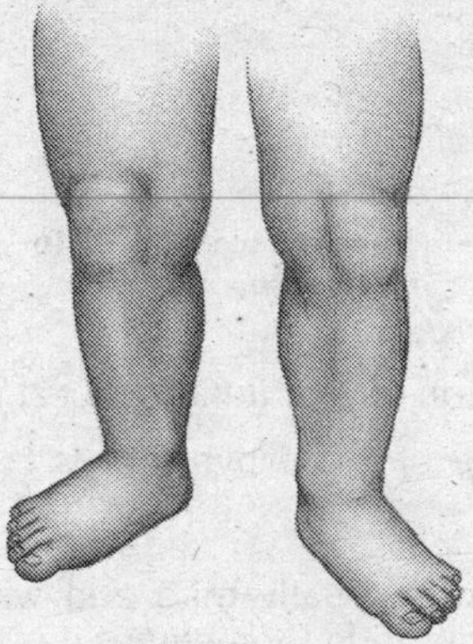

arthritis. This rigid type of flat foot is seldom seen in an infant or very young child. (More often, rigid flat feet develop during the teen years and should be evaluated by your child's pediatrician.)

Symptoms that should be checked by a pediatrician include foot pain, sores or pressure areas on the inner side of the foot, a stiff foot, limited side-to-side foot motion, or limited up-and-down ankle motion. For further treatment you should see a pediatric orthopedic surgeon or podiatrist experienced in childhood foot conditions.

PIGEON TOES (INTOEING)

Babies whose feet turn in are described as being "pigeon-toed" or having "intoeing." This is a very common condition that may involve one or both feet, and it occurs for a variety of reasons.

Intoeing During Infancy Infants are sometimes born with their feet turning in. This turning occurs from the front part of their foot, and is called metatarsus adductus (see figure below). It most commonly is due to being positioned in a crowded space inside the uterus before the baby is born.

You can suspect that metatarsus adductus may be present if:

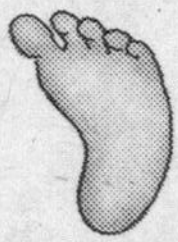

Appearance of foot in metatarsus adductus

- The front portion of your infant's foot at rest turns inward.
- The outer side of the baby's foot is curved like a half-moon.

This condition is usually mild and will resolve before your infant's first birthday. Sometimes it is more severe, or is accompanied by other foot deformities that result in a problem called clubfoot. This condition requires a consultation with a pediatric orthopedist and treatment with early casting or splinting.

Intoeing in Later Childhood When a child is intoeing during her second year, this is most likely due to inward twisting of the shinbone (tibia). This condition is called internal tibial torsion (see figure on page 695). This condition tends to run in families.

Treatment

Some experts feel no treatment is necessary for intoeing in an infant under six months of age. For severe metatarsus adductus in infancy, early casting may be useful.

Studies show that most infants who have metatarsus adductus in early infancy will outgrow it with no treatment necessary. If your baby's intoeing persists after six months, or if it is rigid and difficult to straighten out, your doctor may refer you to a pediatric orthopedist who may recommend a series of casts applied over a period of three to six weeks. The main goal is to correct the condition before your child starts walking.

Intoeing in early childhood often corrects itself over time, and usually requires no treatment. But if your child has trouble walking, discuss the condition with your pediatrician

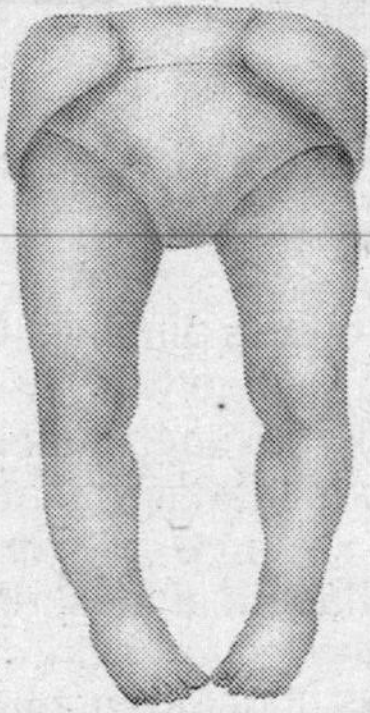

Internal tibial torsion

who may refer you to an orthopedist. A night brace (special shoes with connecting bars) was used in the past for this problem, but it hasn't proven to be an effective treatment. Because intoeing often corrects itself over time, it is very important to avoid nonprescribed "treatments" such as corrective shoes, twister cables, daytime bracing, exercises, shoe inserts, or back manipulations. These do not correct the problem and may be harmful because they interfere with normal play or walking.

Nevertheless, if a child's intoeing remains by the age of nine or ten years old, surgery may be required to correct it.

29

SKIN

Skin problems in babies often get the attention—and sometimes raise the anxiety levels—of parents. After all, these skin conditions are immediately visible, and while the overwhelming majority are not serious, they can still become a source of worry. In this chapter, you'll find an alphabetical description of common skin problems. Other related skin conditions (specifically eczema, hives, and insect bites and stings) are discussed in Chapter 13, *Allergies*.

BIRTHMARKS AND HEMANGIOMAS

Dark-Pigmented Birthmarks (Nevi or Moles)

Nevi, or moles, are either congenital (present at birth) or acquired. Composed of so-called nevus cells, these spots are often dark brown or black.

Congenital Nevi Small nevi (less than three inches in diameter) appear at birth and are relatively common, occurring in about 1 out of every 100 newborns. They tend to grow with the baby and usually don't cause any problems. Rarely, however, these moles may develop into a type of serious skin cancer (melanoma) at some later time. Therefore, while you don't have to worry about them right away, it's a good idea to watch them carefully and have them checked by your pediatrician at regular intervals or if there is any change in appearance (color, size, or shape). She may refer you to a pediatric dermatologist who will advise you on removal and any follow-up care.

A much more serious type of nevus is a large congenital one that varies in size from 3 inches to as large as this book. It might be flat or raised, may have hair growing from it (although small, insignificant nevi sometimes also have hair), and can be so large that it covers an arm or a leg. Fortunately, these nevi are very rare (occurring in 1 out of every 20,000 births). However, they are much more likely than the smaller ones to develop into a melanoma, so early consultation with a pediatric dermatologist is advisable.

Acquired Nevi, or Moles Most Caucasian people develop ten to thirty pigmented nevi, or moles, throughout the course of their lives. They usually occur after the age of five, but sometimes develop earlier. These acquired moles are seldom a cause for worry. However, if your child develops one that's irregularly shaped (asymmetrical), has multiple colors within its structure, and is larger than a pencil eraser, ask your pediatrician to examine it.

One final note: Probably the most common acquired dark spots on the skin are freckles. They can appear as early as ages two to four years, are found more often on parts of the body exposed to the sun, and tend to run in families. They often become darker or larger during the summer and are less prominent in the winter. They represent no danger and should not cause concern when they occur in children.

Blood Vessel Birthmarks on the Skin (Hemangiomas of Infancy)

Your young infant has a red raised bump growing rapidly on his forehead and a flat dark-red patch on one arm. They're unsightly, but are they harmful?

These birthmarks occur when a certain area of the skin develops an abnormal blood supply before birth. This, in turn, causes the tissue to enlarge over the course of several weeks or months and become reddish blue. When the condition involves only the capillaries (the smallest blood vessels), the birthmark is called a "hemangioma of infancy" (or, more simply, "hemangioma"). When the blood vessels are larger, they may be of a different type and have a different appearance.

Flat Angiomata (Stork Bites) These most common blemishes on the skin appear most often on the eyelids or back of the neck. They usually disappear over the first months to years of life and are not serious.

Hemangiomas of Infancy Hemangiomas of infancy (which used to be called strawberry patches) are found in at least 2 of every 100 babies born. Although frequently they are not noticeable at birth, they appear within the first or second month of life as a red patch or raised dot. They can occur on any area of the body, but are seen most commonly on the head, neck, and trunk. Usually a child has just a single hemangioma, but occasionally these marks will be scattered over several parts of the body.

If your infant develops a hemangioma, have your pediatrician examine it so he can follow its course from the start. During the first six months of life, hemangiomas usually grow very rapidly, which can be quite alarming. But they soon stop enlarging and often flatten or even disappear by the time the child is nine years old.

Quite often, the large reddish-purplish appearance of these birthmarks so upsets parents that they want to have them removed immediately. However, since the vast majority will gradually reduce in size over the second to third year of life, it's generally best to leave them alone. Studies have shown that when this type of hemangioma is left untreated, few complications or cosmetic problems result.

At times, hemangiomas may need to be treated or removed—namely, when they occur close to vital structures, such as the eye, throat, or mouth; when they seem to be growing much faster than usual; or when they are likely to bleed profusely or become infected. Such conditions are uncommon, but require careful evaluation and management by your pediatrician and pediatric dermatologist. In some cases, hemangiomas on the face are removed in infancy because of the social stigma from having this facial birthmark and because of only minor scarring that occurs in this age group; this is a decision that can be made with your pediatrician and pediatric dermatologist, as well as with the plastic surgeon who would perform the procedure.

Very rarely, hemangiomas are found in large numbers on the face and upper trunk. On such occasions, hemangiomas also may be located on organs inside the body. If this is suspected, your pediatrician may need to conduct further tests.

Port Wine Stains Port wine stains are flat malformations of small blood vessels, usually present at birth. They are dark red and often found on the face or limbs (usually only on one side of the body), although they may occur anywhere. Unlike hemangiomas, port wine stains don't go away, although they sometimes fade. Even so, they rarely cause any problems. On occasion, however, if they are found on the upper eyelid and/or forehead, there is a chance of a related problem in the underlying brain structures (a disorder called Sturge-Weber syndrome). If the birthmark is located immediately around the eye, there is a possibility that glaucoma may develop in that eye.

Port wine stains should be examined from time to time to evaluate their size, location, and appearance. If your child is very unhappy with this birthmark, a special covering makeup can be used. Laser treatment has been successful in many cases, but other types of surgery are rarely recommended. (See also *How Your Newborn Looks,* page 152.)

CHICKENPOX

Chickenpox was once one of the most common childhood illnesses. But thanks to the varicella vaccine, far fewer children now get this disease. Chickenpox is a highly contagious infection causing an itchy, blisterlike rash that can cover most of the body. Children often get a mild fever along with the rash.

After your baby has been exposed to the virus that causes chickenpox, the rash usually begins twelve to fourteen days later. Small blisters, which may have a red area around them, will begin to appear on the body and scalp, then spread to the face, arms, and legs. There may be as many as 250 to 500 of these blisters. Normally the blisters will crust over and then heal, but tiny sores and possibly small scars may develop if your baby scratches them and they become infected. The skin around some of the blisters may become darker or lighter, but this change in coloring will disappear gradually after the rash is gone.

Treatment

From your own childhood, you may remember just how itchy chickenpox can be. You should try to discourage your baby from scratching, because that can cause additional infection. Acetaminophen (in the appropriate dose for your child's age and weight) may decrease the discomfort from the rash or fever. Trimming her fingernails and bathing her daily with soap and water also can help prevent secondary bacterial infection. Oatmeal baths, available without prescription from your pharmacy, will ease the itch. Antihistamines can be used to decrease the itch. (Be sure to follow the dosing instructions carefully.) A prescription medicine (acyclovir) also can decrease the severity of the symptoms if started within twenty-four hours of the onset of the disease. This medicine, while not needed by everyone, is especially valuable for babies with weakened immune systems or eczema (a skin disorder).

Do not give your baby aspirin or any medication that contains aspirin or salicylates when she has chickenpox. These products increase the risk of Reye syndrome, a serious illness that involves the liver and brain. You also should avoid steroids and any medicines that interfere with the immune system. If you are not sure about what medications you can safely use at this time, ask your pediatrician for advice.

Incidentally, the doctor probably won't need to see your child unless she develops a complication such as a skin infection, trouble breathing, or if her temperature rises above 102 degrees Fahrenheit (38.9 degrees Celsius) or lasts longer than four days. Let the pediatrician know if areas of the rash become very red, warm, or tender; this may indicate a bacterial infection. Be sure to call your pediatrician *immediately* if your child develops any signs of Reye syndrome or encephalitis: vomiting, nervousness, confusion, convulsions, lack of responsiveness, increasing sleepiness, or poor balance.

Your baby may be contagious one to two days before the rash starts and for twenty-four hours after the last new blister appears (usually five to seven days). In some cases, the contagious period lasts until all the blisters are dry and crusted over. Only individuals who have never had chickenpox (or the chickenpox vaccine) are susceptible. After she's recovered from the chickenpox, your child usually will be immune to it for the rest of her life.

Prevention

A vaccine to protect against chickenpox is recommended for all healthy children between twelve and fifteen months of age who have never had the disease, plus a booster dose given between four and six years of age. Until your baby has received this vaccine, the only sure way to protect her is to avoid exposure to the chickenpox virus. Protection from exposure is important for newborn infants, especially premature babies, in whom the disease can be more severe (but rarely fatal).

Most infants whose mothers have had chickenpox are immune to the disease for the first few months of life since mothers pass short-lived protective antibodies to their infants. Susceptible children who have diseases affecting the immune system (i.e., cancer) or who are using certain drugs (i.e., cortisone) also must avoid being exposed to chickenpox. If these children or normal adults are exposed, they may be given a special medication to provide immunity to the disease for a limited period. It's important to remember that since the varicella vaccine is a live virus vaccine, babies who have a weakened immune system may not have a normal response to it and generally should not be vaccinated.

Cradle Cap and Seborrheic Dermatitis

Your beautiful one-month-old baby has developed scaliness and redness on his scalp. You're concerned and think maybe you shouldn't shampoo as usual. You also notice some redness in the creases of his neck and armpits and behind his ears. What is it and what should you do?

When this rash occurs on the scalp alone, it's known as cradle cap. But although it may start as scaling and redness of the scalp, it also can be found later in the other areas just mentioned. It can extend to the face and diaper area, too, and when it does, pediatricians call it seborrheic dermatitis (because it occurs where there are the greatest number of oil-producing sebaceous glands). Seborrheic dermatitis is a noninfectious skin condition that's very common in infants, usually beginning in the first weeks of life and slowly disappearing over a period of weeks or months. Unlike eczema or contact dermatitis (see pages 470–473), it's rarely uncomfortable or itchy.

No one knows for sure the exact cause of this rash. Some doctors have speculated that it may be influenced by the mother's hormonal changes during pregnancy, which stimulate the infant's oil glands. This overproduction of oil may have some relationship to the scales and redness of the skin.

Treatment

If your baby's seborrheic dermatitis is confined to his scalp (and is, therefore, just cradle cap), you can treat it yourself. Don't be afraid to shampoo the hair; in fact, you should wash it (with a mild baby shampoo) more frequently than before. This, along with soft brushing, will help remove the scales. Stronger medicated shampoos (antiseborrhea shampoos containing sulfur and 2 percent salicylic acid) may loosen the scales more quickly, but since they also can be irritating, use them only after consulting your pediatrician.

Some parents have found using petroleum jelly or ointments beneficial. But baby oil is not very helpful or necessary. In fact, while many parents tend to use unperfumed baby oil or mineral oil and do nothing else, doing so allows scales to build up on the scalp, particularly over the soft spot on the back of the head, or fontanelle. Instead, your doctor also might prescribe a cortisone cream or lotion, such as 1 percent hydrocortisone cream. Once the condition has improved, you can prevent it from recurring, in most cases, by continuing with frequent hair washing with a mild baby shampoo.

Sometimes yeast infections occur on the affected skin, most likely in the crease areas rather than on the scalp. If this occurs, the area will become extremely reddened and quite itchy. In this case, your pediatrician might prescribe a medication such as an antiyeast cream.

Rest assured that seborrheic dermatitis is not a serious condition, or an infection. Nor is it an allergy to something you're using, or due to poor hygiene. It will go away without any scars.

Hair Loss (Alopecia)

Almost all newborns lose some or all of their hair. This is normal and to be expected. The baby hair falls out before the mature hair comes in. So hair loss occurring in the first six months of life is not a cause for concern.

Very commonly, a baby loses her hair where she rubs her

scalp against the mattress or as a result of a head-banging habit. As she starts to move more and sit up or outgrow this head-rubbing or -banging behavior, this type of hair loss will correct itself. Many babies also lose hair on the back of the scalp at age four months as their hair grows at varying times and rates.

In very rare cases, babies may be born with alopecia (hair loss), which can occur by itself or in association with certain abnormalities of the nails and the teeth. Later in childhood, hair loss may be due to medications, a scalp injury, or a medical or nutritional problem.

Because alopecia and other types of hair loss can be a sign of other medical or nutritional problems, bring these conditions to your pediatrician's attention whenever they occur after the first six months of age. The doctor will look at your child's scalp, determine the cause, and prescribe treatment. Sometimes, a referral to a pediatric dermatologist is necessary.

MEASLES

Thanks to vaccinations, cases of measles are uncommon in America today. During the first six months of 2008, the national Centers for Disease Control and Prevention reported 131 measles cases. Most cases that occur now are imported from other countries and occur in children who have never been vaccinated or are too young to receive the vaccine. If your child has never been immunized or had the measles, he can get them if he is exposed. The measles virus is passed through the air droplets transmitted by an infected person. Anyone who breathes the droplets and is not immune to the disease can become infected.

Signs and Symptoms

For the first eight to twelve days after being exposed to the measles virus, your child probably will have no symptoms; this is called the incubation period. Then he may develop an illness that seems like a common cold, with a cough, runny nose, and pinkeye (conjunctivitis; see page 255). The cough may be severe at times and will last for about a week, and your child probably will feel miserable.

During the first one to three days of the illness, the cold-like symptoms will become worse, and he'll develop a fever that may run as high as 103 to 105 degrees Fahrenheit (39.4–40.5 degrees Celsius). The fever will last until two to three days after the rash first appears.

After two to four days of illness, the rash will develop. It usually begins on the face and neck, and spreads down the trunk and out to the arms and legs. It starts as very fine red bumps, which may join together to form larger splotches. If you notice tiny white spots, like grains of sand, inside his mouth next to his molars, you'll know the rash will follow soon. The rash will last five to eight days. As it fades, the skin may peel a little.

Treatment

Although there is no treatment for the disease, it is important that the pediatrician examine your child to determine that measles is, in fact, the cause of the illness. Many other conditions can start in the same way, and measles has its own complications (see below) that the doctor will want to watch for. When you call, describe the fever and rash, so that the doctor knows that you suspect measles. When you visit the office, the pediatrician will want to separate your child from other patients, so that the virus is not transmitted to them.

Your child is contagious from several days before the rash breaks out until the fever and rash are gone. During this period he should be kept at home (except for the visit to the doctor) and away from anyone who is not immune to the illness.

At home, make sure your child drinks plenty of fluids and give acetaminophen in the proper dose if your child is uncomfortable due to the fever. The conjunctivitis that accompanies measles can make it painful for the child to be in bright light or sunshine, so you may want to darken his room to a comfortable level for the first few days.

Sometimes bacterial infections develop as a complication of the measles. These most often include pneumonia (see page 505), middle ear infection (see page 557), or encephalitis (inflammation of the brain). In these cases, your child must be seen by the pediatrician, who may prescribe antibiotic treatment or admit your child to the hospital.

Prevention

Almost all children who receive two doses of the MMR (measles, mumps, rubella) vaccine after their first birthday are protected against measles for life. Because up to 5 percent of children may not respond to the initial vaccination, a second (booster) dose is recommended later in childhood. Your pediatrician will tell you what is best for your child. (See Chapter 27, *Immunizations.*)

If your unimmunized child has been exposed to someone who has the measles, or if someone in your household has the virus, notify your pediatrician at once. The following steps can help keep your child from getting sick.

1. If he is under one year old or has a weakened immune system, he can be given immune globulin (gamma globulin) up to six days following exposure. This may temporarily protect him from becoming infected, but will not provide extended immunity.
2. An infant six to eleven months of age may receive the measles vaccine alone if he is exposed to the disease or if he is living in a community where exposure is highly likely or in an epidemic situation. If doses are given during these months, your child still may need additional doses to be fully immunized.

MRSA Infections

MRSA (methicillin-resistant *Staphylococcus aureus*) is the name of a "staph" bacterium that can cause infections not only on the surface of the skin, but also into the soft tissue where a boil or abscess can form. In recent years, MRSA has become a major public-health problem because this bacterium has become resistant to antibiotics called beta-lactams, which include methicillin and other commonly prescribed antibiotics (such as penicillin and amoxicillin). This resistance has made treating these infections more difficult. While MRSA was once limited to hospitals and nursing homes, it has spread into the community in schools, households, and child care centers, among other places. It can be transmitted from person to person through skin-to-skin contact, particularly through cuts and abrasions.

If your baby has a wound that appears to be infected—specifically, if it is red, swollen, hot, and draining pus—have it checked by your pediatrician. He may drain the infection and prescribe antibiotics. The most serious MRSA infections may cause pneumonia and bloodstream infections. Even though MRSA infections are resistant to some antibiotics, they are treatable with other medications.

To prevent your baby from getting MRSA at a child care facility or other public places, the following strategies can be helpful:

- **Follow good hygiene** practices. Your baby should have his hands washed frequently with soap and warm water, or use alcohol-based hand sanitizers.
- **Use a clean** dry bandage to cover any cuts, scrapes, or breaks in your baby's skin. These bandages should be changed at least daily.
- **Don't let your** baby share towels, washcloths, or other personal items (including clothing) with anyone else.
- **Frequently clean surfaces** that your baby touches.

Roseola Infantum

Your ten-month-old doesn't look or act very ill, but she suddenly develops a fever between 102 degrees Fahrenheit (38.9 degrees Celsius) and 105 degrees Fahrenheit (40.5 degrees Celsius). The fever lasts for three to seven days, during which time your child may have less appetite, mild diarrhea, a slight cough, and a runny nose, and seems mildly irritable and a little sleepier than usual. Her upper eyelids may appear slightly swollen or droopy. Finally, *after her temperature returns to normal,* she gets a slightly raised, spotty pink rash on her trunk, which spreads only to her upper arms and neck and fades after just twenty-four hours. What's the diagnosis? Most likely it's a disease called roseola—a contagious viral illness that's most common in children under age two. Its incubation period is seven to fourteen days. The key to this diagnosis is that the rash appears *after* the fever is gone. We now know that a specific virus causes this condition.

Treatment

Whenever your infant or young child has a fever of 102 degrees Fahrenheit (38.9 degrees Celsius) or higher for twenty-four hours, call your pediatrician, even if there are no other symptoms. If the doctor suspects the fever is caused by roseola, he may suggest ways to control the temperature and advise you to call again if your child becomes worse or the fever lasts for more than three or four days. For a child who has other symptoms or appears more seriously ill, the doctor may order a blood count, urinalysis, or other tests.

Since illnesses that cause fever can be contagious, it's wise to keep your child away from other children, at least until you've conferred with your pediatrician. Once she is diagnosed as having roseola, don't let her play with other children until her fever subsides. Once her fever is gone for twenty-four hours, even if the rash has appeared, your child can return to child care or preschool, and resume normal contact with other children.

While your child has a fever, dress her in lightweight clothing. If she is very uncomfortable because of the fever, you can give her acetaminophen in the appropriate dose for her age and weight. (See Chapter 23, *Fever.*) Don't worry if her appetite is decreased, and encourage her to drink extra fluids.

Although this disease rarely is serious, be aware that early in the illness, when fever climbs very quickly, there's a chance of convulsions (see *Seizures, Convulsions, and Epilepsy,* page 666). There may be a seizure regardless of how well you treat the fever, so it's important to know how to manage convulsions even though they're usually quite mild and occur only briefly, if at all, with roseola.

Rubella (German Measles)

Although some of today's parents had rubella, or German measles, during their childhood, it is a rare illness now, thanks to an effective vaccine. Even when it was prevalent, however, rubella was usually a mild disease.

Rubella is characterized by a mild fever (100–102 degrees Fahrenheit [37.8–38.9 degrees Celsius]), swollen glands (typically on the back of the neck and base of the skull), and a rash. The rash, which varies from pinhead size to an irregular redness, is raised and usually begins on the face. Within two to three days it spreads to the neck, chest, and the rest of the body as it fades from the face.

Once exposed to rubella, a baby usually will develop the disease in fourteen to twenty-one days. The contagious period for rubella begins several days before the rash appears and continues for five to seven days after it develops. Because the disease can be so mild, it goes unrecognized in about half the children who contract it.

Before the rubella vaccine was developed, this illness tended to occur in epidemics every six to nine years. Since the vaccine was introduced in 1968, there have been no significant epidemics in the United States. Even so, the disease still occurs. Fortunately, except for causing fever, discomfort, and occasional pain in the joints, these small epidemics are of little consequence.

The situation is quite different when rubella infects an unvaccinated, susceptible woman in the first three months of her pregnancy. In this case it can cause severe, irreversible damage to the unborn fetus. Babies born with this form of rubella (congenital rubella) may have eye disorders (cataracts, glaucoma, small eyes), heart problems, deafness, severe mental retardation, and other evidence of central nervous system damage.

What You Can Do

If your pediatrician diagnoses rubella in your baby, you may be able to make him more comfortable by giving him extra fluids, bed rest (if he's fatigued), and acetaminophen if he has a fever. Keep him away from other children or adults unless you are sure that they're immunized. As a general rule, children with rubella should not be in child care or any other group setting for seven days after the rash first appears. In particular, make a special effort not to expose pregnant women to a child with rubella.

If your baby is diagnosed as having the congenital form of rubella, your pediatrician can advise you on the best way to manage his complex and difficult problems. Infants born with congenital rubella are often infectious for a year after birth and therefore should be kept out of any group child care setting, where they could expose other susceptible children or adults to the infection.

When to Call the Pediatrician

If your baby has a fever and a rash and appears uncomfortable, discuss the problem with your pediatrician. If rubella is diagnosed, follow the guidelines suggested earlier for treatment and isolation.

Prevention

Being immunized is the best way to prevent German measles. The vaccine usually is administered as part of a three-in-one shot called MMR (measles, mumps, rubella), given when the baby is twelve to fifteen months old. A booster dose needs to be given. (See Chapter 27, *Immunizations.*)

There are relatively few adverse reactions to the rubella vaccine. Occasionally babies will get a rash and a slight fever. *An infant can be immunized even if his mother is pregnant at the time.* However, a susceptible pregnant woman should not be immunized herself. She also should be extremely careful to avoid contact with any child or adult who may be infected with the virus. After delivery, she should be immunized immediately.

SUNBURN

While those with darker skin coloring tend to be less sensitive to the sun, everyone is at risk for sunburn and its associated disorders. Babies especially need to be protected from the sun's burning rays, since most sun damage occurs in childhood. Like other burns, sunburn will leave the skin red, warm, and painful. In severe cases it may cause blistering, fever, chills, headache, and a general feeling of illness.

Your baby doesn't actually have to be burned, however, in order to be harmed by the sun. The effects of exposure build over the years, so that even moderate exposure during childhood can contribute to wrinkling, toughening, freckling, and even cancer of the skin in later life. Also, some medications can cause a skin reaction to sunlight, and some medical conditions may make people more sensitive to the sun.

Treatment

The signs of sunburn usually appear six to twelve hours after exposure, with the greatest discomfort during the first twenty-four hours. If your baby's burn is just red, warm, and painful, you can treat it yourself. Apply cool compresses to the burned areas or bathe the infant in cool water. You also can give acetaminophen to help relieve the pain. (Check the package for appropriate dosage for her age and weight.)

If the sunburn causes blisters, fever, chills, headache, or a general feeling of illness, call your pediatrician. Severe sunburn must be treated like any other serious burn, and if it's very extensive, hospitalization sometimes is required. In addition, the blisters can become infected, requiring treatment with antibiotics. Sometimes extensive or severe sunburn also can lead to dehydration (see *Diarrhea,* page 440, for signs of dehydration) and, in some cases, fainting (heatstroke). Such cases need to be examined by your pediatrician or the nearest emergency facility.

Prevention

Many parents incorrectly assume that the sun is dangerous only when it's shining brightly. In fact, it's not the visible light rays but rather the invisible ultraviolet rays that are harmful. Your baby actually may be exposed to more ultraviolet rays on foggy or hazy days because she'll feel cooler and therefore stay outside for a longer time. Exposure is also greater at higher altitudes. Even a big hat or an umbrella is not absolute protection because ultraviolet rays reflect off sand, water, snow, and many other surfaces.

Try to keep your baby out of the sun when the peak ultraviolet rays occur (between 10 a.m. and 4 p.m.). In addition, follow these guidelines.

- **Always use a** sunscreen to block the damaging ultraviolet rays. Choose a sunscreen made for babies with a sun protection factor (SPF) of at least 15. (Check the label.) Apply the protection half an hour before going out. Keep in mind that *no* sunscreens are truly waterproof, and thus they need to be reapplied every one and a half to two hours, particularly if your child spends a lot of time in the water. Consult the instructions on the bottle.

- **Dress your infant** in lightweight cotton clothing with long sleeves and long pants.
- **Use a beach** umbrella or similar object to keep her in the shade as much as possible.
- **Have her wear** a hat with a wide brim.
- **Babies under six** months of age should be kept out of direct sunlight. If adequate clothing and shade are not available, sunscreen may be used on small areas of the body, such as the face and the backs of the hands.

(See also *Burns,* page 573.)

WARTS

Warts are caused by a virus—the human papillomavirus (HPV). These firm bumps (although they also can be flat) are yellow, tan, grayish, black, or brown. They usually appear on the hands, toes, around the knees, and on the face, but can occur anywhere on the body. When they're on the soles of the feet, doctors call them plantar warts. Although warts can be contagious, they appear infrequently in children under the age of two.

Treatment

Your pediatrician can give you advice on treating warts. Sometimes he will recommend an over-the-counter medication that contains salicylic acid or even treat them in the office using a liquid nitrogen–based solution or spray. If any of the following are present, he may refer you to a dermatologist.

- Multiple, recurring warts
- A wart on the face or genital area
- Large, deep, or painful plantar warts (warts on the soles of the feet)
- Warts that are particularly bothersome to your baby

Some warts will just go away by themselves. Others can be removed using prescription or nonprescription preparations. However, surgical removal by scraping, cauterizing, or freezing is sometimes necessary with multiple warts, those that continue to recur, or deep plantar warts. Although surgery usually has a good success rate, it can be painful and results in scarring. Laser treatment may help. The earlier the warts are treated, the better the chance of permanent cure, although there is always the possibility that they will recur even after treatment that is initially successful.

If a wart comes back, simply treat it again the way you did the first time, or as directed by your pediatrician. Don't wait until it becomes large, painful, or starts to spread.

West Nile Virus

The West Nile virus has received plenty of attention in recent years. It is spread to humans through the bite of an infected mosquito. The first outbreak occurred in the United States in 1999. Although some children have become ill when infected with the virus, in most cases the symptoms are mild.

Mosquitoes become carriers of the virus by feeding on infected birds. Although other animals have been infected with the virus—including horses, bats, squirrels, and domestic animals—birds are the most common reservoir. Once the virus has been transmitted to a human through a bite, it can multiply in an individual's bloodstream and in some cases cause illness. However, even if your baby is bitten, she'll probably have only mild symptoms or none at all. Among people who have been bitten and contracted the infection, about one in five develop mild flulike symptoms (i.e., a fever, headaches, and body aches) and at times a skin rash. These symptoms tend to last only a few days. In less than 1 out of 100 infections, a severe illness can occur (so-called West Nile encephalitis or meningitis), with symptoms such as a high fever, a stiff neck, tremors, muscle weakness, convulsions, paralysis, and loss of consciousness.

Prevention

Like all people, your own baby's risk of West Nile virus comes mostly from mosquito bites. She cannot catch the disease from an infected playmate or from touching or kissing a person with the infection (or even by touching a bird infected with the virus).

There is no vaccine to protect your baby from the West Nile virus. But you can reduce her likelihood of developing the disease by taking steps to reduce the chance that she will be bitten by a mosquito that could be carrying the virus. Here are some strategies to keep in mind. (Some of them are described in the *Insect Bites and Stings* section on page 481.)

- **Apply insect repellent** to your baby, using just enough to protect her exposed skin.
- **The concentrations of** DEET vary significantly from product to product—ranging from less than 10 percent to over 30 percent—so be sure to read the label before you buy. The higher the concentration of DEET, the longer the action and the greater the effectiveness of the product. Effectiveness peaks at 30 percent, which is also the maximum concentration recommended for children. Check the label for this percentage because some products can have concentrations much higher than 30 percent. DEET's safety does not appear to be related to its level of concentration, however; a prudent approach is to select the lowest effective concentration for the amount of time your child spends outdoors.
- **Avoid products that** include DEET in a sunscreen because the sunscreen needs to be applied frequently, while the DEET should be used just once a day. More frequent applications of DEET may be associated with toxicity. Also be sure to wash the DEET off with soap and water at the end of the day. Even older children should not apply DEET-containing repellents more than once a day.
- **Do not use** DEET preparations on infants under two months of age. In older children, apply it sparingly around the ears, and don't use it on the mouth or the eyes. Don't put it over cuts.
- **An alternative to** DEET, called Picaridin, has had wider use in Europe, but has recently been marketed for use in the United States. It is a pleasant-smelling product without

the oily residue of DEET. It is used in concentrations of 5 to 10 percent.

- **Whenever possible, dress** your baby in long sleeves and long pants while she's outside. Use mosquito netting over a baby's infant carrier.
- **Keep your baby** away from locations where mosquitoes are likely to congregate or lay their eggs, such as standing water (e.g., in birdbaths and pet water dishes).
- **Because mosquitoes are** more likely to bite humans at certain times of day—most commonly at dawn, dusk, and in the early evening—consider limiting the amount of time your baby is outdoors during those hours.
- **Repair any holes** in your screens.

30

YOUR BABY'S SLEEP

Sleep is an essential, healthy part of your baby's life. In the same way that good nutrition is important for the development of his body, sleep is crucial for the development of his brain. As your baby establishes and maintains a regular sleep schedule, he is more likely to sleep longer and less likely to awaken during the night, with all the health benefits of that kind of sound sleep.

No wonder many parents worry about the sleep habits and behaviors of their child. "Is he getting too little sleep? Or too much? How important are naps, and how many hours of napping are enough? Should I let him cry himself to sleep at night, or should I pick him up when he's in tears? Why does he seem to go to sleep later—or earlier—than other children of the same age?"

Even though many parents are anxious about their baby's sleep patterns, the good news is that many of their concerns can easily be addressed. Many moms and dads may be unclear about the optimal sleep schedule for a child at different ages. Even when they ask questions and get some clarification from their pediatrician, they still may be left frustrated with general advice that may be applicable to babies at large, but not necessarily to their own child. After all, infants aren't alike, and there are normal variations from one child to another; some babies may develop regular sleep rhythms in the first six to eight weeks of life, and they may sleep for many hours at a time; others, however, may have unpredictable sleep behaviors that stay that way for many months—or longer. It's reasonable to discuss with your pediatrician the specific questions you have and to review your own family's routines, problems, and challenges that may affect your baby's sleep patterns.

In fact, although some parents may ask their doctor questions like "How many hours should my baby sleep at night?", there's no universal answer that applies to

SCENARIO #1

The mother of a four-month-old baby complained to friends that while her infant had slept extremely well in the first week of his life, his sleep patterns seemed to have unraveled after that. More than anything, his sleep times were erratic and unpredictable. She conceded that she tried to keep her baby awake well into the evening so her husband could play with the infant upon returning home from work between 8:00 and 8:30 p.m. But before his arrival, her baby would often fuss and cry. Even though he seemed drowsy at times, she would try keeping him awake for a little while longer, awaiting her husband's arrival. But more often than not, the infant had become so overtired that he just couldn't be consoled.

Mother and father were conflicted over what to do: Dad seemed comfortable with the baby crying until he arrived home, while Mom worried that they were being heartless. Sometimes, she would try putting him down for a brief nap in the very late afternoon, but he would still become cranky later that night, and tension escalated between husband and wife.

They decided to ask their pediatrician for advice. The doctor explained the importance of being respectful of the baby's evolving sleep schedule. For a typical four- to eight-month-old, a healthy nightly bedtime is between 6 and 8 p.m. But keeping the infant up longer to greet his father would leave him overtired and out of sync with his own biological rhythms.

Always be mindful of your baby's sleep needs. His biological clock is evolving, and when he feels the need to sleep, he should be allowed to do so. If his sleep-wake schedule is artificially disrupted, he will probably become moody and less attentive when he is awake. If he goes to bed earlier, he may get up a *little* earlier, but his total night sleep will be longer. This will allow more time for a working parent to spend with their infant in the morning. If any adjustments in schedules need to be made, they should begin with Mom and Dad, who should find a way to be available to their baby when he's awake and alert.

every child. In the first two years of life in particular, your infant's unique genetics have a powerful influence on sleep; whether he takes long naps or short ones, his genetic makeup may be the reason. Or his distinctive temperament could be influencing his sleep behavior. Also, family circumstances can vary, affecting when, how long, and how well a baby sleeps. An infant whose parents are divorced may encounter markedly differing sleep environments when he's sleeping at the home of one parent during the week, and the other on weekends. If the parent works at night and sleeps during the day, this can also affect the baby's sleep schedule.

Getting Sleep in Sync

Despite parental concerns—or in some cases, perhaps because of them—moms and dads sometimes unknowingly disrupt the sleep of their children. For example, even though parents want to do what's healthy for their baby, they don't always appreciate the effect that their own busy schedules and family decision making may have on their infant's sleep.

Most commonly, parents may not recognize the importance of adopting a lifestyle that keeps their baby in sync with his emerging biological system. Timing is everything (or at least it's pretty close). Because the timing of sleep is critical, it is important to understand that *when* your children sleep is probably more important than *how long* they sleep. The quality of a baby's sleep, which can restore alertness and maintain an even temperament, depends largely on when sleep occurs. That means encouraging him to sleep in rhythm with his own biological clock.

Pay attention to your baby, and you'll find that, just like adults, he has "drowsy times" during the day. If he sleeps during these drowsy periods, the quality of that sleep will be greater than sleep that occurs out of phase with his biological cycles. But if you wait to put him down for sleep until well after he's shown signs of drowsiness, he's likely to be overtired by then, which will make it more difficult for him to fall asleep.

As a parent, you need to nurture and support your infant's need to sleep. As much as possible, encourage him to sleep during those times of the day when he's likely to benefit the most from it. However, adopting an optimal sleep schedule won't happen overnight. It takes a while for a baby's biological (circadian) rhythms to develop, with your ultimate goal of getting his sleep patterns to match his internal mechanisms. Give it time, and it will develop naturally. Your challenge as a parent is to be sensitive to those moments when his body is telling him (and you) that he's ready for sleep. Otherwise, you may be putting him down in his crib way too early or way too late, and the ease with which he falls asleep—and the restorative capacity of that sleep—will be affected.

For clues on whether your baby is getting enough sleep—particularly quality sleep—observe him at the end of the day. Is he sweet, adaptable, friendly, cooperative, independent, and engaging? Or is he whiny, crabby, excitable, wired, and irritable? He may be running out of steam as the day draws to a close, all because of mild but chronic sleep deprivation. So if he's consistently melting down, you may need to make some adjustments in the times in which you put him to sleep.

Establishing a Sleep Schedule—and Dealing with Crying

Some babies cry every night when they're placed in their crib for sleep; others almost never do. For many parents, it can be gut-wrenching when a child cries in his crib for long periods of time. As a baby wails and pleads for your attention, your heart may be breaking, and it can be anguishing to keep your distance while you wait for him to fall asleep. Or you might feel frustration or anger at his apparent unwillingness or inability to quiet down and sleep. Even just a few minutes of tears can seem like an eternity.

Often concerned about why their baby is crying, parents may wonder whether the infant is simply letting off steam, is feeling lonely, or whether he's really in distress. Many parents just give in, rushing to their infant's crib side, unable to bear the sound of the sobs.

Not surprisingly, some of the most common questions asked of pediatricians are "Should I let my baby cry himself to sleep, or should I pick him up and comfort him?", as well as the more fundamental question "How much sleep should he really be getting?" To a large degree, the answers to these questions depend on the age of the child.

- *The first weeks of life.* During this period, your baby will spend most of his time asleep. When you put him down to sleep, or when he awakens, try to avoid letting him cry. Instead, respond to those tears, and do whatever you can to soothe your baby, such as singing quietly, talking to him quietly, playing soft music, keeping the lights dim, and/or rocking him gently. Pick him up if necessary, putting him down again five to ten minutes later. By minimizing his discomfort in whatever way works, you'll maximize his sleep time and its quality. (For additional information about soothing a crying baby, see pages 721 and 723 later in this chapter.)

  When is an infant of this age ready for sleep, whether or not he's in tears? In general, after he has been awake for one to two hours, he needs sleep. Sometimes he may need to fall asleep even before an hour goes by and rarely he may stay awake for three hours. No matter what the circumstances, he will begin to show signs of being overtired and irritable if he doesn't get his nap when he needs it. So start soothing him to sleep. After he's been awake for an hour or two, he may need to be soothed. Put him down in his crib when he's drowsy but still awake (this approach will be particularly helpful for daytime napping). If you wait too long, he's likely to become cranky, and have even more difficulty falling asleep.

- *After about six weeks of age (counting from the due date).* Your baby's sleep-wake schedule will begin to settle into more of a routine at this time. He will begin to sleep longer at night, and exhibit signs of drowsiness (and perhaps some crying) earlier. For example, while he may have once been ready for sleep between 9 and 11 p.m., some children start to need sleep somewhat earlier—perhaps between 6 and 8 p.m. His longest sleep period will be in the evening, lasting for three to five hours.

Variations exist, of course, so be sensitive to your own baby's needs and anticipate that he may require an earlier bedtime—no longer at 11 p.m. but rather at 8 p.m. So to minimize crying, put your child to sleep earlier, spend some time soothing him if needed (although if he fusses a little, it won't cause any harm), and let his own biological rhythm dictate whether it will turn into a thirty-minute nap or a four-hour snooze.

As you and your baby get in tune with his rhythms, he'll gradually learn to soothe himself to sleep when you put him down. As that happens, there will be little or no crying. By about three months of age, most babies sleep six to eight hours through the night without disruption. If he awakens too early, you might be able to encourage him to go back to sleep by soothing him, and keeping the lights off and the shades drawn.

- *Four to twelve months of age.* With a four-month-old, and continuing into the weeks and months ahead, keep working at being sensitive to your baby's bodily rhythms, which will minimize episodes of crying. From four months through the rest of the first year of life, most infants need at least two naps—one at midmorning and the other at midday; some children may nap a third time later in the afternoon. Try to get him on a schedule of napping at about 9 a.m. then at 1 p.m., and finally a late afternoon nap if he needs it. Let him nap for as long as he wishes unless he has difficulty falling asleep at night; in that case, talk to your pediatrician about awakening him from his afternoon nap a little earlier than he might wake up on his own. By about nine months of age, try to dispense with late afternoon naps so he'll be ready for bedtime for the night at an earlier time than if those late afternoon naps continued.

  At this age, a baby's nighttime sleep will be his longest sleep period of the day, and by about eight months old, it should last from ten to twelve hours without him awakening for a nighttime feeding. But if an infant of this age seems overtired and he cries at the mere sight of his bed, his naps may be too short (less than thirty minutes long),

SCENARIO #2

A mother and father brought their five-month-old daughter to the pediatrician, and explained that her napping (or lack of it) had become a serious problem that affected the entire family. They would put their baby down for a daytime nap, but she would awaken about thirty-five to forty minutes later, ready to continue her day, at least for a while. They agreed that their baby needed lengthier naps, but were frustrated in their attempts to make them longer. They had tried leaving their baby in her crib for twenty more minutes after awakening, but she would cry nonstop and resisted returning to sleep.

Their pediatrician explained that in infants four to five months old, it can be challenging to initiate a regular nap schedule because their biological rhythms are continuing to change and mature, and thus nap times may not become well established for about another month or two. The doctor suggested that they could try extending the naps by responding promptly when the baby first makes noises or calls out for attention. When that happens, they can try gently patting their baby, giving her a massage, or offering breastfeeding for a short time. With this approach, many infants will fall back asleep for another twenty to thirty minutes, providing a truly restorative nap that leads to greater alertness and attention spans later in the day.

As a child becomes older, however, these particular approaches can become more stimulating than soothing in some children, and thus become counterproductive. After discussing the matter further with the parents, the pediatrician felt there were a couple of factors at play. The baby's bedroom might not be dark enough and the apartment might not be quiet enough to encourage sleep. But more important, the timing of the infant's naps were likely not in sync with her natural rhythms. He recommended that they adjust the sleep environment to make it more conducive to napping, and to be patient until their baby's biological rhythms made her body more agreeable to predictable daytime napping.

or perhaps you're putting him to bed too late at night. In the latter case, place him in bed much earlier, at least temporarily—perhaps at 5:30 or 6 p.m.—to respond to his excessive tiredness. If he cries, check on him and console him with a few comforting words. Change his diaper if needed, make sure he is comfortable, but keep the lights dim and don't arouse him more fully by picking him up and walking with him. Then leave the room quietly. As the days and weeks pass, gradually give him less attention at night, which will help him stop anticipating that you'll show up whenever he cries or calls out for you, and he'll be more likely to learn self-soothing.

It's important to keep in mind that there are times when you may need to let your baby cry himself to sleep; it won't cause any harm and there's no need to worry about the possible messages behind those tears. Remember, you have all day to show your infant how much you love him and care for him. At night, he'll get the message that nighttime is for sleeping, and on those nights when you let him cry, you're helping him learn to soothe himself. He won't be thinking that you're abandoning him or that you don't love him anymore; he knows by your daytime behaviors that this isn't the case at all. In other words, there's no need to worry.

- *At about ages ten to twelve months,* the baby's morning nap will begin to taper off in the minority of infants. Around twelve months of age, some babies may drop their morning nap. As that happens, you can start moving his nighttime bedtime somewhat earlier (perhaps by about twenty to thirty minutes); the afternoon nap can be started a little sooner, too. The time when you put your baby down for nighttime sleep may vary for a while, depending on factors such as how tired your infant seems, and the quality of his daytime napping.

SCENARIO #3

Many parents recognize the importance of bedtime routines—but for some parents, these routines don't always work. One mother tried out many of those that she had heard about, including bathing her baby, massaging him after the bath, singing soft lullabies, and swaddling the baby, but none was effective. In fact, her baby often became *more* irritable as these approaches were used.

When this mother expressed her frustration to her pediatrician, he offered some pointers to make these bedtime routines more effective. He told her to begin using them early, *before* the baby is already overtired and becoming crabby. He also urged her to be consistent, using the same bedtime routines day after day until the infant begins to associate them with sleep. He stressed persistence, explaining that changes don't happen overnight, and that routines need to be relied on over time to have a positive effect.

The pediatrician had another suggestion. He asked the parents to put their infant down for a nap about twenty to thirty minutes *before* they thought the nap should actually begin. As the baby relaxed in her crib, she almost always had a bowel movement within ten to twenty minutes, which prompted her to cry. But then once her diaper was changed, she was now in the correct biological time frame for her nap to begin. Her parents soothed her, and she fell asleep for a lengthy nap.

Getting the Most Out of Sleep

So how do you prepare and soothe your infant to sleep? Soothing techniques may vary based on the age of your baby. Some gentle rubbing of his back can help at almost any age. For young infants, so can touching your own cheek to his in a rhythmic pattern that coincides with his own breathing. Patting him, kissing his forehead, or encouraging sucking behavior with a pacifier or finger, for example, may also be useful for young infants.

Bedtime routines can start as early as four to six months of age, and they'll help get your baby ready for rest, particularly as he starts to associate them with sleep. Try reading him a story. Or give him a warm bath or a massage, sing him a lullaby, or play soothing music. Cut down on your playtime with him right before bedtime, close the curtains, dim the lights, and unplug the phones.

More important than your choice of a specific routine or ritual, you need to continue to stay in rhythm with your child's circadian clock. Remember, timing is the key to healthy sleep. So while it's fine to sit quietly with your child for ten minutes and sing him a lullaby, what you choose to do is usually of less importance than the time you choose to do it.

With this in mind, many mothers and fathers try to change their own behaviors to encourage better sleep in their babies. Yes, modern parents lead very busy lives. But whenever possible, they'll arrange to be at home when their baby needs to nap, rather than shopping or running errands. They'll make sure that their infant naps in his own crib, rather than hoping that he'll doze off in a baby carrier at a noisy restaurant while Mom or Dad is having lunch with friends. On vacations or holidays, they'll try to minimize the disruptions that may keep a baby awake long past the time he would have been napping or in bed for the night. In short, they become as protective as possible of their infant's sleep time, even if it limits and requires adjustment of their own activities. When it's time to sleep, they'll keep their baby away from situations where there is a lot of stimulation, which can lead to crankiness and make sleep difficult. Family activities with the baby before bedtime should be low-key, so as not to overstimulate him.

If your infant is in child care during the first year of life, ask his caregivers to keep him on a regular napping schedule as much as possible. It should be the same schedule that you follow at home to minimize disruptions. Of course, many (but not all) child care facilities are willing and able to make the timing of napping a priority. However, depending on where your child is being cared for, there may not be a dark, quiet room for napping, which can make sleeping difficult. Your baby may be ready for a nap between 9 and 10 a.m., and then again between 1 and 3 p.m.—but the child care environment may not be conducive to napping at those times. There might be too much light, or lots of noise (including crying) from other children. As a result, he may not get the sleep he needs at the time when he most needs it. When that happens, he could be overtired when you pick him up at the end of your workday, and it may be particularly hard to keep him on a regular schedule. In cases like these, work with the staff members of the child care center to maintain consistent napping routines. Their willingness to adapt to your own preferences for napping may be an important factor when you're choosing a facility.

Even with a cooperative child care staff, however, the situation can become mixed up on weekends. If your baby has been in child care all week while you've been at your job, you'll probably be eager to spend as much time as possible with him on Saturday and Sunday. You may give in to his crying or demands to play because of your own guilt about being away so much, and good quality naps may fall by the wayside. Then, after the weekend, the child care workers won't need a calendar to tell that it's Monday—they'll know just by how irritable your infant is from a change in his weekday sleep routines.

Nevertheless, some disruptions in sleep schedules are inevitable. Holidays, vacations, or a family gathering for Grandma's birthday can keep your baby from napping or getting to bed on time. Because the temperament of children varies, some are much more adaptable to changes like these than others; while one child will adjust to changing circumstances very easily, others may not.

As much as possible, respect your infant's nature, and try to maintain normal sleep routines. At the same time, if you know that a disruption of his sleep schedule is on the horizon, he will fare better and adapt more successfully, and have a cheerier disposition, if he is more rested ahead of time. So when you look ahead to a family party, for example, try to keep your baby well rested in the preceding day or two so that this intrusion into his sleep schedule will unfold as smoothly as possible. The more rested your infant is, the better his temperament and the more adaptable he

SCENARIO #4

A father called the family's pediatrician with a problem that he and his wife were trying to solve. They understood the value of keeping their nine-month-old infant on a sleep schedule. At the same time, however, they had two older children with activities that didn't always fit in with the parents' commitment to be protective of their baby's need to nap.

Their pediatrician recommended that the parents work hard at finding a balance between the older children's social needs, and the baby's biologic requirement to nap during the day. Noting that they may not always find the perfect solution that meets the needs of everyone, the doctor added that compromises may be necessary. "Sometimes," he said, "you may have to tell an older child, 'You'll be a little late to your playdate because we're going to wait a few extra minutes until Owen finishes sleeping.' But other times, when the older child has a special event, you may decide to wake up the infant to make sure the older brother or sister gets to where he needs to go on time."

It's true that, in most cases, you should try to avoid awakening a sleeping baby. But a slightly shorter nap now and then won't cause harm, as long as it doesn't become a regular pattern.

will be to changes in his environment—and the better he will sleep.

Dealing with Other Sleep Concerns

You and your spouse should work on other issues that could be disrupting your baby's sleep. Do you have trouble setting limits with him? Is there marital discord between you and your partner that you're just too tired to address, but that is creating tension in the household? Do money worries or other problems create stress that makes it difficult for you to devote energy to establishing sleep routines? If you're not dealing effectively with problems like these, your baby's sleep may pay the price.

Also, does your infant have health issues that make sleeping difficult, such as colic? (Colic is a frequent cause of sleep-disrupting fussiness in very young babies; see page 190 for more information and guidance.) Or your baby could have a short-term health problem like an ear infection that is causing pain and keeping him awake; tend to his immediate needs, following your pediatrician's instructions on how to manage the problem and ease your infant's discomfort.

Putting Sleep in Perspective

When it comes to your baby's sleep, do the best you can, but don't feel bad if things don't always go smoothly. Yes, make a concerted effort to get your infant to bed on time for naps and at night. But as a parent, you also need to set aside any anxiety and blame you might feel if you aren't doing everything perfectly. Inevitably, there will be days and nights when your baby doesn't sleep well, perhaps because you've been too lax in keeping him in sync with his internal rhythms. Or if your baby spends time at child care or with a nanny, and you're simply not present to put him to sleep at nap time, forgive yourself and just make sure that his caretakers understand and are trying to comply with your own preferences about your infant's sleep schedule.

At home, don't beat yourself up if your baby goes to bed a little late for a night or two (or more). Just get back on track as soon as possible, and help him return to a normal sleeping routine. Dealing effectively with your infant's sleeping problems is important, not only for your baby but also because his sleep difficulties can interfere with your own need to rest. Meeting your own sleep needs (as well as those of your partner) is important to effectively care for your baby and the rest of your family. Chronically overtired parents also have a greater risk of becoming depressed.

Keep in mind that helping your baby sleep can be one of parenting's biggest challenges. But it can have an enormous payoff in terms of your infant's health, now and in the future. Many adults are chronically poor sleepers because of patterns that often began during their own childhood and continued on. Sleeping poorly is a learned behavior, and when a baby doesn't get quality sleep, he may not learn how to sleep well. In many cases, such sleep issues are likely to become part of his life for many years. The younger your infant is when you begin to deal with his sleep problems, the more likely you are to resolve them. Remember that your pediatrician can be an ongoing source of support, advice, and reassurance. Additionally, many pediatric medical centers have individuals who specialize in helping babies sleep better.

APPENDIX

The information and policies in the Appendix, such as first-aid procedures for the choking child and cardio-pulmonary resuscitation (CPR), are constantly changing. Ask your pediatrician or other qualified health professional for the latest information on these procedures.

Recommendations for Preventive Pediatric Healthcare

Bright Futures/American Academy of Pediatrics

Each child and family is unique; therefore, these **Recommendations for Preventive Pediatric Healthcare** are designed for the care of children who are receiving competent parenting, have no manifestations of any important health problems, and are growing and developing in satisfactory fashion. **Additional visits may become necessary** if circumstances suggest variations from normal.

	INFANCY							
AGE[1]	PRENATAL[2]	NEWBORN[3]	3-5 d[4]	By 1 mo	2 mo	4 mo	6 mo	9 mo
HISTORY								
Initial/Interval	●	●	●	●	●	●	●	●
MEASUREMENTS								
Length/Height and Weight		●	●	●	●	●	●	●
Head Circumference		●	●	●	●	●	●	●
Weight for Length		●	●	●	●	●	●	●
Body Mass Index								
Blood Pressure[6]		★	★	★	★	★	★	★
SENSORY SCREENING								
Vision		★	★	★	★	★	★	★
Hearing		●[7]	★	★	★	★	★	★
DEVELOPMENTAL/BEHAVIORAL ASSESSMENT								
Developmental Screening[8]								●
Autism Screening[9]								
Developmental Surveillance[8]		●	●	●	●	●	●	
Psychosocial/Behavioral Assessment		●	●	●	●	●	●	●
Alcohol and Drug Use Assessment								
PHYSICAL EXAMINATION[10]		●	●	●	●	●	●	●
PROCEDURES[11]								
Newborn Metabolic/Hemoglobin Screening[12]		◄—	●	——	—►			
Immunization[13]		●	●	●	●	●	●	●
Hematocrit or Hemoglobin[14]						★		
Lead Screening[15]							★	★
Tuberculin Test[17]				★			★	
Dyslipidemia Screening[18]								
STI Screening[19]								
Cervical Dysplasia Screening[20]								
ORAL HEALTH[21]							★	★
ANTICIPATORY GUIDANCE[23]	●	●	●	●	●	●	●	●

KEY

● = to be performed ★ = risk assessment to be performed, with appropriate action to follow, if positive ◄—●—► = range during which a service may be provided, with the symbol indicating the preferred age

American Academy of Pediatrics
DEDICATED TO THE HEALTH OF ALL CHILDREN™

Bright Futures.
prevention and health promotion for infants, children, adolescents, and their families™

Developmental, psychosocial, and chronic disease issues for children and adolescents may require frequent counseling and treatment visits separate from preventive care visits.

These guidelines represent a consensus by the American Academy of Pediatrics (AAP) and Bright Futures. The AAP continues to emphasize the great importance of **continuity of care** in comprehensive health supervision and the need to avoid **fragmentation of care.**

EARLY CHILDHOOD						MIDDLE CHILDHOOD						ADOLESCENCE										
5 mo	18 mo	24 mo	30 mo	3 y	4 y	5 y	6 y	7 y	8 y	9 y	10 y	11 y	12 y	13 y	14 y	15 y	16 y	17 y	18 y	19 y	20 y	21 y
●	●	●	●	●	●	●	●	●	●	●	●	●	●	●	●	●	●	●	●	●	●	●
●	●	●	●	●	●	●	●	●	●	●	●	●	●	●	●	●	●	●	●	●	●	●
●	●	●																				
●	●																					
		●	●	●	●	●	●	●	●	●	●	●	●	●	●	●	●	●	●	●	●	●
★	★	★	★	●	●	●	●	●	●	●	●	●	●	●	●	●	●	●	●	●	●	●
★	★	★	★	●	●	●	●	★	●	★	●	★	●	★	★	●	★	★	●	★	★	★
★	★	★	★	★	●	●	●	★	●	★	●	★	★	★	★	★	★	★	★	★	★	★
	●		●																			
	●	●																				
●		●		●	●	●	●	●	●	●	●	●	●	●	●	●	●	●	●	●	●	●
●	●	●	●	●	●	●	●	●	●	●	●	●	●	●	●	●	●	●	●	●	●	●
												★	★	★	★	★	★	★	★	★	★	★
●	●	●	●	●	●	●	●	●	●	●	●	●	●	●	●	●	●	●	●	●	●	●
●	●	●	●	●	●	●	●	●	●	●	●	●	●	●	●	●	●	●	●	●	●	●
	★	★		★	★	★	★	★	★	★	★	★	★	★	★	★	★	★	★	★	★	★
	★	● or ★[16]		★	★	★	★															
	★	★		★	★	★	★	★	★	★	★	★	★	★	★	★	★	★	★	★	★	★
		★			★		★		★		★	★	★	★	★	★	★	★	←		●	→
												★	★	★	★	★	★	★	★	★	★	★
												★	★	★	★	★	★	★	★	★	★	★
	● or ★[21]	● or ★[21]	● or ★[21]	●[22]			●[22]															
●	●	●	●	●	●	●	●	●	●	●	●	●	●	●	●	●	●	●	●	●	●	●

The recommendations in this statement do not indicate an exclusive course of treatment or standard of medical care. Variations, taking into account individual circumstances, may be appropriate.

1. If a chld comes under care for the first time at any point on the schedule, or if any items are not accomplished at the suggested age, the schedule should be brought up to date at the earliest possible time.
2. A prenatal visit is recommended for parents who are at high risk, for first-time parents, and for those who request a conference. The prenatal visit should include anticipatory guidance, pertinent medical history, and a discussion of benefits of breastfeeding and planned method of feeding per AAP statement "The Prenatal Visit" (2001) [URL: http://aappolicy.aap publications.org/cgi/content/full/pediatrics:107/6/1456].
3. Every infant should have a newborn evaluation after birth, breastfeeding encouraged, and instruction and suppport offered.
4. Every infant should have an evaluation within 3 to 5 days of birth and within 48 to 72 hours after discharge from the hospital, to include evaluation for feeding and jaundice. Breastfeeding infants should receive formal breastfeeding evaluation, encouragement, and instruction as recommended in AAP statement "Breastfeeding and the Use of Human Milk" (2005) [URL: http://aappolicy.aappublications.org/cgi/content/full/pediatrics:115/2/496]. For newborns discharged in less than 48 hours after delivery, the infant must be examined within 48 hours of discharge per AAP statement "Hospital Stay for Healthy Term Newborns" (2004) [URL: http://aappolicy.aappublications.org/cgi/content/full/pediatrics:113/51/1434].
5. Blood pressure measurement in infants and children with specific risk conditions should be performed at visits before age 3 years.
6. If the patient is uncooperative, rescreen within 6 months per the AAP statement "Eye Examination in Infants, Children, and Young Adults by Pediatricians" (2007) [URL: http://aappolicy.aappublications.org/cgi/contents/full/pediatrics;111/4/902].
7. All newborns should be screened per AAP statement "Year 2000 Position Statement:" Principles and Guidelines for Early Hearing Detection and Intervention Programs" (2000) [URL: http://aappolicy.aappublications.org/cgi/contents/full/pediatrics;106/4/798]. Joint Committee on Infant Hearing Year 2007 position statement: principles and guidelines for early hearing detection and intervention programs. *Pediatrics*. 2007; 120:898–921.
8. AAP Council on Children With Disabilities, AAP Section on Developmental Behavorial Pediatrics. AAP Bright Futures Steering Committee, AAP Medical Home Initiatives for Children With Special Needs Project Advisory Committee. Identifying infants and young children with developmental disorders in the medical home: an algorithm for developmental surveillance and screening. *Pediatrics*. 2006:118:405–420 [URL: http://aappolicy.aappublications.org/cgi/contents/full/pediatrics;118/1/405].
9. Gupta VB, Hyman SL, Johnson, CP, et al. Identifying children with autism early? *Pediatrics*. 2007;119:152–153 [URL: http://pediatrics.aap publications.org/cgi/contents/full/119/1/152].
10. At each visit, age-appropriate physical examination is essential, with infant totally unclothed, older child undressed and suitably draped.

11. These may be modified, depending on entry point into schedule and individual need.
12. Newborn metabolic and hemoglobinopathy screening should be done according to state law. Results should be reviewed at visits and appropriate retesting or referral done as needed.
13. Schedules per the Committee on Infectious Diseases, published annually in the January issue of *Pediatrics*. Every visit should be an opportunity to update and complete a child's immunizations.
14. See AAP *Pediatric Nutrition Handbook*, 5th Edition (2003) for a discussion of universal and selective screening options. See also Recommendations to prevent and control iron deficiency in the United States. *MMWR*. 1998:47(RR-3):1–36.
15. For children at risk of lead exposure, consult the AAP statement "Lead Exposure in Children: Prevention, Detection, and Management" (2005) [URL: http://aappolicy.aappublications.org/cgi/contents/full/pediatrics;116/4/1036]. Additionally, screening should be done in accordance with state law where applicable.
16. Perform risk assessments or screens as appropriate, based on universal screening requirements for patients with Medicaid or high prevalence areas.
17. Tuberculosis testing per recommendations of the Committee on Infectious Diseases, published in the current edtion of *Red Book: Report of the Committee on Infectious Diseases*. Testing should be done on recognition of high-risk factors.
18. "Third Report of the National Cholesterol Education Program (NCEP) Expert Panel on Detection, Evaluation, and Treatment of High Blood Cholesterol in Adults (Adult Treatment Panel III) Final Report" (2002) [URL: http://circ.ahajournals.org/cgi/content/full/106/25/3143] and "The Expert Committee Recommendations on the Assessment, Prevention, and Treatment of Child and Adolescent Overweight and Obesity." Supplement to *Pediatrics*. In press.
19. All sexually active patients should be screened for sexually transmitted infections (STIs).
20. All sexually active girls should have screening for cervical dysplasia as part of a pelvic examination beginning within 3 years of onset of sexual activity or age 21 (whichever comes first).
21. Referral to dental home, if available. Otherwise, administer oral health risk assessment. If the primary water source is deficient in fluoride, consider oral fluoride supplementation.
22. At the visit for 3 years and 6 years of age, it should be determined whether the patient has a dental home. If the patient does not have a dental home, a referral should be made to one. If the primary water source is deficient in fluoride, consider oral fluoride supplementation.
23. Refer to the specific guidance by age as listed in Bright Futures Guidelines. (Hagan JF, Shaw JS, Duncan PM, eds. *Bright Futures: Guidelines for Health Supervision of Infants, Children, and Adolescents*. 3rd ed. Elk Grove Village, IL: American Academy of Pediatrics; 2008).

Recommended Immunization Schedule for Persons Aged 0 Through 6 Years—United States • 2009

For those who fall behind or start late, see the catch-up schedule

Vaccine ▼ Age ▶	Birth	1 month	2 months	4 months	6 months	12 months	15 months	18 months	19–23 months	2–3 years	4–6 years
Hepatitis B	HepB	HepB				HepB					
Rotavirus			RV	RV	*RV*						
Diphtheria, Tetanus, Pertussis			DTaP	DTaP	DTaP		DTaP				DTaP
Haemophilus influenzae type b			Hib	Hib	*Hib*	Hib					
Pneumococcal			PCV	PCV	PCV	PCV				PPSV	
Inactivated Poliovirus			IPV	IPV		IPV					IPV
Influenza								Influenza (Yearly)			
Measles, Mumps, Rubella						MMR					MMR
Varicella						Varicella					Varicella
Hepatitis A								HepA (2 doses)		HepA Series	
Meningococcal										MCV	

Range of recommended ages

Certain high-risk groups

This schedule indicates the recommended ages for routine administration of currently licensed vaccines, as of December 1, 2008, for children aged 0 through 6 years. Any dose not administered at the recommended age should be administered at a subsequent visit, when indicated and feasible. Licensed combination vaccines may be used whenever any component of the combination is indicated and other components are not contraindicated and if approved by the Food and Drug Administration for that dose of the series. Providers should consult the relevant Advisory Committee on Immunization Practices statement for detailed recommendations, including high-risk conditions: http://www.cdc.gov/vaccines/pubs/acip-list.htm. Clinically significant adverse events that follow immunization should be reported to the Vaccine Adverse Event Reporting System (VAERS). Guidance about how to obtain and complete a VAERS form is available at http://www.vaers.hhs.gov or by telephone, 800-822-7967.

The Recommended Immunization Schedules for Persons Aged 0 Through 18 Years are approved by the Advisory Committee on Immunization Practices (www.cdc.gov/vaccines/recs/acip), the American Academy of Pediatrics (http://www.aap.org), and the American Academy of Family Physicians (http://www.aafp.org).

DEPARTMENT OF HEALTH AND HUMAN SERVICES • CENTERS FOR DISEASE CONTROL AND PREVENTION

CS103164

For more information from the American Academy of Pediatrics about vaccines, including vaccine safety, go to www.aap.org/immunization.

Catch-up Immunization Schedule for Persons Aged 4 Months Through 6 Years Who Start Late or Who Are More Than 1 Month Behind—United States • 2009

The table below provides catch-up schedules and minimum intervals between doses for children whose vaccinations have been delayed. A vaccine series does not need to be restarted, regardless of the time that has elapsed between doses. Use the section appropriate for the child's age.

CATCH-UP SCHEDULE FOR PERSONS AGED 4 MONTHS THROUGH 6 YEARS

Vaccine	Minimum Age for Dose 1	Minimum Interval Between Doses			
		Dose 1 to Dose 2	Dose 2 to Dose 3	Dose 3 to Dose 4	Dose 4 to Dose 5
Hepatitis B	Birth	**4 weeks**	**8 weeks** (and at least 16 weeks after first dose)		
Rotavirus	6 wks	**4 weeks**	**4 weeks**		
Diphtheria, Tetanus, Pertussis	6 wks	**4 weeks**	**4 weeks**	**6 months**	**6 months**
***Haemophilus influenzae* type b**	6 wks	**4 weeks** if first dose administered at younger than age 12 months **8 weeks** (as final dose) if first dose administered at age 12-14 months **No further doses needed** if first dose administered at age 15 months or older	**4 weeks** if current age is younger than 12 months **8 weeks** (as final dose) if current age is 12 months or older and second dose administered at younger than age 15 months **No further doses needed** if previous dose administered at age 15 months or older	**8 weeks** (as final dose) This dose only necessary for children aged 12 months through 59 months who received 3 doses before age 12 months	
Pneumococcal	6 wks	**4 weeks** if first dose administered at younger than age 12 months **8 weeks** (as final dose for healthy children) if first dose administered at age 12 months or older or current age 24 through 59 months **No further doses needed** for healthy children if first dose administered at age 24 months or older	**4 weeks** if current age is younger than 12 months **8 weeks** (as final dose for healthy children) if current age is 12 months or older **No further doses needed** for healthy children if previous dose administered at age 24 months or older	**8 weeks** (as final dose) This dose only necessary for children aged 12 months through 59 months who received 3 doses before age 12 months or for high-risk children who received 3 doses at any age	
Inactivated Poliovirus	6 wks	**4 weeks**	**4 weeks**	**4 weeks**	
Measles, Mumps, Rubella	12 mos	**4 weeks**			
Varicella	12 mos	**3 months**			
Hepatitis A	12 mos	**6 months**			

Note: For more information from the American Academy of Pediatrics about vaccines, including vaccine safety, go to www.aap.org/immunization.

Boys, birth to 36 months

Name ____________

LENGTH FOR AGE AND WEIGHT FOR AGE PERCENTILES

Record # ________

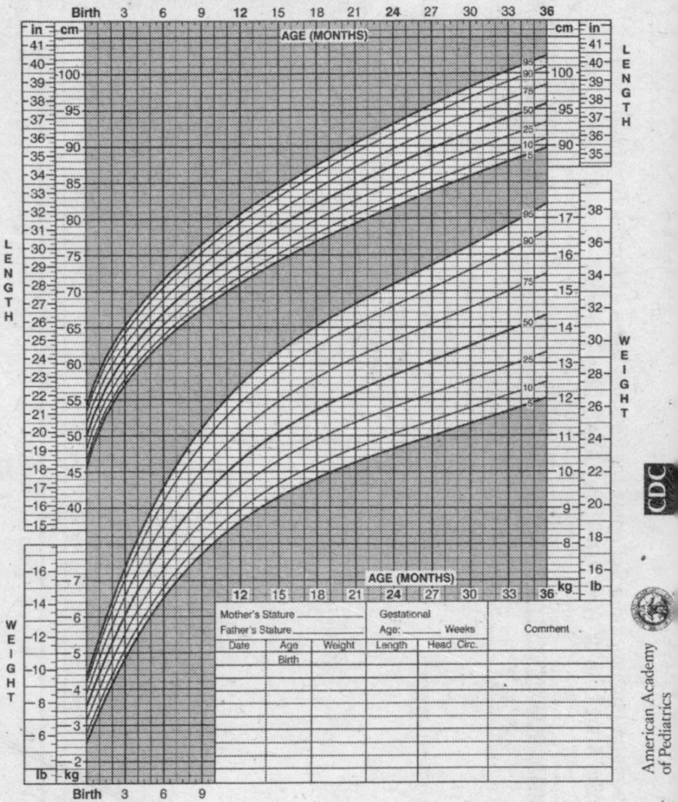

Source: Developed by the National Center for Health Statistics in collaboration with the National Center for Chronic Disease Prevention and Health Promotion (2000) http://www.cdc.gov/growthcharts

Reprinted by the American Academy of Pediatrics

The recommendations in this publication do not indicate an exclusive course of treatment or serve as a standard of medical care. Variations, taking into account individual circumstances, may be appropriate.

Additional copies are available for purchase in quantities of 100.

To order, contact:
American Academy of Pediatrics
141 Northwest Point Blvd
Elk Grove Village, IL 60007-1098
Web site — http://www.aap.org. Minimum order 100.

Girls, birth to 36 months

Name ____________

LENGTH FOR AGE AND WEIGHT FOR AGE PERCENTILES

Record # ______

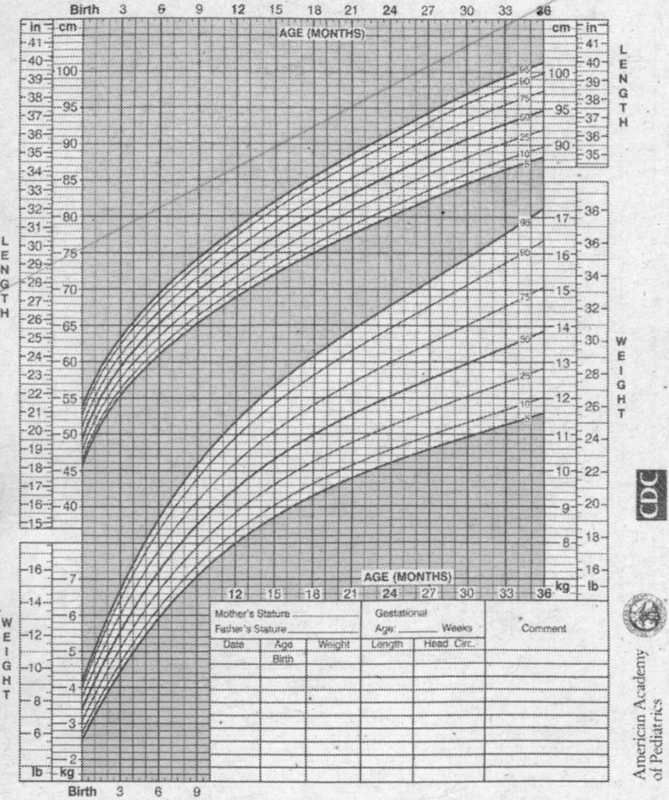

CDC

American Academy of Pediatrics
DEDICATED TO THE HEALTH OF ALL CHILDREN

Source: Developed by the National Center for Health Statistics in collaboration with the National Center for Chronic Disease Prevention and Health Promotion (2000). http://www.cdc.gov/growthcharts

Reprinted by the American Academy of Pediatrics

The recommendations in this publication do not indicate an exclusive course of treatment or serve as a standard of medical care. Variations, taking into account individual circumstances, may be appropriate.

Additional copies are available for purchase in quantities of 100.

To order, contact:
American Academy of Pediatrics
141 Northwest Point Blvd
Elk Grove Village, IL 60007-1098
Web site — http://www.aap.org. Minimum order 100.

Boys, birth to 36 months

Name ______________________

HEAD CIRCUMFERENCE FOR AGE AND WEIGHT FOR LENGTH PERCENTILES

Record # ________

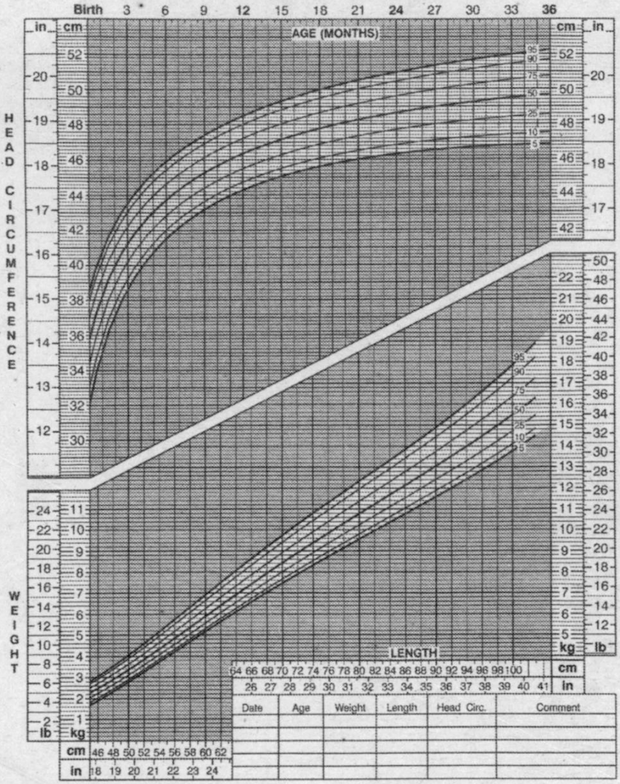

Source: Developed by the National Center for Health Statistics in collaboration with the National Center for Chronic Disease Prevention and Health Promotion (2000). http://www.cdc.gov/growthcharts

Reprinted by the American Academy of Pediatrics

The recommendations in this publication do not indicate an exclusive course of treatment or serve as a standard of medical care. Variations, taking into account individual circumstances, may be appropriate.

9-7/REP-107

Additional copies are available for purchase in quantities of 100.

To order, contact
American Academy of Pediatrics
141 Northwest Point Blvd
Elk Grove Village, IL 60007-1098
Web site — http://www.aap.org. Minimum order 100.

HE0302

CDC

American Academy of Pediatrics

Girls, birth to 36 months

Name _____

AD CIRCUMFERENCE FOR AGE AND WEIGHT FOR LENGTH PERCENTILES

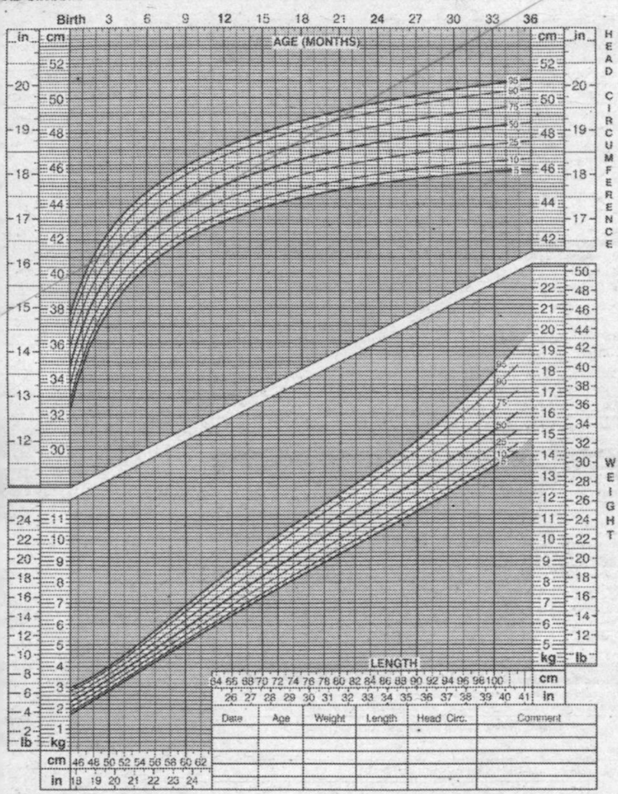

Record # _____

Source: Developed by the National Center for Health Statistics in collaboration with the National Center for Chronic Disease Prevention and Health Promotion (2000).
http://www.cdc.gov/growthcharts

Reprinted by the American Academy of Pediatrics.

The recommendations in this publication do not indicate an exclusive course of treatment or serve as a standard of medical care. Variations, taking into account individual circumstances, may be appropriate.

©2009 American Academy of Pediatrics

Additional copies are available for purchase in quantities of 100.
To order, contact:
American Academy of Pediatrics
141 Northwest Point Blvd
Elk Grove Village, IL 60007-1098
Web site — http://www.aap.org. Minimum order 100.
Source: Developed by the National Center for Health Statistics in collaboration with the National Center for Chronic Disease Prevention and Health Promotion (2000).

American Academy of Pediatrics

DEDICATED TO THE HEALTH OF ALL CHILDREN®

Is This the Right Place for My Child?

(Make a copy of this checklist to use with each program you visit.)

Place a check in the box if the program meets your expectations.	
Will my child be supervised?	
	Are children watched at all times, including when they are sleeping?
	Are adults warm and welcoming? Do they pay individual attention to each child?
	Are positive guidance techniques used? Do adults avoid yelling, spanking, and other negative punishments?
	Are the caregiver/teacher-to-child ratios appropriate and do they follow the recommended guidelines: ▶ One caregiver per 3 or 4 infants ▶ One caregiver per 3 or 4 young toddlers ▶ One caregiver per 4 to 6 older toddlers ▶ One caregiver per 6 to 9 preschoolers
Have the adults been trained to care for children?	
	If a center: ▶ Does the director have a degree and some experience in caring for children? ▶ Do the teachers have a credential*** or Associate's degree and experience in caring for children? **If a family child care home:** ▶ Has the provider had specific training on children's development and experience caring for children?
	Is there always someone present who has current CPR and first aid training?
	Are the adults continuing to receive training on caring for children?
	Have the adults been trained on child abuse prevention and how to report suspected cases?
Will my child be able to grow and learn?	
	For older children, are there specific areas for different kinds of play (books, blocks, puzzles, art, etc.)?
	For infants and toddlers, are there toys that "do something" when the child plays with them?
	Is the play space organized and are materials easy-to-use? Are some materials available at all times?
	Are there daily or weekly activity plans available? Have the adults planned experiences for the children to enjoy? Will the activities help children learn?
	Do the adults talk with the children during the day? Do they engage them in conversations? Ask questions, when appropriate?
	Do the adults read to children at least twice a day or encourage them to read, if they can read?
Is this a safe and healthy place for my child?	
	Do adults and children wash their hands (before eating or handling food, or after using the bathroom, changing diapers, touching body fluids or eating, etc.)?
	Are diaper changing surfaces cleaned and sanitized after each use?
	Do all of the children enrolled have the required immunizations?
	Are medicines labeled and out of children's reach?
	Are adults trained to give medicines and keep records of medications?
	Are surfaces used to serve food cleaned and sanitized?
	Are the food and beverages served to children nutritious, and are they stored, prepared, and served in the right way to keep children growing and healthy?
	Are cleaning supplies and other poisonous materials locked up, out of children's reach?
	Is there a plan to follow if a child is injured, sick or lost?

Notes:

Is This the Right Place for My Child? 38 Research-Based Indicators of High-Quality Child-Care

Place a check in the box if the program meets your expectations.	
	Are first aid kits readily available?
	Is there a plan for responding to disasters (fire, flood, etc.)?
	Has a satisfactory criminal history background check been conducted on each adult present? ▶ Was the check based on fingerprints?
	Have all the adults who are left alone with children had background and criminal screenings? **In a center:** ▶ Are two adults with each group of children most of the time? **In a home:** ▶ Are family members left alone with children only in emergencies?
	Is the outdoor play area a safe place for children to play? ▶ Is it checked each morning for hazards before children use it? ▶ Is the equipment the right size and type for the age of the children who use it? ▶ In center-based programs, is the playground area surrounded by a fence at least 4 feet tall? ▶ Is the equipment placed on mulch, sand, or rubber matting? ▶ Is the equipment in good condition?
	Is the number of children in each group limited? ▶ In family child care homes and centers, children are in groups of no more than** ■ 6-8 infants ■ 6-12 younger toddlers ■ 8-12 older toddlers ■ 12-20 preschoolers ■ 20-24 school-agers
Is the program set up to promote quality?	
	Does the program have the highest level of licensing offered by the state?
	Are there written personnel policies and job descriptions?
	Are parents and staff asked to evaluate the program?
	Are staff evaluated each year; do providers do a self-assessment?
	Is there a written annual training plan for staff professional development?
	Is the program evaluated each year by someone outside the program?
	Is the program accredited by a national organization?
Does the program work with parents?	
	Will I be welcome any time my child is in care?
	Is parents' feedback sought and used in making program improvements?
	Will I be given a copy of the program's policies?
	Are annual conferences held with parents?

Notes:

These questions are based on research about child care; you can read the research findings on the NACCRRA website under "Questions for Parents to Ask" at http://www.naccrra.org. Research-based indicators can only describe quality. Parents should base their decisions on actual observations.

These are the adult-to-child ratios and group sizes recommended by the National Association for the Education of Young Children. Ratios are lowered when there are one or more children who may need additional help to fully participate in a program due to a disability, or other factors.

* Group sizes are considered the maximum number of children to be in a group, regardless of the number of adult staff.

** Individuals working in child care can earn a Child Development Associate credential.

For help finding child care in your area, contact Child Care Aware, a Program of NACCRRA at 1-800-424-2246 or www.childcareaware.org.

For information about other AAP publications visit: www.aap.org

Endorsed by:

American Academy of Pediatrics
DEDICATED TO THE HEALTH OF ALL CHILDREN™

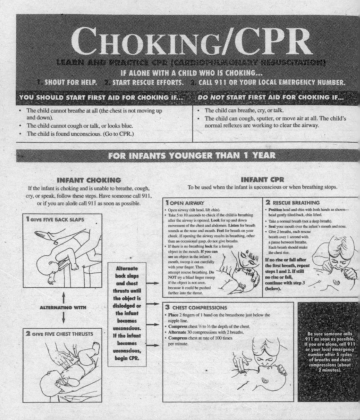

CHOKING/CPR

LEARN AND PRACTICE CPR (CARDIOPULMONARY RESUSCITATION)

IF ALONE WITH A CHILD WHO IS CHOKING...

1. SHOUT FOR HELP. 2. START RESCUE EFFORTS. 3. CALL 911 OR YOUR LOCAL EMERGENCY NUMBER.

YOU SHOULD START FIRST AID FOR CHOKING IF...

- The child cannot breathe at all (the chest is not moving up and down).
- The child cannot cough or talk, or looks blue.
- The child is found unconscious. (Go to CPR.)

DO NOT START FIRST AID FOR CHOKING IF...

- The child can breathe, cry, or talk.
- The child can cough, sputter, or move air at all. The child's normal reflexes are working to clear the airway.

FOR INFANTS YOUNGER THAN 1 YEAR

INFANT CHOKING

If the infant is choking and is unable to breathe, cough, cry, or speak, follow these steps. Have someone call 911, or if you are alone call 911 as soon as possible.

1 GIVE FIVE BACK SLAPS

ALTERNATING WITH

2 GIVE FIVE CHEST THRUSTS

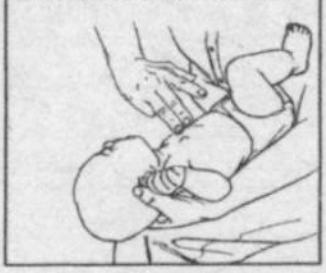

Alternate back slaps and chest thrusts until the object is dislodged or the infant becomes unconscious. If the infant becomes unconscious, begin CPR.

INFANT CPR

To be used when the infant is unconscious or when breathing stops.

1 OPEN AIRWAY

- Open airway (tilt head, lift chin).
- Take 5 to 10 seconds to check if the child is breathing after the airway is opened. **Look** for up and down movement of the chest and abdomen. **Listen** for breath sounds at the nose and mouth. **Feel** for breath on your cheek. If opening the airway results in breathing, other than an occasional gasp, do not give breaths.
- If there is no breathing **look** for a foreign object in the mouth. **If you can see** an object in the infant's mouth, sweep it out carefully with your finger. Then attempt rescue breathing. **Do NOT** try a blind finger sweep if the object is not seen, because it could be pushed farther into the throat.

2 RESCUE BREATHING

- **Position** head and chin with both hands as shown—head gently tilted back, chin lifted.
- Take a normal breath (not a deep breath).
- **Seal** your mouth over the infant's mouth and nose.
- Give 2 breaths, each rescue breath over 1 second with a pause between breaths. Each breath should make the chest rise.

If no rise or fall after the first breath, repeat steps 1 and 2. If still no rise or fall, continue with step 3 (below).

3 CHEST COMPRESSIONS

- **Place** 2 fingers of 1 hand on the breastbone just below the nipple line.
- **Compress** chest ⅓ to ½ the depth of the chest.
- **Alternate** 30 compressions with 2 breaths.
- **Compress** chest at rate of 100 times per minute.

Be sure someone calls 911 as soon as possible. If you are alone, call 911 or your local emergency number after 5 cycles of breaths and chest compressions (about 2 minutes).

If at any time an object is coughed up or the infant/child starts to breathe, call 911 or your local emergency number.

Ask your pediatrician for information on choking/CPR instructions for children older tha[n] 8 years and for information on an approved first aid or CPR course in your community.

To download a copy of this chart, please visit www.healthychildren.org/cpr

Index

Page numbers of illustrations appear in italics.